Handbook on Positive Development of Minority Children and Youth

Natasha J. Cabrera · Birgit Leyendecker
Editors

Handbook on Positive Development of Minority Children and Youth

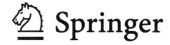
Springer

Editors
Natasha J. Cabrera
Department of Human Development and
  Quantitative Methodology
University of Maryland
College Park, MD
USA

Birgit Leyendecker
Fakultät für Psychologie
Ruhr-Universität Bochum
Bochum
Germany

ISBN 978-3-319-43643-2   ISBN 978-3-319-43645-6 (eBook)
DOI 10.1007/978-3-319-43645-6

Library of Congress Control Number: 2016952814

Printed on acid-free paper

This Springer imprint is published by Springer Nature
The registered company is Springer International Publishing AG
The registered company address is: Gewerbestrasse 11, 6330 Cham, Switzerland

Contents

Part I Conceptual and Methodological Approaches
Frosso Motti-Stefanidi

**Positive Youth Development Among Minority Youth:
A Relational Developmental Systems Model** 5
Richard M. Lerner, Jun Wang, Rachel M. Hershberg,
Mary H. Buckingham, Elise M. Harris, Jonathan M. Tirrell,
Edmond P. Bowers, and Jacqueline V. Lerner

**A Resilience Perspective on Immigrant Youth Adaptation
and Development** 19
Frosso Motti-Stefanidi and Ann S. Masten

Measuring Positive Development I: Multilevel Analysis 35
Jens B. Asendorpf

**Equivalence in Research on Positive Development
of Minority Children: Methodological Approaches** 53
Fons J.R. van de Vijver and Jia He

Part II Individual Level Influences
Robert H. Bradley

**Parental Sensitivity and Attachment in Ethnic
Minority Families** 71
Maike Malda and Judi Mesman

**Conceptualizing Variability in U.S. Latino Children's
Dual-Language Development** 89
Kelly Escobar and Catherine S. Tamis-LeMonda

**An International Perspective on Parenting
and Children's Adjustment** 107
Jennifer E. Lansford

Cultural Identity Development as a Developmental Resource . . . 123
Paul Vedder and Mitch van Geel

**Differential Susceptibility in Minority Children:
Individual Differences in Environmental Sensitivity** 139
Elham Assary and Michael Pluess

Part III   Family/Parenting Level Influences
Marc H. Bornstein

Parenting and Families in the United States and Canada......   157
Catherine Costigan, Joelle Taknint, and Sheena Miao

**Family Resources for Promoting Positive Development
Among Minority Children: European Perspectives**..........   175
Sabine Walper and Birgit Leyendecker

**Minority Fathers and Children's Positive Development
in the United States**...............................   197
Natasha J. Cabrera, Elizabeth Karberg, and Catherine Kuhns

**Language and Parenting: Minority Languages
in North America**   217
Allyssa McCabe

**Minority Language Parenting in Europe
and Children's Well-Being**...........................   231
Annick De Houwer

Part IV   Peers and Friendship Level Influences
Christiane Spiel

Interethnic Friendship Formation.....................   249
Peter F. Titzmann

**The Friendships of Racial–Ethnic Minority
Youth in Context**..................................   267
Leoandra Onnie Rogers, Erika Y. Niwa, and Niobe Way

**Minority and Majority Children's Evaluations of Social
Exclusion in Intergroup Contexts**......................   281
Aline Hitti, Kelly Lynn Mulvey, and Melanie Killen

**Children's Social–Emotional Development in Contexts
of Peer Exclusion.**................................   295
Tina Malti, Antonio Zuffianò, Lixian Cui, Tyler Colasante,
Joanna Peplak, and Na Young Bae

**Positive Youth Development of Roma Ethnic Minority
Across Europe.**...................................   307
Radosveta Dimitrova and Laura Ferrer-Wreder

Part V   Early Childhood and School Level Influences
Allan Wigfield

**Promoting Positive Self-Esteem in Ethnic Minority Students:
The Role of School and Classroom Context**   325
Jochem Thijs and Maykel Verkuyten

**Parental Educational Involvement and Latino Children's
Academic Attainment**   343
Rosario Ceballo, Rosanne M. Jocson, and Francheska Alers-Rojas

**Using Self-Regulated Learning as a Framework for Creating
Inclusive Classrooms for Ethnically and Linguistically
Diverse Learners in Canada**.   361
Nancy Perry, Nikki Yee, Silvia Mazabel, Simon Lisaingo,
and Elina Määttä

Part VI   Policies/Prevention/Programs
Nancy Gonzalez

**Documentation Status and Child Development
in the U.S. and Europe**   385
Natalia Rojas and Hirokazu Yoshikawa

**Research on Positive Youth Development in Boys of Color:
Implications for Intervention and Policy**.   401
Noni K. Gaylord-Harden, Cynthia Pierre, Latriece Clark,
Patrick H. Tolan, and Oscar A. Barbarin

**Civic Engagement as an Adaptive Coping Response
to Conditions of Inequality: An Application
of Phenomenological Variant of Ecological
Systems Theory (PVEST)**.   421
Elan C. Hope and Margaret Beale Spencer

**Developing an Ethnic-Racial Identity Intervention
from a Developmental Perspective: Process, Content,
and Implementation of the Identity Project**.   437
Adriana J. Umaña-Taylor and Sara Douglass

**Children's Centres: An English Intervention for Families
Living in Disadvantaged Communities**   455
Maria Evangelou, Jenny Goff, Kathy Sylva, Pam Sammons,
Teresa Smith, James Hall, and Naomi Eisenstadt

**Instructional Practice with Young Bilingual Learners:
A Canadian Profile**   471
Roma Chumak-Horbatsch

Editors and Contributors

About the Editors

Natasha J. Cabrera is Professor of Human Development at the University of Maryland and was a Society for Research in Child Development, Executive Branch Fellow at the National Institute of Child Health and Human Development (NICHD). Dr. Cabrera's research, funded by NICHD, focuses on father involvement and children's social development; adaptive and maladaptive factors related to parenting; ethnic and cultural variations in fathering and mothering behaviors; family processes in a social and cultural context and children's development; and the mechanisms that link early experiences to children's school readiness. Cabrera has published in peer-reviewed journals on policy, methodology, theory and the implications of fathering and mothering behaviors on child development in low-income minority families. She is the co-editor of the Handbook of Father Involvement: Multidisciplinary Perspectives, Second Edition (Taylor & Francis 2013) and Latina/o Child Psychology and Mental Health: Vol 1: Early to Middle Childhood: Development and Context and Vol 2: Adolescent Development (Praeger 2011). Dr. Cabrera is the Associate Editor of ECRQ and Child Development and the recipient of the National Council and Family Relations award for Best Research Article regarding men in families in 2009. In 2015 The National Academy of Sciences appointed her to its committee supporting the parents of young children and she is a 2015–2016 Visiting Scholar at the Russell Sage Foundation.

Birgit Leyendecker is Professor for Developmental Psychology at the Ruhr-University Bochum. Her research focus is on cultural perspectives on child development and parenting, cultural and psychosocial adaptation of immigrant children and their families, and on resilience, particularly on the role of internal and external resources on children's developmental pathways. She is the Principal Investigator of an international study on the development of resilience among immigrant children and their families. In 2016, she started a funded project on refugee children and their families in Germany.

Contributors

Francheska Alers-Rojas is a doctoral student in the developmental psychology program at the University of Michigan (Ann Arbor, MI). Ms. Alers-Rojas received her B.A. in Pre-Law and J.D. from the University of Puerto Rico (Rio Piedras, PR). She is broadly interested in the intersections of socioeconomic context, race and ethnicity and child development. Her current research examines factors that determine Latina mothers' knowledge and awareness of their children's exposure to community violence. A second line of research employs community-based participatory research methods to develop and test the efficacy of mHealth sexual risks and substance use preventive interventions for youth.

Jens B. Asendorpf is retired Professor of Psychology at the Department of Psychology, Humboldt University, Berlin, and served as head of the department from 2008 to 2010. He spent 12 years at the Max Planck Institute for Psychological Research, Munich, where he cooperated in a major German longitudinal study on personality development (LOGIC), and was a faculty member of the International Max Planck Research School LIFE at the Max Planck Institute for Human Development in Berlin. Since 2008 he is involved in two longitudinal studies on minority adolescents in Greece. He (co)authors more than 150 publications in the areas of personality and developmental psychology.

Elham Assary is a Ph.D. student in the field of behavioral genetics at Queen Mary University of London, UK. In 2009, having spent several years developing her career in the financial sector, she decided to transition away from the world of finance and pursue her interest in psychology and human behavior; starting with a B.Sc. in psychology at Birkbeck, University of London, followed by a M.Sc. in Genes, Environment and Development at Kings' College London. She is broadly interested in exploring the mechanisms and factors that contribute to individual differences in response to positive and negative environmental exposures that shape the trajectory of psychological development. More specifically, she is interested in examining the inter-individual characteristics that contribute to this variation in psychological outcomes, focusing on environmental sensitivity, conceptualized as a personality trait. The main aim of her Ph.D. project is to explore the genetic and environmental factors that contribute to individual differences in environmental sensitivity.

Na Young Bae is a Ph.D. student at the University of Toronto. Her research areas focus on the development of moral emotions, including respect and sympathy, and its effects on children's prosocial behavior. She is interested in investigating the role of moral emotions in promoting children and youth's positive mental health and social outcomes amidst negative social environments, such as peer exclusion and victimization. E-mail: ny.bae@mail.utoronto.ca

Dr. Oscar A. Barbarin is the Elkins Distinguished Professor and Chair of the African American Studies Department and Professor of Psychology, University of Maryland, College Park. His research has focus on mental health, early childhood and boys of color. His research has been honored by the Society for Research in Child Development and the American Orthopsychiatric Association.

Marc H. Bornstein is Senior Investigator and Head of Child and Family Research at the Eunice Kennedy Shriver National Institute of Child Health and Human Development. He holds a B.A. from Columbia College, M.S. and Ph.D. degrees from Yale University, and an honorary doctorate from the University of Padua. Bornstein has held faculty positions at Princeton University and New York University as well as academic appointments in Munich, London, Paris, New York, Tokyo, Bamenda, Seoul, Trento, Santiago, Bristol, and Oxford. Bornstein is President-elect of the SRCD and a past member of the SRCD Governing Council Executive Committee of the ICIS. Bornstein was named to the Top 20 Authors for Productivity in Developmental Science by the AERA. Bornstein has administered both Federal and Foundation grants, sits on the editorial boards of several professional journals, and consults for governments, foundations, universities, publishers, scientific journals, the media, and UNICEF. Bornstein is Editor Emeritus of Child Development and founding Editor of Parenting: Science and Practice. He is author or editor of numerous scholarly volumes and several children's books, videos, and puzzles and has published widely in experimental, methodological, comparative, developmental, and cultural science as well as neuroscience, pediatrics, and aesthetics. Visit www.cfr. nichd.nih.gov and www.tandfonline.com/HPAR.

Edmond P. Bowers is Assistant Professor of Youth Development Leadership at Clemson University. His research focuses on the influence of formal and natural mentors in promoting the Five Cs of Positive Youth Development.

Robert H. Bradley, Ph.D. is Director of the Family and Human Dynamics Research Institute at ASU. He is a member of the HHS/HRSA Advisory Committee on Maternal, Infant and Early Childhood Home Visitation Program Evaluation and on the editorial boards of Parenting: Science and Practice, Journal of Developmental and Behavioral Pediatrics, and Early Childhood Research Quarterly) and was associate editor for both Child Development and Early Childhood Research Quarterly. He has more than 350 publications dealing with parenting, early education, fathers, child care, and the relation between home environments and children's health and development. Dr. Bradley is one of the developers of the HOME Inventory.

Mary H. Buckingham is a doctoral student at the Institute for Applied Research in Youth Development at Tufts University. Her research interests involve the study of empathy and parent–youth relationships.

Rosario (Rosie) Ceballo, Ph.D. is Professor of Psychology and Women's Studies at the University of Michigan (Ann Arbor, MI). Dr. Ceballo is a clinical and developmental psychologist whose research investigates how contextual aspects of living in poverty, such as exposure to community violence, influence children's academic and psychological functioning. In particular, she relies on a resiliency framework to study how parenting, family processes, and cultural values may buffer adolescents from the negative effects of community violence. Presently, Dr. Ceballo serves as Chair of the Women's Studies Department at the University of Michigan and is a member of the American Psychological Association's (APA) Committee on Socioeconomic Status.

Roma Chumak-Horbatsch is Associate Professor in the School of Early Childhood Studies at Ryerson University in Toronto, Canada, where she teaches courses in language development, cognitive development and childhood bilingualism. She has a background in applied linguistics and early language and literacy development. Her research focuses on multilingual pedagogy and the bilingual potential of newcomer children. In her book, Linguistically Appropriate Practice: A Guide for Working With Young Immigrant Children (2012: University of Toronto Press) Dr. Chumak-Horbatsch profiles the language reality of children who arrive in early learning programs with limited (or no) proficiency in the classroom language and presents a research-based, field-tested practice that helps teachers transform their classrooms into multilingual and multi-literate environments where languages and literacy come to life.

Latriece Clark is a graduate student in the Depth Psychology Ph.D. program with Specialization in Community Psychology, Liberation Psychology, & Ecopsychology at Pacifica Graduate Institute. She received her B.S. in psychology from Loyola University Chicago. Her interests include community-based social justice research that is focused on understanding inequalities within our society and using research to improve the lives of individuals from underprivileged backgrounds. She is interested is using research to improve and inform policy.

Tyler Colasante is a Developmental Science Ph.D. student at the Department of Psychology in the University of Toronto. His research concerns the development and interrelations of moral emotions, emotion regulation skills, and both aggressive and prosocial behaviors. In the long term, he aims to translate his research into effective interventions to promote positive socio-emotional and behavioral development in children and adolescents. E-mail: tyler.colasante@mail.utoronto.ca

Catherine Costigan, Ph.D. is Associate Professor and Director of Clinical Training at the University of Victoria in the Department of Psychology. Her research focuses on individual adjustment and family relationships in the context of immigration, including identity formation, acculturation, enculturation, and realignments of parent–child, marital, and sibling dynamics. Her recent work has focused on immigrant Chinese families. Catherine Costigan, Department of Psychology, University of Victoria, Victoria, BC, Canada, V8W 3P5; E-mail: costigan@uvic.ca

Lixian Cui, Ph.D. is Assistant Professor of Psychology at New York University Shanghai. His research focuses on emotion temporal dynamics and psychophysiology during social interactions. He also has a strong interest in emotion socialization in familial, school, and cultural contexts, and its roles in children's and adolescents' developmental psychopathology and positive development.

Annick De Houwer, Ph.D. is Professor of Language Acquisition and Multilingualism at the University of Erfurt in Germany. Her research specialty concerns early child bilingualism. Her work on the topic is used as teaching material all over the world. Dr. De Houwer's recent research focuses on the role of input in bilingual acquisition and on bilingual families' well-being.

Radosveta Dimitrova is a Docent of Psychology at Stockholm University, Sweden and Japan Society for Promotion of Science International Fellow at Hiroshima University, Japan. Her research interests regard identity, well-being, migration, positive youth development, marginalized ethnic minority communities (Roma), adaptation of instruments in different cultures.

Sara Douglass is a postdoctoral research scholar in the T. Denny Sanford School of Social and Family Dynamics at Arizona State University. She received her doctorate in Applied Developmental Psychology from Fordham University. Her research interests include adolescent ethnic/racial identity development, peer interactions as they relate to race and ethnicity, and the influence of diversity on everyday experiences for minority youth.

Naomi Eisenstadt is an Honorary Research Fellow at the University of Oxford, attached to the Department of Education and the Department of Social Policy and Intervention. She became the first Director of the Sure Start Unit in 1999. The unit was responsible for delivering the government's commitment to free nursery education places for all three- and four-year olds, the national childcare strategy, and programs aiming to reduce the gap in outcomes between children living in disadvantaged areas and the wider child population. After Sure Start, Naomi spent 3 years as the Director of the Social Exclusion Task Force working across government to identify and promote policies to address the needs of traditionally excluded groups. She is currently the Independent Advisor on Poverty and Inequality for the Scottish Government.

Kelly Escobar received her Master's degree in Experimental Psychology from Villanova University, Villanova, PA, USA. She is currently pursuing her doctorate in Developmental Psychology at New York University's Steinhardt School of Culture, Education, and Human Development. Her research is focused on bilingual language development in U.S. Latino children throughout infancy and early childhood. Specifically, she is interested in contextual influences of bilingualism, including caregivers, siblings, and peers, and the role that important others play throughout a child's early language development. She emphasizes the variable nature of bilingualism

among Latino children from different ethnic backgrounds, noting that
bilingualism is emergent and context-dependent.

Maria Evangelou is Associate Professor at the Department of Education,
University of Oxford. Her research focuses on the evaluation of early
childhood interventions; the language and literacy development of early
years; parenting education and support; and the role of evidence-based
practices in education. She has led many large grants evaluating parenting
programs including the Evaluation of the Parent Early Education Partnership
Project (PEEP), and the Early Learning Partnership Project (ELPP). *Maria*
was awarded the Brian Simon Educational Research Fellowship from BERA
for 2006/2007 for the project: *A systematic review on 'hard-to-reach' families.* During 2009 she led the literature review on children's cognitive and
socio-emotional development that informed the review of the Early Years
Foundation Stage Curriculum in 2010. She led the parenting strand of the
Evaluation of Children's Centres in England.

Laura Ferrer-Wreder is Associate Professor, Deputy Head of the Division
for Personality, Social, and Developmental Psychology, Department of
Psychology, Stockholm University. Dr. Ferrer-Wreder has published widely
including an authored book on the prevention and positive youth development field. She is active as an investigator and leader of externally funded
research projects in the United States and Sweden. Her current research
interests and/or areas of specialization include: Applied developmental science; positive youth development; and prevention science; child, adolescent,
and emerging adult development; self and identity development; the design,
implementation, and evaluation of school and community supported positive
youth development and prevention interventions; the sustainability of intervention outcomes; and university–community alliances.

Noni K. Gaylord-Harden is Associate Professor of Psychology and
Director of the Parents and Children Coping Together (PACCT) Research
Lab at the Department of Psychology in Loyola University Chicago. Her
primary research interests are in the investigation of stressors, such as
community violence and racial discrimination, on the psychosocial functioning of African American youth and families in under-resourced urban
communities. She has also focused on the role of modifiable protective
factors, such as coping strategies, future orientation, and supportive parenting, among youth in high-risk contexts. Her recent work, funded by the
National Institutes of Health, examines the impact of community violence
exposure on emotional desensitization outcomes in male adolescents of color,
the coping strategies used by youth to manage violence exposure, and the
family factors that encourage more adaptive coping strategies.

Jenny Goff holds a first class honors degree in Psychology from the
University of Reading. She worked as a senior Research Officer at the
University of Oxford and is a member of the *Families, Effective Learning,
and Literacy* (FELL) research group at the Department of Education. She has
been involved in various education projects in Oxford over the past 8 years,
investigating children's early learning and carrying out qualitative research

with young people regarding their use of technology for informal learning. In her last role at Oxford she worked as a research co-ordinator for a project evaluating Children's Centres in England (The Evaluation of Children's Centres in England: ECCE) which was funded by the Department for Education. Most recently, she has taken up a post as an Evaluation Officer at the Open University.

Nancy Gonzales is Foundation Professor of Psychology at Arizona State University. Her research examines cultural and contextual influences on the social, academic, and psychological development of Latino youth across the lifespan. A broad focus of her research is to study the interplay of culture and developmental processes at multiple levels and, especially, to understand how processes of dual cultural adaptation (acculturation and enculturation) unfold over time to impact risk and resilience. The ultimate aims of her research are to translate finding into effective interventions to simultaneously promote positive development and reduce health disparities for Latinos and other vulnerable youth.

James Hall is a research fellow at the Department of Education in the University of Oxford where he teaches graduate courses in education and in research methods. His research lies at the intersection of developmental psychology and education and focuses on developmental risk and resilience. More specifically, the psychosocial mechanisms by which children's development is placed at-risk, and the educational practices that can mitigate the consequences of this. He has published on the neurological and psychological mechanisms underpinning perinatal risks for internalizing disorders, the potential for preschool to function as an Early Intervention, how protected early skills promote long-term outcomes, and the statistical techniques that scientists use to investigate these.

Elise M. Harris is a doctoral student in the Eliot-Pearson Department of Child Development. She earned her M.A. in Human Development and Social Intervention from New York University in 2013 and her B.S. in Psychology from Xavier University in 2010. Broadly, her research interests include understanding the processes that maintain racism within educational contexts and how these contexts affect the sociopolitical development of Black and Brown youth and young adults.

Jia He is a Humboldt postdoc researcher in the German Institute for International Educational Research, Germany. She obtained her Ph.D. degree (*cum laude*) in Cross-Cultural Psychology from Tilburg University, the Netherlands. Her current research involves data comparability in large-scale international surveys, using innovative design of item formats and sophisticated psychometric methods. She is also interested in modern research methods such as structural equation modeling and multilevel analysis.

Rachel M. Hershberg is Assistant Professor of Applied Developmental Psychology and Community-Based Research in the School of Interdisciplinary Arts & Sciences at the University of Washington, Tacoma. Hershberg's research focuses on community-university collaborations as a means for examining and promoting PYD and critical consciousness in diverse groups of adolescents in the U.S.

Aline Hitti is currently a Visiting Scholar at the Department of Psychology, Tulane University and as of 2017 will be Assistant Professor at the Department of Psychology at the University of San Francisco. She received her doctoral degree in Human Development and Quantitative Methodology from the University of Maryland. Her research focuses on children's and adolescents' social cognitive and moral development in intergroup contexts. She has authored and co-authored several chapters on social exclusion and intergroup peer relations, highlighting how morality is applied in these social contexts and across development. Her research has been funded by grants from the Society for Research on Adolescence (SRA) and the Society for the Psychological Study of Social Issues (SPSSI). She has also collaborated on research funded by the National Science Foundation and the Department of Education. Publications of her work can be found in journals, such as, *Child Development*, *Social Development*, *Journal of Educational Psychology* and *Developmental Psychology*.

Dr. Elan C. Hope is Assistant Professor in the Department of Psychology at North Carolina State University. Dr. Hope takes an assets-based approach to explore individual and contextual factors that promote well-being for racially marginalized adolescents and emerging adults. She uses a critical consciousness and PVEST frameworks to examine psychosocial factors related to civic engagement and civic commitment among racially marginalized youth. Hope also investigates racial identity and discrimination in relation to academic outcomes and the transition to and through college for Black and Latino students.

Rosanne M. Jocson, M.S. M.A. is a Ph.D. candidate in Developmental Psychology at the University of Michigan (Ann Arbor, MI). Her research examines pathways through which contextual risks associated with poverty, such as neighborhood conditions, housing contexts, and community violence exposure, influence parents and children. She incorporates international perspectives in her research, with the goal of identifying individual-, familial-, and community-level protective factors that promote resilience among parents and children across different cultural contexts.

Elizabeth Karberg, Ph.D. is a research scientist in the area of reproductive health and family formation at Child Trends (Bethesda, MD). Dr. Karberg received her doctorate in Human Development and Quantitative Methodology from the University of Maryland. She broadly studies parenting with a particular focus on fathers and the family, social, and cultural factors that impact parents and children. She has studied immigrant Latino parents to explore what cultural and parenting factors Latino immigrants implement to help their children's social, linguistic, and regulatory development. She also has a specific interest in and has conducted research on how family formation patterns (e.g., when parents break up and re-partner) influence fathering and children's social development. Her current work includes healthy marriage and responsible fatherhood evaluations.

Melanie Killen, Ph.D. is Professor of Human Development and Quantitative Methodology, Professor of Psychology (Affiliate), and the Director of the NICHD Training Program in Social Development at the University of Maryland. She received her Ph.D. (1985) from the University of California, Berkeley. She is the author of *Children and Social Exclusion: Morality, Prejudice and Group Identity* (2011), co-editor of *Social Development in Childhood and Adolescence: A Contemporary Reader* (2011), and Editor of the *Handbook of Moral Development* (2006, 2014). She was appointed Distinguished Scholar-Teacher by the Provost's office, University of Maryland, and is a Fellow of the Association for Psychological Science, the American Psychological Association, and the Society for the Study of Psychological Issues. Dr. Killen has received funding from the *National Science Foundation* (NSF) and the *National Institute of Child Health and Human Development* (NICHD) for her research on social exclusion, moral reasoning, and intergroup attitudes.

Catherine Kuhns is a doctoral student at the Department of Human Development and Quantitative Methodology in the University of Maryland. She received her M.S. in Teaching English to Speakers of Other Languages from Fordham University and her B.S. in Human Development and Family Studies from Penn State University. She is broadly interested in parent child relationships in low-income and ethnic minority families. She has studied parental control and child compliance in low-income Latino immigrants and is particularly interested in the cultural context these interactions develop in.

Jennifer E. Lansford is Research Professor at Duke University. She received her doctorate in developmental psychology from the University of Michigan. Her major research interests include the development of aggression and other behavior problems in children and adolescents, with an emphasis on how family and peer contexts contribute to or protect against these outcomes.

Dr. Jacqueline V. Lerner is Professor of Applied Developmental and Educational Psychology in the Lynch School of Education at Boston College and studies the positive development of children and adolescents. Her current work involves researching and educating the field about the meaning and measurement of strength-based, rather than deficit-based models of adolescent development. She is now conducting a longitudinal study on the role of intentional self-regulation and moral exemplars in the character development of adolescents.

Richard M. Lerner is the Bergstrom Chair in Applied Developmental Science and the Director of the Institute for Applied Research in Youth Development at Tufts University. He received his Ph.D. in developmental psychology from the City University of New York. His work integrates the study of public policies and community-based programs with the promotion of positive youth development and youth contributions to civil society.

Simon Lisaingo is completing M.A. degree in the Department of Educational and Counselling Psychology and Special Education at the University of British Columbia, Canada. His research examines the motivational beliefs and processes that enable students to overcome challenges they face at home and school. He is currently on a School Psychology internship in Nanaimo, BC, where he supports diverse learners.

Elina Määttä, Ph.D. recently (June 2015) graduated from the Learning and Educational Technology Research Unit, University of Oulu, Finland. Her research interests include studying the development of SRL in primary grade children and developing research tools that enable them to express the ways in which they think about and enact strategies that lead to experiences of success. Currently she is Head of Educational Programs at the Turku Complex Systems Institute in Vancouver, Canada, and raising two immigrant learners.

Maike Malda is Assistant Professor at the Department of Clinical Child and Adolescent Studies in Leiden University. She obtained her Ph.D. in Cross-Cultural Psychology at Tilburg University (2009). Her Ph.D. research took place in India and South Africa and addressed cultural bias in cognitive tests. Dr. Malda received the Ph.D. thesis award by the European Association of Psychological Assessment. As a postdoctoral researcher at the North-West University in Potchefstroom, she studied reading and cognitive skills of South African children from diverse language groups. At Leiden University, Dr. Malda was involved as a postdoctoral researcher in a project on the resilience of Turkish minority children in the Netherlands, Germany, and Norway. Currently, Dr. Malda addresses the well-being of adolescents from diverse cultural backgrounds and she teaches courses on (inter)cultural aspects of parenting and development, and statistics.

Tina Malti, Ph.D. is Associate Professor of Developmental and Clinical Psychology in the Department of Psychology at the University of Toronto. Her research areas of expertise include socio-emotional development in the context of peer exclusion and victimization and the design, implementation, and evaluation of developmental assessment tools and intervention practices in school settings. E-mail: tina.malti@utoronto.ca

Ann S. Masten, Ph.D. Regents Professor of Child Development at the University of Minnesota, studies processes that promote competence, support resilience, and prevent problems in human development. She directs the Project Competence research on risk and resilience, including studies of children and youth exposed to homelessness, war, natural disasters, and migration. She is a recipient of the Bronfenbrenner Award for Lifetime Contributions to Developmental Psychology in the Service of Science and Society from the American Psychological Association and author of the book, Ordinary Magic: Resilience in Development.

Silvia Mazabel is a doctoral student at the Department of Educational and Counselling Psychology and Special Education in the University of British Columbia, Canada. Her research and professional interests include the promotion of SRL and strategic learning practices in language minority learners and in post-secondary settings, with a particular focus on students with learning disabilities.

Allyssa McCabe, Ph.D. is Professor of Psychology at University of Massachusetts Lowell. She studies how oral personal narrative develops with age, how parents can facilitate narrative development, and cultural differences in narration. She is coauthor of a theoretical approach to early literacy called the Comprehensive Language Approach, which looks at ways that various strands of oral and written language affect each other in acquiring full literacy. She founded a journal, Narrative Inquiry, published since 1991.

Judi Mesman, Ph.D. is a Full Professor of Diversity in Parenting and Development at Leiden University in the Netherlands. She specializes in research on culture and gender in relation to early parent–child interactions from an attachment perspective, combined with insights from cognitive theories. Mesman has published widely on the topic of attachment-related parenting themes, with a special focus on parental sensitivity, both theoretically and empirically, in mothers and fathers and across cultures. Her research in migrant populations has focused mostly on the Turkish minority population in the Netherlands.

Sheena Miao, M.Sc. is a doctoral student in the Clinical Psychology program at the University of Victoria. Sheena is primarily interested in immigrant families' adjustment after settling in a new country. In her master's thesis research, she investigated the longitudinal associations between acculturation stress and the parenting behaviors of immigrant Chinese mothers and fathers. Sheena Miao, Department of Psychology, University of Victoria, Victoria, BC, Canada, V8W 3P5; E-mail: smiao@uvic.ca

Frosso Motti-Stefanidi is Professor of Psychology, Department of Psychology, University of Athens, Greece. She is Former President of the European Association of Developmental Psychology and the European Association of Personality Psychology. Currently, she is elected member of the Governing Council of the Society for Research in Child Development (SRCD). She studies immigrant youth adaptation from a risk and resilience perspective and also studies the effect of the great economic recession on Greek and immigrant youth's adaptation.

Kelly Lynn Mulvey, Ph.D. is Assistant Professor in the Department of Educational Studies at the University of South Carolina. She completed her Ph.D. (2013) in the Department of Human Development and Quantitative Methodology at the University of Maryland. Her undergraduate and masters degrees are from Duke University. Prior to completing her doctorate, she was a public school teacher and received certification by the National Board of Professional Teaching Standards. Her research interests include social-cognitive development, in particular moral and social development in intergroup contexts. She conducts research examining gender stereotypes, theory of mind, social exclusion, and group dynamics, including when children challenge peer group norms. Her work examines the influence of children's bias, prejudice and stereotypes on their intergroup relations. Her research has been published in journals including *Cognition, Child Development, Developmental Science, Developmental Psychology, the Journal of Youth and Adolescence, the Journal of Social Issues, Social Development, Psychological Science* and *Human Development.*

Erika Y. Niwa is Assistant Professor in both the Psychology Department and the Children and Youth Studies Program at Brooklyn College. She is also affiliated with the Human Development doctoral program at the CUNY (City University of New York) Graduate Center. Her work examines how culture and context shape the developmental pathways of diverse children and youth, with a specific focus on inequality, discrimination, and political violence.

Joanna Peplak is a Master's student of Developmental Psychology at the University of Toronto. Her research focuses on how children's moral and emotional development influences their aggressive behavior and peer relations. Specifically, her work examines the independent and combined effects of various (a) moral emotions, such as sympathy and respect, on children's proactive and reactive aggression, and social exclusion. E-mail: j.peplak@mail.utoronto.ca

Nancy Perry is Professor in the Department of Educational and Counselling Psychology, and Special Education at the University of British Columbia, Canada. Her research examines how classroom tasks, instructional practices, and interpersonal relationships can support self-regulation in children and youth. She holds the Dorothy Lam Chair in Special Education in UBC's Faculty of Education and is currently President of Division 15, Educational Psychology, in the American Psychological Association.

Cynthia Pierre is a Postdoctoral Fellow at Christian Sarkine Autism Treatment Center at Indiana University School of Medicine/Riley Hospital, in Indianapolis, IN. She received her Ph.D. in Clinical Psychology from Loyola University Chicago. Her research interests include contextual risk factors of mental health and psychosocial outcomes among ethnic minority youth from low-income communities, such as stress and community violence. Her research work examines the impact of exposure to community violence on psychosocial outcomes and the benefits and limitations of support seeking as a coping strategy among African American male adolescents.

Michael Pluess, Ph.D. is a chartered psychologist and Associate Professor in Developmental Psychology at the Department of Biological and Experimental Psychology at the School of Biological and Chemical Sciences, Queen Mary University of London. He is also a visiting fellow at the London School of Economics (LSE). Initially trained in chemistry and music he spent several years working in the lab and on stage before pursuing his interests in psychology. Michael spends most of his day researching how environmental experiences shape the course of psychological development across the life course. More specifically, Dr. Pluess investigates individual differences in the capacity for environmental sensitivity as a function of different individual characteristics—including genetic and personality traits—a notion brought forward in the differential susceptibility and vantage sensitivity frameworks. Dr. Pluess is also interested in the concept of positive development in contrast to developmental psychopathology. This includes the design and empirical evaluation of intervention programs aimed at fostering positive development and the investigation of genetic and psychological moderation of such intervention effects. Dr. Pluess' research has been published in the leading journals of the field.

Leoandra Onnie Rogers is an assistant professor of psychology and faculty fellow of the Institute for Policy Research at Northwestern University. Dr. Rogers' research lies at the intersection of psychology, human development, and education. She is interested in social and educational inequities and the mechanisms through which macro-level disparities are both perpetuated and disrupted at the micro-level of identities and relationships. Her research investigates identity development among racially diverse children and adolescents in urban contexts. She asks how our social groups—and the cultural stereotypes that accompany them—shape how we see ourselves and interact with others. She received her PhD in developmental psychology from New York University's Steinhardt School of Culture, Education, and Human Development and holds a BA in psychology and educational studies from the University of California, Los Angeles (UCLA).

Natalia Rojas is a doctoral student in the Psychology and Social Intervention program at New York University. Previously, she received her BA from New York University. After graduating, she worked at MDRC, a non-profit social policy research organization, as a research associate, working to implement and evaluate two large-scale randomized control trials of early childhood interventions focused on socio-emotional and math skills in low-income preschoolers. Broadly, her research interests include the intersection between research and social policy, specifically she is interested in exploring programs and policies that impact low-income children and families, especially immigrant-origin children, early childhood policies, and designing and testing interventions at improving these settings and informing policy. She currently works with Hiro Yoshikawa and Pamela Morris

Pam Sammons is Professor of Education at the Department of Education, University of Oxford and a Senior Research Fellow at Jesus College, Oxford. Previously she was Professor at the School of Education, University of Nottingham (2004–2009) and at the Institute of Education University of London (1993–2004). Her research interests are school effectiveness and improvement, teaching effectiveness, the early years and promoting equity and inclusion in education. She was a Principal Investigator of the longitudinal Effective Provision of Pre-school Primary and Secondary Education study (1996–2014) and is leading the Impact strand of the Evaluation of Children's Centres in England (2009–2015). She has provided policy briefings for Ministers under successive governments and contributed to various enquiries and reviews. She is working with Oxford University Press on its Oxford School Improvement Pathways resources.

Teresa Smith works in the Department of Social Policy and Intervention in the University of Oxford, where she was Head of Department 1997–2005. Her research focuses on community, family and childcare, and the evaluation of community-based programs for young children and their families. Recent research includes the feasibility studies for the DfES for the evaluation of Sure Start (1999), the national evaluation of the Neighbourhood Nurseries Initiative (2007), and the evaluation of the Early Learning Partnership Project (2008). She was a specialist advisor to the House of Commons Children Schools and Families Select Committee (2004–2010) during their inquiries into children's centers and social work training. Recent publications include Smith, G, Peretz, E and Smith T (2014) *Social Enquiry, Social Reform and Social Action*: *one hundred years of Barnett House,* DSPI.

Margaret Beale Spencer, Ph.D. is Marshall Field IV Professor of Urban Education and Chair of the Department of Comparative Human Development at the University of Chicago. Spencer's phenomenological variant of ecological systems theory (P-VEST) has been used by researchers around the globe both for assisting basic research strategies as well as implementation efforts to support youth resiliency.

Christiane Spiel is Professor of Bildungs-Psychology and Evaluation and Head of Department of Applied Psychology: Work, Education, Economy at the Faculty of Psychology, University of Vienna. Her research topics are on bullying und victimization, lifelong learning, integration in multicultural school classes, evaluation and intervention research, implementation science, and quality management in the educational system. In various projects Christiane Spiel worked together with different Federal Ministries in Austria. She has got several awards for research, university teaching, and university management, has published more than 250 original papers and headed about 40 third party funded projects. Christiane Spiel is and has been chair and member of various international advisory and editorial boards as e.g., president of the European Society for Developmental Psychology, president of the Austrian Psychology Association, and president of the DeGEval– Society for Evaluation (in Germany and Austria). She was founding dean of the Faculty of Psychology at the University of Vienna and is vice-chair of the board of directors of the Wuppertal University in Germany. Currently she is one of the key authors of the International Panel on Social Progress and member of the board of directors of the Global Implementation Initiative.

Kathy Sylva is Professor of Educational Psychology at the University of Oxford. She has conducted large-scale studies on the effects of early education on children's development, including the Effective Pre-school and Primary Education study (EPPE/EPPSE). She co-leads the national Evaluation of Children's Centres in England. She conducted RCTs to evaluate parenting interventions to improve children's behavior and literacy. She was specialist adviser to the UK Parliamentary Select Committee on Education 2000–2009; in 2014/2015 she was specialist advisor to the House of Lords

'Affordable Childcare' enquiry. Currently Kathy is researching the early childhood curriculum across Europe, funded by the EU. She received the Nisbett Award in 2014 from the British Research Association for 'lifetime achievement in educational research' and an OBE in 2008 for services to children and families.

Joelle Taknint, M.Sc. is a doctoral student in the Clinical Psychology program at the University of Victoria, department of psychology. Joelle's research interests broadly address the adjustment and acculturation experiences of individuals from immigrant communities. Her most recent research has focused on experiences of discrimination and identity among immigrant adolescents and adults. E-mail: jtaknint@uvic.ca

Catherine S. Tamis-LeMonda received the Ph.D. degree in Experimental/Developmental Psychology from New York University, New York City, NY, USA. She is currently Professor of Developmental Psychology at New York University's Steinhardt School of Culture, Education, and Human Development, as well as Director of the Center for Research on Culture, Development, and Education at NYU. Her research is focused on infants' developing language, cognition, and social understanding across the first four years of life. Her research highlights the social and cultural contexts of early learning and development within the U.S. and internationally. She has been funded by the National Science Foundation, National Institute of Child Development, National Institute of Mental Health, Administration for Children, Youth and Families, the Ford Foundation, and the Robinhood Foundation.

Jochem Thijs is Assistant Professor at the Faculty of Social and Behavioral Sciences at Utrecht University in the Netherlands. He is also a researcher at the European Research Centre on Migration and Ethnic relations (ERCO-MER) at Utrecht University. His research interests include (ethnic) relations in children and adolescents, and the educational adjustments of ethnic minority children.

Jonathan M. Tirrell is a doctoral student in the Eliot-Pearson Department of Child Study and Human Development at Tufts University. His research is focused on moral development and character education, with a particular interest in forgiveness as a virtue that promotes adaptive social relationships and thriving in human development. He works as a doctoral research assistant in the Institute for Applied Research in Youth Development with Richard M. Lerner, and as managing editor of the Journal of Character Education with Marvin Berkowitz.

Peter F. Titzmann is Professor for Psychology at the University of Education, Weingarten, Germany. During his academic career he was research associate at the Friedrich-Schiller University Jena, Germany, and Assistant Professor for Life Course and Competence Development in Childhood and Adolescence at the Jacobs Center for Productive Youth Development, University of Zürich, Switzerland. His general research interest relates to the interplay between normative development and migration-related adaptation among adolescents with immigrant background. He investigated this interplay in various developmental outcomes, such as experiences of stress, delinquent behavior, friendships, autonomy development, and changes in the family hierarchy and interaction. His often interdisciplinary and longitudinal work is published in various edited volumes, book sections, and peer-reviewed journals, among them are Child Development, Developmental Psychology, Journal of Cross-Cultural Psychology, and the Journal of Youth and Adolescence.

Patrick H. Tolan is Professor at the University of Virginia in the Curry School of Education and in the Department of Psychiatry and Neurobehavioral Sciences in the School of Medicine. He is director of the cross-university multidisciplinary center, Youth-Nex: The U.Va. Center to Promote Effective Youth Development, a transdisciplinary, nexus, focusing on the capabilities of young people in connection to health, communities, schools, and relationships. Over the past 30 years, Prof. Tolan has conducted many research studies on youth development, programs to affect youth development and prevent problems, and to understand and affect youth violence. He has conducted several large-scale randomized trials of violence prevention based in promoting family and neighborhood protective processes. He also leads the 24-year longitudinal study of development of young men residing in inner city Chicago, the Chicago Youth Development Study. His latest book is, *Disruptive Behavior Disorders*, part of the *Advances in Development and Psychopathology,* a volume in the Brain Research Foundation Symposium Series he edits. (Springer, 2013).

Adriana J. Umaña-Taylor is Foundation Professor at Arizona State University in the T. Denny Sanford School of Social and Family Dynamics. She received her Ph.D. in Human Development and Family Studies from the University of Missouri-Columbia. Her research focuses on ethnic-racial identity formation, familial socialization processes, and culturally informed risk and protective factors. Her expertise lies primarily in the developmental period of adolescence, and her work is guided by an ecological framework, with an emphasis on understanding how individual and contextual factors interact to inform adolescent development and adjustment. Dr. Umaña--Taylor currently serves as Associate Editor for the *Journal of Research on Adolescence.* She previously served as a member of the Executive Council of the *Society for Research on Adolescence* and as a member of the Board of Directors for the *National Council on Family Relations.*

Fons J.R. van de Vijver is Professor at the Tilburg University, the Netherlands, at North-West University, South Africa, and the University of Queensland, Australia. He has (co-)authored over 450 publications, mainly in the domain of cross-cultural psychology. The main topics in his research involve bias and equivalence, psychological acculturation and multiculturalism, cognitive similarities and differences, response styles, translations and adaptations. He is the 2013 recipient of the International Award of the

American Psychological Association (for contributions to international cooperation and to the advancement of knowledge of psychology) and the 2014 recipient of the IAAP Fellows Award (of the International Association of Applied Psychology for contributions to applied psychology) and the 2014 Sindbad Award of the Dutch Psychological Association (for contributions to intercultural psychology).

Mitch van Geel is Assistant Professor of Clinical Child and Adolescent Studies at Leiden University in the Netherlands. His research focusses on social processes among adolescents.

Paul Vedder is Professor of Clinical Child and Adolescent Studies at Leiden University in the Netherlands. His research focusses on youth's inter- and intra-generational relationships in acculturation contexts and how these affect their learning and development.

Maykel Verkuyten is Professor in Interdisciplinary Social Science at Utrecht University. He is also the academic director of the European Research Centre on Migration and Ethnic Relations (ERCOMER) at Utrecht University. He has published many papers in international journals on ethnic identity, well-being and interethnic relations. He has also written two monographs; "The social psychology of ethnic identity" (Psychology Press), and "Identity and cultural diversity" (Routledge).

Sabine Walper is Research Director at the German Youth Institute and Professor of Education at the Ludwig-Maximilians-University in Munich, Germany. In 1986 she received her Ph.D. in psychology at the Technical University Berlin. Her research interests focus on children's and adolescents' well-being and social development as well as family issues like parenting and parents' involvement in children's education, effects of poverty and family diversity. She is president of the German League for the Child and member of the Scientific Board of the Federal Ministery of Women, Family, the Elderly, and Youth in Germany.

Jun Wang is Research Assistant Professor at the Institute for Applied Research in Youth Development at Tufts University. Her research focuses on the positive development of children and adolescents from diverse cultural backgrounds.

Dr. Niobe Way Professor of Developmental Psychology at New York University, is an internationally recognized leader in the field of adolescent development. She is also the co-director of the Center for Research on Culture, Development, and Education at NYU and the past President for the Society for Research on Adolescence. Dr. Way received her doctorate from Harvard University in Human Development and Psychology and was an NIMH postdoctoral fellow in the Psychology Department at Yale University. Her work focuses on the social and emotional development of adolescents and the impact of culture and context on health and human development. Her most recent book is "Deep Secrets: Boys' Friendships and The Crisis of Connection" (Harvard University Press, 2011). In addition to her numerous journal publications and award-winning books, she writes blogs for the Huffington Post, The Washington Post, and other media outlets.

Allan Wigfield is Professor, Distinguished-Scholar Teacher, and Director of Human Development Graduate Studies in HDQM. He also is an Honorary Faculty Member in Psychology at the University of Heidelberg, Germany. He received his Ph.D. in Educational Psychology from the University of Illinois, and then went to the University of Michigan on a postdoctoral fellowship in developmental psychology. His research interests concern the development of children's achievement motivation, children's motivation for reading and how it is influenced by different reading instructional practices, and gender differences in achievement motivation. Dr. Wigfield has authored more than 130 peer-reviewed journal articles and book chapters on children's motivation and other topics, including the chapter on the development of motivation in the Handbook of Child Psychology (6th and 7th editions). He was Associate Editor of the Journal of Educational Psychology from 2000 to 2002 and Associate Editor of Child Development from 2001 to 2005. He was editor of the teaching, learning, and human development section of the American Educational Research Journal from 2007–2010.

Nikki Yee is a doctoral student at the Department of Educational and Counselling Psychology and Special Education in the University of British Columbia. She is currently Project Manager for Perry's longitudinal study of children developing self-regulation for learning (SRL). Her research relates to the integration of SRL and decolonizing pedagogies, particularly as they relate to supporting Indigenous learners.

Hirokazu Yoshikawa is the Courtney Sale Ross Professor of Globalization and Education and the Co-Director of the Global TIES for Children Center at New York University. He conducts research on programs and policies related to early childhood development, poverty reduction and immigration in the United States and in low- and middle-income countries.

Antonio Zuffianò, Ph.D. is a postdoctoral research fellow at the Department of Psychology in the University of Toronto and at the Fraser Mustard Institute for Human Development at the University of Toronto. His research focuses on the developmental antecedents and outcomes of both prosocial and aggressive behaviors in children and adolescents. E-mail: antonio.zuffiano@utoronto.ca

Introduction

Over the last decade, social scientists have seen a gradual shift away from research focused exclusively on children's risk and problem behaviors to research more balanced and focused on positive development (Dodge 2011; Guerra et al. 2011). Attention to how parents raise healthy children and how children develop skills and behaviors needed to be successful members of society is timely and necessary for all children, especially in minority families. Although children from minority families are from all social strata, a sizable percentage grow up with limited financial and social resources due to their parents' lower socioeconomic status (SES). Many minority children and their families are often faced with challenges unknown to those from the majority population, such as learning two languages and navigating two or more sets of cultural norms, values, and expectations. These experiences might be challenging but might also confer cognitive and social advantages. Thus, research on the positive development of children living in minority families is essential in order to identify multiple sources and pathways of adaptation. This research sheds light on (a) the linkages among social and cognitive competence, ecological resources, and risk and protective factors; (b) how children develop socially and cognitively, as well as how they forge a sense of identity in a bi-cultural, bilingual environment; and (c) the multiple pathways of adaptation and well-being through interactions with families, peers, schools, and the neighborhoods/communities. For purposes of this *Handbook*, we define minority children as children whose family of origin identify themselves with an ethnic group different from the numeric majority. Children in minority families vary in terms of socioeconomic, race, and immigration (native vs. foreign-born) status.

Although research on minority children in the U.S. and Canada has a long tradition, research on minority families, especially immigrants, has only recently become mainstream research in Europe. The demographic shifts in European societies, as in North American, are especially visible in preschool and school-age children. These demographic shifts in the U.S. have resulted in a population that is quite diverse. Although 22% of children in the U.S. are born to immigrant parents, most of these children are native-born. Similar changes in Europe have dramatically increased the diversity of these countries. In Europe, the percentage of children from immigrant families has increased rapidly and varies from 10% in Italy, 26% in Germany to 39% in Switzerland (Hernandez 2012). Currently, these numbers are increasing as thousands of families flee from war and extreme poverty to Europe. As a result, all European countries now face the challenges of integrating children from diverse ethnic and linguistic backgrounds and facilitating their access to comprehensive education. Despite this, research on minority children is still scarce in many European countries.

To date, the bulk of the extant research on the development of minority children has primarily focused on socio-emotional problem behaviors or on the lack of academic success, which has been useful to advance effective prevention and treatment programs. In comparison, research on the positive adaptive outcomes of children living in minority families is very limited. Nevertheless, there are notable efforts that have called attention to and begun to document positive adaptation. First, the January 2000 Special Edition of the *American Psychologist* focused on individuals' positive and optimal experiences, optimism and happiness, and the association between positive emotions and physical health (Seligman and Csikzentmihalyi 2000). However, with one exception (Larson 2000), the main focus of this special issue was on adults. Minorities and immigrant children were not included. Second, increased efforts to understand the role of resilience in child development have been central to asking pivotal questions such as why do some children who grow up in high-risk environments are able to cope with these challenges successfully while others are not, and what are the protective systems of an individual and of the social, cultural, and religious contexts (Masten and O'Dougherty Wright 2010). But this research paradigm has not always included minority children. Research on resilience provides important insights on adaption ("doing okay/above expectations") of high-risk populations (e.g., homeless children) or of populations exposed to severe threats and adversity (e.g., war). While minority children may be faced with more and other challenges than majority children, they are not necessarily experiencing severe risks and adversity. Therefore, the resilience framework is important, but perhaps less suitable as a general framework to understand the positive development of minority children, all of whom may not experience adversity. Third, in the U.S., we know more about the factors that are related to the decline of positive outcomes than we know about the factors that promote and sustain positive development and adaptation. For example, research on whether, and under what conditions, becoming an American (acculturation) is a risk factor has shown that second or third generation children have worse behavioral and educational outcomes than their less acculturated parents but does not show which children in acculturated families do better (Garcia Coll et al. 2012). Fourth, an emerging body of research has focused on one aspect of adaptation of minority children: the effects of bilingualism on cognitive processes (Adesope et al. 2010; Engel de Abreu et al. 2012) during the early childhood education period (Han 2012; Stoessel et al. 2011). However, less attention has been paid to other domains of development, such as social development, an area where many minority children have shown strengths (Galindo and Fuller 2010). Fifth, in February 2012, the Society for Research in Child Development held its first themed meeting in Tampa, Florida on *Positive Development of Minority Children*. The conference was well received and attended by the research community and featured numerous talks and posters on theoretical, methodological, and empirical issues related to this topic.

Finally, in September 2013, *Positive Development of Minority Children* was the topic of the SRCD Social Policy Report.

The efforts to highlight positive adaptation of minority children make it clear that this is an important area of research that has been growing slowly but is not well synthesized. Thus it is difficult to discern what gains have been made and what areas of research are ready for further exploration. This *Handbook* addresses this gap by providing a forum for researchers from across the U.S., Canada, and Europe to share research on children in minority families and to clearly and succinctly offer a synthesis of where the field is and where it needs to go. The *Handbook* answers a call to the field articulated at the Tampa conference to include international scholars. In an area of globalization and increased migration and immigration, international research is critical to understand what aspects of children growing up in minority families are universal across context and what aspects are more context-specific. More specifically, the *Handbook* addresses the following central questions: (1) What individual, family, peers, neighborhood/policy factors protect children and promote positive adaptation; (2) what factors support children's social integration (e.g., the development of their cultural competencies and their sense of belonging), psychosocial adaptation (e.g., subjective well-being and social and behavioral competence), and external functioning (e.g., doing well in school, being motivated, and developing broad interests), and, (3) what are the mechanisms that explain why social adaptation occurs.

Structure of the Handbook

We organized the *Handbook* by using an ecological perspective that nests the child in a complex network of interconnected systems. Consistent with an ecological framework, there are individual, family, peers and friends, neighborhood and community, and policy factors that separately and collectively contribute to the positive developmental pathways of minority children across developmental periods. The *Handbook* is organized by parts. The authors invited to participate in each part are selected by the section editor in collaboration with the editors. Following an ecological model, the parts address specific levels of influence: individual, family/parenting, peers/friendships, early childhood education and schools. Within each part, chapters focus on specific countries, whenever possible. Given the dearth of data, this was not possible for all topics. Each part starts with an introduction written by a part editor whose expertise shaped the selection of authors as well the content area covered in that part. The part introduction alerts readers to the rationale for inclusion of topics/chapters and offers an integrative summary of the chapters in the part. The part editor, in collaboration with the editors, selected the countries and topics covered in each part. This selection was based on the scholarship available for a particular country (e.g., Albanian Families in Greece) or specific ethnic groups (e.g., Roma Families in Europe). We made great efforts to include scholars from Europe, the U.S., and Canada, but this was not always possible.

Our original intent was to have all chapters organized with a *common structure* with parallel subheadings. Given the nature of the field and the fact that some areas of research are not mature enough, most chapters, but not all, follow a common structure. This general approach enhances the readability and integration across countries and topics. Each chapter is organized according to the following headings: (1) Historical Overview and Theoretical Perspectives; (2) Current Research Questions; (3) Research Measurement and Methodology; (4) Empirical Findings; (5) Universal vs. Culture-specific Mechanisms; (6) Policy Implications; and (7) Future Directions. Reflecting the state of the field, some chapters are no more than a research agenda, others are more focused in scope. This uneven coverage highlights the areas of research that are understudied and ready for future investigation. The goal of Part V is to identify universal vs. cultural-specific mechanisms that can enable researchers to consider the ways in which their findings might be outcome-specific, culture-specific, domain-specific, or universal. The chapters conclude with Future Directions that forms the basis for the next generation of studies on children in minority families. Authors addressed the following questions: What are the questions and topics that need to be addressed in future studies? What can we do to identify the potential of minority children, and how can we measure positive development, what are the important predictors of positive adaptive outcomes? Overall, this structure leads to a discussion of where the field has come from and build up to the current state of theory, questions, methods, and research findings.

Part I: Conceptual and Methodological Approaches. The chapters in this part focus on theoretical approaches to measure children's positive development; measurement issues and indicators of positive development; and the broader ecological context. Measurement issues will are relevant to positive development of all children but also address the question whether instruments are suitable and ecologically valid for minority children. The chapter on the ecological context in which positive development unfolds focuses on the interactions between the home environment and the social support provided by neighborhoods, social relationships and connections within the community. This part addresses question of how key protective factors such as connections to prosocial competent peers, as well as to competent caring teachers and other adults, along with available resources in the neighborhood, daycare, and schools influence children's adaptation and well-being (Masten and Obradovic 2006).

Frosso Motti-Stefanidi of the University of Athens in Greece is the editor of the first part on conceptual and methodological approaches. This part addresses two core issues: (1) who among minority children and youth adapts well or even thrives and (2) why these children adapt and thrive. Richard Lerner and his colleagues examine individual strengths in a developmental context and discuss research that supports the positive youth development (PYD) model. They also examine gaps in research regarding minority youth. Frosso Motti-Stefanidi and Ann Masten present the resilience perspective. While PYD stresses competence and optimal functioning, the resilience perspective focuses on positive patterns of adaptation in the context of adversity—doing "ok" or better than expected. The final two chapters of this part address methodological issues. Jens Asendorpf provides a non-technical introduction to multilevel statistical analysis and Fons van de Vijver and Jia He propose a systematic classification on equivalence research on positive development of minority children.

Part II: Individual Level Influences. The chapters in this part, edited by Robert H. Bradley, address the question of how children's adaptive systems (e.g., language, self-regulation, and social skills) as well as their attachment relationships to their parents or caregivers facilitate their positive developmental pathways. Bradley introduces his part by emphasizing, "Humans are active self-regulating agents functioning within self-regulating interconnected systems" and asks what positive development actually means. As with the questions posed by Motti-Stefanidi and Masten, this question asks whether we are talking about the absence of a negative outcome, about "doing ok" or better than expected in light of severe adversity, or about children and youth who thrive. In addition, Bradley questions the extent to which research in the West can be transferred to research on minority children with a non-Western background. All chapters in this part address the notion of understanding child development in context. Elham To address this issue, Assary and Michael Pluess employ the differential susceptibility and vantage sensitivity framework; Maike Malda and Judi Mesman focus on parental sensitivity and attachment relationships; Kelly Escobar and Catherine S. Tamis LeMonda focus on language competence; Paul Vedder and Mitch van Geel examine the developmental resource of cultural identity; and, Jennifer Lansford discusses parenting and children's adjustment. Both Parts I and II emphasize the relationship between person and environment and consequently the view that positive development of minority children requires a supportive environment provided by parents and other responsible adults.

Part III: Family/Parenting Level Influences. The chapters in this part focus on the role parents, siblings, and other close relatives have on children's development—how do key characteristics of parents, such as their parenting cognitions, ethnic identity, religious orientation, and acculturation, as well as languages spoken at home influence children's everyday experiences in the family context? The chapters in this part illuminate the prevalence and diversity of children in minority families highlighting family processes, the role of family cohesion, family structure (e.g., marriage vs. co-habitation, single parenthood, number of children/children out of wedlock, stability/dissolution of marriages, interethnic marriages), as well the role of cultural membership and other factors and its relationship to identity.

Families are central to children's positive development. As part editor Marc H. Bornstein points out, all authors in this part emphasize the importance of firmly rooting children in their families' cultural heritage while encouraging them to selectively adopt the values of the majority society. Catherine Costigan, Joelle Taknint and Sheena Miao conclude that children who have strong relationships with their parents and at the same time navigate successfully both cultures have the best chances to use the available resources to adapt successfully. Sabine Walper and Birgit Leyendecker write from a European perspective and point out the importance of the legal status of minority and of immigrant families. While the law protects many indigenous minority groups and parents are encouraged to speak their language and to pass on their culture, immigrant families are also expected to integrate or even to assimilate into the receiving countries. Immigrant parents have little legal support and have many difficulties in fostering their children's cultural heritage. Natasha Cabrera, Elizabeth Karberg, and Catherine Kuhns provide evidence from research on fathers in minority families showing the unique influences of minority fathers on their children's positive development. The final two chapters of this part by Allyssa McCabe and by Annick De Houwer focus on language. McCabe focus is on the importance of bilingualism and emphasizes that growing up bilingually provides a unique advantage for minority children. De Houwer supports this view and emphasizes the importance of bilingualism for children's and parent's socio-emotional well-being.

Part IV: Peers and Friendship Level Influences. The chapters in this part examine the buffering influence of peers on the association between environmental inputs and child outcomes, across developmental periods. This part headed by Christiane Spiel focuses on peers and friendship level influences on development. How does being integrated in a community and having friends support children's positive development? Peter Titzmann addresses effects of homophile and friendships for immigrant and native peers on their social adjustment. In contrast, Leonadra Onnie Rogers, Erika Y. Niwa and Niobe Way examine the ways in which the macro-context shapes the micro-context of friendships. Chapter "Minority and Majority Children's Evaluations of Social Exclusion in Intergroup Contexts" Aline Hitti, Kelly Lynn Mulvey, and Melanie Killen examine social exclusion in intergroup contexts while Tina Malti, Antonio Zuffianò, Lixian Cui, Tyler Colasante, Joanna Peplak, and Na Young Bae discuss the risks associated with peer exclusion. Rosveta Dimitrova and Laura Ferrer-Wreder review the existing literature on Roma children and youth and point to the importance of peer and family as a resource for the positive development of this particularly vulnerable group in Europe

Part V: Early Childhood and School Level Influences. The chapters in this part edited by Allan Wigfield focus on the impact of early childhood education and schools on the development of children's well-being, self-esteem, achievement motivation, academic outcomes, and on the mutually influential person-context relations. Nancy Perry, Nikki Yee, Mazabel-Ortega, Simon Lisaingo, and Elina Määttää compare the education experiences of immigrant, Aboriginal, and language minority children in Canadian schools. They describe how educational strategies and practices that match the educational needs of these students can foster their academic achievements. Jochem Thijs and Maykel Verkuyten focus on the direct and indirect influences of children classroom composition, degree of perceived support, discrimination and multicultural education on minority children's developmental outcomes such as self-esteem. Rosario Ceballo, Rosanne M. Jocson, and Francheska Alers-Rojas discuss how children's SES, school attendance, and experiences of discrimination contribute to the achievement outcomes of many Latino children. Parents who want to become involved in (under-resourced) schools are likely to face barriers. Ceballo and her colleagues discuss the potential of raising parents' academic awareness and of facilitating their involvement in their children's schools.

Part VI: Policies/Prevention/Programs. Finally, at the macro level, the chapters in this part edited by Nancy Gonzalez focus on the short- and long-term impact that social policies can have on children's levels of adaptation. In her introduction to this part, Gonzalez sets the tone of this part by stating that "It is not that 'at-risk' youth need special treatment for their deficits; what is needed rather, is to ensure the basic conditions for positive development are made accessible and equitable for all children and youth". The chapters by Natalie Rojas and Hiro Yoshikawa, Noni Gaylor-Harden, Oscar Barbarin, and Pat Tolan, and Maria Evangelou, Jenny Goff, Kathy Sylva, Pam Sammons, Teresa Smith, James Hall and Naomi Eisenstad address the need for translational research: what are the policy changes that will actually make a difference in the life of minority children and youth? Adriana Umana-Taylor and Sara Douglass and Roma Chumak-Horbatsch make the case for the development of curricula that work for all students regardless of their cultural background. Chumak-Horbatsch introduces her model for instructional practice for young bilingual learners. Elan C. Hope and Margaret Beale Spencer focus on civic engagement as an adaptive coping strategy that can facilitate the positive development of children and youth.

This unprecedented collection of cutting-edge research offers the best science available on the positive development of ethnic minority children. It offers a comprehensive view of the advances in the way we conceptualize, measure and research the challenges but more importantly the assets and opportunities of this population. In so doing, it offers a clear set of research recommendations for researchers, practitioners, and policymakers interested in improving the lives of these families. The message of this Handbook is simple: it is not enough to understand the adversity and challenges that ethnic minority families face, to clearly understand the development of ethnic minority children, we must also just as fiercely study the assets and strengths that shape their development.

Natasha J. Cabrera
Birgit Leyendecker

References

Adesope, O. O., Lavin, T., Thompson, T., & Ungerleider, C. (2010). A systematic review and meta-analysis of the cognitive correlates of bilingualism. *Review of Educational Research, 80*(2), 207–245.

Dodge, K. A. (2011). Context matters in child and family policy. *Child Development, 82,* 433–442.

Engel de Abreu, P. M. J., Cruz-Santos, A., Tourinho, C. J., Martin, R., & Bialystok, E. (2012). Bilingualism enriches the poor: Enhanced cognitive control in low income minority children. *Psychological Science, 23*(11), 1364–1371.

Galindo, C., & Fuller, B. (2010). The social competence of Latino kindergartners and growth in mathematical understanding. *Developmental Psychology, 46*(3), 579–592.

Guerra, N. G., Graham, S., & Tolan, P. H. (2011). Raising healthy children: Translating research into practice. *Special Issue of Child Development on Raising Healthy Children, 82*(1), 7–16.

Han, W. -J. (2012). Bilingualism and academic achievement. In C. Garcia Coll & A. K. Marks (Eds.), *The immigrant paradox in children and adolescents. Is becoming American a developmental risk?* (pp. 161–184). Washington, DC: American Psychological Association.

Hernandez, D. (2012). Resources, strengths, and challenges for children in immigrant families in eight affluent countries. In A. Masten, K. Liebkind, & D. J. Hernandez (Eds.), *Realizing the potential of immigrant youth* (pp. 17–40). New York: Cambridge University Press.

Larson, R. W. (2000). Towards a psychology of positive youth development. *American Psychologist, 55*, 170–183.

Marks, A. K. & Garcia Coll, G. (Eds) (2012). *The immigrant paradox in children and adolescents: Is becoming an American a developmental risk?* Washington, DC: American Psychological Association.

Masten, A., & O'Dougherty Wright, M. (2010). Resilience over the lifespan. Developmental perspectives on resistance, recovery, and transformation. In J. W. Reich, A. J. Zautra, & J. Stuart Hall (Eds.), *Handbook of adult resilience* (pp. 213–237). New York: The Guilford Press.

Masten, A., & Obradovic, J. (2006). Competence and resilience in development. *Annals of the New York Academy of Science, 1094*, 13–27.

Seligman, M. E. P., & Csikszentmihalyi, M. (2000). *Positive psychology: An introduction.* American Psychologist, Vol 55(1), Jan 2000, 5–14.

Stoessel, K., Titzmann, P. F., & Silbereisen, R. K. (2011). Children's psychosocial development following the transitions to kindergarten and school: A comparison between natives and immigrants in Germany. *International Journal of Developmental Science, 5* (1–2), 41–55. doi:10.3233/DEV-2011-11077.

Part I

Conceptual and Methodological Approaches

Conceptual and Methodological Issues in the Study of Minority Youth: Adaptation and Development

Frosso Motti-Stefanidi

University of Athens, Athens, Greece

During the last decade research on the well-being of children and youth has gradually shifted from a deficit view, focusing on symptoms and disorders, towards a strength-based view, focusing on positive adaptation, competence, and resilience. The positive youth development perspective (Lerner et al. 2015) and the resilience developmental framework (Masten 2014a) largely express this shift in focus that dominated developmental science for decades. Research on minority children and youth has followed the zeitgeist, and has also increasingly focused on positive patterns of adaptation and development and positive factors and processes that can account for these positive outcomes (see Cabrera 2013; Motti-Stefanidi et al. 2012; Motti-Stefanidi and Masten 2013).

Minority children and youth, like all children and youth, face the developmental challenges of their time and age. However, they are also exposed to challenges that stem from their minority status. Often minority families are embedded in the lower social strata of societies. In addition to lower socioeconomic status, minority families also have to deal with experiences of prejudice and discrimination, as well as with the fact that they have to learn to navigate between at least two cultures. In spite of these challenges, significant diversity in

their adaptation and development is observed. Some minority children and youth are following pathways towards positive adjustment and mental health, whereas others are following pathways towards adaptation difficulties and/or psychological problems. A central question that research on minority youth adaptation and development currently addresses is: "Who among minority youth adapts well or even thrives and why?" These issues are at the core of this part on conceptual and methodological approaches to positive development of minority children.

In Chapter "Positive Youth Development Among Minority Youth: A Relational Developmental Systems Model", Lerner, Wang, Hershberg, Buckingham, Harris, Tirell, Bowers, and Lerner first present core constructs and principles of the positive youth development (PYD) perspective as well as empirical support for this model. PYD examines individual strengths in developmental context and focuses on the continual bidirectional interactions between individuals and their unfolding environments in understanding which interactions promote development and which have a preventive effect and lead to risk and other problem behaviors. PYD stresses the importance of the alignment of youth's strengths with the resources for positive adaptation found in their ecological settings, as well as of the plasticity of human development. However, to date, limited scientific information exists as to what positive youth development may look like for minority youth. The authors present the extant evidence regarding the application of this conceptual model to understanding minority youth positive development and end with a discussion of gaps in our knowledge and a clearly articulated set of suggestions regarding conceptual and methodological issues concerning the study of PYD in minority youth.

In Chapter "A Resilience Perspective on Immigrant Youth Adaptation and Development", Motti-Stefanidi and Masten examine group and individual differences in immigrant youth adaptation and development through the lens of a resilience developmental framework that incorporates acculturation and social psychological variables. They propose that positive adaptation in immigrant youth is judged based on how well they are doing with respect to developmental and acculturative tasks and on their psychological well-being. They address two key questions. The first asks whether immigrant status is a risk factor for youth's adaptation and development. The second concerns the identification of processes that protect immigrant youth who are doing well in spite of the challenges that they face. This integrative conceptual framework allows for a developmental, differentiated, contextualized, and multilevel approach to explaining the diversity in immigrant youth adaptation.

It should be noted that both PYD and the resilience frameworks have their basis on a developmental systems, dynamic approach to human behavior and development. However, these two developmental models have some important differences in emphasis (Masten 2014b), which are consequential for understanding minority youth development. First, they focus on different indices of positive adaptation. PYD focuses on indexes of thriving among youth, that is, the "Five Cs" (competence, confidence, character, connection, and caring) (see Lerner et al. 2016). These are attributes of the individual that are linked to youth doing well in a particular context. Resilience researchers define positive adaptation as doing

well with respect to age-salient developmental tasks across the life course in the context of risk. The integrative model presented in the chapter by Motti-Stefanidi and Masten, proposes two additional criteria for judging positive adaptation, namely adaptation with respect to acculturative tasks (e.g., learning the characteristics of the receiving society in addition to those of the home culture and developing positive ethnic and national identities) and psychological well-being. Second, PYD stresses indexes of optimal functioning, whereas resilience investigators often define positive adaptation as doing adequately well or "okay". Third, resilience researchers, unlike PYD researchers, are particularly interested in individual-context interactions and adaptive function at the high end of a continuum of risk and adversity. The definition of resilience actually requires evidence of positive adaptation under conditions of risk or adversity. Positive adaptation under low-risk conditions is considered to reflect competence and not resilience.

The next two chapters focus on methodological issues related to the study of minority youth development. Asendorpf, based on the argument that children's lives are embedded in a hierarchy of nested social systems, provides a step by step non-technical introduction to multilevel statistical analysis, an important tool for understanding social embeddedness, that allows us to disentangle the influences of different levels of context and of individual attributes, as well as of their interaction, on minority youth adaptation and development. He starts with two- and three-level models and ends with the topic of longitudinal mediation. He argues that understanding how these models are developed and tested is not only required for avoiding biased results but also helps sharpen one's thinking with respect to influences on youth's adaptation at different levels of context and analysis and to psychological mechanisms explaining these phenomena.

In Chapter "Equivalence in Research on Positive Development of Minority Children: Methodological Approaches", van de Vijver and He argue that the study of minority youth inevitably brings to the fore the appropriateness of measurement and of the comparability of one minority group either to another or to the majority group. They propose a systematic classification of bias and equivalence, and describe, using empirical examples, how to handle these methodological issues. They continue with a presentation of issues arising from participants' response styles, which may vary in different cultural groups. They end the chapter with a presentation of mixed methods approaches to the study of minority youth adaptation. They discuss the method of triangulation, which involves the different ways quantitative and qualitative approaches may be combined. These approaches are complementary but have their strengths and weaknesses. They argue that when existing research instruments may fail to cover relevant aspects of the phenomenon under study in a particular group, an open approach may provide rich and new information.

Together, these four chapters present the conceptual and methodological tools that enable us to organize the extant evidence on positive minority youth development with the purpose of identifying gaps in our knowledge, guiding our research questions, and developing the appropriate methods to study such complex, longitudinal and multilevel phenomena. Lerner et al (this book) quoted Lewin (1952) in saying that "There is nothing so practical as a good theory". On the other hand, as van de Vijver and He (this book) argue, adequately designed, conducted,

and analyzed studies are often easier to interpret and more insightful since they allow us to deal with cultural factors more adequately.

References

Cabrera, N. J. (2013). Positive development of minority children. *SRCD Social Policy Report, 27*(2).

Lerner, R. M., Lerner, J.V., Bowers, E., & Geldhof, G. J. (2015). Positive youth development: A relational developmental systems model. In W.F. Overton, & P. C. Molenaar (Eds.), *Handbook of child psychology and developmental science. Vol. 1: Theory and method* (7th ed.). (pp. 607–651). Editor-in-chief: R. M. Lerner. Hoboken, NJ: Wiley.

Lewin, K. (1952). *Field theory in social science: Selected theoretical papers*. London: Tavistock.

Masten, A. S. (2014a). Global perspectives on resilience in children and youth. *Child Development, 85*(1), 6–20.

Masten, A. S. (2014b). Invited Commentary: Resilience and positive youth development frameworks in developmental science. *Journal of youth and adolescence, 43*(6), 1018–1024.

Motti-Stefanidi, F., & Masten, A. S. (2013). School success and school engagement of immigrant children and adolescents. *European Psychologist, 18*, 126–135. doi: 10.1027/1016-9040/a000139

Motti-Stefanidi, F., Berry, J., Chryssochoou, X., Sam, D. L., & Phinney, J. (2012). Positive immigrant youth adaptation in context: Developmental, acculturation, and social psychological perspectives. In A. S. Masten, K. Liebkind, & D.J. Hernandez (Eds.), *Realizing the potential of immigrant youth*. pp. 117–158. New York, NY: Cambridge University Press.

Positive Youth Development Among Minority Youth: A Relational Developmental Systems Model

Richard M. Lerner, Jun Wang, Rachel M. Hershberg,
Mary H. Buckingham, Elise M. Harris, Jonathan M. Tirrell,
Edmond P. Bowers and Jacqueline V. Lerner

Abstract

We present an overview of the positive youth development (PYD) perspective and the relational developmental systems (RDS) metatheory that frames this perspective. We describe the Lerner and Lerner model of PYD, and some of the findings from the 4-H Study of PYD regarding how thriving can be promoted among America's diverse youth. We also address limitations of this research, including the lack of a representative sample of minority youth participants in this study. We discuss how further RDS-based PYD research may be designed with the explicit goal of addressing some of the limitations of past work. We present implications for applying what we have learned from PYD research to programs that aim to promote thriving among minority youth in the U.S. and internationally.

Interests in the strengths of youth, the relative plasticity of human development (the potential for systematic change in the structure and function of development; Lerner 1984), and the concept of resilience (Masten 2014) coalesced in the 1990s to foster the development of the concept of positive youth development (PYD; Lerner et al. 2015). As discussed by Hamilton (1999), the concept of PYD was understood in at least three interrelated ways: 1. as a developmental process; 2. as a philosophy or approach to youth programming; and 3. as instances of youth programs and organizations focused on fostering the healthy or positive development of youth.

In the decade following Hamilton's (1999) discussion of PYD, several different models of the developmental process believed to be involved in PYD were used to frame descriptive, explanatory, or intervention/optimization research across childhood and adolescence (e.g., Benson et al. 2011; Catalano et al. 2002; Damon 2008; Eccles 2004; Eccles and Gootman 2002; Flay 2002; Larson 2000; Lerner et al. 2005, 2015; Masten 2001, 2014; Spencer 2006). However, all of these models of the developmental process involved in

R.M. Lerner (✉) · J. Wang · R.M. Hershberg
M.H. Buckingham · E.M. Harris · J.M. Tirrell
Tufts University, Medford, MA, USA
e-mail: Richard.Lerner@tufts.edu

E.P. Bowers
Clemson University, Clemson, SC, USA

J.V. Lerner
Boston College, Chestnut Hill, MA, USA

© The Editor(s) 2017
N.J. Cabrera and B. Leyendecker (eds.), *Handbook on Positive Development of Minority Children and Youth*, DOI 10.1007/978-3-319-43645-6_1

PYD reflect ideas associated with what is termed relational developmental systems (RDS) metatheory (e.g., Overton 2015).

In this chapter, we first provide an overview of the RDS metamodel and then briefly discuss, as a sample case of RDS-based PYD models, the formulation of such models that has the most extensive empirical support (Heck and Subramaniam 2009), the Five Cs Model of PYD (Lerner et al. 2015). We then point to what we know and what remains to be discerned about PYD among minority youth, that is, youth defined in this chapter as young people of non-European American/White and/or of Hispanic backgrounds (Cabrera and The SRCD Ethnic Racial Issues Committee 2013). As we will explain, at this writing, knowledge of PYD among minority youth is characterized by conceptual, methodological, and substantive limitations. Although research and practice aimed at promoting PYD among minority youth is growing (e.g., Cabrera and The SRCD Ethnic Racial Issues Committee 2013; Hope and Jagers 2014; Travis and Leech 2014), a key limitation is the absence of longitudinal studies with samples that represent the current U.S. sociodemographic landscape (Spencer and Spencer 2014). Accordingly, we conclude this chapter by pointing to important issues to be addressed in future research.

The Relational Developmental Systems Metatheory: An Overview

From the late 1960s through the first half of the second decade of the twenty-first century, the study of human development evolved from a field dominated by split, reductionist (psychogenic or biogenic) approaches to a multidisciplinary (and, in regard to aspirations of many developmental scientists, an interdisciplinary) scholarly domain. The goal of this scholarship is to integrate variables from biological through cultural and historical levels of organization across the life span into a synthetic, coactional system (e.g., Elder

et al. 2015; Ford and Lerner 1992; Gottlieb 1998; Lerner 2012). Prior, reductionist accounts of development that adhered to a Cartesian dualism pulled apart (or split) facets of the integrated developmental system (Overton 2015). For instance, reductionist views typically elevated the importance of such split formulations as nature versus nurture, continuity versus discontinuity, stability versus instability, and basic versus applied science (Overton 2015).

Split approaches are rejected by proponents of theories derived from RDS metatheory which, in turn, are derived from a process-relational paradigm (Overton 2015). Overton (2015) explains that, as compared to a Cartesian worldview, the process-relational paradigm focuses on process, becoming, holism, relational analysis, and the use of multiple perspectives and explanatory forms. Within the process-relational paradigm, the organism is seen as inherently active, self-creating (autopoietic), self-organizing, self-regulating (agentic), nonlinear/complex, and adaptive (Overton 2015).

In turn, within the RDS metatheory, the integration of different levels of organization frames the understanding of life-span human development (Overton 2015). The conceptual emphasis in RDS-based theories is placed on mutually-influential relations between individuals and contexts, on individual ↔ context relations. These relations vary across place and time (Elder et al. 2015); the "arrow of time," or temporality, represents history, which is the broadest level within the ecology of human development. History imbues all other levels with change. Such change may be stochastic (e.g., non-normative life or historical events; Baltes et al. 2006) or systematic, and the potential for systematic change constitutes a potential for (at least relative) plasticity across the life span.

As explained by Lerner (1984), the concept of plasticity was emphasized by developmental scientists who were interested in countering the idea of fixity in human development, for instance a fixity purportedly imposed by genetic inheritance or neuronal "hard wiring." Accordingly, the idea of plasticity arose to denote the capacity in human development for systematic and relatively continuous changes, as compared to stochastic (random) and short-term changes. Such relatively permanent and systematic change can arise through individual ↔ context relations that are either ontogenetically or historically normative or from non-normative life or historical events (Baltes et al. 2006).

Theories derived from an RDS metatheory focus on the "rules" or processes that govern, or regulate, exchanges between (the functioning of) individuals and their contexts. Brandtstädter (1998) termed these relations "developmental regulations" and noted that, when developmental regulations involve mutually-beneficial individual ↔ context relations, these developmental regulations are adaptive. To understand what makes developmental regulations adaptive, one needs both conceptual and empirical criteria. Conceptually, developmental regulations are adaptive when, and only when, they are beneficial to the maintenance of positive, healthy functioning of the components of a bidirectional relation (e.g., both individual and context).

As we have noted, there are several models associated with RDS-based ideas that have been used to study processes pertinent to, or explicitly about, PYD (e.g., see Lerner et al. 2015, for a review). However, the central research question in all of these RDS-based models is: Can youth thriving be promoted through aligning the strengths of young people with the resources for positive development found in their ecological settings? Because the Lerner and Lerner (Lerner et al. 2015) model has more data pertinent to it than any other model, we use it as a sample case to discuss what is and what is not known in response to this central question, especially in regard to PYD among minority youth. Accordingly, we describe several investigations from the 4-H Study of PYD—the research testing the Lerner and Lerner model. We highlight findings that may be most pertinent to research on PYD among minority youth. However, the limitations of the 4-H Study sample preclude findings from

these investigations being generalized to minority youth, a point we emphasize below (Spencer and Spencer 2014). Nevertheless, we provide this brief review as a starting point for discussing future longitudinal research about PYD among minority youth.

The Five Cs Model of PYD

Research on minority youth has often been framed within a deficit conception of their development (Cabrera and The SRCD Ethnic Racial Issues Committee 2013; Travis and Leech 2014). However, as is the case with all RDS-based PYD models, the Lerner and Lerner conception is a strength-based model of development that seeks to understand and enhance the lives of diverse youth through engagement with key contexts in their ecology (e.g., families, schools, peer groups, and out of school programs). Indeed, a major focus of the Lerner and Lerner PYD research has been the study of the latter setting. There is considerable research assessing if and how the lives of diverse youth can be enhanced through engagement with community-based youth-development programs, especially if these programs align features of both youth and program strengths (as occurs when theoretical models, such as the person-stage-environment-fit model, are used to frame program design; Eccles 2004).

The model of the PYD process constructed by Lerner, Lerner, and their colleagues explicitly has drawn on the RDS individual ↔ context conception as its foundation. This model has been elaborated in the context of the longitudinal study of PYD conducted by Lerner, Lerner, and colleagues: the 4-H Study of PYD (e.g., Bowers et al. 2014; Lerner et al. 2005, 2009a, b, 2010, 2011). This research seeks to identify the individual and ecological relations that may promote thriving and, as well, that may have a preventive effect in regard to risk/problem behaviors. Within the 4-H Study, thriving is understood as the growth of attributes that mark a flourishing, healthy young person. These characteristics are termed the "Five Cs" of PYD—competence, confidence, character, connection, and caring.

Consistent with the central research question in all RDS-based models of PYD, the core theory of change tested in this approach to the developmental process of PYD involved in youth programs is that, if: 1. the strengths of youth (e.g., a young person's cognitive, emotional, and behavioral engagement with the school context, having the "virtue" of hope for the future, or possession of intentional self-regulation (ISR) skills such as Selection [S], Optimization [O], and Compensation [C]); can 2. be aligned with the resources for positive growth found in youth development programs, for example, the "Big Three" attributes of youth development programs (i.e., positive and sustained adult-youth relationships, skill-building activities, and youth leadership opportunities); then 3. young people's healthy development will be optimized (e.g., Lerner et al. 2009a, b, 2013; Lerner 2004). He or she will manifest the Five Cs and, as well,

demonstrate other positive attributes of behavior reflecting adaptive developmental regulations—most fundamentally, a Sixth "C," youth contributions to self, family, community, and civil society. In other words, if positive development rests on mutually-beneficial relations between the youth and his/her ecology, then thriving youth should be positively engaged with and act to enhance their world. Further, the youth should be less prone to engage in risk/problem behaviors.

Figure 1 presents an illustration of the Lerner and Lerner conception of the PYD developmental process. The figure illustrates, as well, that these adaptive developmental regulations and their positive and problematic sequelae exist within the broader ecology of human development. This ecology includes families, schools, community institutions, and culture. As well, historical (temporal) variation introduces change at all levels of organization within the relational developmental system.

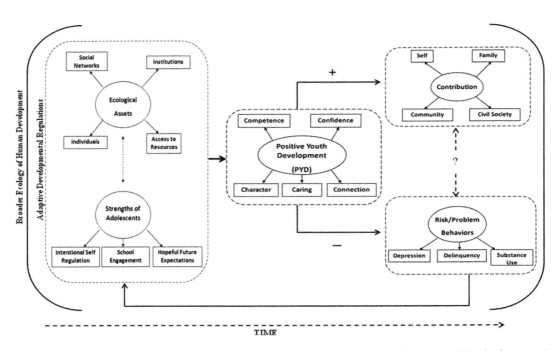

Fig. 1 A relational, developmental systems model of the individual ↔ context relations involved in the Lerner and Lerner conception of the PYD developmental process

Tests of the Lerner and Lerner PYD Model

To test the ideas presented in Fig. 1, researchers at the Institute for Applied Research in Youth Development (IARYD) at Tufts University launched the 4-H Study of PYD, a longitudinal study beginning at Grade 5 and ending at Grade 12. Overall, across eight waves of the study, approximately 7000 youth and 3500 of their parents from 42 states were surveyed. At all eight waves, the sample varied in race, ethnicity, socioeconomic status, family structure, rural-urban location, geographic region, and program participation experiences (Lerner et al. 2015). The research identified the resources, or developmental assets, which existed in the key settings of youth, that is, families, schools, and community-based youth programs. In addition, through obtaining information about the young person's strengths (e.g., ISR, school engagement, and hopeful future expectations) the study assessed the individual strengths of adolescents. Patterns of participation in out-of-school time (OST) activities were also assessed in this study. These activities included Youth Development programs, such as 4-H, Boy Scouts, Girl Scouts, YMCA, Boys & Girls Clubs, and Big Brothers/Big Sisters, sports, arts and crafts, interest clubs, religious clubs, performing arts organizations, or service organizations. Information about civic engagement/civic contribution, future aspirations and expectations, relationships with parents, friends, and other adults, and values were also measured. In addition, parents were asked about the nature and composition of their household, education, employment, and neighborhood.

The findings of the 4-H Study have been reported in more than 100 publications (see Lerner et al. 2015, for a review). Here, we summarize some of the key findings bearing on the Lerner and Lerner theory presented in Fig. 1. IARYD researchers studied youth development programs as settings for/sources of the key ecological assets linked to positive developmental outcomes. These ecological assets were categorized into four categories—other individuals such as parents, peers, mentors, and teachers; community institutions, including youth development programs; collective activity between youth and adults, including program leaders; and access to the prior three types of assets. Theokas and Lerner (2006) found that, in all settings, assets represented by other individuals were the most potent predictors of PYD. Family assets such as parental involvement, autonomy granting, communication, and problem solving, were most important in the lives of youth. One of the strongest predictors of PYD was eating dinner together as a family. Subsequent analyses (Urban et al. 2010) of the youth from Theokas and Lerner's work indicated that dimensions of the neighborhood coact with adolescent youth development programs involvement to predict PYD, depressive symptoms, and risk behaviors—findings consistent with the theory of change model shown in Fig. 1.

In addition, several studies have also used the 4-H Study data set to examine possible interactions between self-regulatory processes and youth development program participation. For example, Urban et al. (2010) found that both the strengths of youth, represented by ISR, and the resources of their contexts are involved in thriving. However, youth ISR abilities moderated the effect of participation in youth development programs on PYD among adolescents living in neighborhoods with relatively low levels of ecological assets. Youth in these settings who had the greatest capacity to self regulate benefitted the most from involvement in youth development programs, in terms of PYD, depressive symptoms, and risk behaviors. These relations were particularly strong for girls.

Moreover, emotions, such as hope for one's future, along with the cognitive and behavioral skills that youth need to activate ISR skills to achieve future goals, may also play important roles in the development of civic engagement. For example, using data collected from youth participants in Grades 7, 8, and 9 of the 4-H Study, Schmid and Lopez (2011) assessed the role of a hopeful future orientation in predicting growth trajectories of positive and negative developmental outcomes, including PYD, contribution, risk behaviors, and depressive symptoms. Hopeful future orientation was a stronger predictor than ISR for each of the outcomes assessed.

The 4-H Study data have also been used to examine the ecological assets of parenting and youth programs in relation to variables reflecting civic engagement. For example, using data from youth in Grades 5 through 8 from the 4-H Study, Lewin-Bizan et al. (2010) found a developmental cascade, wherein positive parenting (indexed by warmth and monitoring) was a key contextual asset predicting subsequent ISR; in turn, ISR predicted subsequent scores for PYD which, in turn, positively predicted later youth Contribution scores.

Using data from Grades 8 through 11, Zaff et al. (2010, 2011) derived a measure of active and engaged citizenship (AEC) from items within the measures used in the 4-H Study. AEC involved four first-order latent constructs: civic participation, civic duty, civic self-efficacy, and neighborhood connection. These four factors indexed the second-order latent construct of AEC. Consistent with the model presented in Fig. 1, engagement with the ecological developmental assets represented by community-based institutions and programs (which, in the Zaff et al. 2011 study involved youth development programs and religious institutions) was associated positively with AEC.

In sum, findings from tests of the model shown in Fig. 1 conducted with data from the 4-H Study of PYD support the idea that links among the strengths of young people and the ecological assets in their families, schools, and communities predict their thriving and, in turn, their contributions to, and active and engaged citizenship within, their communities. However, there have also been tests of the model that have been inconsistent with expectations. For instance, the predicted inverse relation between indices of civic engagement and risk/problem behaviors was not, as was expected, present for all participants at all ages. That is, some trajectories of high, positive civic engagement were coupled with trajectories involving increasingly higher levels of risk/problem behaviors for different youth across different portions of adolescence (Lewin-Bizan et al. 2010; Phelps et al. 2007). Therefore, the overall strength and valence of the relation represented in the model between civic engagement and risk/problem behaviors remain uncertain in any general sense (and is represented by a "?" in Fig. 1).

Additional theory and research will be required to identify the individual and ecological conditions moderating the valence of this relation for specific youth or groups of adolescents. Moreover, future research will need to address other methodological issues that arise when using RDS-based models to study the development of PYD, particularly among minority youth.

Limitations of the 4-H Study Vis-à-Vis Understanding PYD Among Minority Youth

All research has limitations. For instance, in the 4-H Study there were limitations of design and measurement that have been discussed in prior summaries of this work (e.g., Bowers et al. 2014; Lerner et al. 2015) and will in part be returned to again in this chapter. However, the primary limitation of the 4-H Study, at least in regard to understanding PYD among minority youth, pertains to sampling (Spencer and Spencer 2014). Overall, the 4-H Study participants were part of a convenience sample (Bowers et al. 2014). Moreover, across the eight ways of testing, about two-thirds of this sample was White and less than 10 % of the group was Black; similarly less, then 10 % was Latino. Other youth of color were represented in even lower frequencies. In turn, a little more than a third of the sample lived in rural areas and about 25 % in suburban locales. Less than a fifth of the sample lived in urban settings. In addition, the participants came from relatively highly educated families and middle-to-above socioeconomic statuses.

The absence of sufficient, representative numbers of youth from diverse racial and ethnic groups and from urban settings limits the generalizability of the 4-H data set, particularly in regard to minority youth. Spencer and Spencer (2014) underscore these limitations of the 4-H Study data set. They note that the 4-H Study Five Cs model is limited in its ability to illuminate what positive youth development may look like for America's minority youth. Here, sampling shortcomings combine with issues of measurement and design to constrain what can be derived from the data set in regard to PYD among minority youth. Spencer and Spencer (2014) also noted that the 4-H study has a problem of data sufficiency for obtaining and analyzing within-group, ethnic/racial-group findings. Not only does the 4-H study contain a relatively small sample of minority youth, but the sample that does exist is not large enough to establish measurement invariance across age for different racial/ethnic groups. As such, Spencer and Spencer (2014) conclude that the study is not generalizable to non-European American youth. We agree.

In addition, Spencer and Spencer (2014) point to a design limitation of the 4-H Study vis-à-vis minority youth. They note that minority youth in the United States face structural challenges (e.g., institutional racism) and contextual problems (e.g., lack of adequate access to health care) that must be considered when empirically studying this population. By failing to consider the unique contextual challenges that minority youth face, and by defining PYD perhaps too narrowly for these youth (i.e., in regard to the Five Cs), there may be an underestimation of the potentially unique and creative ways in which minority youth utilize perhaps unconventional contextual assets (e.g., "entrepreneurial, but not criminal, gangs;" Taylor 2003) to cope with their settings and thrive, particularly when faced with exceptional circumstances (Spencer 2006).

Certainly, to address these limitations of sampling, measurement, and design, future research should be conducted with more diverse, representatively sampled groups of youth than are present in the 4-H Study data set. These groups must be large enough to establish measurement invariance across race, ethnicity, socioeconomic status, and areas of residence (as well as gender, religion, etc.). Moreover, it may

well be that the survey approach used in the 4-H Study needs to be triangulated with qualitative methods in order to afford understanding of what Spencer and Spencer (2014) believe may be the distinct meaning of PYD among minority youth and, as well, to describe what also may be the distinct assets for coping that exist in their settings.

We believe that adaptive developmental regulations are a fundamental part of thriving for both majority and minority youth, that is, the *process* of PYD is the same for all youth. However, the content of these relations may vary. What minority youth bring to these individual ↔ context exchanges, what the context provides to them, and how thriving may be actualized in minority youth—has not been elucidated adequately in the 4-H Study. We do not know, therefore, if or the extent to which the Lerner and Lerner model can be applied to minority youth, at least in regard to the manifest variables involved in their thriving.

Some scholars have recently begun to examine if and how facets of the PYD model may be applied in research and practice for minority youth (Travis and Leech 2014; Williams et al. 2014). How may sound developmental research proceed to provide this information? We address this question next.

Methodological Issues in the Further Testing of RDS-Based Models Among Minority Youth

Conducting research that derives from the RDS metatheory requires that theoretical ideas about development be actualized through methodological approaches involving change-sensitive research designs, measurements, and data analysis methods. This obligation is an essential feature of "good science—selecting features of one's methodology based on the nature of the (theoretically predicated) questions asked" (Lerner and Overton 2008, p. 250).

Similarly, and as described in detail in Spencer's (2006) Phenomenological Variant of Ecological Systems Theory (PVEST), as individuals actively engage in and experience their worlds, their perceptions of the world, including particular actors in their worlds (e.g. teachers, police officers) may change. Such changes may influence their subsequent actions, interactions, and development (Spencer 2006). Moreover, no two individuals experience and perceive their worlds in the same way, and these individual differences may be especially pronounced when comparing, for example, the experiences of majority, European-American youth to minority youth in the U.S.

Thus, a focus on how individuals produce their own development, and on the specific course of their changes in PYD, must characterize RDS-based research. In addition, a focus on individual differences, both between and within groups of youth, in regard to their PYD, must continue to characterize developmental science. This diversity oriented and person-centered requirement has profound implications for the future study of the development of PYD among minority youth.

Molenaar (2014) explained that the standard approach to statistical analysis in the social and behavioral sciences is not focused on change but is, instead, derived from mathematical assumptions regarding the constancy of phenomena across people and, critically, time. He noted that these assumptions are based on the ergodic theorems. These theorems indicate that 1. all individuals within a sample may be treated as the same (this is the assumption of homogeneity); and 2. all individuals remain the same across time, that is, all time points yield the same results (this is the assumption of stationarity). The postulation of ergodicity leads, then, to statistical analyses placing prime interest on the population level. Interindividual variation, rather than intraindividual change, is the source of this population information (Molenaar 2014).

If the concept of ergodicity is applied to the study of PYD among minority youth, then within-individual variation in PYD across time would either be ignored or treated as error variance. In addition, any sample (group) differences in PYD would be held to be invariant across time

and place. However, within the process-relational paradigm (Overton 2015), development is non-linear and characterized by autopoietic (self-constructing) and, hence, idiographic intraindividual change, features of human functioning that violate the ideas of ergodicity. As such, interindividual differences in trajectories of PYD (i.e., in the course of intraindividual changes in thriving) are important foci for research and, as well, for program and policy applications aimed at enhancing PYD among minority youth across time and place. That is, developmental processes have time-varying means, variances, and/or time-varying sequential dependencies and, therefore, the structure of interindividual variation at the population level is not equivalent to the structure of intraindividual variation at the level of the individual (Molenaar 2014). Developmental processes are, therefore, non-ergodic.

How, then, should research proceed to study PYD among minority youth? One answer is provided by Bornstein (2006), who proposed a "specificity principle," which involves researchers asking multi-part "what" questions when conducting programmatic research exploring the function, structure, and content of development across the life span. Accordingly, to test RDS-based ideas about the ontogenetically changing structure of PYD among minority youth —i.e., to test empirically the process-relational conception of intraindividual change (Overton 2015)—the task for developmental researchers is to undertake programs of research to gain insights into the following multi-part "what" question: (1) What individual-context relations in regard to PYD emerge; that are linked to (2) What antecedent and consequent adaptive developmental regulations (i.e., what trajectories of individual $\leftrightarrow$ context relations); at (3) What points in development; for (4) What minority youth; living in (5) What contexts; across (6) What historical periods?

Gaining greater understanding of this complex, multi-part question will enable developmental scientists to understand the content and course of adaptive developmental regulations linked to the development of PYD among and across different groups of minority youth and, as well, within any member of a sample of minority youth. Using such multi-part "what" questions as a frame would enable developmental scientists to address several still unanswered questions about the application of the PYD model to minority youth[1]:

1. Would the definition of "thriving" need reexamination in the case of minority youth?
2. Similarly, may any of the Five Cs need redefinition?
3. Could the unique contextual challenges that minority youth face (Spencer 2006), which mostly refer to perceived discrimination that these youth often confront, and their effect on positive adaptation and development, be examined through this model?
4. Do the contexts and the "mutually-beneficial relations" between minority youth and their ecology also need special attention? (Minority youth need to learn to navigate between at least two different worlds: one defined by their minority culture, such as family and their own ethnic group; and the other by the majority culture, such as schools, and youth development programs.)
5. How do we define what are mutually-beneficial relations between minority youth and their ecology?

Answers to these questions may provide the evidentiary base for applications of developmental science aimed at enhancing PYD among diverse individuals across diverse contexts.

From Research to Application in the Service of Promoting PYD Among Minority Youth

Among the many split conceptions maintained by viewing the study of development through a Cartesian lens (Overton 2015) is the split between basic and applied research. However,

within models of PYD derived from the ideas of the RDS metatheory, this split joins other ones (e.g., nature–nurture or continuity–discontinuity) in being rejected. When one studies the embodied individual within the developmental system, then explanations of how changes in the individual $\leftrightarrow$ context relation (at Time 1) may eventuate in subsequent changes in this relation (at Time 2, Time 3, etc.) are tested by altering the Time 1 person $\leftrightarrow$ context relation. When such alterations are conducted in the ecologically valid setting of the individual, these assessments constitute tests of the basic relational process of human development and, at the same time, applications (e.g., interventions) into the course of human development (Lerner 2004). Indeed, depending on the level of analysis, aggregation, and time scale at which these interventions are implemented, such changes in the ecology of the individual $\leftrightarrow$ context relation may involve relationships between individuals (e.g., mentoring relationships), community-based programs, or social policies (e.g., Bronfenbrenner 2005).

The rationale for applying developmental science to enhance PYD is predicated on the presence of relative plasticity in human development, a concept that we have explained is derived from RDS-based ideas, such as bidirectionally-influential individual $\leftrightarrow$ context relations. The relative plasticity of human development is a fundamental strength in, and the basis of optimism about, youth development. Developmental scientists can be hopeful that there are combinations of youth and contexts that can be identified or created (through programs or policies) to enhance PYD of all individuals and groups. In other words, developmental scientists may act to change the course of developmental regulations, or individual $\leftrightarrow$ context relations, in manners aimed at optimizing the opportunities for individual and group trajectories across life to reflect greater and more positive development.

However, this optimism must be tempered by the above-noted unaddressed questions regarding the applicability of the PYD model to minority youth and, as well, in recognition of the constraints that may exist in implementing the PYD model among diverse youth and communities.

---

[1]We are grateful to Editor Frosso Motti for suggesting these key conceptual issues to us.

As Spencer and Spencer (2014) have explained (see too Taylor 2003), insufficient information exists about how these constraints place conceptual and theoretical limits on the PYD model. To address fully the diversity of America's youth, important new research directions must be taken. For instance, most work studying the links between PYD and youth development program participation is currently focused on adolescents who are reasonably accessible—such as youth who will volunteer to participate in studies and from whom consent will be provided by their parents. However, future research needs to move beyond a focus on these portions of the nation's population of youth.

Developmental scientists need to know more about youth at the lower end of the SES distribution. The hardest-to-reach youth have not been adequately involved in extant research, and no existing research examines whether the model shown in Fig. 1 applies to youth from challenged ecological circumstances (i.e., from low SES, highly-disorganized, and crime-ridden communities), or to youth who move with a high frequency, are emancipated from their parents, or live in places that are not readily accessible to researchers (e.g., homeless youth).

Even less is known about what PYD is like for youth in other parts of the world. What does positive development mean for children in Syria or adolescents in Honduras—with their current refugee crises—or youth in West Africa where the Ebola epidemic rages on? The model in Fig. 1 may need to be reconfigured to accommodate the lives of these youth. According to the 2010 National Census in mainland China, the child population aged 0–17 in China was 279 million and spanned 56 ethnicities (UNICEF 2013). The size of this youth population is larger than the national population of most countries in the world. Little research has examined how the PYD model could be implemented among these youth (Wen et al. 2015). There is also little research accounting for the influence of their ethnic status on their development within China. Until the multi-part "what" question is addressed in the United States and internationally, we need to be exceedingly humble about what we know of PYD.

Conclusions and Future Directions

Developmental scientists have, in the repertoire of models and methods in their intellectual "tool box," the means to promote more active and positively engaged civic lives and contributions among young people. Furthermore, through enhancement of the adaptive developmental regulations between individual and context, developmental scientists may afford diverse individuals the opportunities needed to maximize their aspirations and actions by engaging with social institutions that support individual agency, freedom, liberty, civil society, and social justice (Fisher et al. 2013; Lerner 2002, 2004; Lerner and Overton 2008). In order to contribute significantly to creating a developmental science aimed at promoting such social justice-oriented outcomes, scholars need to identify the means with which to alter individual ↔ context relations in ways that enhance the probability that all individuals, no matter their individual characteristics or contextual circumstances, have greater opportunities for PYD (e.g., see Fisher et al. 2013).

The theoretical orientations and interests of contemporary cohorts of developmental scientists, the aspiration to produce scholarship that matters in the real world, and the needs for evidence-based means to address the challenges to freedom, liberty, and democracy in the twenty-first century have coalesced to make Kurt Lewin's (1952, p. 169) quote, that "There is nothing so practical as a good theory," an often-proven empirical reality. The scientific and societal merits upon which developmental science will be judged in the future will be based on whether its theoretical and methodological tools accurately reflect the diversity and dynamism of human development and are centered on promoting thriving among the youth of all nations.

Acknowledgments The writing of this chapter was supported in part by grants from the John Templeton Foundation.

References

Baltes, P. B., Lindenberger, U., & Staudinger, U. M. (2006). Lifespan theory in developmental psychology. In R. M. Lerner (Ed.), *Handbook of child psychology. Vol.1: Theoretical models of human development* (6th ed., pp. 569–664). Editors-in-chief: W. Damon & R. M. Lerner. Hoboken, NJ: Wiley.

Benson, P. L., Scales, P. C., & Syvertsen, A. K. (2011). The contribution of the developmental assets framework to positive youth development theory and practice. In R. M. Lerner, J. V. Lerner, & J. B. Benson (Eds.), *Advances in child development and behavior: Positive youth development: Research and applications for promoting thriving in adolescence* (pp. 195–228). London, UK: Elsevier.

Bornstein, M. H. (2006). Parenting science and practice. In K. A. Renninger & I. E. Sigel (Vol. Eds.), *Handbook of child psychology. Vol. 4: Child psychology and practice* (6th ed., pp. 893–949). Editors-in-Chief: W. Damon & R. M. Lerner. Hoboken, NJ: Wiley.

Bowers, E. P., Geldhof, G. J., Johnson, S. K., Lerner, J. V., & Lerner, R. M. (2014). Elucidating the developmental science of adolescence: Lessons learned from the 4-H Study of Positive Youth Development. *Journal of Youth and Adolescence, 43* (6) (Whole Issue).

Brandtstädter, J. (1998). Action perspectives on human development. In W. Damon (Series Ed.) & R. M. Lerner (Vol. Ed.), *Handbook of child psychology. Vol. 1: Theoretical models of human development* (5th ed., pp. 807–863). New York: Wiley.

Bronfenbrenner, U. (2005). *Making human beings human: Bioecological perspectives on human development*. Thousand Oaks, CA: Sage.

Cabrera, N. J., & The SRCD Ethnic Racial Issues Committee. (2013). Positive development of minority children. *Social Policy Report, 27*(2), 3–22.

Catalano, R. P., Hawkins, J. D., Berglund, M. L., Pollard, J. A., & Arthur, M. W. (2002). Prevention science and positive youth development: Competitive or cooperative frameworks? *Journal of Adolescent Health, 31*, 230–239.

Damon, W. (2008). *The path to purpose: Helping our children find their calling in life*. New York: Simon and Schuster.

Eccles, J. S. (2004). Schools, academic motivation, and stage-environment fit. In R. M. Lerner & L. Steinberg (Eds.), *Handbook of adolescent psychology* (Vol. 2, pp. 125–153). Hoboken, NJ: Wiley.

Eccles, J. S., & Gootman, J. A. (Eds.). (2002). *Community programs to promote youth development/committee on community-level programs for youth*. Washington, DC: National Academy Press.

Elder, G. H., Jr., Shanahan, M. J., & Jennings, J. A. (2015). Human development in time and place. In M. H. Bornstein & T. Leventhal (Eds.), *Handbook of child psychology and developmental science* (7th ed.), Volume 4: *Ecological settings and processes in developmental systems.* (pp. 6–54). Editor-in-chief: R. M. Lerner. Hoboken, N.J.: Wiley.

Fisher, C. B., Busch, N. A., Brown, J. L., & Jopp, D. S. (2013). Applied developmental science: Contributions and challenges for the 21st century. In R. M. Lerner, M. A. Easterbrooks, & J. Mistry (Eds.), *Handbook of psychology. Vol. 6: Developmental psychology* (2nd ed., pp. 516–546). Editor-in-chief: I. B. Weiner. Hoboken, N.J.: Wiley.

Flay, B. R. (2002). Positive youth development requires comprehensive health promotion programs. *American Journal of Health Behavior, 26*(6), 407–424.

Ford, D. H., & Lerner, R. M. (1992). *Developmental systems theory: An integrative approach*. Newbury Park, CA: Sage.

Gottlieb, G. (1998). Normally occurring environmental and behavioral influences on gene activity: From central dogma to probabilistic epigenesis. *Psychological Review, 105*, 792–802.

Hamilton, S. (1999). A three-part definition of youth development. Unpublished manuscript, College of Human Ecology, Cornell University, Ithaca, NY.

Heck, K. E., & Subramaniam, A. (2009). *Youth development frameworks. [Monograph]*. Davis, CA: 4-H Center for Youth Development, University of California.

Hope, E. C., & Jagers, R. J. (2014). The role of sociopolitical attitudes and civic education in the civic engagement of black youth. *Journal of Research on Adolescence, 24*(3), 460–470.

Larson, R. W. (2000). Towards a psychology of positive youth development. *American Psychologist, 55*, 170–183.

Lerner, R. M. (1984). *On the nature of human plasticity*. New York, NY: Cambridge University Press.

Lerner, R. M. (2004). *Liberty: Thriving and civic engagement among America's youth*. Thousand Oaks, CA: Sage.

Lerner, R. M. (2012). Essay review: Developmental science: Past, present, and future. *International Journal of Developmental Science, 6*, 29–36.

Lerner, R. M., & Overton, W. F. (2008). Exemplifying the integrations of the relational developmental system: Synthesizing theory, research, and application to promote positive development and social justice. *Journal of Adolescent Research, 23*, 245–255.

Lerner, R. M., Lerner, J. V., von Eye, A., Bowers, E. P., & Lewin- Bizan, S. (2011). Individual and contextual bases of thriving in adolescence: A view of the issues. *Journal of Adolescence, 34*(6), 1107–1114.

Lerner, J. V., Phelps, E., Forman, Y., & Bowers, E. P. (2009a). Positive youth development. In R. M. Lerner & L. Steinberg (Eds.), *Handbook of adolescent psychology: Vol. 1 Individual bases of adolescent development* (3rd ed., pp. 524–558). Hoboken, NJ: Wiley.

Lerner, R. M., von Eye, A., Lerner, J. V., & Lewin-Bizan, S. (2009b). Exploring the foundations and functions of adolescent thriving within the 4-H study of positive youth development: A view of the issues. *Journal of Applied Developmental Psychology, 30*(5), 567–570.

Lerner, R. M., Lerner, J. V., Bowers, E., & Geldhof, G. J. (2015). Positive youth development: A relational developmental systems model. In W. F. Overton, & P. C. Molenaar (Eds.), *Handbook of child psychology and developmental science. Vol. 1: Theory and method* (7th ed.). (pp. 607–651). Editor-in-chief: R. M. Lerner. Hoboken, NJ: Wiley.

Lerner, R. M., von Eye, A., Lerner, J. V., Lewin-Bizan, S., & Bowers, E. P. (2010). Special issue introduction: The meaning and measurement of thriving: A view of the issues. *Journal of Youth and Adolescence, 39*(7), 707–719.

Lerner, J. V., Bowers, E. P., Minor, K., Lewin-Bizan, S., Boyd, M. J., Mueller, M. K., et al. (2013). Positive youth development: Processes, philosophies, and programs. In R. M. Lerner, M. A., Easterbrooks, & J. Mistry (Eds.), *Handbook of psychology, volume 6: developmental psychology* (2nd edn). Editor-in-chief: I. B. Weiner. (pp. 365–392). Hoboken, NJ: Wiley.

Lerner, R. M., Lerner, J. V., Almerigi, J. B., Theokas, C., Phelps, E., Gestsdottir, S., et al. (2005). Positive Youth Development, Participation in community youth development programs, and community contributions of fifth-grade adolescents: Findings from the first wave of the 4-H study of Positive Youth Development. *Journal of Early Adolescence, 25*(1), 17–71.

Lewin, K. (1952). *Field theory in social science: Selected theoretical papers*. London: Tavistock.

Lewin-Bizan, S., Bowers, E. P., & Lerner, R. M. (2010). One good thing leads to another: Cascades of positive youth development among American adolescents. *Development and Psychopathology, 22*, 759–770.

Masten, A. S. (2001). Ordinary magic: Resilience processes in development. *American Psychologist, 56*, 227–238.

Masten, A. S. (2014). Global perspectives on resilience in children and youth. *Child Development, 85*(1), 6–20.

Molenaar, P. C. M. (2014). Dynamic models of biological pattern formation have surprising implications for understanding the epigenetics of development. *Research in Human Development, 11*, 50–62.

Overton, W. F. (2015). Process and relational developmental systems. In W. F. Overton, & P. C. Molenaar (Eds.), *Handbook of child psychology and developmental science. Vol. 1: Theory and method* (7th ed.).

(pp. 9–62). Editor-in-chief: R. M. Lerner. Hoboken, NJ: Wiley.

Phelps, E., Balsano, A., Fay, K., Peltz, J., Zimmerman, S., & Lerner, R. M. (2007). Nuances in early adolescent development trajectories of positive and problematic/risk behaviors: Findings from the 4-H Study of Positive Youth Development. *Child and Adolescent Psychiatric Clinics of North America, 16* (2), 473–496.

Schmid, K. L., & Lopez, S. (2011). Positive pathways to adulthood: The role of hope in adolescents' constructions of their futures. In R. M. Lerner, J. V. Lerner, & J. B. Benson (Eds.), *Advances in Child Development and Behavior: Positive Youth Development* (Vol. 41, pp. 72–89). London, England: Academic Press.

Spencer, M. B. (2006). Phenomenology and ecological systems theory: Development of diverse groups. In W. Damon & R. M. Lerner (Eds.), *Handbook of child psychology, Vol. 1: Theoretical models of human development* (6th ed., pp. 829–893). Hoboken, NJ: John Wiley & Sons.

Spencer, M. B., & Spencer, T. R. (2014). Exploring the promises, intricacies, and challenges to Positive Youth Development. *Journal of Youth and Adolescence, 43*, 1027–1035.

Taylor, C. (2003). Youth gangs and community violence. In R. M. Lerner, F. Jacobs, & D. Wertlieb (Eds.), *Handbook of applied developmental science: Promoting positive child, adolescent, and family development through research, policies, and programs* (Vol. 2, pp. 65–80). Enhancing the life chances of youth and families: Public service systems and public policy perspectives Thousand Oaks, CA: Sage.

Theokas, C., & Lerner, R. M. (2006). Observed ecological assets in families, schools, and neighborhoods: Conceptualization, measurement, and relations with positive and negative developmental outcomes. *Applied Developmental Science, 10*(2), 61–74.

Travis, R., & Leech, T. G. (2014). Empowerment-Based Positive Youth Development: A New Understanding of Healthy Development for African American Youth. *Journal of Research on Adolescence, 24*(1), 93–116.

UNICEF. (2013). Census data about children in China: Facts and Figures 2013. Retrieved December 29, 2014, from http://www.unicef.cn/en/index.php?m= content&c=index&a=show&catid=59&id=2040

Urban, J. B., Lewin-Bizan, S., & Lerner, R. M. (2010). The role of intentional self regulation, lower neighborhood ecological assets, and activity involvement in youth developmental outcomes. *Journal of Youth and Adolescence, 39*(7), 783–800.

Wen, M., Su, S., Li, X., & Lin, D. (2015). Positive youth development in rural China: The role of parental migration. *Social Science and Medicine, 132*, 261–269. doi:10.1016/j.socscimed.2014.07.051

Williams, J. L., Anderson, R. E., Francois, A. G., Hussain, S., & Tolan, P. H. (2014). Ethnic identity and positive youth development in adolescent males: A culturally integrated approach. *Applied Developmental Science, 18*(2), 110–122.

Zaff, J. F., Boyd, M., Li, Y., Lerner, J. V., & Lerner, R. M. (2010). Active and engaged citizenship: Multi-group and longitudinal factorial analysis of an integrated construct of civic engagement. *Journal of Youth and Adolescence, 39*(7), 736–750.

Zaff, J. F., Kawashima-Ginsberg, K., Lin, E. S., Lamb, M., Balsano, A., & Lerner, R. M. (2011). Developmental trajectories of civic engagement across adolescence: Disaggregation of an integrated construct. *Journal of Adolescence, 34*(6), 1207–1220.

A Resilience Perspective on Immigrant Youth Adaptation and Development

Frosso Motti-Stefanidi, and Ann S. Masten

Abstract

Immigrant youth comprise a sizable and integral part of contemporary societies. Their successful adaptation is a high-stakes issue for them, their families and for society. In spite of the challenges they face, most of them adapt well in their new countries. However, considerable diversity in their adaptation has been reported. This chapter examines the question: "Who among immigrant youth adapt well and why?" To address this question, first, we propose a definition for positive immigrant youth adaptation. Second, we present extant knowledge on group and individual differences in immigrant youth adaptation from the perspective of a resilience developmental framework, which incorporates acculturative and social psychological variables. Third, we examine whether immigrant status and related social challenges place immigrant youth adaptation at risk. Finally, we review social and personal resources that promote and/or protect positive immigrant youth adaptation. In conclusion, we argue that focusing on strengths and resilience, instead of on weaknesses and psychological symptoms, among immigrant youth has significant implications for policy and practice.

Introduction

In the past two decades European Union countries have experienced a rapid surge in immigration. The number of children living in families with a least one-immigrant parent has geometrically increased. Consequently, the integration of immigrant youth in receiving societies has become a pressing issue. Events, such as the riots that took place this past decade in many European cities, were at least partially linked to frustrated immigrant youth protesting about their

F. Motti-Stefanidi (✉)
Department of Psychology, National and Kapodistrian University of Athens, Athens, Greece
e-mail: frmotti@psych.uoa.gr
URL: http://www.frossomotti.com/index.html

A. S. Masten
Institute of Child Development, University of Minnesota, Minneapolis, MN, USA

© The Editor(s) 2017
N.J. Cabrera and B. Leyendecker (eds.), *Handbook on Positive Development of Minority Children and Youth*, DOI 10.1007/978-3-319-43645-6_2

experiences of discrimination, economic marginalization, and social exclusion (Migration Policy Institute 2013). Adding to this highly politicized and polarized situation, the large and increasing influx of Syrian refugee families has created a humanitarian crisis. Nonetheless, it is important to the economic and political future of both receiving societies and immigrants, that the former treat immigrants with fairness and dignity and promote their positive adaptation and well-being (Commission of the European Communities 2003).

According to a 2012 report from the Organization for Economic Co-operation and Development (OECD 2012), the best way to measure how well immigrants are integrated into a society is to assess how well their children are doing. Considerable group and individual differences in the adaptation of immigrant youth have been reported (Masten et al. 2012). Adaptation among immigrant youth varies as a function of ethnic group and features of the receiving society, as well as individual differences in personality, social resources, or other attributes, with some young immigrants doing quite well in spite of the challenges they face.

To account for these group and individual differences in immigrant youth adaptation, it is important to use a developmental lens because immigrant youth, like all youth, are developing individuals. Development always emerges from interactions of organisms with their contexts (Lerner et al., this volume; Overton 2015). As a result, immigrant youth adaptation needs to be examined in developmental context, taking into account normative developmental processes (e.g., cognitive, social, emotional), and the socioecological contexts (e.g., family, school, neighborhood) in which their life is embedded. Additionally, immigrant youth also face unique contextual influences, not faced by their non-immigrant peers. Immigrant status and culture, and related social variables such as discrimination, also are expected to contribute to their adaptation. Thus, to explain group and individual differences in immigrant youth adaptation, it is important to integrate developmental, acculturative and social psychological approaches (Motti-Stefanidi et al. 2012a).

The purpose of this chapter is to address the question: "Who among immigrant youth adapt well and why?" We examine extant knowledge on group and individual differences in immigrant youth adaptation from the perspective of a resilience developmental framework, which incorporates acculturative and social psychological variables (Motti-Stefanidi et al. 2012a). This integrative framework allows for a differentiated, longitudinal, contextualized and multi-level approach to understanding immigrant youth adaptation.

The chapter is organized in three main sections. After the introduction, the second section focuses on the above-mentioned theoretical perspective and on methodology related to the study of group and individual differences in immigrant youth adaptation. This section has two subsections. The first subsection examines core concepts of the resilience developmental framework and the second subsection presents the main ideas of an integrative model that was developed to account for the diversity in immigrant youth adaptation. The third section examines and discusses universal and specific mechanisms accounting for immigrant youth adaptation. This section has three subsections. The first subsection proposes a definition for positive immigrant youth adaptation that incorporates developmental and acculturative perspectives. The second subsection examines whether immigrant status and related social challenges place immigrant youth adaptation and development at risk. The third subsection reviews social and personal resources that promote and/or protect positive immigrant youth adaptation.

Theoretical Perspectives and Methodology

The Resilience Developmental Framework

Resilience refers to the capacity for adaptation to challenges that threaten the function or development of a dynamic system, manifested in pathways and patterns of positive adaptation during or following exposure to significant risk or adversity (Masten 2014). The study of resilience phenomena is an integral part of the discipline of developmental psychopathology (Cicchetti and Rogosch 2002; Masten and Cicchetti 2016). Developmental psychopathologists are interested in the interface between normal and abnormal, which they consider mutually informative. They focus on the full range of functioning among individuals exposed to conditions of adversity, and are committed to discovering which young people at risk for problems are following trajectories towards mental health and/or positive adaptation, and which, in contrast, are following trajectories towards psychological symptoms and/or adaptation difficulties, and why.

Resilience in an individual is inferred from two fundamental judgments about the individual's adaptation: First, the person must be, or have been, challenged by exposure to significant risk or adversity, and second, he/she must be "doing ok"—functioning or developing well in spite of exposures to adversity or risk (Masten 2014). Over decades of resilience science, researchers have used a variety of criteria to define and measure these two components of resilience (Masten and Cicchetti 2016).

Positive adaptation in young people often is defined based on how well they are doing with respect to age-salient developmental tasks (Masten 2014; McCormick et al. 2011; Sroufe et al. 2005). These tasks reflect the expectations and standards for behavior and achievement that parents, teachers, and societies set for individuals over the life span in a particular context and time in history. As they grow older, children usually (though not always) come to share these criteria and evaluate their own success by these expected accomplishments. Adaptive success is multidimensional and developmental in nature.

Developmental tasks vary over the life course of the individual. Each developmental period is characterized by a group of salient developmental tasks that provide criteria for judging who is doing well. Early in childhood, individuals are expected to form attachment bonds with their caregivers, learn to walk, and begin to communicate in the language of the family. Later in development, children often are expected to go to school, get along with other children, follow the rules of society, and practice the religion of the family.

These tasks wax and wane in significance across development and across contexts. School success, for example, becomes important in most societies during the expected years of school attendance and then decreases in salience as young people enter adult roles of work and family.

Families and societies value and attend to achievements in salient developmental tasks because these accomplishments are widely assumed to forecast future success. Developmental evidence from numerous longitudinal studies over the years has corroborated those expectations (Masten and Cicchetti 2016).

Developmental tasks can be organized in broad domains: individual development, relationships with parents, teachers, and peers, and functioning in the proximal environment and in the broader social world (Sroufe et al. 2005). Positive adaptation with respect to developmental tasks may be judged based on external behavior, such as success in school, having close friends/being liked by peers, knowing or obeying the laws of society, civic engagement, or on internal adaptation, such as development of self-control or establishment of a cohesive, integrated and multifaceted sense of identity (e.g., Motti-Stefanidi 2014a, b). Success in these developmental tasks does not mean that youth should exhibit "ideal" or "superb" effectiveness, but rather they should be "doing adequately well."

To identify resilience, there also must be evidence of past or present threat, trauma, or negative life experiences in the life of the individual. Such hazards often co-occur or pile up in the lives of individuals or families and as risk levels rise the level of average problems or symptoms often increases as well, suggesting a cumulative risk (or dose) gradient (Evans et al. 2013; Obradovic et al. 2012). In the absence of risk or adversity, positive adaptation is not considered an expression of resilience but rather of competence. The resilience literature includes studies of many different kinds of risks, such as high-risk status variables (e.g., immigrant status, low SES, single parent family), exposure to traumatic and stressful experiences (e.g., maltreatment, community violence, war), or biological risk markers (e.g., low birth weight, physical illness).

The goal of resilience research is not only to identify who is well-adapted in spite of adversity, but also to identify the processes that explain how positive adaptation was achieved. To account for group and individual differences in adaptation in the context of risk, potential predictors of positive adaptation have been examined at multiple levels of context and analysis (Masten 2014). Two broad types of influences that counteract or mitigate the potential effects of adversity on adaptation and development have been described. The first type of influence or effects is called promotive (Sameroff 2000), referring to factors that have a generally positive effect on adaptation independent of risk level. Promotive factors reflect "main effects" in statistical terms and these effects are sometimes described as assets, resources, compensatory effects, or social and human capital. Such promoters support positive adaptation independently of risk or adversity in the individual's life, with observable effects both in low and high adversity. The second type of influence or effect is conditional, with greater effects under more adverse conditions. These influences reflect moderating influences on risk or adversity, suggesting protective roles. Protective factors have a special function when conditions are adverse or risky, and they reflect interaction (risk X moderator) effects in adaptation.

It needs to be emphasized that these different effects are functional in nature, defined in part by the context. The same characteristic of an individual or a family can serve different functions depending on the domain of adaptation under consideration, the context, or the nature of the threat. In the context of maltreatment or war, for example, fearfulness and vigilance may well be adaptive and protective, whereas in a safe and supportive context, the same behaviors could be maladaptive. Similarly, parents who monitor their children closely in a dangerous environment may be viewed as "overprotective" in a safe context.

Integrative Conceptual Framework for Immigrant Youth Adaptation

An integrative multilevel framework was developed to explain the diversity in immigrant youth adaptation by Motti-Stefanidi et al. (2012a). This framework was influenced by theory from multiple fields, but especially the following perspectives: the resilience developmental framework (Masten 2014), Bronfenbrenner's bioecological model of human development (Bronfenbrenner and Morris 2006); Berry's cultural transmission model (Berry et al. 2006); and the three-level model of immigrant adaptation proposed by Verkuyten (2005), a social psychologist studying issues of ethnicity and migration.

Based on this integrative framework, individual and group differences in immigrant youth adaptation are examined in developmental and acculturative contexts, taking into account multiple levels of analysis (Motti-Stefanidi et al. 2012a; Motti-Stefanidi & Masten 2013). The backbone of the framework consists of three levels. The individual level concerns individual differences in personality, cognition, and motivation. The level of interaction is focused on interactions that shape the individual life course of immigrants, and that take place in contexts, such as the school and the family. These contexts serve the purpose both of development and acculturation, and are divided into those representing the home culture (family, ethnic peers, ethnic group) and into those representing the host culture (school, native peers). Finally, the societal level is focused on variations in cultural beliefs, social representations, and ideologies, as well as variables that reflect power positions within society (e.g., social class, ethnicity) that have been shown to have an impact on immigrants' adaptation. The three levels of the model are viewed as interconnected and embedded within each other.

No precedence is given either to the individual as sole agent, or to society as sole determinant of individual differences in immigrant youth's adaptation. Instead, it is argued that both the individual and society, that is, both sociocultural circumstances and structures, and human agency play a central role in the adaptive processes that contribute to youth adaptation. Moreover, from a developmental systems perspective, reciprocal influences are expected from the interactions of individuals with their contexts over time.

The levels of this integrative model refer to system levels of context. However, the concept of levels can also refer to levels of analysis, or scientific explanation. The influence of each of the levels of context (individual, level of inter-action, societal) on adaptation can be examined at different levels of scientific explanation. These two conceptions of levels are interrelated, yet distinct. For example, the influence of socioeconomic status, a societal level variable, on adaptation can be examined at the individual level of analysis, by assigning to each study participant a score reflecting the SES status of the family, or at the level of interaction, by assigning a score on mean SES to schools or classrooms.

Influences at each of these three levels may contribute independently, or in interaction with each other, to group and individual differences in immigrant youth's adaptation. Furthermore, variables from these three levels of context may promote, or may instead present challenges and obstacles, for their adaptation. Thus, influences stemming from each of these different levels of context could function either as risk, as promotive or as protective factors for immigrant youth's adaptation.

Universal Versus Culture-Specific Mechanisms

Criteria for Positive Adaptation

The integrative model of immigrant youth resilience offers a conceptual framework for judging positive adaptation in immigrant youth (Motti-Stefanidi et al. 2012a; Motti-Stefanidi & Masten 2013). Their adaptation can be judged based on how well they are doing with respect to developmental and acculturative tasks, as well as in terms of their psychological well-being.

Immigrant youth, like all youth, face the developmental tasks of their time and age (Motti-Stefanidi et al. 2012a, b). However, their adaptation takes place in the context of multiple cultures, which may have conflicting developmental task expectations and standards. Immigrant parents' working models of culture, that is, their beliefs, attitudes, values and practices were formed in their culture of origin (Kuczynski and Navara 2006). They bring from their home country a conceptual model of the characteristics and achievements of a successful adult and of how to raise a child that will eventually become a competent adult. However, socialization agents in the receiving country may have different ideas on who is a successful adult and relatedly on the appropriate childrearing practices (Bornstein and Cote 2010). Thus, parental ethnotheories, which refer to the values and beliefs that parents consider important for their children's positive adaptation in their culture (Harkness and Super 1996), and which often guide their child-rearing practices (Ogbu 1991), may be at odds with the criteria for positive adaptation set by teachers and the majority culture.

It becomes clear that immigrant youth do not only face developmental challenges but they also have to deal with the acculturative challenges of living and growing in the context of at least two cultures (Motti-Stefanidi et al. 2012a; Motti-Stefanidi & Masten 2013). Numerous scholars have suggested and evidence broadly supports the hypothesis that learning and maintaining both ethnic and national cultures is linked to better developmental outcomes and psychological well-being (Berry et al. 2006; Oppedal and Top-pelberg 2016; Phinney et al. 2001). Immigrant youth have to develop cultural competence, which involves the acquisition of the knowledge and skills of both ethnic and national cultures (Oppedal and Toppelberg, 2016). From this perspective, culturally competent immigrants would be able to communicate effectively in ethnic and national languages, have friends from both their own and other groups, know the values and practices of both groups, code-switch between languages and cultures as necessary, and also make sense of and bridge their different worlds. They also would be expected to develop positive ethnic and national identities (Phinney et al. 2001).

Developmental and acculturative tasks are intertwined. Thus, the criteria for judging immigrant youth positive adaptation may involve a combination of developmental and acculturative tasks. Furthermore, performance with respect to such criteria may reflect both how development and how acculturation are proceeding. For example, being liked by peers and having friends, independently of the ethnicity of these peers, is an important developmental task that forecasts future adaptation (Rubin et al. 2015). On the other hand, being liked by and having friends among both ethnic and national peers is an important acculturative task that plays a fundamental role in the acculturation process (Titzmann 2014). Thus, immigrant adolescents, like all adolescents, need to be liked and accepted by their peers, independently of the ethnicity of these peers, but they also need to learn to navigate successfully between intra- and inter-ethnic peers. Thus, evaluations about the adaptation of immigrant youth with respect to peer relations would rest on both these criteria (Motti-Stefanidi et al. 2012b).

Civic engagement is another task that youth face which in the case of immigrant youth reflects not only how development is proceeding, but also how they are adapting in the receiving society. Civic engagement, which includes community-oriented and political participation goals, is an emerging task of adolescence and early adulthood that becomes more salient later in development (Obradovic and Masten 2007). It involves different forms of civic and political participation such as volunteering, campaigning, voting, protesting, and participation in social organizations at school. It is positively linked to other developmental tasks such as youth's identity, positive peer and family relations, as well as to youth's adjustment (e.g., Crocetti et al. 2012; Pancer 2015). Both immigrants' ethnic group and receiving society are possible contexts for civic engagement. Immigrant youth may contribute to

both cultures. Being civically engaged can signify for all youth that development is proceeding well (Obradovic and Masten 2007). For immigrant youth, it may also reflect how well they are dealing with important acculturative tasks, such as their involvement in the host society, as well as how well they negotiate the relation between their home and host societies (Motti-Stefanidi et al. 2012a).

Developmental and acculturative tasks are also intricately linked over time. The acquisition of acculturative tasks is in some cases expected to precede the acquisition of developmental tasks. For example, immigrant youth's proficiency in the national language, a key acculturative task, is essential for doing well academically in the schools of the receiving nation, which is a developmental task (e.g., Suárez-Orozco et al. 2008). However, most studies examining the relation between developmental and acculturative tasks are cross-sectional, fewer are longitudinal, and very few examine the direction of effects between the two types of tasks. To examine the direction of effects between developmental and acculturative tasks, one cross-lagged study examined the longitudinal interplay between immigrant youth's orientation towards the host culture, an acculturative task, and their self-efficacy, a developmental task (Reitz et al. 2013). Results indicated that immigrant youth's orientation towards the host culture predicted changes in self-efficacy, not vice versa, and this finding held for both time windows. Thus, the acquisition of the acculturative task functioned as a significant resource over time for immigrant youth's success in this developmental task.

It has been argued that the acculturative task of acquiring bi-cultural competence may actually be considered an additional developmental task for ethnic minority youth (Oppedal and Toppelberg 2016). For example, the formation of ethnic identity and learning the national language, in addition to the ethnic language, are developmental tasks triggered by the acculturation process(e.g., see Umaña-Taylor et al. 2014). They reflect expectations of immigrant parents and society, respectively. However, becoming bi-culturally competent may not be a developmental task as such. First, it does not necessarily reflect the actual expectations of receiving societies, schools and/or immigrant families. Second, the acquisition of bi-cultural competence does not always follow a normative developmental timetable. These points are further developed below.

As was mentioned previously, developmental tasks reflect the expectations that society, schools and families have regarding the behavior and performance of developing individuals. Conceiving the acquisition of bi-cultural competence as a developmental task implies that immigrant youth are expected by the receiving society, schools, and families to develop cultural competence in both cultures. In particular, acquiring the ability to code-switch between languages and cultures and to make sense of and bridge their different worlds require that immigrant youth achieve an integration of their ethnic and the national cultures. The achievement of this integration partly depends on society's expectations regarding the acculturation of immigrants (Bourhis et al. 1997), and necessitates that receiving societies respect cultural diversity and have adopted a multicultural ideology. However, receiving societies often follow an assimilationist ideology, as evidenced by the observation that in many cases they do not recognize different ethnic groups' uniqueness and specific needs and do not adapt their institutions to accommodate these needs (Berry 2006). Schools and the school system are a case in point, since they often clearly express the assumptions or preferences of a society for assimilation (Phinney et al. 2001; Vedder and Motti-Stefanidi 2016). On the other hand, even though immigrant parents differ in their degree of involvement in the new culture, often they have dissimilar levels of acculturation with their children. Their main goal in the new sociocultural context may be to protect the transmission to their children of the ethnic culture, which may result in an extensive negotiation process with their children as they develop (Kwak 2003).

Developmental tasks follow a normative developmental timetable that reflects both the developing cognitive, social and emotional capacities of the young person and the developmental goals and milestones set by the culture or community. Acculturative tasks do not necessarily follow a developmental timetable. The timing of migration may play a significant role in the odds of migrating children to achieve developmental tasks related to acculturation. Whether, when, how and to what degree immigrant youth will acquire different dimensions of bi-cultural competence may be linked to the age of the child at migration. Research in Canada suggests, for example, that the likelihood of non-English speaking children to acquire strong English proficiency diminished for migrants arriving after age 7 and the likelihood of high school graduation diminished with arrival after age 9 (Corak 2012). Beyond these ages the probability that immigrant children will achieve these milestones decreases significantly every year. Language acquisition of English proficiency is easier at younger ages and plays a critical role in academic success and the odds of graduation. Similarly, migrating before the age of 5 seems to yield distinct social, language and psychological acculturation processes for the child, especially with regard to language and ethnic identity, educational attainment and aspirations, patterns of social mobility, outlooks and frames of reference, and even their propensity to sustain transnational attachments over time, compared with youth who migrate when they are 13 years old or older (Portes and Rumbaut 2006).

Two important issues have emerged regarding developmental tasks among immigrant youth (Motti-Stefanidi et al. 2012a; Motti-Stefanidi and Masten 2013). One is whether to compare the behavior and successes of immigrant youth with ethnic or nonimmigrant peers and the other concerns the value judgments for evaluating adaptive outcomes, that is, whether to use the values of receiving society or the family or ethnic community.

Comparing the behavior and achievements of immigrant youth to that of their nonimmigrant peers may lead to the conclusion that immigrant youth are inferior in some way, which holds the risk of mistaken attributions to genetic, behavioral, or cultural "deficiencies". This "deficit" approach to the study of minority group adaptation has been resoundingly denounced; instead, it has been argued that the adaptation of minority children needs to be examined in its own right, and not always in comparison to the standards of the majority society (e.g., McLoyd 2006; Motti-Stefanidi et al. 2012b).

We propose that the criteria for judging the quality of immigrant youth's adaptation be differentiated depending on the domain. This argument follows the distinction made in the acculturation literature between the public (functional, utilitarian) domain and the private (social-emotional, value-related) domain (Arends-Tóth and van de Vijver 2006). It is reasonable to judge immigrant youth's current behavior and performance that has consequences for their future adaptation in the receiving society by comparing their accomplishments to those of nonimmigrant youth, with the caveat that the role of socioeconomic differences also may need to be considered (Motti-Stefanidi and Masten 2013). For example, doing adequately well in school presupposes receiving grades that are comparable to the normative performance of nonimmigrant students and not dropping out early, since these are indices of present positive adaptation and forerunners of future adaptation in society for both immigrant and nonimmigrant youth.

On the other hand, immigrant youth adaptation with respect to certain domains may involve private values that are related to linguistic and cultural activities, to religious expression, and to the domestic and interpersonal domains of the family (Bourhis et al. 1997). The appropriate criteria for success in this case may be complex, involving neither the adoption of the public values of the receiving society nor that of the values of youth's ethnic culture. Instead, young immigrants need to develop unique working models of culture that integrate these values (Kuczynski and Navara 2006; Oppedal and Toppleberg 2016).

Internal psychological adaptation, evaluated by indices of perceived well-being versus distress, is also a significant marker of positive adaptation for all youth. The presence of self-esteem and life satisfaction and the absence of emotional symptoms are common markers of psychological well-being used by developmental and acculturative researchers (e.g., Berry et al. 2006; Masten 2014). Psychological well-being and successful adaptation with respect to developmental and acculturative tasks are interrelated, influencing each other concurrently and across time (Motti-Stefanidi et al. 2012a).

Risks for Immigrant Youth Adaptation

Is immigrant status a risk factor for youth's adaptation? The results from studies conducted in different European countries and in North America are mixed. Significant diversity has been observed in the quality of adaptation of immigrant youth, revealing a mixture of risk and advantage. Some studies have found evidence for what has been termed the "immigrant paradox" wherein immigrant youth adaptation is more positive than expected and in some cases, better than the adaptation of their nonimmigrant peers (Berry et al. 2006), or first-generation immigrants are found to be better adapted than later generation immigrants (Garcia-Coll and Marks 2012; Marks et al. 2014), whose adaptation converges with that of their nonimmigrant peers (Sam et al. 2008). The immigrant paradox literature focuses on indices of adaptation that are related to developmental tasks, such as academic achievement, school engagement and conduct, as well as on youth's psychological well-being.

These results were not expected because first generation immigrant youth often are overrepresented in the low SES strata of host societies and less acculturated, with less competence in the national language, than later-generation immigrant youth. However, the immigrant paradox has not been observed consistently. The immigrant paradox phenomenon seems to depend to a large extend on the domain of adaptation, the host society, and the ethnic group (Garcia-Coll and Marks 2012; Sam et al. 2008).

A significant number of studies conducted mainly in the USA and Canada comparing first-with second-generation immigrants provide evidence in favor of the immigrant paradox (see Garcia-Coll and Marks 2012). First-generation immigrant children exhibit fewer risky behaviors, such as substance use and abuse, unprotected sex, and delinquency, have more positive attitudes towards school, and present fewer internalizing problems than their second-generation counterparts. In a comparative study including 5 European countries, Sam et al. (2008) found some support for the immigrant paradox in two of these countries (Sweden and Finland), particularly for adaptation with respect to developmental tasks, such as is school adjustment and conduct, but not with respect to psychological well-being. In contrast to expectations, second-generation immigrant youth reported better psychological well-being compared both to their first-generation counterparts and to national peers. However, a meta-analysis based on 51 studies conducted across the European continent revealed that being an immigrant was a risk factor for academic adjustment, externalizing and internalizing problems (Dimitrova et al. 2016). Immigrant status has been linked not only to worse academic achievement, but also to worse school engagement, and conduct (Motti-Stefanidi 2014a, b, 2015). Furthermore, at the classroom level of analysis, classrooms with a higher concentration of immigrants may be a risk factor for all students' academic achievement (e.g., OECD 2010).

In this regard, an OECD (2010) review of reading performance of immigrant youths at age 15, based on data from 20 countries, reported that in most countries (except Australia, Canada, Ireland, and New Zealand) immigrant students have on average lower reading performance compared to nonimmigrant students. According to this report, in most European countries, immigrant students, independently of generation, have lower reading performance scores than nonimmigrant students, and second generation immigrant students have higher reading performance scores than first generation.

Longitudinal patterns of the academic achievement, school engagement, and conduct of immigrant and nonimmigrant early adolescents seem to follow similar declining paths (Motti-Stefanidi et al. 2012b; Suárez-Orozco et al. 2010; Wigfield et al. 2006). The decline in school engagement over the middle school years has been found to be steeper for immigrant youth (Motti-Stefanidi et al. 2014c). It is not clear whether these declines reflect purely developmental change or can be attributed to acculturation on the developmental change, and, thus, entail risk for immigrant youth's adaptation. One would need to study a third group—youth of same ethnicity as the immigrants but who remained in their home country—to clarify this issue (Fuligni 2001). However, in the cases where the decline over time is steeper for immigrants, one could argue that immigrant status is a risk factor for change in adaptation over the middle school years.

Positive peer relations are important for immigrant youth's development and acculturation. At first contact in the classroom, as would be expected based on the homophily phenomenon (McPherson et al. 2001), immigrant youth seem to be less liked and to have fewer friends compared to their nonimmigrant classmates (see Motti-Stefanidi 2014a, b; Titzmann 2014). However, the classroom context differentiates these results. When immigrants are the majority in the classroom, they are more liked and have more friends than the students who are the minority. Similarly, Jackson, Barth, Powell and Lochman (2006) found that Black students in U.S. classrooms receive more positive nominations when they are the majority in a classroom. Over time, through intergroup contact (Pettigrew and Tropp 2006), immigrant students who were the minority in their classrooms became increasingly more liked by their nonimmigrant classmates (see Motti-Stefanidi 2014a, b; Titzmann 2014).

Immigrants often have to deal with the challenges of adapting to a new culture in a context replete with prejudice and discrimination. Even though discrimination is a very real experience for minority group members, it is difficult to measure objectively. Therefore, a distinction has been drawn between objective discrimination and perceived discrimination. Another important distinction is drawn in the social psychological literature between perceived discrimination against one's ethnic group and perceived discrimination against the self.

Perceived discrimination has been shown to have deleterious consequences on immigrants' adaptation, psychological well-being, and mental health (Liebkind et al. 2012; Vedder and Motti-Stefanidi 2016). However, most studies that have included measures of both perceived group and personal discrimination converge on the finding that perceived discrimination against the self has a stronger negative effect than perceived discrimination against the group on these outcomes (e.g., Verkuyten 1998). In the case of immigrant youth, it has been shown, for example, that perceived discrimination against the self is a risk factor for depression, stress, behavioral problems (e.g., Brody et al. 2006), self-esteem (e.g., Verkuyten 1998), academic achievement and, generally, school adjustment (e.g., Liebkind et al. 2004; Wong et al. 2003). Perceived personal discrimination has also been shown to be a risk factor for immigrant youth's national identity and commitment to the new culture and for harmonious intergroup relations (e.g., Berry et al. 2006). In contrast, it is linked to stronger ethnic identity.

Immigrant youth's proximal context also may present challenges for their adaptation. Immigrant adolescents and their parents have different experiences of cultures and different future expectations (Kwak 2003). This acculturation gap between parents and their children may result in conflicts within the family (Vedder and Motti-Stefanidi 2016). The underlying assumption regarding this conflict is that immigrant children acquire the prevailing values and norms of their settlement society, which often stress the need for the development of autonomy, much faster than their parents do, who often emphasize more the need for relatedness (Birman 2006). The acculturation gap and the resulting parent-adolescent conflict have been found to be significant risk factors for immigrant adolescents'

adaptation and psychological well-being (e.g., Kwak 2003; Motti-Stefanidi et al. 2011).

Resilience for Immigrant Youth Adaptation

In the previous section, we examined whether immigrant status and social challenges encountered by immigrant youth function as risk factors for their adaptation. While evidence indicates risk, significant variation is reported both at the group and at the individual level in the quality of immigrant youth adaptation. This variation suggests that some youth show resilience in multiple domains and other youth show resilience in some domains. These patterns of variation raise an important set of questions about promotive and protective resources and processes for immigrant youth: What makes the difference for youth who do well in spite of the social challenges that they face?

Resources for youth's positive adaptation and development, just as risks, may stem from factors situated within individuals (genetic and hormonal systems, personality, intelligence), as well as in the proximal (e.g., family and school) and distal contexts (societal, cultural, institutional levels) in which their lives are embedded (Masten 2014). At the group level, research on the immigrant paradox stresses the role of family values, which involve a sense of family cohesion, closeness and obligation, high parental aspirations for education, and an emphasis on education, to promote the positive adaptation of first-generation immigrant youth as compared to their later-generation counterparts. First-generation immigrant youth, many of whom share their family's values and attitudes, are academically motivated and invest energy in school and learning, characteristics that are also connected to positive adaptation (e.g., Garcia-Coll and Marks 2012; Kwak 2003; Suárez-Orozco et al. 2008).

However, it should be noted that immigrant families differ significantly in their ability to help their children translate their aspiration into success in the educational system (Garcia-Coll and Marks 2012). Therefore, Garcia-Coll and Marks (2012), summarizing the results of studies focusing on the academic achievement of immigrant children and adolescents, pointed out that the immigrant paradox is more consistently found in educational attitudes and behavior, such as time spent preparing homework, than in grades and test scores. However, higher levels of parental education, more financial resources, and better information and access regarding educational resources and opportunities are promotive for immigrant youth's academic achievement.

Youth's social context and their individual attributes do not only contribute to group differences in adaptation, such as between first and second generation immigrants, but also to individual differences within these groups. Their regular interactions with people in their proximal environment have been viewed as the primary engines for their development (Bronfenbrenner and Morris 2006) and their acculturation (Oppedal and Toppelberg 2016; Vedder and Motti-Stefanidi, 2016). Two key social contexts that contribute to individual differences in immigrant youth adaptation are the family and schools.

Immigrant youth's relationship with their parents and the functioning of the immigrant family play an important role in their life and in their well-being. Immigrant parents need not only to acculturate their children to their home culture, but must also support them in getting along in the culture of the receiving society and in succeeding in society at large, and, furthermore, to help them understand and teach them how to deal with issues of discrimination and prejudice (Phinney and Chavira 1995). Key to positive immigrant adolescent-parent relationships is that parents show flexibility and the ability to negotiate and embrace their child's developmental changes and demands for more autonomy instead of imposing high expectations of family embeddedness (Kwak 2003). It has been found that better family functioning and lower parent-adolescent conflict contribute to better adaptation. For example, cross-lagged analyses revealed that well-functioning families positively influenced changes in developmental (self-efficacy) and acculturative (ethnic identity) tasks (Reitz et al. 2014). In contrast, after reaching a threshold in parent-adolescent conflict, immigrant youth's psychological symptoms and conduct problems increased, and self-esteem decreased, exponentially (Motti-Stefanidi et al. 2011).

Schools are also a key social context for immigrant youth. They contribute both to their development and their acculturation (Vedder and Motti-Stefanidi 2016). Schools that respect their students' fundamental needs for competence, autonomy, and relatedness are expected to promote their self-determined behavior, intrinsic motivation, sense of belonging to their school, as well as their engagement with the learning process (Roeser et al. 1998). For example, meaningful and relevant curricula, related to students' own interests and goals, promote greater school engagement and intrinsic motivation in all students, but may be especially important for immigrant youth who need to navigate between at least two cultures. Similarly, caring relationships with teachers have been shown to be particularly important for immigrant youth, supporting them to better adapt to the new country, language, and educational demands (Suárez-Orozco et al. 2009).

Even though contexts play a preponderant role for immigrant youth adaptation, they are clearly not its sole determinant. Young immigrants are active agents in their development and acculturation (Kuczynski and Navara 2006). Youth process first the influences emanating from the contexts in which their lives are embedded, before they translate them into behavior. Thus, the meaning they attribute to experience functions as a mediator between the actual context and their behavior and adaptation in that context (see Motti-Stefanidi et al. 2012a). They actively construct working models of culture (see also Oppedal and Toppelberg 2016), which accommodate the information and demands that their parents, teachers, peers, as well as the media and the broader social context present them with. As development proceeds, youth are able to better self-regulate and to decide which values and demands of the family and of the host society they want to accept and incorporate into their identity and which they want to reject. However, immigrant youth living in multicultural societies and growing up in families that promote both the enculturation and their acculturation would be expected to be better able to become bi-cultural, and to integrate into their working models of culture both host and ethnic cultures.

Self-efficacy and locus of control are central mechanisms of personal agency. Self-efficacy refers to people's beliefs in their capabilities to regulate their functioning, and to manage environmental demands in order to achieve desired outcomes. Internal locus of control refers to the extent to which individuals believe they can control events affecting them. They both have been shown to differentially predict immigrant youth adaptation with respect to developmental tasks and psychological well-being (e.g., Motti-Stefanidi et al. 2012b).

Each of these contexts and personal attributes contribute to immigrant youth adaptation. Consistently with the resilience literature, youth who are equipped with and bring to the experience solid, normative human resources are better adapted with respect to developmental tasks and to psychological well-being, whether they live in low- or high-risk circumstances, than those who did not possess such social and personal capital (Masten 2014).

However, influences stemming either from context or from the individual may contribute, in accordance with the specificity principle in acculturation (Bornstein, in press), to immigrant youth's adaptation in interaction with each other. The effect of social challenges, such as discrimination or low SES, often facing immigrant youths and their families, may be moderated by characteristics of the young people and by other contextual features, the presence of which may modify in a positive direction the expected outcome. For example, it has been found that positive connections to their ethnic group moderate the negative association between perceived discrimination and academic achievement for adolescents. In this case, feelings of positive connection function as a protective factor for adaptation (Brown and Chu 2012; Wong et al. 2003).

Over and above the independent contribution of different contextual and personal resources to immigrant youth's adaptation, the congruence between individual attributes and social contexts are also important determinants of the quality of their adaptation (see Motti-Stefanidi et al. 2012a). In the case of immigrant youth, the match between the needs of developing and acculturating youth and the opportunities afforded them by their proximal environments significantly predicts adaptation. For example, the schools that offer immigrant students the opportunity to experience their learning environment as relevant and meaningful promote better adaptation (Roeser et al. 1998). Along the same line, the quality of interactions between people in children's proximal contexts may also meet, or fail to meet, the latter's developmental and acculturative needs. For example, parents and teachers who support the missions of school and the family are likely to have a positive influence on children's adaptation (Coatsworth et al. 2000). Similarly, the degree of congruence, or the cultural distance, between the social contexts of immigrant youth is also an important predictor of their adaptation. For example, for immigrant groups who value strong family embeddedness and delayed autonomy, migrating to an individualistic society may put a strain on parent–child relations, as adolescents demand autonomy sooner than parents are ready to grant it to them (Kwak 2003).

Brown and Chu (2012) showed in an interesting study the importance of the person-context congruence for immigrant youth's adaptation. They found that for Latino children, who had positive ethnic identity perception, and were enrolled in a predominantly Latino school, higher perceived peer discrimination was associated with greater sense of school belonging. They argued that peer discrimination, for children who feel positively about their ethnicity and are embedded in a context in which most other peers are from the same ethnic group, is associated with feeling like one fits in more, possibly reflecting an agreed upon group norm.

Finally, in addition to current influences, immigrant youth's adaptive history with respect to developmental and acculturative tasks may also function as a resource (or as risk) for current adaptation (Motti-Stefanidi et al. 2012a). Adaptive functioning with respect to developmental tasks is coherent and shows continuity over time (Sroufe et al. 2005). Thus, positive adaptation with respect to earlier stage developmental tasks increases the probability of subsequent successful adaptation. For example, in a recent study of immigrant students those who were shown to follow the high-stable school engagement pathway in adolescence had as young adults more years of schooling, earned a higher academic degree and had better mental health (Hao and Woo 2012).

Future Directions for Research and Policy Implications

Traditionally, researchers studying immigrant youth adaptation and mental health followed a risk approach focused on maladaptive processes and negative outcomes. Acculturative stress was assumed to increase the risk of immigrant youth for psychological problems and adaptation difficulties. However, research over the past decade has shown that most immigrant youth, in spite of the many developmental, acculturative and social challenges that they encounter, adapt to their new reality and actually do quite well. A growing focus on resilience has shifted attention from negative to positive outcomes and processes.

The framework presented to account for resilience in immigrant youth adaptation and development integrates developmental, acculturative, and social psychological processes (Motti-Stefanidi et al. 2012a; Motti-Stefanidi & Masten 2013). This expanded integrative framework guides the formulation of research questions taking into account the dynamic, transactional, contextualized and multilevel nature of immigrant youth's adaptation. Thus, it aims to capture the complexity inherent in describing and accounting for group and individual differences in the adaptation and development of immigrant youth.

An increasing number of studies on immigrant youth adaptation adopt within-subjects, longitudinal designs. Such designs facilitate the

disentangling of developmental and acculturative influences on adaptation outcomes. However, most of these studies are conducted in North America. Longitudinal research in more diverse cultural, political and economic contexts could expand the evidence base on developmental and acculturative processes involved in immigrant youth resilience. The longitudinal tracking of immigrant youth adaptation from different ethnic groups and living in different host societies could shed light on social, as well as individual, factors and processes that promote and/or protect their adaptation, concurrently and over time in the new country.

More multilevel studies conducted in diverse host societies are also needed. They allow researchers to disentangle the effect of contextual influences, examined at different levels of analysis, on immigrant youth adaptation and development. Immigrant youth's low socio-economic status and/or perception of being discriminated against are important risk factors for their adaptation and well-being. However, the mean socio-economic status and/or degree of perceived discrimination of the students at the level of the classroom/school may explain additional variance in adaptation outcomes.

Finally, we know significantly more about patterns of immigrant youth adaptation than we know about the processes explaining resilience phenomena (Marks et al. 2014). To tackle research questions regarding explanatory processes we need to adopt a mediation modeling approach. However, mediation implies change over time and, thus, also requires the adoption of time-varying, within subjects designs (e.g., see Maxwell and Cole 2007). Analyses of longitudinal mediation will provide better insights about processes that cause or explain group and individual differences in immigrant youth adaptation.

In conclusion, we would like to stress the translational value of research on positive immigrant youth adaptation and related adaptive processes. A focus on strengths and resilience among immigrant youth instead of on weaknesses and psychological symptoms has significant implications for policy and practice as well as public and private perceptions of the potential of immigrant youth. It generates interest, first, in finding out what may be helpful in reducing exposure to risk. For example, reducing discrimination requires the adoption of policy and program initiatives that promote a positive public attitude towards immigrants. It also generates interest in promoting positive adaptation and development. For example, we know that policies and practices that enhance teaching immigrant youth the language of instruction and training teachers and school leaders to treat diversity as a resource rather than an obstacle for successful teaching and learning are expected to promote the concurrent and long-term positive adaptation of immigrant youth in the host country (OECD 2010). This approach is likely to garner greater support from immigrant youth and their families for participating in society as well as research, and could influence aspirations among immigrant youth. Finally, and perhaps most importantly, the focus on strengths and positive adaptation can contribute to changes in public perceptions of immigrant youth, boosting recognition that immigrant youth have enormous potential to contribute to the economic and social capital of receiving societies.

References

Arends-Tóth, J. V., & van de Vijver, F. J. R. (2006). Issues in conceptualization and assessment of acculturation. In M. H. Bornstein & L. R. Cote (Eds.), *Acculturation and parent-child relationships: Measurement and development* (pp. 33–62). Mahwah: Lawrence Erlbaum.

Berry, J. W. (2006). Contexts of acculturation. In D. L. Sam & J. W. Berry (Eds.), *Handbook of acculturation* (pp. 27–42). New York: Cambridge University Press.

Berry, J. W., Phinney, J. S., Sam, D. L., & Vedder, P. (Eds.). (2006). *Immigrant youth in cultural transition: Acculturation, identity and adaptation across national contexts.* Mahwah, NJ: Lawrence Erlbaum Associates.

Birman, D. (2006). Acculturation gap and family adjustment findings with Soviet Jewish refugees in the United States and implications for measurement. *Journal of Cross-Cultural Psychology, 37*(5), 568–589.

Bornstein, M. H., & Cote, L. (2010). Immigration and acculturation. In M. H. Bornstein (Ed.), *Handbook of cultural developmental science.* New York: Psychology Press.

Bornstein, M. H. (in press). The specificity principle in Acculturation science. Perspectives on Psychological Science.

Bourhis, R. Y., Moïse, L. C., Perreault, S., & Senécal, S. (1997). Towards an interactive acculturation model: A social-psychological approach. *International Journal of Psychology, 32*(6), 369–386.

Brody, G. H., Chen, Y., Murry, V. M. B., Ge, X., Simons, R. L., Gibbons, F. X., et al. (2006). Perceived discrimination and the adjustment of African American youths: A five year longitudinal analysis with contextual moderation effects. *Child Development, 77*, 1129–1520.

Bronfenbrenner, U., & Morris, P. A. (2006). The bioecological model of human development. In R. M. Lerner (Ed.), *Handbook of child psychology: Vol. 1. Theoretical models of human development* (6th ed., pp. 793–828). Hoboken, NJ: Wiley.

Brown, C. S., & Chu, H. (2012). Discrimination, ethnic identity, and academic outcomes of Mexican immigrant children: The importance of school context. *Child Development, 83*(5), 1477–1485.

Cicchetti, D., & Rogosch, F. A. (2002). A developmental psychopathology perspective on adolescence. *Journal of Consulting and Clinical Psychology, 70*, 6–20.

Coatsworth, J. D., Pantin, H., McBride, C., Briones, E., Kurtines, W., & Szapocznik, J. (2000). Ecodevelopmental correlates of behavior problems in young Hispanic females. *Applied Developmental Science, 6* (3), 126–143.

Commission of the European Communities. (2003). *Communication on immigration, integration and employment, COM (2003) 336.* Brussels: Author.

Corak, M. (2012). Age at immigration and the education outcomes of children. In A. S. Masten, K. Liebkind, & D. J. Hernandez (Eds.), *Capitalizing on migration: The potential of immigrant youth.* Cambridge: Cambridge University Press.

Crocetti, E., Jahromi, P., & Meeus, W. (2012). Identity and civic engagement in adolescence. *Journal of Adolescence, 35*(3), 521–532.

Dimitrova, R., Chasiotis, A. & van de Vijver, F. J. R. (2016). Unfavorable adjustment outcomes of immigrant children and youth in Europe: A meta-analysis. *European Psychologist, 21*(2), 150–162. doi: 10.1027/1016-9040/a000246

Evans, G. W., Li, D., & Whipple, S. S. (2013). Cumulative risk and child development. *Psychological Bulletin, 139*(6), 1342–1396. doi:10.1037/a0031808

Fuligni, A. J. (2001). A comparative longitudinal approach to acculturation among children from immigrant families. *Harvard Educational Review, 71*, 566–578.

Garcia-Coll, C., & Marks, A. K. (2012). *The immigrant paradox in children and adolescents: Is becoming American a developmental risk?.* Washington, DC: American Psychological Association.

Hao, L., & Woo, J. (2012). Distinct trajectories in the transition to adulthood: Are children of immigrants advantaged? *Child Development, 83*, 1623–1639. doi:10.1111/j.1467-8624.2012.01798.x

Harkness, S., & Super, C. M. (Eds.). (1996). *Parents' cultural belief systems: Their origins, expressions, and consequences*. New York: Guilford Press.

Jackson, M. F., Barth, J. M., Powell, N., & Lochman, J. E. (2006). Classroom contextual effects of race on children's peer nominations. *Child Development, 77*(5), 1325–1337.

Kuczynski, L., & Navara, G. (2006). Sources of change in theories of socialization, internalization and acculturation. In M. Killen & J. Smetana (Eds.), *Handbook of moral development* (pp. 299–327). Mahwah, NJ: Erlbaum.

Kwak, K. (2003). Adolescents and their parents: A review of intergenerational family relations for immigrant and non-immigrant families. *Human Development, 46*(2–3), 115–136. doi:10.1159/000068581

Liebkind, K., Jasinskaja-Lahti, I., & Mähönen, T. A. (2012). Specifying social psychological adaptation of immigrant youth: Intergroup attitudes, interactions, and identity. In A. S. Masten, K. Liebkind, & D. J. Hernandez (Eds.), *Realizing the potential of immigrant youth* (pp. 117–158). New York, NY: Cambridge University Press.

Liebkind, K., Jasinskaja-Lahti, I., & Solheim, E. (2004). Cultural identity, perceived discrimination, and parental support as determinants of immigrants' school adjustment: Vietnamese youth inFinland. *Journal of Adolescent Research, 19*, 635–656.

Marks, A. K., Ejesi, K., & García Coll, C. (2014). Understanding the US immigrant paradox in childhood and adolescence. *Child Development Perspectives, 8*(2), 59–64. doi:10.1111/cdep.12071

Masten, A. S. (2014). *Ordinary magic: Resilience in development*. New York, NY: Guilford Press.

Masten, A. S., & Cicchetti, D. (2016). Resilience in development: Progress and transformation. In D. Cicchetti (Ed.), *Developmental Psychopathology* (3rd ed.). Volume 4: Risk, Resilience and Intervention (pp 271–333). New York: Wiley.

Masten, A. S., Liebkind, K., & Hernandez, D. J. (Eds.). (2012). *Capitalizing on migration: The potential of immigrant youth*. Cambridge: Cambridge University Press.

Maxwell, S. E., & Cole, D. A. (2007). Bias in cross-sectional analyses of longitudinal mediation. *Psychological Methods, 12*(1), 23.

McCormick, C. M., Kuo, S. I., & Masten, A. S. (2011). Developmental tasks across the lifespan. In K. L. Fingerman, C. Berg, J. Smith, & T. C. Antonucci (Eds.), *The handbook of lifespan development* (pp. 117–140). New York: Springer.

McLoyd, V. (2006). The legacy of child development's 1990 special issue on minority children: An editorial retrospective. *Child Development, 77*, 1142–1148.

McPherson, M., Smith-Lovin, L., & Cook, J. M. (2001). Birds of a feather: Homophily in social networks. *Annual Review of Sociology, 27*, 415–444.

Migration Policy Institute. (2013). http://www.migrationpolicy.org/research

Motti-Stefanidi, F., Pavlopoulos, V., Tantaros, S. (2011). Parent-adolescent conflict and adolescents' adaptation: A longitudinal study of Albanian immigrant youth living in Greece. [Special Issue], *International Journal of Developmental Science, 5*(1–2), 57–71.

Motti-Stefanidi, F. (2014a). Identity development in the context of the risk and resilience framework. In M. Syed & K. McLean (Eds.), *Oxford handbook of identity development* (pp. 472–489). New York, NY: Oxford University Press.

Motti-Stefanidi, F. (2014b). Immigrant youth adaptation in the Greek school context: A risk and resilience perspective. *Child Development Perspectives, 8*(3), 180–185.

Motti-Stefanidi, F. (2015). Risks and resilience in immigrant youth adaptation: Who succeeds in the Greek school context and why? *European Journal of Developmental Psychology, 12*(3), 261–274.

Motti-Stefanidi, F., Asendorpf, J. B., & Masten, A. S. (2012b). The adaptation and psychological well-being of adolescent immigrants in Greek schools: A multilevel, longitudinal study of risks and resources. *Development and Psychopathology, 24*(02), 451–473.

Motti-Stefanidi, F., Berry, J., Chryssochoou, X., Sam, D. L., & Phinney, J. (2012a). Positive immigrant youth adaptation in context: Developmental, acculturation, and social psychological perspectives. In A. S. Masten, K. Liebkind, & D. J. Hernandez (Eds.), *Realizing the potential of immigrant youth* (pp. 117–158). New York, NY: Cambridge University Press.

Motti-Stefanidi, F., & Masten, A. S. (2013). School success and school engagement of immigrant children and adolescents. *European Psychologist, 18*, 126–135. doi:10.1027/1016-9040/a000139

Motti-Stefanidi, F., Masten, A., & Asendorpf, J. B. (2014c). School engagement trajectories of immigrant youth: Risks and longitudinal interplay with academic success. *International Journal of Behavioral Development,*. doi:10.1177/0165025414533428

Obradović, J., & Masten, A. S. (2007). Developmental antecedents of young adult civic engagement. *Applied Developmental Science, 11*(1), 2–19.

Obradović, J., Shaffer, A., & Masten, A. S. (2012). Risk in developmental psychopathology: Progress and future directions. In L. C. Mayes & M. Lewis (Eds.), *The Cambridge handbook of environment of human development: A handbook of theory and measurement* (pp. 35–57). New York, NY: Cambridge University Press.

OECD. (2010). *Closing the gap for immigrant students: Policies, practice, and performance*. Paris: OECD.

OECD. (2012). *Untapped skills: Realising the potential of immigrant students*. Retrieved from http://www.oecd.org/edu/Untapped%20Skills.pdf

Ogbu, J. (1991). Immigrant and involuntary minorities in comparative perspective. In M. Gibson & J. Ogbu (Eds.), *Minority status and schooling: A comparative study of immigrant and involuntary minorities* (pp. 3–33). New York: Garland.

Oppedal, B., & Toppelberg, C. O. (2016). Acculturation and development. In D. L. Sam & J. Berry (Eds.), *Cambridge handbook of acculturation psychology* (2nd ed.). Cambridge: Cambridge University Press.

Overton, W. F. (2015). Process and relational developmental systems. In W. F. Overton & P. C. Molenaar (Eds.), *Handbook of child psychology and developmental science. Vol. 1: Theory and method* (7th ed.). (pp. 9–62). Editor-in-chief: R.M. Lerner. Hoboken, NJ: Wiley.

Pancer, S. M. (2015). The psychology of citizenship and civic engagement. USA: Oxford University Press.

Pettigrew, T. F., & Tropp, L. (2006). A meta-analytic test of intergroup contact theory. *Journal of Personality and Social Psychology, 90*, 751–783. doi:10.1037/0022-3514.90.5.751

Phinney, J. S., & Chavira, V. (1995). Parental ethnic socialization and adolescent coping with problems related to ethnicity. *Journal of Research on Adolescence, 5*, 31–53.

Phinney, J. S., Horenczyk, G., Liebkind, K., & Vedder, P. (2001). Ethnic identity, immigration and well-being: An interactional perspective. *Journal of Social Issues, 57*, 493–510.

Portes, A., & Rumbaut, R. G. (2006). *Immigrant America: A portrait*. Berkeley: University of California Press.

Reitz, A. K., Motti-Stefanidi, F., & Asendorpf, J. B. (2013). Mastering developmental transitions in immigrant adolescents: The longitudinal interplay of family functioning, developmental, and acculturative tasks. *Developmental Psychology, 50*(3), 754–765. doi:10.1037/a0033889

Reitz, A. K., Motti-Stefanidi, F., & Asendorpf, J. B. (2014). Mastering developmental transitions in immigrant adolescents: The longitudinal interplay of family functioning, developmental and acculturative tasks. *Developmental Psychology, 50*(3), 754.

Roeser, R. W., Eccles, J. S., & Sameroff, A. J. (1998). Academic and social functioning in early adolescence: Longitudinal relations, patterns, and prediction by experience in middle school. *Development and Psychopathology, 10*, 321–352.

Rubin, K. H., Bukowski, W. M., & Bowker, J. C. (2015). Children in peer groups. In R. M. Lerner, M.H. Bornstein, & T. Leventhal (Eds.), *Handbook of child psychology and Developmental Science: Vol. 4. Ecological settings and processes* (7th ed., pp. 175–222). Hoboken, NJ: John Wiley.

Sam, D. L., Vedder, P., Liebkind, K., Neto, F., & Virta, E. (2008). Immigration, acculturation and the paradox of adaptation in Europe. *European Journal of Developmental Psychology, 5*, 138–158. doi:10.1080/17405620701563348

Sameroff, A. J. (2000). Developmental systems and psychopathology. *Development and Psychopathology, 12*(03), 297–312.

Sroufe, L. A., Egeland, B., Carlson, E. A., & Collins, W. A. (2005). *The development of the person: The Minnesota study of risk and adaptation from birth to adulthood*. New York: Guilford.

Suárez-Orozco, C., Pimentel, A., & Martin, M. (2009). The significance of relationships: Academic engagement and achievement among newcomer immigrant youth. *Teachers College Record, 111*, 712–749.

Suarez-Orozco, C., Gaytan, F. X., Bang, H. J., Pakes, J., O'Connor, E., & Rhodes, J. (2010). Academic trajectories of newcomer immigrant youth. *Developmental Psychology, 46*, 602–618.

Suárez-Orozco, C., Suárez-Orozco, M., & Todorova, I. (2008). *Learning a new land. Immigrant students in American society*. Cambridge, MA: Harvard University Press.

Titzmann, P. F. (2014). Immigrant adolescents' adaptation to a new context: Ethnic friendship homophily and its predictors. *Child Development Perspectives, 8*(2), 107–112. doi:10.1111/cdep.12072

Vedder, P. H., & Motti-Stefanidi, F. (2016). Children, families, and schools. In D. L. Sam & J. Berry (Eds.), *Cambridge handbook of acculturation psychology* (2nd ed.). Cambridge: Cambridge University Press.

Umaña-Taylor, A. J., Quintana, S. M., Lee, R. M., Cross, W. E., Rivas-Drake, D., Schwartz, S. J., ... & Seaton, E. (2014). Ethnic and racial identity during adolescence and into young adulthood: An integrated conceptualization. *Child Development, 85*(1), 21–39.

Verkuyten, M. (1998). Perceived discrimination and self-esteem among ethnic minority adolescents. *The Journal of Social Psychology, 138*, 479–493.

Verkuyten, M. (2005). *The social psychology of ethnic identity*. New York: Psychology Press.

Wigfield, A., Eccles, J. S., Schiefele, U., Roeser, R. W., & Davis-Kean, P. (2006). Development of achievement motivation. In W. Damon, R. M. Lerner, & N. Eisenberg (Eds.), *handbook of child psychology: Vol. 3. Social, emotional, and personality development* (6th ed., pp. 933–1002). Hoboken, NJ: Wiley.

Wong, C. A., Eccles, J. S., & Sameroff, A. (2003). The influence of ethnic discrimination and ethnic identification on African American adolescents' school and socioemotional adjustment. *Journal of Personality, 71*, 1197–1232.

Measuring Positive Development I: Multilevel Analysis

Jens B. Asendorpf

Abstract

This chapter presents multilevel analysis as a useful tool for analyzing data where individuals are nested in varying social contexts such as classrooms, schools, or neighborhoods; time points are nested in individuals (longitudinal analyses); or situations are nested in individuals (diaries). Discussed are two-level models where individuals are nested in social contexts, time points, or situations, and three-level models where longitudinal changes or diary data are studied in varying social contexts. These models are illustrated with data from a longitudinal study of immigrant adolescents and their native classmates in varying classrooms and neighborhoods. More advanced topics such as multilevel moderation, multilevel mediation, and multilevel structural equation modeling are also covered, and statistical software options for these analyses are described.

Why We Sometimes Need Multilevel Analysis

Children develop in a nested world. For example, children become part of classrooms that are nested in schools which are nested in neighborhoods which are nested in communities which are nested in a society. Thus a major part of children's environment can be reconstructed as a *hierarchy of nested social systems* (see Bronfenbrenner 1977, for a seminal theory of nested environments).

Although psychologists focus on the level of individuals and their immediate environment, there are often good reasons to consider more distant environments that influence the individuals indirectly through their immediate or proximal environments. The study of minority children's adaptation and development requires consideration of both their proximal home culture contexts and the distant dominant culture contexts, which are both influenced by political, ideological, cultural, and economic characteristics of the society at

Chapter prepared for: Cabrera, N. J., & Leyendecker, B. (Eds.), *Handbook of positive development of minority children.* Amsterdam, NL: Springer.

J.B. Asendorpf (✉)
Department of Psychology, Humboldt University Berlin, Berlin, Germany
e-mail: asendorpf@gmail.com

© The Editor(s) 2017
N.J. Cabrera and B. Leyendecker (eds.), *Handbook on Positive Development of Minority Children and Youth*, DOI 10.1007/978-3-319-43645-6_3

35

large (see Motti-Stefanidi et al. 2012b, Fig. 5.1). In addition to normative developmental contexts, minority youth also face unique circumstances such as immigrant/minority status and their culture of origin, and related social variables such as discrimination, which significantly contribute to their adaptation. Furthermore, youth's personal attributes also influence their adaptation and development. The influences are bidirectional suggesting that all levels of contexts and individual attributes have an impact on each other. That is, causal influence can run both ways; lower-order units influence higher-order ones through membership, and higher-order ones can influence lower-order ones directly or indirectly.

This nested world poses two main problems for the statistical analysis of psychological data. First, if some participants share the same higher-order system, their data can be *statistically dependent*. Statistical dependence violates the assumption of most statistical tests that the units of analysis are independently sampled, and thus biases all significance tests. For example, in a study of children sampled in classrooms, the data of all children in a classroom on a particular outcome can be dependent because they share teachers and most often also the neighborhood of the school. Consequently, any statistical test about group differences, correlations, regressions, paths in structural equation models etc. is biased to the extent that classmates are more similar to each other than to children in other classrooms.

This similarity is often measured in terms of the *intraclass correlation* that compares the variance of higher-order units with the overall variance. The higher the intraclass correlation is, the greater the problem of statistical dependency. In a study of children in classrooms, an intraclass correlation of 0.30 for some outcome variable of interest indicates that 30 % of the variance in the outcome concerns differences between classrooms whereas 70 % concerns differences within classrooms; an intraclass correlation of zero indicates that there are no classroom differences in the outcome. The intraclass correlation can be also interpreted as the expected correlation between two randomly chosen lower-order units of the same higher-order unit. If we randomly choose one pair of children from each classroom, the outcome is expected to correlate zero between the paired children if there are no classroom differences (thus, if the intraclass correlation is zero). If however the intraclass correlation is 0.30, even randomly chosen pairs from the classrooms are expected to show some similarity due to the differences between classrooms, and indeed the correlation between the paired children is 0.30.

If all classrooms have the same distribution of the outcome variable, the intraclass correlation is zero and statistical dependency is not a problem. If all classmates have identical values in the outcome variable, but the outcome is different across classrooms, the intraclass correlation is 1 and the analysis should be done at the classroom level only. In most cases, the intraclass correlation is not large but substantial such that ignoring the nested structure of the data leads to biased significance tests. This first problem of nested data (often the alternative term *clustered data* is used) can be completely resolved by adjusting the standard errors for the statistical tests. Many statistical packages such as R, SAS, or MPlus provide simple adjustment procedures for clustered data. It is *not* necessary to conduct a multi-level analysis if one only wants to control statistical dependencies in nested data.

The second problem of nested data is more consequential because it requires more than a correction of standard errors. Often, one is interested in effects of higher-order units on lower-order units (*cross-level effects*). For example, does individual math achievement, or the difference between minority and majority children in math achievement, depend on the teaching style of the math teacher? Teaching style is a variable at the classroom level, not at the individual level, because all children in a classroom share it (its intraclass correlation is 1).

Whenever cross-level effects are interesting, *multilevel analysis* is required. If the effects can be described by linear regressions, *multilevel linear regression models* can be applied (also called *hierarchical linear models* or *random coefficient regression models*). In essence, these are multiple regression models where the regression coefficients obtained at a lower level are assumed to vary across higher-order units ("random coefficients"), and therefore can be regressed at the higher level on characteristics of the higher-order units. For example, within each classroom, children's math achievement can be regressed on their math anxiety. Classrooms may vary in the extent to which achievement depends on anxiety, and this variation may be predictable by the teaching style of the math teacher.

Such cross-level effects could be tested without applying multilevel models. One could simply regress within each classroom achievement on anxiety, record the intercepts and slopes, and regress them in a second step on teaching style. However, the advantage of multilevel models is that they simultaneously estimate all effects within one model and weight the lower-order regressions according to their reliability. It is intuitively clear that the within-classroom regressions are better estimated in larger classrooms than in smaller classrooms such that the larger classroom results should get a higher weight in the between- classroom regressions (similar to the weighting of large versus small studies in meta-analysis). Multilevel models include such weighting and have additional advantages from an estimation point of view (see Hox 2010, or Raudenbush and Bryk 2002, for overviews).

In the reminder of this chapter, I provide a step-by-step non-technical introduction to multilevel analysis, starting from simple two-level models and ending with the advanced topic of multilevel mediation. This introduction is meant to help researchers to understand published results of multilevel analyses in the literature, to decide whether multilevel analysis is helpful for answering own research questions, to use multilevel analysis when it it useful, and to avoid it when it is not necessary (the last point is important too because multilevel analysis is right now fashionable and sometimes applied when it is not really necessary).

Study Used for Illustration

Each step of the introduction to multilevel analysis is organized around a particular research question in order to avoid too abstract arguments.

A longitudinal study of adolescent immigrant students and their non-immigrant classmates helps illustrate most of the steps (Motti-Stefanidi et al. 2012a). It was designed within a developmental risk and resilience framework where risks and resources are assumed to operate at both the level of individual adolescents and their environment (families, classrooms, neighborhoods); see Motti-Stefanidi et al. (2012b). In such a framework, individual students are nested in classrooms and neighborhoods. Therefore, individual risks and resources can be statistically dependent, and any study of the impact of risks and resources at the classroom or neighborhood level on individual students requires multilevel analysis.

Motti-Stefanidi et al. (2012a) studied the adaptation and well-being of adolescents from immigrant and non-immigrant families over the first three years of middle school (ages 13–15 years) and related it to individual and environmental risks and resources. The students were sampled from schools in Athens, Greece, in neighborhoods with a high proportion of immigrant families. The proportion of immigrants in a classroom varied strongly across classrooms, with an average of 44 % immigrants. This design made sure that immigrant and non-immigrant children were matched in terms of their school environment. They were even matched in terms of their neighborhood because the students were mandated by law to attend the nearest school in their neighborhood.

The present chapter focuses on academic achievement (grade point average) as the only adaptation variable. It is predicted at the individual level by the risks immigrant status (yes, no) and family social adversity (a cumulative risk index) as well as by resources such as self-efficacy (self-rated by the students) and parental involvement in school issues (teacher-rated). At the classroom level, the average family social adversity in the classroom serves as a good measure of the social adversity of the neighborhood because all children of a classroom shared the same neighborhood.

In the study by Motti-Stefanidi et al. (2012a), students were nested in classrooms and classrooms in schools because in each school multiple first-grade classrooms were assessed. Therefore, in principle, a three-level study design resulted: 1057 students were nested in 49 classrooms that were nested in 12 schools. Although this design suggests analyzing the data with a statistical three-level model, this was not viable because only few schools were assessed. The rule of thumb in multilevel analysis is that approximately 50 units are required for the highest level of analysis because all statistical tests are based on the units at this level (see Hox 2010; Raudenbush and Bryk 2002). Twelve schools are clearly not sufficient (regressions based on only 12 data points could be seriously biased by one outlier). Therefore, only a two-level structure can be modeled in this study, with students nested in classrooms.

Two-Level Models of Adaptation in Context

In this section I consider the probably most common case in research on minority children where multilevel analysis is required: a cross-sectional study of individuals nested in classrooms, schools, or neighborhoods. For illustrative purposes I consider in this section immigrant and non-immigrant students' academic achievement in the first grade of middle school. Were (a) immigrant status and/or family social adversity risks for low achievement, were (b) self-efficacy and parental involvement in school issues resources for high achievement, did (c) risks and resources interact in predicting achievement, were (d) adverse neighborhoods a risk factor for low achievement, and were (e) the above individual risks and resources moderated by the adversity of the neighborhood (e.g., was being an immigrant a stronger risk for low achievement in relatively benign neighborhoods than in relatively adverse neighborhoods?). Questions (a)–(c) concern Level 1 effects, questions (d) and (e) concern cross-level effects.

Is Multilevel Analysis Useful?

The first step in such a two-level analysis is computing the intraclass correlation of the outcome which is the percentage of variance accounted for by the higher-order units, thus, in the present case classrooms (see earlier section in this chapter). If the intraclass correlation is close to zero, between-classroom differences in the outcome are unimportant, analyses of cross-level effects make no sense, multi-level analysis is unnecessary, and data analysis can proceed as usual, only at the individual level. In the two-level case, the intraclass correlation is computed with a two-level model without predictors at both levels (see "Appendix" for statistical software for multilevel analysis). In such an analysis, the variance components for Level 2 and for Level 1 (the residual variance) are determined, the significance of the Level 2 component is computed with a χ^2 test, and the intraclass correlation ICC is directly shown in the output of the software or can be easily computed as

$$ICC = \text{Level 2 component}/(\text{Level 2 component} + \text{residual component})$$

In the present example, the Level 2 (classroom) component was 0.83 ($p < 0.001$) and the residual component was 8.35 such that the intraclass correlation was 0.09; thus, 9 % of the variance in academic achievement was between classrooms and significant such that a multilevel analysis of the data was useful.

Level 1 Effects: Individual Risks and Resources and Their Interactions

Academic achievement was predicted by a sequence of hierarchical regressions. In Step 1a, risks were entered first, followed by resources in Step 2a; in Step 1b, resources were entered first, followed by risks in Step 2b. Thereby, the unique contributions of risks and resources were studied. In Model 3, one Level 1 moderation was analyzed (immigrant status by parental involvement); the interaction term was entered in addition to the main effects of risks and resources (see also later section on multilevel moderation). The results for these models are presented in Table 1 for two different methods of coding group differences with dummy variables (see Hox 2010,

Table 1 Results of two-level regressions predicting academic achievement from risks and resources for two methods of using dummy variables

Fixed effect (Level 2)	Pseudo-R^2	Intercept included	
Step		Yes	No
1a. Risks	0.20		
Level 1 Intercept		14.76(0.18)***	–
Greek (0 = immigrant, 1 = Greek)		–	14.76(0.18)***
Immigrant (0 = Greek, 1 = immigrant)		−2.09(0.27)***	12.67(0.18)***
Adversity (z-score)		−0.56(0.09)***	−0.56(0.09)***
1b. Resources	0.36		
Parental involvement (z-score)		1.66(0.13)***	1.66(0.13)***
Self-efficacy (z-score)		0.58(0.11)***	0.58(0.11)***
2a. Resources controlled for risks	0.43		
Parental involvement (z-score)		1.39(0.15)***	1.39(0.15)***
Self-efficacy (z-score)		0.48(0.11)***	0.48(0.11)***
2b. Risks controlled for resources	0.43		
Greek (0 = immigrant, 1 = Greek)		–	14.40(0.21)***
Immigrant (0 = Greek, 1 = immigrant)		−0.99(0.31)**	13.41(0.19)***
Adversity (z-score)		−0.33(0.09)***	−0.33(0.09)***
3. Risks × resources	0.44		
Greek × parental involvement		–	0.21(0.24)
Immigrant × parental involvement		−0.21(0.24)	–

Reported are the results of two-level linear regression models without predictor at Level 2. Reported are for each model the *Pseudo-R^2* for the explained variance by the model and the unstandardized regression coefficients *b* (*SE* in parentheses) for the included Level 1 predictors. Significances for *b* refer to robust standard errors *SE*
**p < 0.01; ***p < 0.001

Appendix C, for these and more methods of coding group differences).[1]

Group Coding Including Intercept

The first, more common method includes the intercept at Level 1 and dummy-codes immigrant

[1]The results differ somewhat from those reported by Motti-Stefanidi et al. (2012a) in their Table 4 mainly because the latter are estimates for Grade 1 from a longitudinal analysis of Grades 1–3 and were controlled for gender.

status. The advantage is that the significance of the immigrant status effect (which is central here) is directly shown in terms of the effect of the dummy variable. The disadvantage is that the overall mean of the immigrants is not shown although it can be easily computed from the table because the intercept in multilevel models (just as in any multiple regression model) refers to cases with zeros in all predictors. Because all predictors except for the dummy codes were z-scored ($M = 0$, $SD = 1$), the intercept refers to

Greeks with average scores in all other predictors, thus to the estimated mean achievement of Greek students, and the mean achievement of immigrants is the intercept plus the immigrant status effect.

Group Coding Excluding Intercept

Less common is the method of dropping the intercept from the model and including instead dummy variables for *all* groups. In this case, the Greek effect is the mean of the Greeks, and the immigrant effect is the mean of the immigrants. The significance tests are not informative in this case because they refer to a test whether the mean is zero. The advantage of this second method is that the mean of each group is directly shown. The disadvantage is that group differences are not directly shown although they can be simply computed by substracting group means. The significance of the group differences can be tested with appropriate contrasts between the dummy variables. More generally, any two effects can be tested for a significant difference using contrasts, whether the intercept is included in the model or not.

Standardization of Predictors and Outcomes

In models with many continuous predictors as in the present case, it is useful to standardize them because it helps interpreting the intercept and the meaning of the unstandardized regression coefficients b. In general, b indicates the effect on the outcome if the predictor value increases by 1. Thus for standardized variables with $SD = 1$, $b = 1$ indicates the effect on the outcome if the predictor value increases by 1 standard deviation, and the effect size of different predictors can be directly compared with one another in terms of the b values. If the outcome is also standardized, b is a standardized regression coefficient, and the predictor effects can be directly compared between different outcomes.

Explained Variance

Unfortunately, adding a predictor to a multilevel regression model may under certain conditions decrease rather than increase the explained variance such that the incremental explained variance is negative (Hox 2010). These rare cases are due to indirect effects through other levels of the model. Therefore a more cautious approach is in order where the explained variance is called *Pseudo-R^2*, and the significance of a model comparison is interpreted as an overall difference between the models rather than the significance of incremental variance explained by the added predictors.

Random and Fixed Effects

In multilevel analysis, the variance components from which the intraclass correlation and the explained variances are computed are called *random effects*, and the unstandardized regression coefficients b are called *fixed effects*. The standard errors of the fixed effects are either computed based on the assumption of a normal distribution of the outcome variable, or without this assumption (*robust standard errors*). Because the data often violate the normality assumption, it is better to always report robust standard errors. The significance of the fixed effects is computed slightly differently by different statistical software but with only minimal effects on the p values in most cases (see Hox 2010). The analyses reported in this chapter were done with HLM 7 (Raudenbush et al. 2011).

Results

The results are reported in Table 1. In Step 1a achievement is predicted by risks. Adding dummy-coded immigrant status and adversity at Level 1 to the model without predictors reduced the Level 1 residual from 8.35 to 6.64 (not reported in the table), thus explains 20 % of the initial residual variance (*Pseudo-R^2* = 0.20). The significance of this change can be tested by comparing the *deviance scores* of the two models (not shown in the table). The deviance for the model without predictors was 4227 (2 estimated parameters) and for the model in Step 1a 3886 (7 estimated parameters). The difference is tested with a χ^2 test with $df = 7 - 2 = 5$ (the logic is similar to comparing the fit of structural equation models), thus $\chi^2(5) = 4227 - 3886 = 341$, $p < 0.001$.

The model with intercept shows that Greek students achieved a grade point average of 14.76 (because the intercept represents Greek students); that immigrants achieved 2.09 points less, thus 12.67, if adversity was controlled; and that 1 *SD* more in adversity was accompanied by a decrease of achievement of 0.56 points if immigrant status was controlled. Because both the immigrant status and the adversity effects were significant, it can be concluded that both risks uniquely contributed to lower achievement. The model without intercept directly shows the mean for immigrants but the immigrant status effect has to be computed by substracting the mean for Greeks from the mean for immigrants, and testing its significance requires an additional test of the contrast comparing the means of Greeks and immigrants (not shown in the table because the result is identical with the immigrant status effect in the model with intercept).

The alternative model in Step 1b predicts achievement by resources. Resources predicted achievement much more strongly than risks (36 % versus 20 % explained variance) which again can be tested for significance by comparing the deviances of the two models. Parental involvement in school issues strongly predicted achievement when self-efficacy was controlled; as Table 1 shows, a 1 *SD* increase in involvement was associated with a 1.66 increase in grade point average. This prediction was nearly three times as strong as the prediction from self-efficacy when parental involvement was controlled (0.58 increase; the unique effects of the two resources can be directly compared because both refer to standardized variables). The model without intercept shows the same effects because they do not involve the dummy variables.

Step 2a shows the effects of resources when risks are controlled, thus the results for resources in a model with four Level 1 predictors (2 risks and 2 resources). This model explained 43 % of the variance. Compared to Step 1b, the unique effects of both resources decreased slightly due to the control of the risks but remained highly significant. Step 2b shows the effects of the two risks in this model; compared to Step 1a they decreased by approximately 50 % but remained

significant. The decreasing immigrant status effect after controlling for both resources is also reflected in the model without intercept that directly shows the means of Greeks and immigrants. In sum, resources mattered more for achievement than risks.

Finally, Model 3 indicates that the effects of immigrant status and parental involvement on achievement did not show a significant interaction. The interaction effects in the models with/out intercept are identical except for the sign because the dummy variables for Greeks and for immigrants correlate -1. If other interactions between risks and resources are of interest, they should not be added to this model because they would be strongly correlated; instead, they should be tested one by one in separate models.

A comparison of the two methods of using dummy variables shows that the results differ only for variables involving the dummy variables, and that all information of interest can be reconstructed from either method. If the focus is on group differences, the model with intercept is preferable. The model without intercept is more useful for interpreting effects group by group, particularly in the case of more complex models with more than one type of group differences (e.g., if immigrant status and gender are both dummy-coded). In these cases, computing effects for specific groups is tedious such that I recommend using both methods of dummy-coding in order to cross-check results and avoid mistaken interpretations.

Level 2 Effects: Main Effects and Cross-Level Interactions

The models discussed up to now did not include predictors at Level 2 and thus no cross-level effects (main effects of Level 2 predictors and cross-level interactions, i.e., moderation of the Level 1 parameters by a Level 2 predictor). In the present example, classroom characteristics such as the mean social adversity of all students in class or the percentage of immigrants in the classroom may have an effect on achievement and may moderate the effects of risks and/or

Table 2 Results of
two-level regressions
predicting academic
achievement from risks and
resources and their
moderation by mean
adversity in class

Fixed effect (Level 2)	b	SE	p
Level 1 intercept			
Level 2 intercept	14.28	0.21	0.000
Classroom adversity	−0.41	0.16	0.013
Immigrant status			
Level 2 intercept	−0.96	0.30	0.003
Classroom adversity	0.55	0.26	0.044
Adversity			
Level 2 intercept	−0.35	0.09	0.000
Classroom adversity	0.11	0.10	0.320
Parental involvement			
Level 2 intercept	1.46	0.14	0.000
Classroom adversity	−0.17	0.14	0.228
Self-efficacy			
Level 2 intercept	0.47	0.09	0.000
Classroom adversity	0.13	0.11	0.257

Reported are the results of two-level linear regression models. Classroom adversity was standardized across classrooms ($M = 0$, $SD = 1$). Reported are the unstandardized regression coefficients b for the Level 1 predictors. Significances for b refer to robust standard errors SE

resources. Table 2 reports the results of a two-level model with both risks and both resources as Level 1 predictors and mean adversity in class as a Level 2 predictor.

Table 2 reports the results in a format used in many publications of multilevel analyses (Table 1 used a more condensed format which is also possible). The fixed effects are grouped by the parameters at the lowest level (here: Level 1).

Level 2 Main Effect

Note that there are two types of intercepts. The Level 1 intercept (which varies across classrooms) and the Level 2 intercept (the estimated mean across all classrooms). In Table 1, Level 2 intercepts are reported for all Level 1 parameters but this was not made explicit in the table because there were no other Level 2 effects. In Table 2, there are two Level 2 effects: the Level 2 intercept and the Level 2 slope which refers to the effect of the Level 2 predictor classroom adversity (mean adversity across all classmates). Note that adversity is a variable at both Level 1 and Level 2; Level 1 adversity refers to

within-classroom differences, Level 2 adversity refers to between-classroom differences.

The results for the Level 2 intercepts are highly similar to those reported for Step 2a, b in the model including the intercept in Table 1; they are not identical because inclusion of the Level 2 predictor resulted in a more complex model with minor consequences for the Level 2 intercept estimates. New are the effects of classroom adversity. The classroom adversity effect for the Level 1 intercept of $b = -0.41$, $p = 0.013$, indicates that grade point average significantly decreased by 0.41 points for a 1 SD increase in classroom adversity (note that SD refers here to between-classroom differences, not to between-student differences); thus, students in more adverse neighborhoods had lower grades. This is a Level 2 main effect.

Cross-Level Interaction

The classroom adversity effect for immigrant status of $b = 0.55$, $p = 0.044$, indicates that the immigrant status effect on achievement (after controlling for within-classroom adversity, parental involvement, and student self-efficacy) was

Fig. 1 Cross-level effect of classroom adversity on the effect of immigrant status on academic achievement

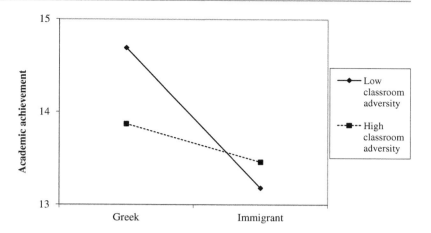

moderated by classroom adversity (a cross-level interaction). Whereas it was $b = -0.96$ for a classroom of average adversity, it was $-0.96 + 0.55 = -0.41$ for a classroom 1 SD above average classroom adversity, and $-0.96 - 0.55 = -1.51$ for a classroom 1 SD below average classroom adversity. Thus, the immigrant status effect became larger in more benign neighborhoods. These cross-level effects can be visualized just as in the case of ordinary moderated regressions by plotting the regression lines for ± 1 SD in the moderator variable (see Fig. 1). Figure 1 indicates that immigrant status had a stronger effect on achievement in more benign neighborhoods and that neighborhood adversity mattered only for Greeks' achievement (two alternative views of the same effect).

Two-Level Models of Development of Adaptation: Longitudinal Data

A second important application of multilevel analysis is the longitudinal study of changes in adaptation. In this case, time points are nested in individuals. Whereas repeated ANOVA designs require that each individual is assessed at the same time points, multilevel models can handle also studies with different numbers and/or different time points of assessment for different individuals. At Level 1, a linear regression is fitted to the available assessments of the outcome for each individual, and at Level 2 the intercept

and slope of these individual developmental functions are predicted by constant characteristics of the individuals such as sex, age, SES, and personality at the beginning of the study. Note that these linear regression models can be adapted easily to measure nonlinear developmental functions by transforming the time scale. For example, if the outcome is regressed on both time and time squared, accelerated or decelerated change (linear plus or minus quadratic) is modeled. Thus, multilevel models are well suited to measure interindividual differences in intraindividual change with great flexibility.

Two Main Assumptions

Standard applications of multilevel analysis to longitudinal data make two important assumptions. First, they assume measurement equivalence across time, that is, the same assessment instrument or different instruments used at different time points have the same validity for each time point. Whereas measurement equivalence can be assumed for short-term studies, it can be of concern in studies covering a large age interval, even if the same instrument is used at all assessments (see van de Vijver & He, this volume, for a discussion of measurement equivalence). Second, standard applications assume uncorrelated measurement errors across time. This assumption is often violated if the assessments are closely spaced in time. For example, if cognitive competence is tested a few days apart with the same test such that many participants remember their answers in the earlier assessment, measurement error can be correlated. One solution is using parallel test versions at assessments close in time. Another solution is modeling the correlated errors within the multilevel model with additional parameters (see Hox 2010; Raudenbush and Bryk 2002).

Centering Time

An important decision in multilevel longitudinal studies concerns centering time. If the longitudinal observation starts or ends at a psychologically meaningful time point (e.g., birth, starting to attend a particular classroom, menarche, starting a job, separation from the partner, death), it is useful to center time at the first or last assessment (thus the first or last assessment is coded as 0). If the observation starts at a more arbitrary point in time (e.g., a study of changes over adolescence between ages 12 and 18 where the participants start puberty at different points in time), it is more useful to center time at the midpoint of the observed interval (thus, a study with 5 yearly assessments is centered at the 3rd assessment). Also, this choice has the advantage that the intercepts are less correlated with the slopes. Similar but not identical is "grand-mean centering" where time is centered at the mean assessment point of all individuals. Due to missing data or different spacing of the assessments, the mean assessment point can be different from the midpoint of the observation such that its interpretation is less obvious. Often not useful is centering time within each individual (often called "group-mean centering" where in the present case "group" refers to individuals) because in this case the individual Level 1 intercepts refer to different time points such that these differences are confounded with other interindividual differences. Group mean centering is only useful if the zero point is psychologically meaningful for each individual (e.g., if data before and after the individually determined onset of puberty is analyzed).

Dealing with Missing Data

Selective Attrition

A frequent point of concern in longitudinal studies is biased results due to selective drop-out of the participants (*selective attrition*). For example, if low-achieving participants drop out from school or refuse to further participate in the study more frequently than high-achieving participants (which is often the case in longitudinal studies), the variance of achievement at later assessments is restricted which leads in ANOVAs or ordinary regressions to an underestimation of effects on later achievement. One approach to avoid such biases is estimating the missing assessments with (multiple) imputation (see Asendorpf et al. 2014). If however the data are analyzed with longitudinal multilevel models, imputation is not necessary because the estimation procedure corrects for selective drop-out as far as it is related to the first assessment (see Hox 2010; Little 1995). Only if drop-out is related to measured variables not included in the multilevel model (*auxiliary variables*) biases due to such selective drop-out are not corrected with the multilevel estimation procedures. In this case, it is useful to use multiple imputation with these variables as predictors. Depending on the multilevel software, multiple imputation is done before the multilevel analysis is run, or there is an auxiliary variables option in the multilevel analysis procedure.

Missing Data at Higher Levels

Although missing data at the lowest level do not present a problem in multilevel analysis in most cases, they do present a problem at higher levels because they reduce the number of included higher-level units *and* all lower-level assessments of these units. In the example in the preceding section, the classroom-level predictor could be computed for all classrooms such that this was not a problem. But assume that observed teaching style is a classroom-level predictor but some teachers refused to cooperate in the study. In this case, the cross-level effect of teaching style can be evaluated only for the students with a cooperative teacher, which may bias the results.

This problem is even stronger in longitudinal studies of adaptation where multiple predictors are studied at the individual level such as in the present example because all individuals with a missing value in *one* of the predictors are excluded from analysis (listwise deletion), just as in ordinary multiple regressions. Therefore it is useful in this case to impute missing values at the individual level, and the best method is multiple imputation using all available individual-level variables, even if they are not included in the model (see Asendorpf et al. 2014, and Graham 2009, for non-technical overviews and practical recommendations). Depending on the multilevel software, multiple imputation is done before the multilevel analysis is run, or it is an option in the multilevel analysis procedure.

Illustration

The study by Motti-Stefanidi et al. (2012a) was a longitudinal study with three yearly assessments (*waves*) of all outcome variables. Therefore it allowed for answering questions about overall (mean) change in academic achievement and about *differential change* for groups (e.g., different change for immigrants versus non-immigrants) and for individuals (e.g., change related to family social adversity or student self-efficacy). The first assessment was psychologically meaningful because it was done in the first year at middle school. Therefore wave was centered at Wave 1. Because neither theoretical considerations nor inspection of the mean change in academic achievement suggested nonlinear change, the three waves were coded as 0, 1, 2 such that linear change was studied. Although individuals were nested in classrooms, this fact is ignored in the present section in order to simplify the issues addressed in this section. Thus developmental changes in academic achievement are studied here with a two-level linear regression model, with time at Level 1 and individuals at Level 2, and the two individual risks and the two individual resources as the Level 2 predictors. Participant drop-out was significantly related to initial low achievement but this selective attrition was corrected by the multilevel estimation

procedure. Missing data at Level 2 was imputed with SPSS 22 (5 imputations), and the multilevel analyses were based on the 5 imputed Level 2 files, using the multiple imputation option in the multilevel software HLM 7.

Random Effects (Variance Components)

A model with wave as the Level 1 predictor and no predictor at Level 2 showed that 88 % of the variance was due to the Level 1 intercepts and 3 % of the variance was accounted by the Level 1 slopes. Because time was centered at Wave 1, the Level 1 intercepts refer to interindividual differences in initial academic achievement, and the slopes refer to interindividual differences in linear change in achievement over 2 years, from Wave 1 to Wave 3. Although the slopes accounted for only 3 % of the overall variance, this variance component was significant ($p < 0.001$).

Fixed Effects for Intercepts and Slopes

The results for the fixed effects are presented in Table 3.

The results for the Level 1 intercept were similar but not identical to those reported in Table 1 for the steps 2a, b for the model including the intercept; the differences are due to the fact that the Level 1 intercept (the initial achievement) was estimated in the developmental model from the full data including Wave 2 and Wave 3. Because the interindividual differences in academic achievement were highly stable across the three waves (see Motti-Stefanidi et al. 2015), the developmental model led to a better estimation of the Level 1 intercepts (the standard errors became smaller and the significance of the intercepts increased).

The results for the Level 1 slopes indicate that academic achievement significantly decreased overall by 0.34 points per year, and that this decrease was not moderated by the Level 2 predictors, particularly not by immigrant status. One reason for the lack of interindividual differences in intraindividual change seems to be that the reliability of the slopes was not high due to the high stability of the interindividual differences in achievement (the year-to-year stability was 0.89 which leaves little room for true differential

Table 3 Results of two-level regressions predicting initial status and change in academic achievement from risks and resources

Fixed effect (Level 2)	Level 1 intercept			Level 1 slope		
	b	SE	p	b	SE	p
Level 2 intercept	14.34	0.13	0.000	−0.34	0.05	0.000
Immigrant (0 = Greek, 1 = immigrant)	−1.45	0.20	0.000	0.01	0.08	0.869
Adversity (z-score)	−0.35	0.08	0.000	0.06	0.03	0.099
Parental involvement (z-score)	1.02	0.10	0.000	−0.05	0.04	0.274
Self-efficacy (z-score)	0.54	0.09	0.000	0.01	0.04	0.847

Reported are the results of two-level linear regression models. Time was centered at the first assessment such that the Level 1 intercept refers to Greeks in grade 1

Reported are the unstandardized regression coefficients b for the Level 1 predictors. Significances for b refer to robust standard errors SE

change; see Motti-Stefanidi et al. 2015). Also, three waves are not optimal for estimating change because two assessments are already needed to estimate a slope; thus even students who participated in all waves contributed only 1 additional assessment for increasing the reliability of the slope. More waves would yield more reliable estimates of change.

Multilevel Versus Growth Curve Modeling

Researchers familiar with growth curve modeling (a particular type of structural equation models where the intercepts and slopes of repeated assessments are modeled) may wonder to which extent the two-level approach discussed in this section is similar to a particular growth curve model. The answer is that it is *identical* with a growth curve model where the residual variances of the outcome variable are constrained to be equal across time (see Hox 2010, chapter 16, for the advantages and disadvantages of growth curve modeling versus multilevel modeling of longitudinal data). The main advantage of multilevel modeling is that the models can be easily expanded to three-level models that include contextual variables such as classrooms or neighborhoods, as will be shown in the next section.

Three-Level Models of Development of Adaptation in Context

The results reported in the preceding section have to be considered with caution because the nested structure of the data (students were nested in classrooms) was ignored to simplify the presentation. Instead a three-level model is appropriate, with time at Level 1, students at Level 2, and classrooms at Level 3. Such three-level models are rarely found in the literature due to their complexity and the lack of longitudinal studies with individuals nested in measured contexts. But their application is a straightforward extension of two-level models to an additional level; there are no issues specific to three-level models except for the fact that there are more parameters for interpretation and more complex tables for presenting the results.

Research Questions

Three-level developmental models answer all questions answered by two-level cross-sectional and by two-level developmental models. In addition, they answer questions about cross-level effects of context on overall change (e.g., does academic achievement change differently in adverse versus benign neighborhoods?) as well as questions about cross-level effects of context on differential change (e.g., is differential change of immigrants versus non-immigrants in academic achievement moderated by neighborhood adversity?). These latter questions concern *moderation of moderation effects* which are in fact anwered by three-way interactions between time, interindividual or between-group differences, and contextual differences. As in ordinary multiple regression analyses, the statistical power for testing the significance of these three-way interactions is often low except for very large samples (see Hox 2010, chapter 12, for power estimation in multilevel models). Thus the lack of significant moderation of moderation effects may be due to insufficient statistical power, and it is difficult to replicate significant moderation of moderation effects in another study. Therefore moderation of moderation effects should be considered with great caution.

But this problem should not distract from the important advantage of three-level developmental models that they correct for biased significance tests if the context matters. Even three-level developmental models without any contextual predictor should be preferred to two-level developmental models if the outcome variable shows significant variation across contexts.

Illustration

Motti-Stefanidi et al. (2012a) used a three-level model for analysis, with time at Level 1, students at Level 2, and classrooms at Level 3. A three-level model for academic achievement with wave as the Level 1 predictor and no predictors at Levels 2 and 3 showed that the variance components for the intercepts and slopes were significant at both Level 2 and Level 3. Thus, there were significant interindividual differences in intraindividual change, and significant classroom differences in intraindividual change. For example, the overall decrease of academic achievement from Wave 1 to Wave 3 (see Table 3) varied significantly between classrooms. Because of these significant classroom differences, the results in the preceding section that ignored that students were nested in classrooms yielded biased results. The results for the fixed effects estimated with the three-level model are presented in Table 4.

The fixed effects were similar but not identical to those reported in Table 3 because they respect now the within-classroom similarity of academic achievement. The standard errors were slightly larger in the three-level model, indicating that the significance tests for the two-level model were somewhat too liberal. In addition to this

Table 4 Results of three-level regressions predicting initial status and change in academic achievement from risks and resources

Fixed effect (Level 3)	Level 1 intercept			Level 1 slope		
	b	SE	p	b	SE	p
Level 2 intercept	14.36	0.18	0.000	−0.36	0.08	0.000
Immigrant (0 = Greek, 1 = immigrant)	−1.38	0.26	0.000	0.02	0.08	0.819
Adversity (z-score)	−0.35	0.08	0.000	0.04	0.03	0.155
Parental involvement (z-score)	1.05	0.13	0.000	−0.01	0.04	0.875
Self-efficacy (z-score)	0.48	0.10	0.000	0.00	0.04	0.954

Reported are the results of three-level linear regression models without predictor at Level 3. Time was centered at the first assessment such that the Level 1 intercept refers to Greeks' achievement in Grade 1

Reported are the unstandardized regression coefficients b for the Level 1 predictors. Significances for b refer to robust standard errors SE correction, the three-level model offers opportunities for studying cross-level effects of classroom characteristics. For example, classroom adversity effects could be studied not only on the initial academic achievement (see Table 2) but also on change in academic achievement (see Motti-Stefanidi et al. 2012a, Table 5).

Multilevel Models of Daily Adaptation

A last important application of multilevel models to research on minority children is the study of changes in daily adaptation over a period of many days (*diary studies*). Nezlek (2012) provides an excellent introduction to diary methods based on multilevel modeling. If the participants report only summary ratings of daily mean levels of adaptation, well-being, or their antecedents and consequences, the data can be analyzed similarly to developmental data, with days at Level 1, individuals at Level 2, and (optionally) context at Level 3. Nevertheless, there are two main specifics of diary data. First, it is often useful to model weekend effects by adding an appropriate contrast as the Level 1 predictor (e.g., Monday through Friday is coded as −1 and Saturday and Sunday is coded as 2.5 such that the sum of all contrast coefficients is zero). The effect of days would then assess long-term trends over the diary period (which are often very small) whereas the contrast would model effects of weekends (which can be large). Similar contrasts can be used to model effects of expected events or interventions that occur during the diary; days before the event could be coded −1, and days including the event and later could be coded 1.

The second specific feature of diary studies is that the assumption of uncorrelated measurements across days is often unrealistic. Instead, lagged influences of the preceding days are often modeled by including lagged variables. For example, the effect of rejection by an outgroup member on next days' aggression against outgroup members can be included as a lagged predictor in addition to the immediate effect of rejection on the same day.

Diary studies are not limited to daily summary reports (*interval sampling* where the interval is one day). If participants report on particular events or situations that may or may not occur during a particular day, or that may occur multiple times per day (*event sampling*, for example stress situations, social interaction situations), these data can also be studied with multilevel models, with situations at Level 1, individuals at Level 2, and (optionally) context at Level 3. In this case, time of day or other characteristics of the situation such as being alone versus dyadic situation versus group situation, or the judged intensity of stress in the situation can be used as Level 1 predictors.

Multilevel Moderation

Two types of moderation can be distinguished in multilevel analysis: within-level moderation and cross-level moderation. Within-level moderation where the effect of a predictor on the outcome is moderated by another predictor is studied exactly as in ordinary regression analysis. Both predictors have to be centered (or standardized), and included in a within-level multiple regression of the outcome on both predictors and their product; the product term assesses the moderation effect (see Table 1, Model 3, where the interaction between immigrant status and parental involvement was studied at Level 1). As in ordinary regression, inclusion of the product term changes the main effects of the predictors such that the main effects should be studied before the product term is added.

Cross-level moderation is any effect of a higher-level predictor on a lower-level predictor (e.g., the classroom adversity effects reported in Table 2, or the effects of individual risks and resources on change in adaptation reported in Tables 3 and 4). Thus, moderation in multilevel analysis is straightforward, and its implementation is not difficult. One can even study the cross-level moderation of a lower-level within-level moderation effect. However, for similar reasons as for moderation of moderation effects, such effects should be considered with great caution because they are in fact three-way interactions that are unreliable unless the sample is very large.

Multilevel Mediation

Multilevel mediation is much more complicated than multilevel moderation because of hidden cross-level effects. For example, it is *not* appropriate to run a mediation analysis at Level 1 of a two-level model by simply computing the mediation effect as in ordinary regression, ignoring the multilevel structure of the data (see Preacher et al. 2010, who present the problems and propose a general solution using multilevel structural equation modeling). The reason is that all Level 1 variables contain Level 2 variation too unless they are *only* measuring differences *within* Level 2 units. For example, the Level 1 immigrant status effect in Table 1 contains also information on effects of between-classroom differences in immigrant status, namely the percentage of immigrants in the classroom which varied widely across classrooms. If one wants to study the mediation of the effect of immigrant status on academic achievement by individual social adversity (all variables are at Level 1), the effects of both the predictor and the mediator vary on both Level 1 and Level 2, and the Level 2 components are included in the Level 1 mediation.

Because the causal effects involved in the Level 2 mediation part and in the Level 1 part can be completely different (in nasty cases they may even cancel each other if they are of equal strength but opposite sign), it is important to distinguish between the "pure" Level 1 part of the mediation and the "pure" Level 2 part of the mediation. Preacher et al. (2010) call them Within effects and Between effects; they are statistically independent by definition. Ordinary applications of multilevel modeling do not distinguish Between effects from Within effects and instead report a single mean estimate that combines the two and thus confounds them. Preacher et al. (2010) show that all possible instances of mediation in two-level models can be decomposed into Within and Between components such that causal interpretation of the effects is improved (within the limits of non-experimental designs).

In a two-level model, 8 different types of mediation are possible; they are labeled by the levels of predictor—mediator—outcome (see Table 5). The case discussed above is a 1-1-1 mediation where all variables involved in the mediation are Level 1 variables. The case of 2-2-2 mediation is unproblematic because all effects are Between effects. The other mediation types involve both Level 1 and Level 2 variables. Because Level 2 variables are silent about Within effects, and part of the mediation is at Level 2, the causal effects are strictly at Level 2 only (see Preacher et al. 2010). Only the 1-1-1 mediation is informative about causal processes at Level 1. These considerations show that it is important to distinguish the level of assessment of a variable from the level of causal processes. Level 1 variables can be involved in processes at both Level 1 and Level 2, Level 2 variables can be involved only in processes at Level 2.

For example, consider the case of a 2-1-1 mediation where the effect of the percentage of immigrants in the classroom on individual academic achievement is mediated by individual social adversity. The 2-1 part is a cross-level

Table 5 Different types of mediation in a two-level model of adaptation in context

Type	Example
1-1-1	Immigrant effect on individual achievement mediated by individual social adversity
1-1-2	Immigrant effect on classroom achievement mediated by individual social adversity
1-2-1	Immigrant effect on individual achievement mediated by neighborhood adversity
1-2-2	Immigrant effect on classroom achievement mediated by neighborhood adversity
2-1-1	% immigrants in class effect on individual achievement mediated by individual social adversity
2-1-2	% immigrants in class effect on individual achievement mediated by individual social adversity
2-2-1	% immigrants in class effect on individual achievement mediated by neighborhood adversity
2-2-2	% immigrants in class effect on classroom achievement mediated by neighborhood adversity

effect, namely the effect of a classroom variable on an individual variable. Only causal processes operating between classrooms can be responsible for this effect; for example, neighborhoods with a higher proportion of immigrants are characterized by higher adversity; consequently, the students in these neighborhoods are also characterized by higher individual adversity on average. This part of the mediation is unproblematic. Now consider the 1-1 part. It is the effect of individual adversity on individual achievement which confounds a Within classroom effect with a Between classroom effect. Only the Between classroom effect is relevant in this case because only the Between classroom effect of the mediator is relevant. Therefore it would be misleading to multiply the 1-1 regression coefficient with the 2-1 regression coefficient as in the case of ordinary mediation. Instead, the Between component of the 1-1 regression coefficient should be multiplied with the 2-1 regression coefficient.

A simple solution would be computing classroom means for the mediator and the outcome and regressing the outcome means on the mediator means. However, if the classroom means are not completely reliable, a more efficient statistical solution is considering the Between component as a latent variable (see Preacher et al. 2010), and this is the point where multilevel structural equation modeling (MSEM) is relevant. The other mediation types are analyzed similarly by considering only the Between effect (see Preacher et al. 2010); MPlus (Muthén and Muthén 1998–2012) scripts for analyzing the most common multilevel mediation models can be found at www.quantpsy.org/medn (retrieved on February 17, 2015).

Multilevel Structural Equation Models (MSEM)

Recent approaches to multilevel mediation use MSEM in order to estimate Between effects as latent variables. Recent advances in MSEM allow for studying two-level structural equation models where the path coefficients at Level 1 vary across the Level 2 units, and paths at Level 2 and cross-level effects are included (such models can be estimated with MPlus; Muthén and Muthén 1998–2012). However, often the research questions do not concern higher-level paths or cross-level effects. In these cases ordinary structural equation models are sufficient for estimating the path coefficients, and the nested structure can be accounted for simply by correcting the standard errors. In MPlus a single line of syntax is sufficient to account for clustering effects. Motti-Stefanidi et al. (2015) used SEM for analyzing cross-lagged effects between teacher-rated school engagement and academic achievement, and Reitz et al. (2014) used SEM for analyzing cross-lagged effects between family functioning, self-efficacy, ethnic identity, and acculturation. When the reported SEM results were compared with SEM results where effects of the clustering in classrooms were corrected, the results were found to be highly similar (note that the correlations and path coefficients are identical in both cases, only the standard errors and thus the significances may vary).

Thinking Clearly About Effects at Multiple Levels

The preceding sections show how multilevel analysis can be applied to answer research questions that concern nested data structures. Application of multilevel analysis is not only required for avoiding biased results but also has an important training effect on one's thinking about psychological mechanisms. Psychologists unfamiliar with multilevel analysis often confuse psychological mechanisms at different levels when they interpret their data. Consider the classic study by Robinson (1950) on reading ability in the USA in 1930. Across all federal states, the mean reading ability in a state correlated 0.53 with the percentage of immigrants in the state, that is, the higher the proportion of immigrants in a state, the better the reading ability in this state. This may seem paradoxical; do immigrants read better than natives? Of course, the opposite was the case; within all states, natives showed a higher reading ability than immigrants. The correlation at the state level resulted from selective immigration; immigrants selected states with better working opportunities for their residence, and the *natives* in these states had a higher reading ability. The seemingly paradoxical result was not paradoxical at all, it was a misinterpretation of the results by confusing the level of states (Level 2) with the level of individuals (Level 1). The 0.53 correlation concerned Level 2 and informs about Between effects; it is silent about correlations at Level 1 that inform about Within effects. Robinson (1950) called this confusion the *ecological fallacy* because the "ecological" correlation involving environmental differences is misinterpreted as a correlation involving interindividual differences.

More common in psychology is the similar confusion between intraindividual and interindividual effects. Consider the classic diary study by Epstein (1983) where the participants reported the intensity of emotions in particular situations. Angriness (the average report of being angry across all situations) and happiness (the average report of being happy across all situations) correlated only slightly negatively because of interindividual differences in the overall tendency to report intense emotions (some "unemotional" participants reported both low angriness and low happiness, some "emotional" participants reported both high angriness and high happiness). In contrast, being angry and being happy correlated strongly negatively across situations *within* persons because situations where one experiences mixed angry-happy emotions are rare. It would be misleading to infer from a correlation at the higher level (sample of participants) the same correlation at the lower level (sample of situations within participants) or vice versa.

The correlations can even have a different sign. For example, Cacioppo et al. (1992) measured students' physiological arousal and facial expressions of fear in multiple situations and reported a positive correlation between students' average frequency of skin conductance responses and the average expression of fear but within most students a negative correlation across situations between skin responses and fear

expression. After correction for attenuation, correlations at the higher level can be expected to be identical with those at the lower level only if the condition of *ergodicity* is met (see Molenaar and Campbell 2009). Ergodicity requires that the intraindividual pattern is the same for all individuals in the sample such that it would suffice to study only one individual (which would then represent the whole population). In psychology, such cases are extremely rare such that ergodicity cannot be assumed. Instead, effects at the intraindividual level have to be clearly distinguished from effects at the interindividual level, and knowledge about multilevel analysis is extremely helpful for making this distinction.

Conclusion

This chapter has shown that multilevel analysis is not only a useful tool for analyzing nested data (individuals in context, individual development, individual development in context) but is also helpful to avoid the misinterpretation of interindividual correlations in terms of intraindividual processes or intraindividual correlations in terms of interindividual effects. Within-level effects including moderations, cross-level effects (cross-level moderations), various types of multilevel mediations, and multilevel structural equation models can be studied although it should be kept in mind that multilevel analysis is unnecessary if higher-level and cross-level effects are not interesting; in these cases, correction for clustering effects is sufficient.

Appendix: Statistical Software for Multilevel Analysis

Numerous software packages can be used for standard multilevel analysis. First, standard statistical software such as R, SAS, or SPSS contains packages or procedures for multilevel analyses (the R package lme4; the SAS procedure PROC MIXED; and the SPSS procedure MIXED). Although this is convenient for experienced users of this software, I recommend to beginners the specialized software HLM (current version HLM 7; Raudenbush et al. 2011) because of its intuitive graphical interface that helps to build more complex models and to avoid confusion of levels. A free student version is available that is only limited in terms of the maximum number of units and effects at different levels. A drawback of all these alternatives is that multilevel mediation using MSEM, and MSEM in general, cannot be done. The software MPlus (Muthén and Muthén 1998–2012) deals with both standard multilevel analysis and MSEM, and many MPlus scripts are available for more advanced models including multilevel mediation (see e.g. www.quantpsy.org/medn, retrieved on February 17, 2015).

I recommend to methodologically more advanced researchers to begin with running a few standard models with HLM, apply MPlus to the same models until the results are consistent, and then continue with MPlus (note that the results may show minor differences due to different estimation procedures and significance tests). HLM requires that special data files are prepared before the analyses can be done, and if not all variables are included, these data files have to be prepared once more. MPlus is more flexible in computing additional variables not included in the original data set (e.g., standardized variables or interaction terms for within-level moderation analyses), and allows for using auxiliary variables for the imputation of missing values.

References

Asendorpf, J. B., van de Schoot, R., Denissen, J. J. A., & Hutteman, R. (2014). Reducing bias due to systematic attrition in longitudinal studies: The benefits of multiple imputation. *International Journal of Behavioral Development, 38*, 453–460.

Bronfenbrenner, U. (1977). Toward an experimental ecology of human development. *American Psychologist, 32*, 513–531.

Cacioppo, J. T., Uchino, B. N., Crites, S. L., Snydersmith, M. A., Smith, G., Berntson, G. G., et al. (1992). Relationship between facial expressiveness and sympathetic activation in emotion. *Journal of Personality and Social Psychology, 62*, 110–128.

Epstein, S. (1983). A research paradigm for the study of personality and emotions. In M. M. Page (Ed.), *Personality: Current theory and research. 1982 Nebraska Symposium on Motivation* (pp. 91–154). Lincoln, NE: University of Nebraska Press.

Hox, J. J. (2010). *Multilevel analysis: Technique and applications* (2nd ed.). New York, NY: Routledge.

Little, R. J. A. (1995). Modeling the drop-out mechanism in repeated measures studies. *Journal of the American Statistical Association, 90*, 1112–1121.

Motti-Stefanidi, F., Asendorpf, J. B., & Masten, A. (2012a). The adaptation and well-being of adolescent immigrants in Greek schools: A multilevel, longitudinal study of risks and resources. *Development and Psychopathology, 24*, 451–473.

Motti-Stefanidi, F., Berry, J., Chryssochoou, X., Sam, D. L., & Phinney, J. (2012b). Immigrant youth adaptation in context: Developmental, acculturation, and social-psychological perspectives. In A. S. Masten, K. Liebkind, & D. J. Hernandez (Eds.), *Realizing the potential of immigrant youth* (pp. 117–158). New York, NY: Cambridge University Press.

Motti-Stefanidi, F., Masten, A. S., & Asendorpf, J. B. (2015). School engagement trajectories of immigrant youth: Risks and longitudinal interplay with academic success. *International Journal of Behavioral Development, 39*, 32–42.

Molenaar, P. C. M., & Campbell, C. G. (2009). The new person-specific paradigm in psychology. *Current Directions in Psychological Science, 18*, 112–117.

Muthén, L. K., & Muthén, B. O. (1998–2012). *Mplus version 7* [Computer program]. Los Angeles, CA: Author.

Nezlek, J. B. (2012). *Diary methods for social and personality psychology*. Thousand Oaks, CA: Sage.

Preacher, K. J., Zyphur, M. J., & Zhang, Z. (2010). A general multilevel SEM framework for assessing multilevel mediation. *Psychological Methods, 15*, 209–233.

Raudenbush, S. W., & Bryk, A. S. (2002). *Hierarchical linear models* (2nd ed.). Thousand Oaks, CA: Sage.

Raudenbush, S. W., Bryk, A. S., Cheong, Y. F., & Congdon, R. T., Jr. (2011). *HLM for windows (version 7.0)*. Lincolnwood, IL: Scientific Software International.

Reitz, A. K., Motti-Stefanidi, F., & Asendorpf, J. B. (2014). Mastering developmental transitions in immigrant adolescents: The longitudinal interplay of family functioning, developmental and acculturative tasks. *Developmental Psychology, 50*, 754–765.

Robinson, W. S. (1950). Ecological correlations and the behavior of individuals. *American Sociological Review, 15*, 351–357.

Equivalence in Research on Positive Development of Minority Children: Methodological Approaches

Fons J.R. van de Vijver and Jia He

Abstract

We describe methodological challenges in studies of positive development of minority youth. A framework is described that captures the main validity threats in this type of research. The framework involves different types of bias (referring to sources of systematic error in studies of minority youth). If there is bias in a study, the comparability of constructs or scores across minority groups can be challenged. Many procedures have been proposed in the literature to deal with such methodological problems, which affect either the design or the analysis of a study. We review such procedures and pay special attention to two topics that attract much attention in recent studies: response styles and mixed methods. It is concluded that sound methods can help to make study results more robust and replicable.

Researchers studying positive development of minority children face many conceptual and methodological challenges (e.g., Motti-Stefanidi 2014; Spencer 1990). We argue that the combination of a culturally sensitive approach and rigorous research methods is crucial in advancing this research field. Various methodological problems in research on positive development of minority children can be addressed by a careful design and analysis of studies, building on the extensive experience from cross-cultural and developmental psychological studies of the last decades. This chapter focuses on the methodological challenges of comparability and validity in data obtained in different immigrant groups. We first define and review bias and equivalence in cross-cultural research as a theoretical framework to address the comparability and validity issues; we then describe how to deal with bias and equivalence issues, based on empirical examples; we end the chapter with an overview of domains of current research interest and rapid development, and a description of possible future directions.

F.J.R. van de Vijver (✉) · J. He
Department of Culture Studies, Tilburg University,
P.O. Box 90153, 5000 LE Tilburg, The Netherlands
e-mail: fons.vandevijver@tilburguniversity.edu

J. He
e-mail: jamis.he@gmail.com

F.J.R. van de Vijver
North-West University, Potchefstroom, South Africa

F.J.R. van de Vijver
University of Queensland, St. Lucia, Australia

© The Editor(s) 2017
N.J. Cabrera and B. Leyendecker (eds.), *Handbook on Positive Development of Minority Children and Youth*, DOI 10.1007/978-3-319-43645-6_4

Historical Overview and Theoretical Perspectives

The research on minority children inevitably concerns the appropriateness of measurement and/or the comparability of one minority group to another or to the majority group. According to Poortinga (1995), studies with a cross-cultural comparative nature in the 1940s based their findings on two assumptions: firstly, existing, notably Western, conceptualizations of psychological constructs in one culture are applicable to other cultures; secondly, cultural contexts do not affect the processes and outcomes of an assessment. The second assumption was challenged in the 1960s, and since then culturally sensitive tests were promoted. In the 1980s, the pervasive influences of culture on comparative studies could no longer be ignored, therefore various approaches to adapt tests and sophisticated psychometric analysis tools have been developed (e.g., Cronbach and Drenth 1972; Poortinga and Van de Vijver 1987).

Van de Vijver and Leung (1997) put forward a systematic classification of bias and equivalence, which provides the framework to address methodological issues of cross-cultural studies. *Bias* occurs when score differences on the indicators of a particular construct do not correspond to differences in the underlying trait or ability. It refers to systematic errors in data that are expected to be found again were the study to be repeated and that have an impact on the adequacy of the measure for assessing the purported underlying construct or the average scores of at least of one of the cultures studied. *Equivalence* refers to the implications of bias on test score comparability. It is an indicator of the measurement level at which scores obtained in different cultural groups can be compared.

A Taxonomy of Bias

Three types of bias, namely construct, method, and item bias, are distinguished based on the source of invalidity (Van de Vijver 2015; Van de Vijver and Leung 1997; Van de Vijver and Tanzer 2004). *Construct bias* occurs when the construct measured is not identical across cultures, either because the concept or because the elements taken to comprise its measure (e.g., attitudes, behaviors, or cognitions) are not comparable (Van de Vijver and Poortinga 1997). For instance, resilience is defined by Ungar (2008) as the capacity of individuals to navigate their way to health-enhancing resources and the capacity of individuals' physical and social ecologies. The definition may well be universally applicable; yet, its manifestations may vary across cultures. With minority children, resilience can manifest itself in different ways. Drop-out is generally recognized as a negative school outcome and an important indicator of poor resilience (e.g., Masten and Coatsworth 1998); however, dropout was found to be a positive indicator of resilience in a group of African Canadian students to establish dignity, personal efficacy, and independence (Dei et al. 1997). A discussion of the pros and cons of both operationalizations is beyond the scope of this chapter. However, the example illustrates that assessing resilience requires researchers to have a good knowledge of the cultural contexts of their studies and to take culture-specific aspects into consideration (e.g., Masten and Motti-Stefanidi 2009).

Another example of construct bias comes from acculturation research. Before describing findings in the acculturation domain, a caveat on terminology is needed. The literature on positive youth development uses the concept of acculturation in two quite distinct meanings. In the first, acculturation is the same as adjustment; well acculturated children refer then to immigrant children who are well adjusted to their new cultural context (e.g., Riggs 2006). The second meaning, adopted here, is broader and views acculturation as orientations towards both the ethnic and mainstream culture (e.g., Neblett et al. 2012). In the psychological acculturation literature the latter view has become dominant (e.g., Sam and Berry 2006), whereas the former view is common in acculturation literature in sociology (Sakamoto et al. 2009) and public health (Lara et al. 2005). The field of positive youth development would gain in clarity if authors were more explicit about the view on acculturation that they espouse.

It can be argued that these conventional models, notably the view of equating acculturation with adjustment, are increasingly at odds with how acculturation takes place these days. In many contexts youth does not deal with two but with three or even more cultures. An example is "3D-acculturation" which describes how Jamaican immigrants to the US simultaneously negotiate the Jamaican, European American mainstream, and African American cultures (Ferguson et al. 2012). Another example is superdiversity, which refers to neighborhoods where people from many different ethnicities live together (Vertovec 2007); in these neighborhoods acculturation (and identity) processes can no longer be captured in a simple mainstream—immigrant dichotomy but involve multiple allegiances, which can even include cosmopolitanism (as a pan-human identity) (Van de Vijver et al. 2015).

According to Snauwaert et al. (2003), the often employed classification in acculturation orientations (i.e., integration, assimilation, separation, and marginalization; Berry 1997) cannot be taken to refer to immigrant preferences that are the same across all life domains. These authors studied immigrants in Belgium. If acculturation was measured in a contact domain (i.e., perceived desirability of having contacts with both mainstreamers in the country of settlement and immigrants from the same country of origin), integration was preferred; most immigrants find it desirable to have contacts with both groups, which in the conceptual model is taken as evidence in favor of integration. However, if identification with the mainstream and ethnic culture was assessed, Snauwaert and colleagues found support for separation, as identification with the ethnic culture was much stronger than identification with the mainstream culture. These findings are in line with results obtained by Arends-Tóth and Van de Vijver (2003), who found that Turkish-Dutch prefer separation in the private domain and integration in the public domain. These studies suggest that acculturation

orientations vary with personal involvement of the domain and that domains with a strong personal involvement (such as identification and religion) are most resistant to acculturative change. As a consequence, there is no such thing as *the* acculturation orientation of an immigrant or an immigrant group. The common conceptualization of acculturation orientations refers to a domain-independent construct and does not refer to any domain, where such domain dependence may be part and parcel of the construct.

Method bias is a generic term for all forms of systematic errors occurring during the process of assessment. It can derive from sampling, structural features of the instrument, or administration processes. *Sample bias* results from incomparability of samples. Cross-cultural variations in sample characteristics can be related to target measures; confounding sample differences could lead to observed score differences in the target measures that do not involve valid cross-cultural differences. A typical case in point is the confounding of educational quality with IQ in cross-cultural comparisons of IQ scores obtained in very different cultural contexts. A meta-analysis revealed that national expenditure on education, which can be taken as a proxy for educational quality, was a predictor of cross-national differences in scores on the Raven's Progressive Matrices (Brouwers et al. 2009).

Instrument bias refers to incomparability arising from instrument characteristics. In comparing the cognitive performances of children from black and white groups in South Africa, Malda et al. (2010) found that children from both groups performed better when the version of the test was designed for their own group, which illustrates how differences in stimulus familiarity, due to cultural differences, can affect cross-cultural comparisons. Another source of instrument bias is response styles, the systematic tendency to use certain answer anchors on some basis other than the target construct (Cronbach 1950). Okanda and Itakura (2010) reported that 3-year-old Japanese children tended to inappropriately say "yes" to yes–no questions, although they knew the answers to the questions. Comparing different ethnic groups in the Netherlands, He and Van de Vijver (2013) found that Nonwestern immigrants tend to use response moderation strategies such as acquiescent and midpoint responding more than Western immigrants and Dutch mainstreamers.

Administration bias can result from different administration conditions (e.g., paper-and-pencil versus online survey, individual versus group administration), unclear instructions, and communication between test administrator and respondents, such as halo effects. For example, African preschoolers showed higher test scores on the Peabody Picture Vocabulary Test-R when tested by African American field staff than by white field staff (Doucette-Gates et al. 1998).

Item bias, also known as Differential Item Functioning (DIF), means that an item has a different psychological meaning in the cultures studied. Technically, an item is biased if persons with the same trait or ability, but coming from different cultures, are not equally likely to endorse the item (Van de Vijver and Leung 1997). There are multiple sources of item bias, both linguistic (e.g., poor translation, language features) and cultural (e.g., inapplicability of item contents in different cultures, and items with ambiguous connotations). If item bias is observed, it is important to identify explanations for it (e.g., poor translation or inapplicability of an item in a certain context) (Leung and Van de Vijver 2008). In their study of interethnic attitudes of German mainstream children and Turkish children in Germany, Feddes, Noack, and Rutland (2009) administered a four-item scale, asking how many out-group children were friendly, polite, smart, and bad. For Turkish children, the item "bad" showed DIF, as it caused a lower reliability in the Turkish group. The authors speculated that this might be due to children's willingness to attribute less positive traits to one group, but not necessarily also attribute more negative traits to this group. Thus, this item was dropped in their further analysis.

A Taxonomy of Equivalence

Equivalence reflects the level of comparability across cultures. Three levels of equivalence are identified (Van de Vijver and Leung 1997). Whereas bias refers to sources of systematic distortions in cross-cultural comparisons that challenge their validity, equivalence deals with the implications of bias for the comparability of constructs and scores. *Construct equivalence* means that the same theoretical construct is measured in each culture studied. Construct equivalence is a prerequisite for any cross-cultural comparison in any study; without it, no cross-cultural comparison involving the construct would be valid. It is an important first step in the statistical analysis of cross-cultural data to explore the structure of the construct and the adequacy of sampled items. When a construct does not have the same meaning across the cultures, researchers need to acknowledge the incompleteness of conceptualization and can still compare the equivalent facets of the construct (i.e., partial invariance; Byrne et al. 1989). The current Zeitgeist appears to emphasize identity of constructs across cultures. In such a climate the lack of construct equivalence can easily be construed as a reflection of inadequacy of design, sampling, or data administration. This is regrettable as the observation of construct non-equivalence can point to important cross-cultural differences.

Measurement unit equivalence (or *metric equivalence*) indicates that measures of interval or ratio level have the same measurement unit (metric) across cultural contexts, but they have different scale origins. When measures show metric equivalence, scores can be compared within cultural groups (e.g., gender differences can be tested in each group), but scores cannot be compared across groups (means of females in one group cannot be compared to means of females in another group).

Full score equivalence (or *scalar equivalence*) represents the highest level of equivalence, which means that scales in all groups studied have the same measurement unit and origin. Observed scores are then free from any type of bias and can be compared directly within and across cultures. When measures show full score equivalence, analyses of variance and *t* tests to examine cross-cultural differences in means are appropriate for (and only for) this level of equivalence.

Equivalence as a Characteristic of a Cross-Cultural Comparison

Equivalence cannot be assumed, but should be empirically demonstrated (Van de Vijver and Poortinga 1997). Consequently, before means are compared across cultures, the first research question to address in minority children studies should be whether there is equivalence, which is the basis for any meaningful and valid conclusion to be drawn (e.g., Benson et al. 2009; Bodkin-Andrewsa et al. 2010; Buhs et al. 2010). Such an analysis should be routinely conducted in any cross-cultural comparison as a first check, in the same way as internal consistency is reported.

So, cross-cultural studies of immigrant youth should report equivalence and internal consistency. Internal consistency is not an intrinsic characteristic of an instrument, but a characteristic of scores obtained with an instrument in a specific study. The same holds for equivalence. Conclusions about equivalence are based on analyses of data obtained in specific samples. Studies of minority youth are often based on non-probability sampling; as a consequence, generalizability of conclusions about equivalence may be limited. Like internal consistency, equivalence has to be examined and demonstrated in each study.

Research Measurement and Methodology

It requires careful design, implementation, and statistical analysis to ensure equivalence (e.g., Cheung and Rensvold 2002; Van de Vijver and Tanzer 2004). We propose to integrate the strategies at different stages of a study, focusing on best practices in the design and implementation stage and on statistical measures that can empirically test equivalence in the analysis stage.

Design and Implementation Strategies

Choice of Instrument

In the conceptualization and design stage of a study involving minority children, a decision has to be made as to whether an existing instrument will be used or whether a new instrument is to be developed. The choice should depend on more than the availability of an existing instrument. Available instruments have the advantage that they often have been tried and tested, usually in Western groups. Notably when such instruments have shown robust psychometric properties, there may be an expectation that similar characteristics will be found in other cultural groups, although obviously, such characteristics have to be shown. However, it is not a foregone conclusion that instruments applied in their original form can transcend language and culture differences in a new context (e.g., Peña 2007). A major weakness of most existing instruments is that they have not been developed with a cross-cultural target group in mind. Therefore, even if their psychometric properties are favorable, their cultural adequacy may be problematic. It is often all too easily assumed that the instrument may work well and that equivalence analyses can be used to identify possible problems. The development of minority children can be easily construed as "deviant" if majority-based norms are used as starting point (Spencer 1990). Therefore, we argue that the choice of an instrument in studies on minority children and youth should be approached from a broader perspective, balancing substantive and psychometric concentrations.

We argue that three options are available in instrument choice: adoption, adaptation, and assembly (Van de Vijver and Leung 1997). *Adoption* involves the use of the original of a measure (and applying a close translation of an instrument if needed) in another cultural group or context. The main advantages are that the process is simple to implement and it makes a direct comparison of scores possible (assuming that equivalence can be demonstrated); yet, adoption can only be used when the items in the source and target language versions adequately cover the construct measured and the response formats are appropriate in the new contexts (Harkness 2003). *Adaptation* is a combination of a close translation of certain stimuli and modification of other stimuli; an adaptation is preferred when adoption of all stimuli is inadequate for linguistic, cultural, or psychometric reasons. Nowadays, adaptation has become more and more frequently used and the term is often used as the de facto standard in working with tests in multiple contexts. The change of word signifies the change of emphasis in the process of working with multiple language versions. There is a change from a linguistic to a multidisciplinary perspective in which in addition to language, cultural information and psychological knowledge about the target constructs are viewed as essential in preparing stimulus materials for a new cultural context. *Assembly* refers to the compilation of a new measure; it is indicated when neither adoption nor adaptation would be adequate. Assembly can maximize the cultural appropriateness of an instrument, but it renders numerical comparisons of scores across cultures impossible.

The choice for any of the three options should depend on the target cultures and research aims. Adoption is favored if the goal is to compare scores across-cultures directly, whereas adaptation and assembly are better to enhance the suitability of the instrument for the context in which it will be administered. It is important to note that there is no intrinsically superior option; adoption, adaptation, or assembly can be the best choice, given the balance required between psychometric and cultural considerations.

Adoption has long been viewed as the default choice in cross-cultural research; it is often the "quick-and-dirty" choice that combines relatively little effort to create an instrument for a new group with high levels of comparability. However, adopting an existing instrument may conceal interesting cross-cultural differences that are not covered by the items of an existing instrument. When adopting an existing instrument, the question is implicitly or explicitly asked whether this instrument, developed for another group, is adequate in the new group. However, the culturally more appropriate question would be: Is the existing instrument the best possible to measure the target construct in the new cultural group? There is a subtle, yet important difference in perspective between these two questions: in the first perspective one culture is taken as frame of reference whereas in the second perspective there is a balance between the perspectives.

Pretests and Standardization of Procedures

It is recommended to carry out pilot studies and cognitive interviews before the field work (Willis 2005), because they can provide information about the adequacy of the instrument in a specific cultural context, reveal possible design problems, and serve to reduce the likelihood of systematic measurement bias. Pilot studies are particularly important when measures are to be assembled from scratch or transported to locations with a large geographic and cultural distance from the culture in which the original instrument was developed. For example, cognitive interviewing elicits respondents' opinions on the response process, which serves as an effective tool to detect possible bias (e.g., Friborg et al. 2006). The target population should be involved at an early stage for consultation to have assessment of high levels of acceptability and meaningfulness for ethnic minority children (Leff et al. 2006).

When implementing the study, all field workers should abide by a standard protocol, which may include a standardized training for all interviewers. Additional elements aimed to reduce bias, notably method bias, involve the specification of suitable administration conditions (e.g., individual assessment or group assessment) and administration modes (e.g., face-to-face interview, telephone interview, paper-and-pencil survey or online survey) and monitoring the interaction of interviewers and interviewees (in case of halo effects). Other measures such as clear instruction and examples, detailed field work documentation, assessment of response styles, and test-retest comparisons may also contribute to the minimization of biases (Van de Vijver and Tanzer 2004).

Statistical Strategies

After administration, various analytic approaches to detect bias and ensure equivalence in collected data can be applied. In this section, we illustrate the utilization of factor analysis at the scale level and Differential Item Functioning analysis (DIF) at the item level.

Factor Analysis

Both Exploratory Factor Analysis (EFA) and Confirmatory Factor Analysis (CFA) can be used to examine construct bias, whereas it is the advantage of CFA that it can also detect item bias (Vandenberg and Lance 2000). When the underlying structure of a construct is unclear, EFA is preferred in investigating and comparing factor structures. The use of EFA (and various other dimensionality-reducing techniques) to study equivalence is based on a simple reasoning: identical constructs are measured in all groups if the structure of an instrument, as analyzed with these techniques, is the same across cultures. So, identity of factors (or dimensions) is taken as sufficient evidence for equivalence. Comparisons of multiple cultures can be conducted either in a pairwise or in a one-to-all manner (in the latter case each culture is compared with the combined solution; Van de Vijver and Poortinga 2002). Target rotations are employed to compare the structure across cultures and to evaluate factor congruence, often by means of the computation of Tucker's phi coefficient, which tests to what extent factors are identical across cultures. Values of the coefficient above 0.90 are usually considered to be adequate and above 0.95 to be excellent (Van de Vijver and Leung 1997). Yağmur and Van de Vijver (2012) compared self-report acculturation and language orientations of Turkish immigrants in four host countries, and the structural equivalence of all the scales were established by

pairwise target comparisons of factor solutions of each scale in the four countries. Such a procedure ensures comparability across Turkish immigrants across host countries.

CFA, as one application of structural equation modeling procedures, is often employed when the structure of the construct can be derived from theory or previous work. An acceptable fit from the CFA indicates that the hypothesized factor structure can be accepted, and there is evidence for equivalence. CFA can test hierarchical models based on information of covariance matrix. For example, if we set to examine whether the same one-factor model holds in various cultures, a series of nested models are usually tested (Cheung and Rensvold 2002). The *configural invariance model* specifies that the same latent construct with the same indicators are assumed. In the *measurement weights model*, factor loadings on the latent variable are constrained to be equal across cultures. If a multigroup confirmatory factor analysis yields a satisfactory fit, the construct under investigation can be said to have construct equivalence. In the *intercept invariance model*, items are constrained to have the same intercept across cultures. A satisfactory fit of the intercept invariance model provides evidence that there is no item bias. Various additional types of invariance have been proposed; for example, in a *structural covariance model* the covariances of latent factors are identical across groups; a *structural residual model* refers to identity of the error component of the latent variable; a *measurement residuals model* specifies the identity of error component of the items. Although it is quite clear that factor loading and intercept invariance are the most important aspects, there is no agreement in the literature about the importance of the other types of invariance. When full invariance cannot be reached, it is also possible to resort to partial invariance by removing the constraints of equal factor loadings and/or intercepts in non-invariant items (Byrne 2001; Byrne and Van de Vijver 2010).

Model fit in CFA is usually evaluated by χ^2 tests, their significance, and tests of the change in χ^2 values between different models of invariance. Additional and frequently used indices include the Tucker Lewis Index (TLI; acceptable above

0.90 and excellent above 0.95), Root Mean Square Error of Approximation (RMSEA; acceptable below 0.06 and excellent below 0.04), and Comparative Fit Index (CFI; acceptable above 0.90 and excellent above 0.95). Whether or not a more restricted model is acceptable can be established by the change of Comparative Fit Index; changes of values within 0.01 from the less restricted to the more restricted model usually suggest acceptable fit of the latter (Byrne 2001; Van de Vijver and Poortinga 1997).

The technique, combined with other strategies, has been used in research on positive development of minority children, and proven to prolific. Michaels, Barr, Roosa, and Knight (2007) used multigroup CFA to check the equivalence of the five domains of self-esteem among Anglo, Mexican, Africa and Native American youths aged 9–14 years of low-income, inner-city school district in a large metropolitan area in the southwestern United States. Scalar equivalence was reached for the global self-worth and scholastic competence domain, whereas other domains only showed scalar equivalence in some of those groups, indicating that these domains were only meaningful to certain ethnic groups or that items might not adequately represent the construct in all groups. White, Umaña-Taylor, Knight, and Zeiders (2011) investigated the cross-language measurement equivalence of three components of ethnic identity (i.e., exploration, resolution, and affirmation) among Mexican American early adolescents. They reported scalar equivalence of measures of exploration and resolution across language versions and compared full and partial invariance models to draw conclusions on overall comparability. Researchers are encouraged to use these statistic tools to demonstrate comparability of data before making inferences on cultural differences and similarities.

DIF Analysis

DIF (item bias) analysis targets the identification of anomalous items. DIF refers to the problems caused by the differing probabilities of correctly solving or endorsing an item after matching on the underlying ability that the item is intended to measure in different cultures (Zumbo 2007).

With some exceptions, DIF analysis is applicable only to one-dimensional constructs; therefore for multidimensional constructs, DIF analysis should be performed per dimension. There are many models and procedures one can follow to detect uniform and non-uniform item bias, including ANOVA, logistic regression, item response theory, and the Mantel-Haenszel method. Computer programs to conduct tehse procedures to study DIF are widely available; examples are logistic regression using SPSS (Zumbo 1999) and Mantel-Haenszel using EASY-DIF (Gonzalez et al. 2011).

Applications of DIF analyses in the literature on positive youth development tend to be part of invariance testing procedures using structural equation modeling where invariance of intercepts (taken as absence of item bias) is tested. A first example comes from a study on invariance in development (Bowers et al. 2010). Using a longitudinal design, these authors tested whether the structure of measures gauging the Five Cs (i.e., Competence, Confidence, Connection, Character, and Caring; see Lerner this volume) of Positive Youth Development were the same among 920 youth across grades 8, 9, and 10. They found evidence for scalar invariance of the measures across these grades, suggesting that their measure can be used to assess the Five Cs in a comparable manner in this age range. A second example is due to Shek and Ma (2010), who tested the gender invariance of the structure of the Chinese Positive Youth Development Scale in a large sample of lower-secondary school students attending a positive youth development program in Hong Kong. They found evidence of scalar invariance of the 15 basic dimensions of this scale and four higher-order factors (i.e., cognitive-behavioral competencies, prosocial attributes, positive identity and general positive youth development qualities).

Focus Areas of Development

In this section we review specific topics in cross-cultural research methods that are relevant for the study of positive youth development. Each area has the potential to lead to more insights in this development. We discuss (a) response styles and (b) mixed methods. For an overview of recent developments in multilevel modeling, another rapidly evolving field that is relevant for positive youth development, we refer to Asendorpf's chapter in this volume.

Response Styles

Self-reports using a Likert-type response format continue to be important in the study of youth development. It has been argued repeatedly that their advantages (easy to administer and analyze) are offset by their shortcomings, notably their susceptibility to impression management (Paulhus 1986) and common method variance (Podsakoff et al. 2003). Four response styles have been frequently studied: Acquiescent Response Style (tendency to agree irrespective of item content), Midpoint Response Style (tendency to choose the midpoint or scores around the midpoint of the response scale), Extremity Response Style (tendency to choose the extremes of response scales), and Social Desirability (tendency to choose responses that are in line with perceived norms about what is appropriate in a culture) (e.g., Van Vaerenbergh and Thomas 2013). In one of the few studies that used a measure of response styles (more specifically, social desirability), Papacharisis et al. (2005) evaluated the effectiveness of a life skills program, that was administered to adolescent volleyball and soccer players during their regular practice hours. The trained life skills were goal setting, problem solving, and positive thinking. The authors found that a social desirability scale did not show correlations with questionnaire items, such as items about self-beliefs. The authors concluded that it was very unlikely that social desirability would have any influence on their findings. Gilman et al. (2008) administered the Multidimensional Students' Life Satisfaction Scale to 1338 youth adolescents from Ireland, the US, China, and South Korea. In line with literature on the strong response modesty of East

Asians, the authors found that American and Irish adolescents reported more extremity and acquiescence than Chinese and South Koreans did.

In an attempt to integrate response styles, He and Van de Vijver (2013) found in studies of adults from different ethnic groups in the Netherlands that all styles merge in a single factor; this General Response Style factor has Social Desirability and Extremity Response Style as positive indicators and Acquiescent and Midpoint response Style as negative indicators. At the individual level, the General Response Style is related to all Big Five personality traits and several values (such as embeddedness). At country level, the factor is negatively related to countries' socioeconomic development (with less affluent countries showing higher scores on Social Desirability and Extremity Response Style). The existence of more restrictive norms in less developed countries which emphasize conformity and promote amplified self-expression may underlie these higher scores (He et al. 2014). The General Response Style was even found in a large cross-cultural study that used the Occupational Personality Questionnaire (OPQ32), a forced-choice format personality measure designed to be less affected by response styles than regular personality measures.

Taken together, the evidence suggests that response styles are better viewed as communication styles (amplifying versus moderating of responses), internalized as part of the socialization process (Smith 2004), than as deliberate errors or distortions. Much old research into response styles was based on the idea that these styles should be eliminated, notably the influence of social desirability was to be eliminated (Nederhof 1985). However, there is increasing evidence that validity is not increased by correcting for response styles. Ones et al. (1996) demonstrated that job performance is not better predicted after "peeling off" response styles from applicants' self-reports; in the same vein, He and Van de Vijver (2015) found that statistical corrections for the response style did not affect the size or patterning of cross-cultural differences in teacher reports. These findings suggest that we may need to reconceptualize and refine our views on response styles.

Most studies of response styles involved adults; therefore, extending these findings to positive youth development awaits confirmation. Still, the picture that emerges is rather clear. Response styles are real, replicable, and can explain sizeable amounts of variance in cross-cultural studies (we found examples of more than 20 %; He et al. 2014); yet, individual differences in response styles explain considerably more variance than cross-cultural differences do. However, statistical corrections may create a false sense of security as these may not increase the validity and typically cannot statistically "explain away" cross-cultural differences.

Mixed Methods

Scientific progress can be stifled by persistent controversies. The best best-known example in the field of cross-cultural methods is the emic-etic distinction (Pike 1967). The emic perspective is associated with the qualitative approach (understanding a culture from within), whereas the etic perspective is associated with the quantitative approach (comparing samples from different cultural groups). The two camps have long been at loggerheads. Yet, there is good reason for trying to integrate qualitative and quantitative procedures more (Van de Vijver 2015); the strengths and weaknesses of both procedures are complementary, so that they do not only have their own methods but also their own research questions. The richness of qualitative research, with its emphasis on an open approach to reality, has its main strength in exploring new constructs and cultures. The main strength of quantitative procedures is their rigor and allowance to test specific hypotheses. So, qualitative procedures are best in the context of discovery, whereas quantitative procedures are best in the context of justification (Reichenbach 1938).

In the last decades we have witnessed the emergence of so-called mixed methods that combine qualitative and quantitative methods (Tashakkori and Teddlie 2010). The most frequent combination is a study in which in a first phase qualitative methods are used (in cross-cultural studies this is often used to examine the context), followed by a quantitative stage in which a survey is conducted. However, other combinations are possible, such as a quantitative study with a qualitative follow-up (the procedure is described by Onwuegbuzie and Leech 2004). The statistical procedure will yield outliers, which would be adolescents with exceptionally low or high resilience scores, given their parenting style scores. Follow-up interviews with these adolescents are then conducted to identify which factors could have contributed to their extreme scores.

An important and not yet fully developed methodological component of mixed-methods is triangulation (Denzin 2012), which amounts to the question of how the qualitative and quantitative evidence can be combined. If two types of evidence provide convergent information, triangulation is straightforward. As an example, Van de Vijver et al. (2015; see also Blommaert 2013) were interested in the identity of immigrants in a superdiverse area in Oud-Berchem, a suburb of Antwerp, Belgium. Superdiversity refers to the presence of many ethnic groups in a single neighborhood, thereby creating their own mixtures, dynamics, and relationships. The common distinction between ethnic and mainstream culture does not suffice to describe the cultural richness and complexities of such neighborhoods. Using an ethnographic approach, these authors found a rather strong cohesion in the area despite its huge ethnic diversity. This qualitative leg of the study led to the expectation that the immigrant inhabitants would show rather strong Belgian, ethnic, and cosmopolitan identities, which was confirmed in a quantitative survey. The convergence of the qualitative and quantitative results made the results easy to interpret. Suppose now that Belgian and cosmopolitan identity scores would have been low. Triangulation of results could then become problematic unless a clear interpretation of the low scores could be given (e.g., poor measurement or complete lack of coherence in the neighborhood).

Mixed-methods applications in the field of positive youth development have been reported. For example, Henderson et al. (2005) were interested in the influence of organized camp programs on growth and development of youth in the US. They derived quantitative (pre-post surveys) and qualitative evidence (observations) from a total of six camps. The data included pre- and post-questionnaires given to campers (youth) to measure domains, such as positive identity, social skills, positive values, and thinking and physical skills. The qualitative part focused more on camp characteristics and included observations on the structure and delivery of the program. There was some convergence of the main findings of both approaches: the camps that showed significant pre-post differences had also the programs that yielded more favorable qualitative data. Yet, at a more detailed level, it was difficult to link qualitative data about the camps to (quantitative) changes in youth. The latter is a common problem in triangulating quantitative and qualitative data: both types of data often address somewhat different issues (such as a more contextual, qualitative analysis and a more individual-oriented quantitative approach).

A second example uses a very different and common type of triangulation: qualitative evidence is converted to quantitative evidence (or the other way around) so that triangulation takes place within a single data mode. This is easier than cross-mode triangulation. For example, if qualitative data are quantified, regular statistical approaches can be employed to analyze convergence with the other, quantitative data. In a study designed to explore links between perceived family support, acculturation, and life satisfaction, Edwards and Lopez (2006) studied Mexican American adolescents. Qualitative data came from a thematic analysis of open-ended responses to a question about life satisfaction; notably if existing instruments may fail to cover all relevant aspects in a certain group, such an open approach has important advantages. The other constructs were assessed using quantitative instruments. The quantified life satisfaction data were then used as dependent variables in a regression analysis, with perceived support from family and Mexican and Anglo acculturation orientations as predictors. As expected, both independent variables were significant predictors of life satisfaction.

Future Directions

Positive development of minority children is an emerging field; its potential to further promote children's welfare is remarkable, as it has been repeatedly demonstrated that protective factors are at least as important than risk factors in child development (e.g., Motti-Stefanidi et al. 2012). Compared to decades ago, an impressive number of studies have been conducted and we have gained valuable experience informing us what (not) to do in these studies. We argued in this chapter that the quality of research on minority children could be improved by paying more attention to methodological issues. Adequately designed, conducted, and analyzed studies are often easier to interpret, have to deal with fewer alternative score interpretations, and are more insightful as they deal with cultural factors more adequately. If we use the tools and experience reviewed in this chapter, the future of positive development studies on minority children is bright and we can expect to considerably enlarge our insights in the cross-cultural differences and similarities of child development.

References

Arends-Tóth, J. V., & Van de Vijver, F. J. R. (2003). Multiculturalism and acculturation: Views of Dutch and Turkish-Dutch. *European Journal of Social Psychology, 33*, 249–266. doi:10.1002/ejsp.143

Benson, N., Oakland, T., & Shermis, M. (2009). Cross-national invariance of children's temperament. *Journal of Psychoeducational Assessment, 27*, 3–16. doi:10.1177/0734282908318563

Berry, J. W. (1997). Immigration, acculturation and adaptation. *Applied Psychology: An International Review, 46*, 5–68.

Blommaert, J. (2013). *Ethnography, superdiversity and linguistic landscapes: Chronicles of complexity*. Bristol, United Kingdom: Multilingual Matters.

Bodkin-Andrewsa, G. H., Haa, M. T., Cravena, R. G., & Yeunga, A. S. (2010). Factorial invariance testing and latent mean differences for the self-description questionnaire II (Short Version) with indigenous and non-indigenous Australian secondary school students. *International Journal of Testing, 10*, 47–79. doi:10.1080/15305050903352065

Bowers, E. P., Li, Y., Kiely, M. K., Brittian, A., Lerner, J. V., & Lerner, R. M. (2010). The five Cs model of positive youth development: A longitudinal analysis of confirmatory factor structure and measurement invariance. *Journal of Youth and Adolescence, 39*, 720–735. doi:10.1007/s10964-010-9530-9

Brouwers, S. A., Van de Vijver, F. J. R., & Van Hemert, D. A. (2009). Variation in Raven's progressive matrices scores across time and place. *Learning and Individual Differences, 19*, 330–338. doi:10.1016/j.lindif.2008.10.006

Buhs, E. S., McGinley, M., & Toland, M. D. (2010). Overt and relational victimization in Latinos and European Americans: Measurement equivalence across ethnicity, gender, and grade level in early adolescent groups. *Journal of Early Adolescence, 30*, 171–197. doi:10.1177/0272431609350923

Byrne, B. M. (2001). *Structural equation modeling with AMOS: Basic concepts, applications, and programming*. Mahwah, NJ: Lawrence Erlbaum Associates.

Byrne, B. M., & Van de Vijver, F. J. R. (2010). Testing for measurement and structural equivalence in large-scale cross-cultural studies: Addressing the issue of nonequivalence. *International Journal of Testing, 10*, 107–132. doi:10.1080/15305051003637306

Byrne, B. M., Shavelson, R. J., & Muthén, B. (1989). Testing for the equivalence of factor covariance and mean structures: The issue of partial measurement invariance. *Psychological Bulletin, 105*, 456–466. doi:10.1037/0033-2909.105.3.456

Cheung, G. W., & Rensvold, R. B. (2002). Evaluating goodness-of-fit indexes for testing measurement invariance. *Structural Equation Modeling, 9*, 233–255. doi:10.1207/s15328007sem0902_5

Cronbach, L. J. (1950). Further evidence on response sets and test design. *Educational and Psychological Measurement, 10*, 3–31.

Cronbach, L. J., & Drenth, P. J. D. (Eds.). (1972). *Mental tests and cultural adaptation*. The Hague, the Netherlands: Mouton.

Dei, G. J. S., Mazzuca, J., McIsaac, E., & Zine, J. (1997). *Reconstructing "drop-out": A critical ethnography of the dynamics of Black students' disengagement from school*. Toronto, Canada: University of Toronto Press.

Denzin, N. K. (2012). Triangulation 2.0. *Journal of Mixed Methods Research, 6*, 80–88. doi:10.1177/1558689812437186

Doucette-Gates, A., Brooks-Gunn, J., & Chase-Lansdale, P. L. (1998). The role of bias and equivalence in the study of race, class and ethnicity. In V. C. McLoyd & L. Steinberg (Eds.), *Studying minority adolescents: Conceptual, methodological, and theoretical issues* (pp. 211–236). Mahwah, NJ: Erlbaum.

Edwards, L. M., & Lopez, S. J. (2006). Perceived family support, acculturation, and life satisfaction in Mexican American youth: A mixed-methods exploration.

Journal of Counseling Psychology, 53, 279–287. doi:10.1037/0022-0167.53.3.279

Feddes, A. R., Noack, P., & Rutland, A. (2009). Direct and extended friendship effects on minority and majority children's interethnic attitudes: A longitudinal study. *Child Development, 80*, 377–390. doi:10.1111/j.1467-8624.2009.01266.x

Ferguson, G. M., Bornstein, M. H., & Pottinger, A. M. (2012). Tridimensional acculturation and adaptation among Jamaican adolescent-mother dyads in the United States. *Child Development, 83*, 1486–1493. doi:10.1111/j.1467-8624.2012.01787.x

Friborg, O., Martinussen, M., & Rosenvinge, J. H. (2006). Likert-based vs. semantic differential-based scorings of positive psychological constructs: A psychometric comparison of two versions of a scale measuring resilience. *Personality and Individual Differences, 40*, 873–884. doi:10.1016/j.paid.2005.08.015

Gilman, R., Huebner, E. S., Tian, L., Park, N., O'Byrne, J., Schiff, M., et al. (2008). Cross-national adolescent multidimensional life satisfaction reports: Analyses of mean scores and response style differences. *Journal of Youth and Adolescence, 37*, 142–154. doi:10.1007/s10964-007-9172-8

Gonzalez, A., Padilla, J.-L., Hidalgo, M. D., Gomer-Benito, J., & Benitez, I. (2011). EASYDIF: Software for analysing differential item functioning using the Mantel-Haenszel and standardization procedures. *Applied Psychological Measurement, 35*, 490–499. doi:10.1177/0146621610381489

Harkness, J. A. (2003). Questionnaire translation. In J. A. Harkness, F. J. R. Van de Vijver, & P. P. Mohler (Eds.), *Cross-cultural survey methods* (pp. 19–34). New York, NY: Wiley.

He, J., & Van de Vijver, F. J. R. (2013). A general response style factor: Evidence from a multi-ethnic study in the Netherlands. *Personality and Individual Differences, 55*, 794–800. doi:10.1016/j.paid.2013.06.017

He, J., & Van de Vijver, F. J. R. (2015). Effects of a general response style on cross-cultural comparisons: Evidence from the Teaching and Learning International Survey. *Public Opinion Quarterly, 79*, 267–290. doi:10.1093/poq/nfv006

He, J., Bartram, D., Inceoglu, I., & Van de Vijver, F. J. R. (2014). Response styles and personality traits: A multilevel analysis. *Journal of Cross-Cultural Psychology, 45*, 1028–1045. doi:10.1177/0022022114534773

Henderson, K. A., Powell, G. M., & Scanlin, M. M. (2005). Observing outcomes in youth development: An analysis of mixed methods. *Journal of Park and Recreation Administration, 23*, 58–77.

Lara, M., Gamboa, C., Kahramanian, M. I., Morales, L. S., & Hayes Bautista, D. E. (2005). Acculturation and Latino health in the United States: A review of the literature and its sociopolitical context. *Annual Review of Public Health, 26*, 367–397. doi:10.1146/annurev.publhealth.26.021304.144615

Leff, S. S., Crick, N. R., Angelucci, J., Haye, K., Jawad, A. F., Grossman, M., et al. (2006). Social cognition in context: Validating a cartoon-based attributional measure for urban girls. *Child Development, 77*, 1351–1358. doi:10.1111/j.1467-8624.2006.00939.x

Leung, K., & Van de Vijver, F. J. R. (2008). Strategies for strengthening causal inferences in cross cultural research: The consilience approach. *International Journal of Cross Cultural Management, 8*, 145–169. doi:10.1177/1470595808091788

Malda, M., Van de Vijver, F. J. R., & Temane, M. (2010). Rugby versus soccer in South Africa: Content familiarity contributes to cross-cultural differences in cognitive test scores. *Intelligence, 38*, 82–595. doi:10.1016/j.intell.2010.07.004

Masten, A. S., & Coatsworth, J. D. (1998). The development of competence in favorable and unfavorable environments: Lessons from research on successful children. *American Psychologist, 53*, 205–220. doi:10.1037/0003-066X.53.2.205

Masten, A. S., & Motti-Stefanidi, F. (2009). Understanding and promoting resilience in children: Promotive and protective processes in schools. In T. R. Gutkin & C. Reynolds (Eds.), *The handbook of school psychology* (4th ed., pp. 721–738). Hoboken, NJ: Wiley.

Michaels, M. L., Barr, A., Roosa, M. W., & Knight, G. P. (2007). Self-esteem: Assessing measurement equivalence in a multiethnic sample of youth. *Journal of Early Adolescence, 27*, 269–295. doi:10.1177/0272431607302009

Motti-Stefanidi, F., Asendorpf, J. B., & Masten, A. S. (2012). The adaptation and well-being of adolescent immigrants in Greek schools: A multilevel, longitudinal study of risks and resources. *Development and Psychopathology, 24*, 451. doi: 10.1017/S0954579412000090

Motti-Stefanidi, F. (2014). Immigrant youth adaptation in the Greek school context: A risk and resilience developmental perspective. *Child Development Perspectives, 8*, 180–185. doi:10.1111/cdep.12081

Neblett, E. W., Rivas-Drake, D., & Umaña-Taylor, A. J. (2012). The promise of racial and ethnic protective factors in promoting ethnic minority youth development. *Child Development Perspectives, 6*, 295–303. doi:10.1111/j.1750-8606.2012.00239.x

Nederhof, A. J. (1985). Methods of coping with social desirability bias: A review. *European Journal of Social Psychology, 15*, 263–280.

Okanda, M., & Itakura, S. (2010). When do children exhibit a "yes" bias? *Child Development, 81*, 568–580. doi:10.1111/j.1467-8624.2009.01416.x

Ones, D. S., Viswesvaran, C., & Reiss, A. D. (1996). Role of social desirability in personality testing for personnel selection: The red herring. *Journal of Applied Psychology, 81*, 660–679. doi:10.1037/0021-9010.81.6.660

Onwuegbuzie, A. J., & Leech, N. L. (2004). Enhancing the interpretation of "significant" findings: The role of mixed methods research. *The Qualitative Report, 9*, 770–792.

Papacharisis, V., Goudas, M., Danish, S. J., & Theodorakis, Y. (2005). The effectiveness of teaching a life skills program in a sport context. *Journal of Applied Sport Psychology, 17*, 247–254. doi:10.1080/10413200591010139

Paulhus, D. L. (1986). Self-deception and impression management in test responses. In A. Angleitner & J. S. Wiggins (Eds.), *Personality assessment via questionnaire* (pp. 143–165). New York, NY: Springer-Verlag.

Peña, E. D. (2007). Lost in translation: Methodological considerations in cross-cultural research. *Child Development, 78*, 1255–1264. doi:10.1111/j.1467-8624.2007.01064.x

Pike, K. L. (1967). *Language in relation to a unified theory of structure of human behavior* (2nd ed.). The Hague, the Netherlands: Mouton Press.

Podsakoff, P. M., MacKenzie, S. B., Lee, J. Y., & Podsakoff, N. P. (2003). Common method biases in behavioral research: A critical review of the literature and recommended remedies. *Journal of Applied Psychology, 88*, 879–903. doi:10.1037/0021-9010.88.5.879

Poortinga, Y. H. (1995). Cultural bias in assessment: Historical and thematic issues. *European Journal of Psychological Assessment, 11*, 140–146. doi:10.1027/1015-5759.11.3.140

Poortinga, Y. H., & Van de Vijver, F. J. R. (1987). Explaining cross-cultural differences: Bias analysis and beyond. *Journal of Cross-Cultural Psychology, 18*, 259–282. doi:10.1177/0022002187018003001

Reichenbach, H. (1938). *Experience and prediction.* Chicago, IL: University of Chicago Press.

Riggs, N. R. (2006). After-school program attendance and the social development of rural Latino children of immigrant families. *Journal of Community Psychology, 34*, 75–87. doi:10.1002/jccp.20084

Sakamoto, A., Goyette, K. A., & Kim, C. (2009). Socioeconomic attainments of Asian Americans. *Annual Review of Sociology, 35*, 255–276. doi:10.1146/annurev-soc-070308-115958

Sam, D. L., & Berry, J. W. (Eds.). (2006). *The Cambridge handbook of acculturation psychology.* Cambridge, United Kingdom: Cambridge University Press.

Shek, D. T., & Ma, C. M. (2010). Dimensionality of the Chinese positive youth development scale: Confirmatory factor analyses. *Social Indicators Research, 98*, 41–59. doi:10.1007/s11205-009-9515-9

Smith, P. B. (2004). Acquiescent response bias as an aspect of cultural communication style. *Journal of Cross-Cultural Psychology, 35*, 50–61. doi:10.1177/0022022103260380

Snauwaert, B., Soenens, B., Vanbeselaere, N., & Boen, F. (2003). When integration does not necessarily imply integration: Different conceptualizations of acculturation orientations lead to different classifications. *Journal of Cross-Cultural Psychology, 34*, 231–239. doi:10.1177/0022022102250250

Spencer, M. B. (1990). Development of minority children: An introduction. *Child Development, 61*, 267–269. doi:10.1111/j.1467-8624.1990.tb02778.x

Tashakkori, A., & Teddlie, C. (Eds.). (2010). *Sage handbook on mixed methods in social and behavioral research.* Thousand Oaks, CA: Sage Publications.

Ungar, M. (2008). Resilience across cultures. *British Journal of Social Work, 38*, 218–235. doi:10.1093/bjsw/bc1343

Van de Vijver, F. J. R., & Poortinga, Y. H. (2002). Structural equivalence in multilevel research. *Journal of Cross-Cultural Psychology, 33*, 141–156. doi: 10.1177/0022022102033002002

Van de Vijver, F. J. R. (2015). Methodological aspects of cross-cultural research. In M. Gelfand, Y. Hong, & C. Y. Chiu (Eds.), *Handbook of advances in culture & psychology* (Vol. 5, pp. 101–160). New York, NY: Oxford University Press.

Van de Vijver, F. J. R., & Leung, K. (1997). *Methods and data analysis of comparative research*. Thousand Oaks, CA: Sage.

Van de Vijver, F. J. R., & Poortinga, Y. H. (1997). Towards an integrated analysis of bias in cross-cultural assessment. *European Journal of Psychological Assessment, 13*, 29–37. doi:10.1027/1015-5759.13.1.29

Van de Vijver, F. J. R., & Tanzer, N. K. (2004). Bias and equivalence in cross-cultural assessment: an overview. *Revue Européenne de Psychologie Appliquée/European Review of Applied Psychology, 54*, 119–135. doi:10.1016/j.erap.2003.12.004

Van de Vijver, F. J. R., Blommaert, J. M. E., Gkoumasi, G., & Stogianni, M. (2015). On the need to broaden the concept of ethnic identity. *International Journal of Intercultural Relations, 46*, 36–46. doi:10.1016/j.ijintrel.2015.03.021

Van Vaerenbergh, Y., & Thomas, T. D. (2013). Response styles in survey research: A literature review of antecedents, consequences, and remedies. *International Journal of Public Opinion Research, 25*, 195–217. doi:10.1093/ijpor/eds021

Vandenberg, R. J., & Lance, C. E. (2000). A review and synthesis of the measurement invariance literature: Suggestions, practices, and recommendations for organizational research. *Organizational Research Methods, 3*, 4–70. doi:10.1177/109442810031002

Vertovec, S. (2007). Super-diversity and its implications. *Ethnic and Racial Studies, 30*, 1024–1054. doi:10.1080/01419870701599465

White, R. M. B., Umaña-Taylor, A. J., Knight, G. P., & Zeiders, K. H. (2011). Language measurement equivalence of the ethnic identity scale with Mexican American early adolescents. *The Journal of Early Adolescence, 31*, 817–852. doi:10.1177/0272431610376246

Willis, G. B. (2005). *Cognitive interviewing: A tool for improving questionnaire design*. Thousand Oaks, CA: Sage.

Yağmur, K., & Van de Vijver, F. J. R. (2012). Acculturation and language orientations of Turkish immigrants in Australia, France, Germany, and the Netherlands. *Journal of Cross-Cultural Psychology, 43*, 1110–1130. doi:10.1177/0022022111420145

Zumbo, B. D. (1999). *A handbook on the theory and methods of differential item functioning (DIF): Logistic regression modeling as a unitary framework for binary and Likert-Type (ordinal) item scores*. Ottawa, ON: Directorate of Human Resources Research and Evaluation, Department of National Defense.

Zumbo, B. D. (2007). Three generations of DIF analyses: Considering where it has been, where it is now, and where it is going. *Language Assessment Quarterly, 4*, 223–233. doi:10.1080/15434300701375832

The Puzzle of Coaction and the Imbroglio of Paradox

Robert H. Bradley

In their recent recapitulation of Relational Developmental Systems (RDS) theory, Lerner et al. (2015) argued that developmental science is a non-ergodic field. Human development is viewed as an embodied phenomenon that involves ongoing coaction (mutual influences) between an individual and the multiple systems in which the individual is embedded. Humans are active self-regulating agents functioning within active self-regulating interconnected systems. From this perspective, what does positive development mean and how does one come to understand individual differences using such a framework? Each of the chapters in this part, in its own way, takes a shot at answering these two questions—but the authors candidly admit that the information available does not allow one to fully answer either question.

Assary and Pluess immediately confronted the problem of "What does positive development mean?" as applied to minority youth. As they note, for some it means that absence of a likely bad outcome (e.g., psychopathology). For others, including the editors of this volume and Lerner and colleagues (2015), it means more—thriving. The latter perspective has advantages in the sense of appreciating that developmental domains are integrated and that strengths in one domain tend to support strengths in others. The notion about self-productivity in the work of Cunha and Heckman (2007) reflects such a belief. In that regard, the finding that exposure to multiple languages early in life appears to enhance executive functioning (as discussed in the chapter by Escobar and Tamis-LeMonda) seems revealing. On the other hand, the chapters by Lansford and by Vedder and van Geel remind us that it is not yet clear how exposure to different ideas and practices concerning appropriate social behavior within and across family, peer, and community contexts leads to greater social competence, higher achievement, or emotional well-being. Unfortunately, as Lansford aptly noted, most of what we know about individual differences in human characteristics comes from studies done in WEIRD countries (i.e., Western, educated, industrialized, rich, democratic). Most minority children do not live in WEIRD countries; and, even when they do, many occupy a developmental niche that is quite different from majority children in those countries (Super and Harkness 1986). Different cultures (and minorities living in a dominant culture) have both different values regarding what needs to be developed and different ways of promoting children's development (Bornstein 1985). The degree of alignment between the structures, processes, and resources used to promote particular goals for children varies across developmental niches. To the degree that everything in every system connected to a child is "in synch", development in a particular domain is likely to proceed at a good pace. However, things may not always be in good alignment for minority children. If not, it can have profound implications for "what" develops and how fast it develops—and sometimes what emerges seems paradoxical. Interesting in this regard is the discussion of the movement toward radicalization by some Muslim youth in Europe, even though many of them attend excellent schools and receive solid emotional support from family and peers. It is further evidence that to some degree "everything counts" and that there is dynamic interplay between individual and all of the affordances present in the environment.

The notion of person-in-context is addressed in every chapter. It is at the heart of the chapter by Assary and Pluess. The differential susceptibility and vantage sensitivity frameworks address biologically connected dispositions that increase or decrease a person's sensitivity to environmental affordances. These frameworks suggest that positive development will be more likely for minority youth who have certain genetically driven characteristics when those youth have supportive encounters with the environment. Consider as an example Asian minority groups in the US. As noted in the chapters by Lansford, Asian societies often place high value on educational achievement and Asian parents often spend time encouraging academic efforts. A temperamentally reactive Asian child may especially benefit if parents are both supportive and highly encouraging of the child's investment in education. At the same time, positive development will be less likely if those same youth have non-supportive encounters (e.g., acts of discrimination), as was the case with African-American adolescents (Brody et al. 2011). As is noted in every chapter, minority families are frequently faced with a multitude of contextual risks (e.g., poverty, discrimination, household instability, low social support/capital) that decrease the likelihood that minority children will adapt well and show positive development. These same factors also decrease the likelihood of good parenting, positive support from others in the community, and ready access to community resources (i.e., potentially offsetting contextual conditions). In effect, the coaction that occurs between minority youth and the various

aspects of their overall environments often does not bode well for optimal development. That said, as Assary and Pluess make clear, being a member of a minority group does not mean that one faces environmental risks. Indeed, some minority groups enjoy privileged status.

The chapters in this part address a broad range of individual characteristics: attachment relationships (Malda and Mesman); language competence (Esccobar and Tamis-LeMonda); identity development (Vedder & van Geel); achievement, moral development, and social development (Lansford); and maladaptive behavior (Lansford; Assary and Pluess). In addressing what research shows about factors known to impact developmental course, the authors give due consideration to systems theories that view children's development as embedded in layers of interconnected systems: from family to school to community to cultural and political. Several of the authors make note of the fact that the interplay among these systems makes it difficult to isolate how minority status per se "influences" the course of development, independent of factors such as SES, nativity, geography, and community resources. The authors discuss the problems of trying to use standardized measures in studies of minority children. Not only is there the worry that the form some characteristic takes (e.g., respectful behavior towards adults) could be different in different groups (Bornstein 1985); but the assumption of "sameness" across groups with respect to phenomena being measured is questionable (Lerner et al. 2015)—is social savvy even the same thing across groups? In effect, researchers may well be comparing apples to oranges in many studies of minority children or at least comparing two kinds of apples.

The final chapter by Vedder and van Geel would seem to offer an enlightening perspective with which to view the development of minority children and to consider what individual differences in minority children tell us as scientists, practitioners, and policy makers. Their chapter deals with the development of identity—who am I? Forming attachment relationships with key caregivers directly connects to a child's emerging sense of whom she or he is (Malda and Mesman). In a similar way, language skills contribute to one's understanding of self, others, objects and how to engage the environment (Escobar and Tamis-LeMonda). The places where children grow up and the settings they inhabit also gives children a perspective on who they are, what things they should be doing, and how they should react to the people and events they encounter (Lansford). If, as Vedder and van Geel made clear, the messages and structures are fractured or if resources and reinforcements are not optimally aligned, then it can lead to identity diffusion or a decision to identify oneself with a group or a purpose that has negative consequences. As Lerner and colleagues argued, optimal development (which includes a positive, well-consolidated sense of identity) requires ongoing supportive coaction between person and environment, where each brings many mutually supportive assets to ongoing encounters. When this happens, it becomes more likely that a minority child will commit to being someone who contributes not only to his or her own well-being but also to the benefit of the community she or he inhabits.

References

Bornstein, M. H. (1995). Form and function: Implications for studies of culture and human development. *Culture & Psychology, 1*, 123–137.

Brody, G. H., Beach, S. R. H., Chen, Y.-F., Obasi, E., Philibert, R. A., Kogan, S. M., & Simons, R. L. (2011). Perceived discrimination, serotonin transporter linked polymorphic region status, and the development of conduct problems. *Developmental Psychopathology, 23*, 617–627.

Cunha, F., & Heckman, J. J. (2007). The technology of skill formation. *American Economic Review, 97*, 31–47.

Lerner, R. M., Johnson, S. K., & Buckingham, M. H. (2015). Relational developmental systems-based theories and the study of children and families: Lerner and Spanier (1978) revisited. *Journal of Family Theory and Review, 7*, 83–104.

Super, C. M., & Harkness, S. (1986). The developmental niche: A conceptualization at the interface of child and culture. *International Journal of Behavioral Development, 9*, 545–569.

Parental Sensitivity and Attachment in Ethnic Minority Families

Maike Malda and Judi Mesman

Abstract

Attachment is considered a universal human need and, although relevant studies are scarce, it appears that the main tenets of attachment theory (i.e., children becoming attached to one or more particular caregivers, the normativity of secure attachment patterns, and the positive effects of parental sensitivity) are also applicable to non-Western cultural groups, including ethnic minorities. Parental sensitivity and secure attachment appear to occur at a lower rate in ethnic minority than in ethnic majority families, but such differences can generally be ascribed to group differences in socioeconomic status and related social challenges. Attachment-based intervention efforts specifically aimed at enhancing parenting practices among ethnic minorities exist, but there is a scarcity of studies testing their effectiveness. It is also important to pay more attention to the ethnicity of coders in the mostly observational methods of attachment research, as there is evidence that coder ethnicity may influence scoring. Finally, the field would greatly benefit from a more theoretical and more overarching approach to how attachment-related family functioning might vary depending on migration background (e.g., refugee, labor migration, postcolonial migration), and the extent to which they are linguistically, culturally, and religiously (dis)similar to the ethnic majority.

Historical Overview and Theoretical Perspectives

Attachment theory is based on evolutionary and ethological considerations, and was formulated as a universally applicable framework describing the bond between caregivers and infants (Bowlby 1969). Attachment refers to a child's innate tendency to seek proximity to one or more specific caregivers in times of distress or danger.

M. Malda (✉)
Clinical Child and Adolescent Studies, Leiden University, Leiden, The Netherlands
e-mail: m.malda@fsw.leidenuniv.nl

J. Mesman
Centre for Child and Family Studies, Leiden University, Leiden, The Netherlands

© The Editor(s) 2017
N.J. Cabrera and B. Leyendecker (eds.), *Handbook on Positive Development of Minority Children and Youth*, DOI 10.1007/978-3-319-43645-6_5

In a secure child–parent attachment relationship, the use of the parent as a haven of security in times of need is in balance with the child's age-appropriate exploration behavior in non-threatening situations (Ainsworth et al. 1978; Cassidy 2008). The child–parent attachment relationship is viewed from an organizational perspective, meaning that its function is central to its definition, not its context-specific manifestation (Sroufe and Waters 1977). In other words: the function of children's attachment behavior is to be close to one or more preferred caregivers who can provide a safe haven when necessary, but what this behavior looks like may vary across cultures (see also Mesman et al. 2016a). This has also been referred to as universality without uniformity (Schweder and Sullivan 1993).

One of the most researched parenting predictors of a secure child–caregiver relationship is parental sensitivity, defined as a parent's ability to notice child signals, interpret these signals correctly, and respond to these signals promptly and appropriately (Ainsworth et al. 1974). These components of parental behavior refer to universally relevant aspects of caregiving, including proximity to the child (necessary for protection and meeting basic needs) and contingent responding (promoting social development). Consistent with an organization approach to the attachment relationship, the definition focuses on the appropriateness of parental interventions based on the child's responses (emphasizing the function of providing a predictable and safe haven) rather than on a fixed list of specific parenting behaviors (Mesman and Emmen 2013; Mesman et al. 2012a). The assumption that sensitive parenting fosters the development of a secure attachment relationship has been confirmed in two meta-analyses (Bakermans-Kranenburg et al. 2003; De Wolff and Van IJzendoorn 1997). In addition, both parental sensitivity and a secure child–parent attachment relationship have been found to predict positive child outcomes across various domains of functioning, including cognitive competence, language development, and social-emotional well-being (e.g., Bernier et al.

2010; Groh et al. 2014; Sroufe et al. 2005; Tamis-LeMonda et al. 2001). Studies of attachment security as well as parental sensitivity have mostly been done with mothers, although attachment theory and research is increasingly focusing on fathers as well (e.g., Bretherton 2010; Grossmann et al. 2002).

One of the main questions in cross-cultural research in general, and in research addressing ethnic minority populations in particular is whether the major assumptions of attachment theory, developed by Western researchers and tested on Western samples, are applicable to non-Western cultural groups and whether maternal and paternal sensitivity and secure attachment are also beneficial to child development in these groups. Although the formation of an attachment relationship between child and caregiver is expected to be universal, the specific nature of the relationship and its suggested correlates could be culture-specific (Van IJzendoorn and Sagi-Schwartz 2008). Despite the fact that only a limited number of cross-cultural studies have been conducted relative to the total amount of research on attachment, existing data on parenting from a range of countries shows that children use their mothers as a secure base from which to explore the world (Posada et al. 2013). This is also true for fathers (Bretherton 2010), but father–child attachment has been much less studied in countries outside the Western world. Support for the universality and normativeness of the attachment construct has been found in Africa, Israel, Latin America and in East and South-East Asia with mothers (Mesman et al. 2016a). The three primary attachment patterns of secure, avoidant, and ambivalent attachment were found in all studied contexts, and the secure pattern was most common across all groups. In keeping with the notion of universality without uniformity, the specific behaviors that indicate secure attachment do differ between cultural groups. For example, Gusii infants in Kenya are used to being greeted with a handshake by their caregivers. Consistent with this custom, secure infants would reach out to an adult with one arm to receive the expected handshake after a brief separation (as a North-American child would hold up two arms for a hug), whereas the insecure infants would avoid the adult or reach and then pull away after the adult approached (Kermoian and Leiderman 1986).

With regard to maternal sensitivity, a recent study showed strong convergence between maternal beliefs about the ideal mother and attachment theory's description of the sensitive mother across 26 cultural groups from 15 countries (Mesman et al. 2016b). Also, a review of observational studies of sensitivity supports the notion that the construct of sensitivity shows meaningful relations with child outcomes outside the cultural areas in which these instruments were developed (Mesman and Emmen 2013), and some have addressed sensitivity in fathers in cultural minority families in the U.S. as well (e.g., Kelley et al. 1998). Further, a growing number of studies in non-Western countries confirm the beneficial outcomes of sensitive parenting (Mesman et al. 2016a).

Although the above discussed findings confirm the universal relevance of the attachment and sensitivity concepts, their cross-cultural applicability has also been criticized. It has been suggested that the construct of attachment by definition implies independence and autonomy of the child as important values and goals whereas this behavioral pattern is not in line with the values and socialization goals of many non-Western cultural groups with cultural orientations that focus on relatedness emphasizing the social community in which people develop (Otto and Keller 2014). However, the dichotomous view on cultural orientation has been criticized, and it is now more accepted to view cultures on continuous scales, and as containing elements of different cultural models (e.g., Tamis-LeMonda et al. 2007). Further, viewing sensitivity and attachment as uniform without room for cultural variation in their manifestations is also no longer the norm (Mesman et al. 2016a). For example, Posada et al. (2002) examined both the operationalization of the sensitivity construct and the relation with attachment security in the US and Colombia. The overall relations between the constructs were similar, but the specific behavioral content

showed some differences. This is in line with studies describing culture-specific contingency patterns in the interaction between mother and infant (Carra et al. 2014; Kärtner et al. 2010) and reflects the idea that although parenting behaviors may come in different forms (e.g., nursing and rocking), they tend to have a similar function (e.g., comforting a distressed infant) (Bornstein 1995).

Another interesting study comparing Anglo and Puerto Rican infants (matched on SES) showed that maternal physical control (observed use of physical contact to manipulate, limit, or control the infant's movements), was related to insecure attachment in the Anglo sample, but to secure attachment in the Puerto Rican sample (Carlson and Harwood 2003). These results may have something to with the fact that the interactional context can moderate the relation between parenting and child outcomes. For example, high maternal warmth has been found to attenuate the negative effects of maternal intrusiveness (which is similar to control) on child development in African-American families (Ispa et al. 2004). The higher normativeness of controlling behaviors in certain ethnic minorities may result in less negative effects of these behaviors on children depending on other aspects of the quality of parenting. Unfortunately, the samples in the Carlson and Harwood study (2003) were too small to test moderation effects, and too small and homogenous to detect a substantial range in sensitivity scores so that potential effects of this variable were difficult to capture.

Because the current chapter focuses on ethnic minority children rather than on indigenous cultural groups, the ongoing debate about the cross-cultural applicability of the constructs and measures of attachment and maternal sensitivity may be of less relevance. Ethnic minority families live their lives in the context of a majority group with its specific ideas on which parenting and child behaviors are expected and appropriate in public domains, such as school and work settings. Ethnic minority families generally hold on to certain norms and values of their culture of origin, mostly in private settings, and at the same time, these families adopt characteristics of the majority group, mainly in public settings (Arends-Tóth and Van de Vijver 2003). Ethnic minority families generally value what is valued in these public domains by the majority group not only because these families feel pressured to succeed in these domains, but also because they want to succeed (Durgel et al. 2009; Fuligni and Fuligni 2007). However, it was not until the late 1990s and early 2000s that studies on attachment and sensitivity in ethnic minority families emerged in more than negligible numbers, mostly reporting on African Americans (e.g., Bost et al. 1998; Goodman et al. 1998; Ward and Carlson 1995) or Hispanic Americans (Fracasso et al. 1994; Schölmerich et al. 1997). During the 1990s and 2000s, studies focusing on attachment- and sensitivity-related family processes in ethnic minorities in Europe also emerged, such as the Surinamese-Dutch (Riksen-Walraven et al. 1996; Van IJzendoorn 1990) and the Turkish-Dutch (Leseman and Van den Boom 1999; Yaman et al. 2010). However, such studies remain very rare despite the fast growth of the ethnic minority populations in many European countries.

In sum, despite some criticisms and despite variation in manifestations of parenting across countries and cultures, attachment is considered a universal human need and the universality and normativity hypotheses are generally supported. Further, the construct of sensitive parenting appears to be applicable to different cultural contexts and important to positive child development across different cultures both within and between countries. However, studies addressing the specific ways in which sensitivity and attachment occurs in ethnic minority groups are still scarce, whereas this line of research could be very important to understanding and positively influencing ethnic minority family functioning and minority children's development.

Current Research Questions

The types of topics that are currently investigated in attachment research in ethnic minority families are rather basic and reflect the fact that this field of research is still catching up with regard to

ethnic minority populations. Studies in non-majority groups did not emerge until about two decades after the notion of attachment research became current. Nevertheless, basic issues regarding the nature and meaning of sensitivity and attachment in ethnic minority families need to be addressed before moving on to more complex issues. Thus, the literature in this area generally focuses on the following topics (a) comparing ethnic minority families to ethnic majority families to uncover potential mean-level differences and predictors of such differences; (b) examining relations with child outcomes to test whether the same patterns of associations are found as in ethnic majority families; (c) testing the effectiveness of interventions aimed at improving parental sensitivity and/or child attachment security.

Research Measurement and Methodology

The attachment paradigm is characterized by the expert administration of time-intensive standardized observational and interview measures rather than questionnaires. This is a direct consequence of the fact that its main constructs (attachment and sensitivity) are not readily noticed or interpreted correctly by untrained individuals. For instance, the balance between attachment behaviors (e.g., seeking proximity to the caregiver) and exploration behaviors (e.g., examining objects in the wider environment) is crucial to determining attachment security, but can easily be misunderstood. Attachment behaviors are prone to being confused with dependence and exploration behaviors with rejection. Indeed, the use of the Attachment Q-sort (see below) as self-report instruments for parents has been shown to have serious validity problems (Van IJzendoorn et al. 2004). Further, recognizing one's own sensitive parenting skills requires substantial self-reflection and insensitive parents are very unlikely to know that they are indeed insensitive precisely because they lack skills related to reflective functioning. It may even be that sensitive parents are likely to underestimate their own sensitivity, because of their acute awareness of the reality of not always being responsive to all signals in all situations. It is therefore not surprising that self-report measures of sensitivity are practically non-existent. For these reasons we will discuss only standardized and validated observational and interview measures here.

Attachment Measures

Attachment patterns can be categorized according to the Strange Situation procedure (Ainsworth et al. 1978), commonly used with infants between 12 and 20 months of age. The procedure is the most widely known assessment of attachment and focuses on the infant's response to reunions with a parent after brief episodes of separation and of interaction with a stranger. Infants can be classified showing secure, avoidant, ambivalent, or disorganized attachment. Reliability and validity of the instrument is well established in North America and Western Europe, however, studies outside of these areas are limited in number (Solomon and George 2008). Although the applicability of the Strange Situation procedure to non-Western groups has been criticized (Keller 2013), the instrument has been used regularly and successfully used with ethnic minority groups in North America and Western Europe. The Cassidy-Marvin Assessment of Attachment in Preschoolers applies the principles of the Strange Situation procedure to young children (Cassidy and Marvin 1992).

The Attachment Q-sort (AQS; Vaughn and Waters 1990) is used with children aged 1–5 and is composed of 90 items reflecting behaviors associated with a secure base. Trained independent observers sort these cards into 9 stacks reflecting behaviors from least to most descriptive of the child's behavior. Inter-rater reliabilities between .72 and .95 have been reported (Solomon and George 2008). Cross-cultural validity of the AQS is not firmly established. Although there are general similarities in the structure of the responses, correlations between card sorts across contexts were relatively low.

The Adult Attachment Interview (AAI; George et al. 1984) is not only used for adults but also for adolescents and requires the interviewee to describe childhood experiences relating to attachment as well as the effect of these experiences on subsequent development and functioning (Hesse 2008). The resulting narratives are then analyzed and classified according to a coding system into one of three main categories: Secure-Autonomous (F), Insecure-Dismissing (Ds), and Insecure-Preoccupied (E). Incoherent, very short or very long narratives are associated with insecure attachment, rather than the characteristics of the attachment history itself. The AAI has been used with groups from various cultural and linguistic backgrounds (Bakermans-Kranenburg and Van IJzendoorn 2009), yielding results that to a large extent fit with the patterns of non-clinical Caucasian North Americans. The stability and discriminant validity of the AAI have been thoroughly examined, showing good psychometric properties. The Child Attachment Interview (CAI; Target et al. 2003) was developed and validated for children aged 8–13 years, and based on the principles of the AAI. Inter-rater reliability, test–retest reliability, concurrent and discriminant validity are good (Shmueli-Goetz et al. 2008).

Other validated measures of attachment focus on the symbolic representation of attachment, such as the Manchester Child Attachment Story Task which is a doll-play vignette completion method for children aged 5–7 (Green et al. 2000). One doll represents the child and another doll represents the caregiver. A story is initiated by the experimenter (e.g., a child wakes up alone in the middle of the night from a nightmare). The child then completes the story by enacting it with the dolls. The Attachment Script Assessment can be used with older children and adolescents and uses a story titles and a list of 12–14 word prompts with each story title to evoke attachment-relevant stories (Waters and Waters 2006). An example of such a story title is "Doctor's office" with word prompts such as "mother", "Tommy", "bike", "hurry", and "cry". The narratives that are produced are analyzed and scored for the presence of elements of a secure base script (i.e., consistency, coherence, completeness).

Sensitivity Measures

Since the formulation of the sensitivity construct by Ainsworth, many studies on parenting have included a measure of sensitivity or constructs closely related to sensitivity, such as responsiveness. In the nineties, De Wolff and Van IJzendoorn (1997) already reviewed 66 studies describing a many as 55 different constructs reflecting behaviors labeled as sensitive or responsive. Due to the fact that it is extremely difficult to realistically evaluate one's own sensitivity by means of self-report, observational measures seem to provide the most valid indication of the construct (Mesman and Emmen 2013). On the downside, these measures imply expensive and laborious data collections which may lead to feasibility issues.

Mesman and Emmen (2013) performed a systematic review of observational instruments measuring parental sensitivity. Out of at least fifty reported instruments, the authors selected the eight most commonly used measures reported in the literature and described their similarities and differences in comparison to Ainsworth's original Sensitivity-Insensitivity to Infant Signals and Communications observational scale (Ainsworth et al. 1974). Ainsworth formulated nine descriptions of sensitive behaviors, from highly insensitive to highly sensitive based on observations of mother–infant dyads in Uganda. All descriptions address the extent to which the mother notices the child's signals, interprets these correctly, and responds to them appropriately, as derived from the child's response to mother's behavior.

Examples of commonly used scales that are examined by Mesman and Emmen are the Emotional Availability Scales (the EA scales; Biringen 2008), the Erickson scales (Egeland et al. 1990), and the Maternal Behavior Q-sort (MBQS; Pederson et al. 1999). The EA scales have mostly been used to code parental sensitivity in free-play settings. The 3rd edition of this instrument includes one sensitivity scale whereas the 4th edition contains seven sensitivity subscales. The Erickson scales are generally used to code interactions in teaching situations and reflect the constructs of supportive presence, lack of respect for autonomy (later labeled as intrusiveness), hostility, clarity of instruction, sensitivity and timing of instruction, and confidence. The MBQS is generally used as an observational instrument and consists of 90 items describing maternal behaviors associated with sensitive parenting. A trained coder organizes these 90 cards into 9 stacks of cards, reflecting behaviors from least (stack 1) to most (stack 9) descriptive of a particular mother that is being observed when interacting with her child.

Some of the newer observational instruments distinguish various sensitivity subscales that refer to parenting related to sensitivity but not necessarily identical to sensitivity, whereas the Ainsworth scale only contains one global sensitivity rating. The newer instruments also differ in the in- or exclusion of positive affect or warmth as reflecting sensitivity. Although observational data on parent–child interactions obtained in non-Western cultures are relatively rare, six out of the eight reviewed instruments by Mesman and Emmen (2013) were used outside of a Western(ized) context. The generally successful (though still rather limited) use of both attachment and sensitivity measures with a diversity of cultural groups supports the validity of the empirical findings discussed in the next section.

Empirical Findings

Sensitivity Levels and Attachment Classifications

Parental sensitivity encompasses both beliefs and actual behaviors. Beliefs about what constitutes the ideal mother as measured using the MBQS as a self-report have been shown to be highly similar across groups of Dutch, Moroccan and Turkish mothers (convenience samples diverse in SES) living in the Netherlands, regardless of socioeconomic status (Emmen et al. 2012). In addition, the views of the Turkish minority mothers included in this study appeared strongly in line with the beliefs of native Dutch and Turkish health care professionals as well as the views of sensitivity experts (Ekmekci et al. 2014). These findings on the high cross-cultural similarity of sensitivity beliefs correspond with the results of a large international study by (Mesman et al. 2016b) with 26 cultural groups from 15 countries.

A review of studies applying observational measures of parental sensitivity in ethnic minority families in the US, the Netherlands, and Canada (Mesman et al. 2012b) revealed that families in these studies generally show less sensitive parenting (i.e., less appropriate and prompt responding to children's signals) behaviors than majority families.. For example, comparing predominantly low-income samples revealed that African-American mothers were less sensitive towards their children than Latin-American and European-American mothers in free play, teaching, and daily routine activities (Bernstein et al. 2005). Also, low- to middle-class Turkish immigrant mothers in the Netherlands were less sensitively supportive of their children in a problem-solving task than native middle class Dutch mothers, and they were more intrusive and less authoritative (Yaman et al. 2010). However, in their review, Mesman et al. (2012b) note that the discrepancies in sensitivity between ethnic groups are to a large extent caused by discrepancies in socioeconomic status as reflected by income and educational level (with ethnic minority groups being mostly of lower SES than majority groups) and its related stressors (e.g., single parenthood, neighborhood quality) rather than by specific cultural factors. Nevertheless, not all group differences tend to disappear when controlling for SES. A recent study found that low-income European-American mothers showed more positive and less negative mothering than African-American and Latin-American mothers (Fuligni and Brooks-Gunn 2013). Controlling for

remaining SES differences within the already low SES groups did not eliminate the ethnic differences between the European- and African-American mothers. The authors suggested that the ethnic minority families may have a longer history of poverty going back generations than the majority families, which may have a more severe impact on parenting quality. The same is likely to be true for the duration of single parenthood (longer in ethnic minorities than majority groups) and parental problems that may relate to parenting quality such as poor physical and mental health (Fuligni and Brooks-Gunn 2013).

With regard to attachment classifications based on the Strange Situation procedure, similar percentages of children were found in each attachment category for European Americans and immigrants from Central America (Schölmerich et al. 1997). Also, the distributions of attachment classifications were very similar for Surinamese-Dutch and native Dutch participants (Van IJzendoorn 1990). Low SES Hispanic-American children who were not born in the US and African-American children showed higher percentages of insecurely attached children than European-American, Asian-American children, and Hispanic-American children who were born in the US (Huang et al. 2012). In a study with low-SES Hispanic (Puerto Rican and Dominican) infants in New York, about half of the sample was evaluated as insecurely attached (Fracasso et al. 1994). The authors stressed that attachment classifications in lower-class samples tend to differ from middle-class samples. Stressful and demanding living environments and life experiences of the lower-class samples may result in lower levels of maternal sensitivity which may lead to insecure attachment patterns. Another study found that the attachment classifications of low-SES African American preschoolers matched with the general findings for low-SES samples (Barnett et al. 1998). A study examining differences in attachment security between African-American and European-American children with the NICHD Early Childcare Research Network data set and the

AQS (Bakermans-Kranenburg et al. 2004), found that the African-American children were less securely attached, however, this discrepancy was explained by differences in SES.

In sum, parental sensitivity and secure attachment appear to occur at a lower rate in ethnic minority than in ethnic majority families, but such differences can generally be ascribed to group differences in SES and related challenges, such as stress and lack of support. This suggests that these aspects of the parent–child relationship are not so much culturally determined but rather need to be interpreted from the perspective of the Family Stress Model (Conger and Donnellan 2007), which is discussed in the section on universal versus culture-specific mechanisms in this chapter.

Relations with Child Outcomes

According to attachment theory, a secure attachment child–parent relationship would predict positive child functioning across developmental domains, because the securely attached child will feel secure and confident enough to explore the environment, make social contacts, and learn new skills (Cassidy 2008). In addition, sensitive parenting, either through secure attachment or directly, is expected to lead to positive child outcomes, as it models positive and empathic social interactions, and fosters behavioral contingency detection processes that are conducive to learning and behavioral regulation (Lohaus et al. 2005). We now review studies that have examined relations between parental sensitivity and attachment security on the one hand with child outcomes on the other hand.

Outcomes of Parental Sensitivity

With regard to child developmental outcomes, research has generally shown that sensitivity is (moderately) predictive of social-emotional, cognitive, and behavioral outcomes. The review by Mesman et al. (2012b) demonstrates that sensitivity also relates to positive outcomes for ethnic minority groups in North America and the Netherlands, such as secure attachment, lower

levels of problem behaviors, self-regulation, language development, and cognitive competence. For example, maternal sensitivity was found predictive of attachment security of African-American preschoolers in a low-income sample (Goodman et al. 1998). For European-American mothers and lower SES mothers recently immigrated from Central America, mother's contingent responsiveness (i.e., the timing of her behavior relative to her infant's behavior) predicted attachment security (Schölmerich et al. 1997). Mexican-American children of low-income mothers with high sensitivity ratings showed higher responsiveness and involvement over time in free play interactions with their mothers (Howes and Obregon 2009). Maternal sensitive supportiveness assessed in structured play predicted cognitive outcomes in 3 year old children from a mixed sample of low-income immigrant families (Mistry et al. 2008). A higher observed quality of mother–infant interactions was related to infant's higher cognitive test scores in a low-SES Latin-American sample (Cabrera et al. 2006). Maternal responsiveness of Surinamese-Dutch mothers with relatively low SES was predictive of attachment security (Van IJzendoorn 1990). The quality of proximal processes (quality of book reading and problem solving interactions) was associated with Surinamese-Dutch, Turkish-Dutch, and native Dutch children's cognitive competence (Leseman and Van den Boom 1999).

These findings support the cross-cultural importance of sensitivity in fostering children to thrive, although the specific nature of the associations between sensitivity and outcomes may still depend on ethnicity (Huang et al. 2012). In a study with mostly African-American adolescent mothers, sensitivity was not predictive of their children's attachment security (Ward and Carlson 1995). This finding may be partly explained by the multiple caregiving arrangements in this sample (see also the section on universal versus culture-specific mechanisms). Ispa et al. (2004) also found that the relation between (the sensitivity-related construct of) nonintrusiveness and outcomes depended on ethnicity and level of acculturation. For European-American families, intrusiveness related negatively to child outcomes and the interaction with mother. For African-American families, intrusiveness combined with high levels of parental warmth did not result in negative outcomes. For Mexican-American families, intrusiveness was less predictive of outcomes than for the other groups, however, the more acculturated families showed more resemblance with the European-American families in the relations among constructs. For low-SES Hispanic infants in New York, maternal sensitivity was related to secure attachment, but intervening in the child's behavior was related to secure attachment as well (Fracasso et al. 1994). This finding corresponded with valued cultural practices in parenting in these Hispanic groups.

Outcomes of Attachment Security

Several studies on the outcomes of attachment security have been conducted with children and adolescents from ethnic minority groups in the US and the UK. Attachment security was positively predictive of the social network and social competence of 3- and 4-year-old children from mainly African-American origin (Bost et al. 1998). Another study included two American low income cohorts with European Americans, African Americans, Asian Americans, Hispanic Americans, or an ethnic mix (Bosquet Enlow et al. 2014). The first cohort comprised mothers and infants and results showed that mother's post-traumatic stress disorder (PTSD) negatively affected the quality of the attachment relationship between mother and infant as measured by the Strange Situation procedure. The second cohort comprised adolescents, but data from their infancy and childhood was available as well. Results showed that insecure attachment in infancy was predictive of PTSD in adolescence.

In the UK, families from low-income and ethnically diverse backgrounds (black African, Afro-Caribbean, white British, southeast Asian, Indian, Mediterranean, and mixed) in an urban context in England were studied (Futh et al. 2008). Children with a mean age of 5.5 years participated in a play session with a child doll

and caregiver doll and four story themes. The authors found that children's attachment narratives that were indicative of a more secure attachment were predictive of fewer conduct problems as reported by teachers and parents. These narratives were also predictive of more prosocial behavior and higher peer competence. Relations between the constructs showed hardly any variation across the different ethnic groups. For the same sample, observer ratings of parent–child interaction quality during standard interaction tasks were predictive of the quality of children's attachment narratives (Matias et al. 2014). Ethnic background did not moderate this relation.

Thus, the findings in ethnic minority samples—although relatively sparse—confirm one of the basic tenets of attachment theory that sensitive parenting and a secure attachment relationship with a primary caregiver are beneficial to child development.

Interventions

Assessing levels of maternal sensitivity and evaluating the presence of particular attachment patterns are necessary starting points for studying these constructs in an ethnic minority context. However, to assist parents in optimizing their parental behaviors so as to positively affect developmental outcomes in their children requires more than merely descriptive studies. Unfortunately, particular ethnic minority groups are hard to reach for intervention purposes, such as Latin Americans and Asian Americans in the United States and Moroccans and Turks in the Netherlands (Abe-Kim et al. 2007; Zwirs et al. 2006). Nonetheless, various parenting interventions have shown to be successful with ethnic minority families, although only few of them specifically target attachment security and sensitivity.

Bakermans-Kranenburg et al. (2009) conducted a series of meta-analyses on interventions that explicitly focused on improving attachment security and sensitivity and they found that the most effective interventions were the ones that were short-term and that addressed concrete behaviors. Unfortunately, very few of them have been tested with and/or developed for ethnic minority families. An example of an effective intervention targeting attachment is Child–Parent Psychotherapy (CPP; Lieberman and Van Horn 2005) which connects parents' childhood experiences to the interaction with their own children. A therapist observes and addresses the dynamics between parent and child during play and other unstructured interactions. CPP is mainly used with economically disadvantaged and traumatized families with children below the age of five. Several randomized control trial have shown the program's success, with medium to large effect sizes. The CPP program has been applied to families from various ethnic backgrounds in the US (e.g., Weiner et al. 2009). Another effective intervention is the Video-feedback Intervention to promote Positive Parenting and Sensitive Discipline (VIPP-SD; Juffer et al. 2008). The intervention consists of six home visits of which the first four have their own themes with regard to sensitivity and discipline, and the last two sessions are booster sessions to review the themes from the previous sessions (see Mesman et al. 2008 for a full description of the VIPP-SD intervention sessions). Recently, the VIPP-SD has been fine-tuned to suit Turkish minority mothers in the Netherlands, and the resulting VIPP-Turkish Minorities (VIPP-TM) has been successful in improving the sensitivity and non-intrusiveness of mothers in interaction with their toddlers in a randomized control study, with small effect sizes (Yagmur et al. 2014). Cultural-tuning of the VIPP-SD program consisted of replacing certain tasks because some of the original materials were not familiar to the Turkish families (e.g., playing with hand puppets was replaced by playing with clay). Also, the verbal language use of the experimenters was matched with the language of the mother. The appropriateness and effectiveness of intervention programs for ethnic minority families could benefit from sensitivity to parents' linguistic and cultural customs.

Several other attachment interventions have been successfully applied to samples including ethnic minority families, but without specifying the results for these various groups. An example

is the Attachment and Biobehavioral Catch-up (ABC) program, which targets mothers and their infant or toddler exposed to early adversity and consists of 10 home-based sessions that are guided by a trained intervener and uses video recordings of mother–child interactions (Dozier et al. 2005). The program has shown positive behavioral effects (with medium effect sizes) as well as biological effects in both mothers and children in randomized control trials (e.g., Bernard et al. 2014). The Circle of Security (COS) program (Powell et al. 2014) has also shown positive results with a randomized control trial including ethnic minorities (Cassidy et al. 2011). A trained intervener teaches parents about attachment and helps them in examining their own parenting experiences and behaviors. Video materials and graphical depictions of attachment concepts are used. Fewer studies on the effectiveness of COS are available, compared to the three previously discussed intervention programs. Programs such as ABC and COS could benefit greatly from explicitly examining ethnic minority groups, preferably with randomized control designs.

General parenting interventions that tap into, but are not specifically aimed at, improving sensitivity or attachment have been successfully applied to ethnic minority groups. Many studies on the outcomes of (Early) Head Start have presented combined results for various ethnicities in the sample (e.g., Love et al. 2005). However, some studies took a closer look at ethnicity, such as a recent study on the effectiveness of Early Head Start with African-American families (Harden et al. 2012). The results showed that the program positively affected parenting aspects such as supportiveness. Studies with the Incredible Years Parenting Program (Webster-Stratton 2001) have shown increased positive parenting skills (e.g., using more praise, being less critical and more consistent) among various ethnic minority groups in the US, UK, and in the Netherlands. A recent meta-analysis showed that the Incredible Years program was effective in diminishing disruptive behavior and in increasing prosocial behavior in children regardless of ethnic background (Menting et al. 2013). The effectiveness of the program with families from diverse backgrounds may originate from the flexibility of the program to be adjusted to the particular needs of parents.

In sum, although several general parenting interventions have reached ethnic minority parents in the US and Europe, only few programs specifically target sensitivity and attachment security. Programs focusing on these aspects of the parent–child relationship may benefit from testing their effectiveness in ethnic minority groups in studies using randomized control designs.

Universal Versus Culture-Specific Mechanisms

A wide range of factors could affect sensitive parenting and attachment security through a variety of mechanisms. Some of these factors and mechanisms are likely to be universal and therefore applicable across cultures, whereas others may be culture-specific. Socioeconomic status (SES) is an example of a universal factor affecting parenting and developmental outcomes. Two mechanisms have been widely described to explain the processes underlying SES effects (Conger and Donnellan 2007). The Family Stress model suggests that low SES relates to the experience of multiple stressors that increase parenting stress and negatively affect parenting, which in turn takes its toll on child outcomes. The Family Investment Model points out that low SES families generally do not have the means to foster their children's development by educational tools or by otherwise providing an enriching home environment. Group differences ascribed to differences in cultural beliefs or practices can in many cases be ascribed to SES rather than culture (Mesman et al. 2012b). Taking into account SES differences between groups generally leads to a decrease or even a disappearance of group differences.

However, SES-related factors do not suffice to fully explain cross-cultural differences in parenting in all studies (e.g., Yaman et al. 2010). Ethnic minority groups may experience stressors specific to their immigration history and experiences in the country of settlement that significantly affect their thoughts and behaviors which may translate into daily practices such as parenting. Acculturation (i.e., the process of cultural and psychological change that occurs when different cultures are in contact over time; Sam and Berry 2010) and discrimination are examples of such minority-specific experiences. In Turkish families in the Netherlands, the relation between SES and sensitive parenting was not only mediated by general stress, but also by acculturation stress (Emmen et al. 2013). These findings indicate that mechanisms affecting parenting and developmental outcomes cannot be easily generalized across contexts and groups. Not only is it important to be careful in generalizing from majority to minority groups, but also to take into account that ethnic minorities themselves may differ from each other substantially, for example with regard to experiences of acculturation stress or feelings of discrimination.

As mentioned in earlier sections, studies on attachment have been mainly limited to Western majority groups. The few studies that were conducted with non-Western groups provided valuable information on the factors that should be taken into account when testing the boundaries of the attachment construct. One of the cultural lessons learned is to widen the perspective on attachment from a dyadic point of view to include multiple attachment relationships (Jackson 1993; see also Keller 2013). Depending on cultural characteristics, predictors of attachment relations may vary and attachment relations with certain individuals may be more predictive of child outcomes than others. For example, the absence of a relation between maternal sensitivity and attachment security in an African-American sample (Ward and Carlson 1995) could possibly be explained by the mother not being the primary caregiver. However, alternative explanations cannot be ruled out, such as the instability of care provided by caregivers in challenging circumstances. The complex context in which children develop with multiple caregivers with multiple roles may ask for measurements of attachment and sensitivity that take into account this complexity and the multiplicity of input for child development, rather than considering relations among characteristics of a single caregiver and child outcomes as linear (Otto and Keller 2014). However, it needs to be stressed that regardless of the exact nature and number of attachment relationships, the mere availability of care could be limited by disadvantageous circumstances. Even though caregivers may be sensitive to the child's needs, unstable access to these caring adults could result in insecure rather than secure attachment patterns.

Policy Implications

The general conclusion that can be drawn from attachment research in ethnic minority families is that parental sensitivity and a secure child–parent relationship are generally important precursors to more optimal child development, similar to findings in ethnic majority families. Further, there is some evidence that attachment-based parenting interventions can be effective in ethnic minority families and can therefore be an important tool to improve the lives of families in need of support. Policies aimed at supporting struggling families in terms of providing parenting programs should therefore not distinguish between families from different ethnic backgrounds. Attachment-based interventions can be seen as basic groundwork for all struggling families across ethnicities, especially in early childhood, before work on more culturally sensitive issues such as discipline (e.g., Lansford et al. 2005) are addressed. As in many areas of intervention research, very few attachment-based interventions have been tested rigorously with RCT designs. However, the ones that have been shown to be effective in well-designed studies (e.g., VIPP-SD and CPP) deserve special attention when policy-makers decide which support programs to offer to ethnic minority families in need.

Because we do not yet know enough about the importance of the ethnic match (having the same ethnicity) versus the cognitive match (having the same ideas about the goals of the intervention) between parents and professionals in attachment-based parenting interventions, it may be fruitful to explicitly discuss such issues with parents before embarking on a therapeutic relationship that can make or break the intervention's effectiveness. Since research suggests that sensitive parenting and a securely attached child are valued across many cultures, discussing the parents' ideas about these topics might serve as an equalizer, i.e., a way to see past superficial (ethnic or socioeconomic) differences between the professional and the parent and to realize that there can be a common goal to work towards.

The attainment of sensitive parenting is likely to be hampered by daily stressors that go together with economic pressures that are unfortunately all too common in ethnic minority families in many societies. To facilitate the application of newly learned attachment-related skills in daily life, some relief on the economic front would be most helpful. Only when ethnic minority families are not weighed down by disproportionate economic stress will they have the same opportunities as ethnic majority families to build secure attachment relationships that have the potential to set their children on a positive developmental pathway.

Future Directions

Ethnic minority families are a very heterogeneous group with a huge variety of cultural backgrounds and smaller but significant variation in the majority cultural context and the origins of the minority status (e.g., labor migration versus post-colonial migration). It is all too likely that family processes in, for example, African Americans who share a language and religious orientation with the majority culture and often do not have a recent migration background, are very different from those in first-generation Turkish migrants in Norway who speak a different language and have a different religious orientation than their very new host culture, or from those in Somalian refugee families who have come to Europe to escape war and are often traumatized. Exactly how attachment-related family processes develop and show themselves in child function-ing may very well vary according to such dif-ferences in ethnic minority background and characteristics. However, it appears that this has never been investigated either empirically or theoretically and the ways in which such varia-tions might show themselves thus require further study. The field would greatly benefit from a more theoretical and more overarching approach to what it means to be part of an ethnic minority depending on such considerations and how this would affect family functioning in general and attachment-related family functioning in particular.

It is also important to note that the vast majority of research conducted on attachment and sensitivity in ethnic minority families focu-ses solely on mothers. This imbalance is also found in studies on ethnic majority families, but is probably more pronounced in minority populations because of more traditional cultural ideas about the role of men and women in childcare that are less likely to foster fathers' involvement and interest in parenting (such as in Turkish-Dutch families), and because of the absence of fathers as active caregivers (such as in low-income African-American populations). Further, many researchers are inexperienced in recruiting fathers for research and could benefit from expertise on specific strategies to include them in studies on parenting (such as ways of adapting information materials to be more attractive to fathers). However, there are some inspiring examples of studies in ethnic minority fathers (e.g., Cabrera et al. 2011; Caldwell et al. 2014) that do not focus specifically on attach-ment or sensitivity, but that can hopefully con-tribute to the inclusion of fathers in attachment studies in ethnic minorities in the future.

Further, the attachment research field has expanded its area of interest to the neurobiological and genetic underpinnings and consequences of attachment-related family processes (e.g., Fox and Hane 2008; Joosen et al. 2012; Riem et al. 2012). This line of research has yielded some very important and fundamental insights into the mechanisms underlying sensitivity, attachment, and child development. However, this area of study does not appear to have been applied to ethnic minority families yet. Since brain morphology and genetic characteristics are known to differ between ethnic groups (Brickman et al. 2008; Kitayama and Uskul 2011), the inclusion of these factors in studies on attachment and sensitivity in ethnic minority families would be very valuable.

Another important avenue for future research lies in randomized control trials to test the effectiveness of interventions in specific ethnic minority populations. There is some evidence that attachment-based interventions are useful across different ethnic groups, but well-designed intervention studies testing their effectiveness and the role of potential culture-specific adapta-tions to the delivery and content of such inter-ventions are rare. In a related vein, explicitly studying the relative importance of the ethnic match versus cognitive match between parent and professional in attachment-based interven-tions would also be informative and helpful to understanding therapeutic processes that may lead to enhanced parental sensitivity and child attachment security.

Empirical studies of attachment and sensitiv-ity generally employ observational methods, but very few studies address issues of the influence of coder and participant ethnicity on coding processes. This is unfortunate given that there is evidence for biased coding depending on the combination of coder and participant ethnic backgrounds (Melby et al. 2003; Yasui and Dishion 2008). Thus an important future direc-tion in attachment research in ethnic minority families is the careful monitoring of coding bias due to ethnicity, and ideally having all video-tapes double-coded by both matching ethnic minority and ethnic majority researchers (in many cases the latter would have to use trans-lated subtitles). This way, discrepancies between the two types of coders can be uncovered and discussed to provide a more thorough under-standing of culture-specific and culture-general aspects of attachment and sensitivity. It may also be helpful to allow for the coding of sensitivity of more than one caregiver in naturalistic observa-tions, as multiple caregivers are the norm rather than an exception in many cultural groups.

Finally, very few studies have explicitly aimed to elucidate the specific ways in which sensitivity and attachment are manifested across different cultures. The notion of universality without uniformity is informative, but would be much more powerful as a guiding principle in attachment theory and research if there is a broader knowledge base about the 'without uniformity' part of this idea. Filling this gap requires more in-depth analyses of extensive observational data that is likely to be hard to obtain. Nevertheless, the value of such observations and their analyses would by far exceed the efforts needed to obtain them, as they would fill in the blanks that are still present in our understanding of cultural specificity in attachment-related family processes.

References

Abe-Kim, J., Takeuchi, D. T., Hong, S., Zane, N., Sue, S., Spencer, M. S., et al. (2007). Use of mental health-related services among immigrant and US-born Asian Americans: Results from the National Latino and Asian American Study. *American Journal of Public Health, 97*(1), 91–98.

Ainsworth, M. D. S., Bell, S. M., & Stayton, D. J. (1974). Infant–mother attachment and social development: Socialisation as a product of reciprocal responsiveness to signals. In M. P. M. Richards (Ed.), *The introduction of the child into a social world* (pp. 9–135). London: Cambridge University Press.

Ainsworth, M. D. S., Blehar, M. C., Waters, E., & Wall, S. (1978). *Patterns of attachment*. Hillsdale, NJ: Erlbaum.

Arends-Tóth, J., & Van de Vijver, F. J. R. (2003). Multiculturalism and acculturation: Views of Dutch and Turkish-Dutch. *European Journal of Social Psychology, 33*(2), 249–266. doi:10.1002/ejsp.143

Bakermans-Kranenburg, M. J., & Van IJzendoorn, M. H. (2009). The first 10,000 Adult Attachment Interviews: Distributions of adult attachment representations in clinical and non-clinical groups. *Attachment & Human Development, 11*(3), 223–263. doi:10.1080/14616730902814762

Bakermans-Kranenburg, M. J., IJzendoorn, M. H., & Juffer, F. (2003). Less is more: Meta-analyses of sensitivity and attachment interventions in early childhood. *Psychological Bulletin, 129*(2), 195–215. doi:10.1037/0033-2909.129.2.195

Bakermans-Kranenburg, M. J., IJzendoorn, M. H., & Kroonenberg, P. M. (2004). Differences in attachment security between African-American and white

children: Ethnicity or socio-economic status? *Infant Behavior and Development, 27*(3), 417–433. doi:10.1016/j.infbeh.2004.02.002

Barnett, D., Kidwell, S. L., & Leung, K. H. (1998). Parenting and preschooler attachment among low-income urban African American families. *Child Development, 69*(6), 1657–1671. doi:10.1111/j.1467-8624.1998.tb06183.x

Bernard, K., Dozier, M., Bick, J., & Gordon, M. K. (2014). Normalizing blunted diurnal cortisol rhythms among children at risk for neglect: The effects of an early intervention. *Development and Psychopathology, 8*, 1–13.

Bernier, A., Carlson, S. M., & Whipple, N. (2010). From external regulation to self-regulation: Early parenting precursors of young children's executive functioning. *Child Development, 81*(1), 326–339. doi:10.1111/j.1467-8624.2009.01397.x

Bernstein, V. J., Harris, E. J., Long, C. W., Iida, E., & Hans, S. L. (2005). Issues in the multi-cultural assessment of parent–child interaction: An exploratory study from the starting early starting smart collaboration. *Journal of Applied Developmental Psychology, 26*(3), 241–275. doi:10.1016/j.appdev.2005.02.002

Biringen, Z. (2008). *Emotional availability (EA) scales manual (4th ed.): Part 1. Infancy/early childhood version (child aged 0–5 years).*

Bornstein, M. H. (1995). Parenting infants. In M. H. Bornstein (Ed.), *Handbook of parenting* (Vol. 1, pp. 3–39). Mahwah, NJ: Lawrence Erlbaum Associates.

Bost, K. K., Vaughn, B. E., Washington, W. N., Cielinski, K. L., & Bradbard, M. R. (1998). Social competence, social support, and attachment: Demarcation of construct domains, measurement, and paths of influence for preschool children attending Head Start. *Child Development, 69*(1), 192–218. doi:10.1111/j.1467-8624.1998.tb06143.x

Bowlby, J. (1969). *Attachment and loss, Vol. 1: Attachment*. New York, NY: Basic Books.

Bretherton, I. (2010). Fathers in attachment theory and research: A review. *Early Child Development and Care, 180*, 9–23.

Brickman, A. M., Schupf, N., Manly, J. J., Luchsinger, J. A., Andrews, H., Tang, M. X., et al. (2008). Brain morphology in older African Americans, Caribbean Hispanics, and whites from northern Manhattan. *Archives of Neurology, 65*(8), 1053–1061.

Cabrera, N. J., Hofferth, S. L., & Chae, S. (2011). Patterns and predictors of father–infant engagement across race/ethnic groups. *Early Childhood Research Quarterly, 26*(3), 365–375. doi:10.1016/j.ecresq.2011.01.001

Cabrera, N. J., Shannon, J. D., West, J., & Brooks-Gunn, J. (2006). Parental interactions with Latino infants: Variation by country of origin and English proficiency. *Child Development, 77*(5), 1190–1207. doi:10.1111/j.1467-8624.2006.00928.x

Caldwell, C. H., Antonakos, C. L., Assari, S., Kruger, D., De Loney, E. H., & Njai, R. (2014). Pathways to prevention: Improving nonresident African American fathers' parenting skills and behaviors to reduce sons' aggression. *Child Development, 85*(1), 308–325. doi:10.1111/cdev.12127

Carlson, V. J., & Harwood, R. L. (2003). Attachment, culture, and the caregiving system: The cultural patterning of everyday experiences among Anglo and Puerto Rican mother–infant pairs. *Infant Mental Health Journal, 24*(1), 53–73. doi:10.1002/imhj.10043

Carra, C., Lavelli, M., & Keller, H. (2014). Differences in practices of body stimulation during the first 3 months: Ethnotheories and behaviors of Italian mothers and West African immigrant mothers. *Infant Behavior and Development, 37*(1), 5–15. doi:10.1016/j.infbeh.2013.10.004

Cassidy, J. (2008). The nature of the child's ties. In J. Cassidy & P. R. Shaver (Eds.), *Handbook of attachment: Theory, research, and clinical applications* (pp. 3–22). New York: Guilford Press.

Cassidy, J., & Marvin, R. S. (1992). *Attachment organization in preschool children: Procedures and coding manual*. Charlottesville: University of Virginia.

Cassidy, J., Woodhouse, S., Sherman, L., Stupica, B., & Lejuez, C. W. (2011). Enhancing infant attachment security: An examination of treatment efficacy and differential susceptibility. *Development and Psychopathology, 23*(01), 131–148. doi:10.1017/S0954579410000696

Conger, R. D., & Donnellan, M. B. (2007). An interactionist perspective on the socioeconomic context of human development. *Annual Review of Psychology, 58*(1), 175–199. doi:10.1146/annurev.psych.58.110405.085551

De Wolff, M. S., & Van IJzendoorn, M. H. (1997). Sensitivity and attachment: A meta-analysis on parental antecedents of infant attachment. *Child Development, 68*(4), 571–591. doi:10.1111/j.1467-8624.1997.tb04218.x

Dozier, M., Lindhiem, O., & Ackerman, J. P. (2005). Attachment and biobehavioral catch-up. In L. J. Berlin, Y. Ziv, L. Amaya-Jackson, & M. T. Greenberg (Eds.), *Enhancing early attachments: Theory, research, intervention and policy* (pp. 178–194). New York: Guilford Press.

Durgel, E. S., Leyendecker, B., Yagmurlu, B., & Harwood, R. (2009). Sociocultural influences on German and Turkish immigrant mothers' long-term socialization goals. *Journal of Cross-Cultural Psychology,*. doi:10.1177/0022022109339210

Egeland, B., Erickson, M. F., Clemenhagen-Moon, J., Hiester, M. K., & Korfmacher, J. (1990). *24 months tools coding manual: Project steep-revised 1990 from Mother–Child Project scales*. Minneapolis, MN: University of Minnesota, Institute of Child Development.

Ekmekci, H., Yavuz-Muren, H. M., Emmen, R. A. G., Mesman, J., Van IJzendoorn, M. H., Yagmurlu, B., et al. (2014). Professionals' and mothers' beliefs about maternal sensitivity across cultures: Toward effective interventions in multicultural societies. *Journal of Child and Family Studies,*. doi:10.1007/s10826-014-9937-0

Emmen, R. A. G., Malda, M., Mesman, J., Ekmekci, H., & Van IJzendoorn, M. H. (2012). Sensitive parenting as a cross-cultural ideal: Sensitivity beliefs of Dutch, Moroccan, and Turkish mothers in the Netherlands. *Attachment & Human Development, 14*(6), 601–619. doi:10.1080/14616734.2012.727258

Emmen, R. A. G., Malda, M., Mesman, J., Van IJzendoorn, M. H., Prevoo, M. J. L., & Yeniad, N. (2013). Socioeconomic status and parenting in ethnic minority families: Testing a minority family stress model. *Journal of Family Psychology, 27*(6), 896. doi:10.1037/a0034693

Enlow, M. B., Egeland, B., Carlson, E., Blood, E., & Wright, R. J. (2014). Mother–infant attachment and the intergenerational transmission of posttraumatic stress disorder. *Development and Psychopathology, 26*(01), 41–65. doi:10.1017/S0954579413000515

Fox, N. A., & Hane, A. A. (2008). Studying the biology of human attachment. In J. Cassidy & P. R. Shaver (Eds.), *Handbook of attachment: Theory, research, and clinical applications* (pp. 217–240). New York: Guilford Press.

Fracasso, M. P., Busch-Rossnagel, N. A., & Fisher, C. B. (1994). The relationship of maternal behavior and acculturation to the quality of attachment in Hispanic infants living in New York City. *Hispanic Journal of Behavioral Sciences, 16*(2), 143–154. doi:10.1177/07399863940162004

Fuligni, A. S., & Brooks-Gunn, J. (2013). Mother–child interactions in Early Head Start: Age and ethnic differences in low-income dyads. *Parenting, 13*(1), 1–26. doi:10.1080/15295192.2013.732422

Fuligni, A. J., & Fuligni, A. S. (2007). Immigrant families and the educational development of their children. In J. E. Lansford, K. Deater-Deckard, & M. H. Bornstein (Eds.), *Immigrant families in contemporary society* (pp. 231–249). New York, NY: The Guilford Press.

Futh, A., O'Connor, T. G., Matias, C., Green, J., & Scott, S. (2008). Attachment narratives and behavioral and emotional symptoms in an ethnically diverse, at-risk sample. *Journal of the American Academy of Child and Adolescent Psychiatry, 47*(6), 709–718. doi:10.1097/CHI.0b013e31816bff65

George, C., Kaplan, N., & Main, M. (1984). *Adult Attachment Interview protocol*. Berkeley: University of California at Berkeley.

Goodman, G., Aber, J. L., Berlin, L., & Brooks-Gunn, J. (1998). The relations between maternal behaviors and urban preschool children's internal working models of attachment security. *Infant Mental Health Journal, 19*(4), 378–393. doi:10.1002/(SICI)1097-0355(199824)19:4<378::AID-IMHJ2>3.0.CO;2-J

Green, J., Stanley, C., Smith, V., & Goldwyn, R. (2000). A new method of evaluating attachment representations in young school-age children: The Manchester Child Attachment Story Task. *Attachment & Human Development, 2*(1), 48–70. doi:10.1080/146167300361318

Groh, A. M., Fearon, R. P., Bakermans-Kranenburg, M. J., Van IJzendoorn, M. H., Steele, R. D., & Roisman, G. I. (2014). The significance of attachment security for children's social competence with peers: A meta-analytic study. *Attachment & Human Development, 16*(2), 103–136. doi:10.1080/14616734.2014.883636

Grossmann, K., Grossmann, K. E., Fremmer-Bombik, E., Kindler, H., Scheuerer-Englisch, H., & Zimmerman, P. (2002). The uniqueness of the child–father attachment relationship: Fathers' sensitive and challenging play as a pivotal variable in a 16-year longitudinal study. *Social Development, 11*, 301–337. doi:10.1111/1467-9507.00202

Harden, B. J., Sandstrom, H., & Chazan-Cohen, R. (2012). Early Head Start and African American families: Impacts and mechanisms of child outcomes. *Early Childhood Research Quarterly, 27*(4), 572–581. doi:10.1016/j.ecresq.2012.07.006

Hesse, E. (2008). The Adult Attachment Interview: Protocol, method of analysis, and empirical studies. In J. Cassidy & P. R. Shaver (Eds.), *Handbook of attachment: Theory, research, and clinical applications* (pp. 552–598). New York: Guilford Press.

Howes, C., & Obregon, N. B. (2009). Emotional availability in Mexican-heritage low-income mothers and children: Infancy through preschool. *Parenting, 9*(3–4), 260–276. doi:10.1080/15295190902844589

Huang, Z., Lewin, A., Mitchell, S., & Zhang, J. (2012). Variations in the relationship between maternal depression, maternal sensitivity, and child attachment by race/ethnicity and nativity: Findings from a nationally representative cohort study. *Maternal and Child Health Journal, 16*(1), 40–50. doi:10.1007/s10995-010-0716-2

Ispa, J. M., Fine, M. A., Halgunseth, L. C., Harper, S., Robinson, J., Boyce, L., et al. (2004). Maternal intrusiveness, maternal warmth, and mother–toddler relationship outcomes: Variations across low-income ethnic and acculturation groups. *Child Development, 75*(6), 1613–1631.

Jackson, J. F. (1993). Multiple caregiving among African Americans and infant attachment: The need for an emic approach. *Human Development, 36*(2), 87–102.

Joosen, K. J., Mesman, J., Bakermans-Kranenburg, M. J., & Van IJzendoorn, M. H. (2012). Maternal sensitivity to infants in various settings predicts harsh discipline in toddlerhood. *Attachment & Human Development, 14*(2), 101–117. doi:10.1080/14616734.2012.661217

Juffer, F., Bakermans-Kranenburg, M. J., & Van IJzendoorn, M. H. (Eds.). (2008). *Promoting positive parenting: An attachment-based intervention.* Mahwah, NJ: Erlbaum.

Kärtner, J., Keller, H., & Yovsi, R. D. (2010). Mother–infant interaction during the first 3 months: The emergence of culture-specific contingency patterns. *Child Development, 81*(2), 540–554. doi:10.1111/j.1467-8624.2009.01414.x

Keller, H. (2013). Attachment and culture. *Journal of Cross-Cultural Psychology, 44*(2), 175–194. doi:10.1177/0022022112472253

Kelley, M. L., Smith, T. S., Green, A. P., Berndt, A. E., & Rogers, M. C. (1998). Importance of fathers' parenting to African-American toddler's social and cognitive development. *Infant Behavior and Development, 21*(4), 733–744.

Kermoian, R., & Leiderman, P. H. (1986). Infant attachment to mother and child caretaker in an East African community. *International Journal of Behavioral Development, 9*, 455–469.

Kitayama, S., & Uskul, A. K. (2011). Culture, mind, and the brain: Current evidence and future directions. *Annual Review of Psychology, 62*(1), 419–449. doi:10.1146/annurev-psych-120709-145357

Lansford, J. E., Chang, L., Dodge, K. A., Malone, P. S., Oburu, P., Palmérus, K., et al. (2005). Physical discipline and children's adjustment: Cultural normativeness as a moderator. *Child Development, 76*(6), 1234–1246. doi:10.1111/j.1467-8624.2005.00847.x

Leseman, P. P. M., & Van den Boom, D. C. (1999). Effects of quantity and quality of home proximal processes on Dutch, Surinamese-Dutch and Turkish–Dutch pre-schoolers' cognitive development. *Infant and Child Development, 8*(1), 19–38. doi:10.1002/(SICI)1522-7219(199903)8:1<19::AID-ICD187>3.0.CO;2-7

Lieberman, A. F., & Van Horn, P. (2005). *Don't hit my mommy: A manual for child–parent psychotherapy with young witnesses of family violence.* Washington: Zero to Three Press.

Lohaus, A., Keller, H., Lissmann, I., Ball, J., Borke, J., & Lamm, B. (2005). Contingency experiences of 3-month-old children and their relation to later developmental achievements. *The Journal of Genetic Psychology, 166*(4), 365–383. doi:10.3200/GNTP.166.4.365-384

Love, J. M., Kisker, E. E., Ross, C., Raikes, H., Constantine, J., Boller, K., et al. (2005). The effectiveness of early head start for 3-year-old children and their parents: Lessons for policy and programs. *Developmental Psychology, 41*(6), 885–901. doi:10.1037/0012-1649.41.6.885

Matias, C., O'Connor, T. G., Futh, A., & Scott, S. (2014). Observational attachment theory-based parenting measures predict children's attachment narratives independently from social learning theory-based measures. *Attachment & Human Development, 16*(1), 77–92. doi:10.1080/14616734.2013.851333

Melby, J. N., Hoyt, W. T., & Bryant, C. M. (2003). A generalizability approach to assessing the effects of ethnicity and training on observer ratings of family interactions. *Journal of Social and Personal Relationships, 20*(2), 171–191.

Menting, A. T. A., de Castro, B. O., & Matthys, W. (2013). Effectiveness of the incredible years parent training to modify disruptive and prosocial child behavior: A meta-analytic review. *Clinical Psychology Review, 33*(8), 901–913. doi:10.1016/j.cpr.2013.07.006

Mesman, J., & Emmen, R. A. G. (2013). Mary Ainsworth's legacy: A systematic review of observational instruments measuring parental sensitivity. *Attachment & Human Development, 15*(5–6), 485–506. doi:10.1080/14616734.2013.820900

Mesman, J., Oster, H., & Camras, L. (2012a). Parental sensitivity to infant distress: What do discrete negative emotions have to do with it? *Attachment & Human Development, 14*(4), 337–348. doi:10.1080/14616734. 2012.691649

Mesman, J., Stolk, M. N., Van Zeijl, J., Alink, L. R. A., Juffer, F., Bakermans-Kranenburg, M. J., et al. (2008). Extending the video-feedback intervention to sensitive discipline: The early prevention of antisocial behavior. In F. Juffer, M. J. Bakermans-Kranenburg, & M. H. Van IJzendoorn (Eds.), *Promoting positive parenting: An attachment-based intervention*. Mahwah, NJ: Erlbaum.

Mesman, J., Van IJzendoorn, M. H., & Bakermans-Kranenburg, M. J. (2012b). Unequal in opportunity, equal in process: Parental sensitivity promotes positive child development in ethnic minority families. *Child Development Perspectives, 6*(3), 239–250. doi:10.1111/j.1750-8606.2011.00223.x

Mesman, J., Van IJzendoorn, M. H., & Sagi-Schwartz, A. (2016a). Cross-cultural patterns of attachment: Universal and contextual dimensions. In J. Cassidy & P. R. Shaver (Eds.), *Handbook of attachment: Theory, research, and clinical applications* (pp. 852–877). New York: Guilford Press.

Mesman, J., Van IJzendoorn, M. H., Behrens, K., Carbonell, O. A., Cárcamo, R., Cohen-Paraira, I. et al. (2016b). Is the ideal mother a sensitive mother? Beliefs about early childhood parenting in mothers across the globe. *International Journal of Behavioral Development, 40*(5), 385–397. doi: 10.1177/0165025415594030

Mistry, R. S., Biesanz, J. C., Chien, N., Howes, C., & Benner, A. D. (2008). Socioeconomic status, parental investments, and the cognitive and behavioral outcomes of low-income children from immigrant and native households. *Early Childhood Research Quarterly, 23*(2), 193–212. doi:10.1016/j.ecresq.2008.01.002

Otto, H., & Keller, H. (Eds.). (2014). *Different faces of attachment: Cultural variations on a universal human need*. Cambridge, UK: Cambridge University Press.

Pederson, D. R., Moran, G., & Bento, S. (1999). *Maternal behaviour Q-sort*. London, ON: University of Western Ontario.

Posada, G., Jacobs, A., Richmond, M. K., Carbonell, O. A., Alzate, G., Bustamante, M. R., et al. (2002). Maternal caregiving and infant security in two cultures. *Developmental Psychology, 38*(1), 67–78. doi:10.1037/0012-1649.38.1.67

Posada, G., Lu, T., Trumbell, J., Kaloustian, G., Trudel, M., Plata, S. J., et al. (2013). Is the secure base phenomenon evident here, there, and anywhere? A cross-cultural study of child behavior and experts' definitions. *Child Development, 84*(6), 1896–1905. doi:10.1111/cdev.12084

Powell, B., Cooper, G., Hoffman, K., & Marvin, B. (2014). *The circle of security intervention: Enhancing attachment in early parent-child relationships*. New York: Guilford Press.

Riem, M. M. E., Bakermans-Kranenburg, M. J., van IJzendoorn, M. H., Out, D., & Rombouts, S. A. R. B. (2012). Attachment in the brain: Adult attachment representations predict amygdala and behavioral responses to infant crying. *Attachment & Human Development, 14*(6), 533–551. doi:10.1080/14616734. 2012.727252

Riksen-Walraven, J. M., Meij, J. T., Hubbard, F. O., & Zevalkink, J. (1996). Intervention in lower-class Surinam-Dutch families: Effects on mothers and infants. *International Journal of Behavioral Development, 19*(4), 739–756. doi:10.1177/016502549601900404

Sam, D. L., & Berry, J. W. (2010). Acculturation: When individuals and groups of different cultural backgrounds meet. *Perspectives on Psychological Science, 5*(4), 472–481. doi:10.1177/1745691610373075

Schölmerich, A., Lamb, M. E., Leyendecker, B., & Fracasso, M. P. (1997). Mother–infant teaching interactions and attachment security in Euro-American and Central-American immigrant families. *Infant Behavior and Development, 20*(2), 165–174. doi:10.1016/S0163-6383(97)90019-9

Schweder, R. A., & Sullivan, M. A. (1993). Cultural psychology: Who needs it? *Annual Review of Psychology, 44*, 497–523. doi:10.1146/annurev.psych.44.1.497

Shmueli-Goetz, Y., Target, M., Fonagy, P., & Datta, A. (2008). The child attachment interview: A psychometric study of reliability and discriminant validity. *Developmental Psychology, 44*(4), 939–956. doi:10.1037/0012-1649.44.4.939

Solomon, J., & George, C. (2008). The measurement of attachment security and related constructs in infancy and early childhood. In J. Cassidy & P. R. Shaver (Eds.), *Handbook of attachment: Theory, research, and clinical applications* (pp. 383–416). New York: Guilford Press.

Sroufe, L. A., Egeland, B., Carlson, E. A., & Collins, W. A. (2005). *The development of the person*. New York: Guilford Press.

Sroufe, L. A., & Waters, E. (1977). Attachment as an organizational construct. *Child Development, 48*(4), 1184–1199. doi:10.1111/1467-8624.ep10398712

Tamis-LeMonda, C. S., Bornstein, M. H., & Baumwell, L. (2001). Maternal responsiveness and children's achievement of language milestones. *Child Development, 72*(3), 748–767. doi:10.1111/1467-8624.00313

Tamis-LeMonda, C. S., Way, N., Hughes, D., Yoshikawa, H., Kalman, R. K., & Niwa, E. Y. (2007). Parents' goals for children: The dynamic coexistence of individualism and collectivism in cultures and individuals. *Social Development, 17*, 183–209. doi:071124114012002-209

Target, M., Fonagy, P., & Shmueli-Goetz, Y. (2003). Attachment representations in school-age children: the development of the child attachment interview (CAI). *Journal of Child Psychotherapy, 29*(2), 171–186. doi:10.1080/0075417031000138433

Van IJzendoorn, M. H. (1990). Attachment in Surinam-Dutch families: A contribution to the cross-cultural study of attachment. *International Journal of Behavioral Development, 13*(3), 333–344. doi:10.1177/016502549001300306

Van IJzendoorn, M. H., & Sagi-Schwartz, A. (2008). Cross-cultural patterns of attachment: Universal and contextual dimensions. In J. Cassidy & P. R. Shaver (Eds.), *Handbook of attachment: Theory, research, and clinical applications* (pp. 880–905). New York: Guilford Press.

Van IJzendoorn, M. H., Vereijken, C. M. J. L., Bakermans-Kranenburg, M. J., & Marianne R.-W. J. (2004). Assessing attachment security with the attachment Q sort: Meta-analytic evidence for the validity of the observer AQS. *Child Development, 75* (4), 1188–1213. doi:10.1111/j.1467-8624.2004. 00733.x

Vaughn, B. E., & Waters, E. (1990). Attachment behavior at home and in the laboratory: Q-sort observations and strange situation classifications of one-year-olds. *Child Development, 61*(6), 1965–1973. doi:10.1111/j.1467-8624.1990.tb03578.x

Ward, M. J., & Carlson, E. A. (1995). Associations among adult attachment representations, maternal sensitivity, and infant–mother attachment in a sample of adolescent mothers. *Child Development, 66*(1), 69–79. doi:10.1111/1467-8624.ep9503233294

Waters, H. S., & Waters, E. (2006). The attachment working models concept: Among other things, we build script-like representations of secure base experiences. *Attachment & Human Development, 8*(3), 185–197. doi:10.1080/14616730600856016

Webster-Stratton, C. (2001). *The incredible years: Parents and children videotape series: A parenting course (BASIC)*. Seattle, WA: Incredible Years.

Weiner, D. A., Schneider, A., & Lyons, J. S. (2009). Evidence-based treatments for trauma among culturally diverse foster care youth: Treatment retention and outcomes. *Children and Youth Services Review, 31* (11), 1199–1205. doi:10.1016/j.childyouth.2009.08. 013

Yagmur, S., Mesman, J., Malda, M., Bakermans-Kranenburg, M. J., & Ekmekci, H. (2014). Video-feedback intervention increases sensitive parenting in ethnic minority mothers: A randomized control trial. *Attachment & Human Development, 16*(4), 371–386. doi:10.1080/14616734.2014.912489

Yaman, A., Mesman, J., van IJzendoorn, M. H., Bakermans-Kranenburg, M. J., & Linting, M. (2010). Parenting in an individualistic culture with a collectivistic cultural background: The case of Turkish immigrant families with toddlers in the Netherlands. *Journal of Child and Family Studies, 19*(5), 617–628. doi:10.1007/s10826-009-9346-y

Yasui, M., & Dishion, T. J. (2008). Direct observation of family management: Validity and reliability as a function of coder ethnicity and training. *Behavior Therapy, 39*(4), 336–347. doi:10.1016/j.beth.2007.10. 001

Zwirs, B. W. C., Burger, H., Schulpen, T. W. J., & Buitelaar, J. K. (2006). Different treatment thresholds in non-western children with behavioral problems. *Journal of the American Academy of Child and Adolescent Psychiatry, 45*(4), 476–483. doi:10.1097/ 01.chi.0000192251.46023.5a

Conceptualizing Variability in U.S. Latino Children's Dual-Language Development

Kelly Escobar and Catherine S. Tamis-LeMonda

Abstract

Approximately 25 % of the population of children in the United States comes from Latino families, many of whom are immigrants and speak Spanish in the home, and this number is steadily growing. However, research on dual-language learning Latino children is lacking, especially in the field of language development. In order to move toward a framework of positive development of Latino children, it is important to understand the inter- and intra-individual variability that exists within language development of the DLL population in order to highlight their unique skills and advantages that extend beyond the domain of language. Moreover, a focus on variability can prevent negative biases and help researchers and practitioners better support young DLLs in their early education. Accordingly, this chapter presents two main research questions: 1) What does the early language variability of young Latino DLLs look like? 2) What factors might contribute to this variability?

Historical Overview

Approximately one in four children in the United States is Latino, and the majority of these children (71 %) come from immigrant families and live in Spanish-speaking homes (García and Jensen 2009; Zong and Batalova 2015). These children are considered dual-language learners (DLLs): children 0–5 years of age who experience and learn through two distinct languages during a critical developmental period (Castro et al. 2013). Over the last decade, U.S. schools have experienced an enormous increase (105 %) in the number of DLLs, 80 % of who come from Spanish-speaking homes (Collins et al. 2014). Despite growing numbers, Latino DLLs are understudied and underserved in research and early education (Gutiérrez et al. 2010; Tienda and Haskins 2011). It is critical that empirical research addresses the early development and education of U.S. Latino

K. Escobar (✉) · C.S. Tamis-LeMonda
Department of Applied Psychology, Center for Research on Culture, Development and Education, Steinhardt School of Culture, Education and Human Development, New York University, Greene Street, 5th Floor and 410W, New York, NY, USA
e-mail: Kelly.escobar@nyu.edu

© The Editor(s) 2017
N.J. Cabrera and B. Leyendecker (eds.), *Handbook on Positive Development of Minority Children and Youth*, DOI 10.1007/978-3-319-43645-6_6

DLLs to better understand the individual and contextual factors that might shape their future academic success. To do so, research must attend to the variability that exists within the U.S. Latino DLL population, as focusing on global categories of "Latino," "immigrant," or "DLL" children might obscure important variability in children's development within and across these groups (Winsler et al. 2014).

Understanding variability is particularly important in moving toward a framework of positive development for young Latino DLLs. The majority of research on Latino DLL development generally compares DLL's skills to those of monolingual, English-speaking children (Hammer et al. 2014). For example in the domain of language, Spanish-speaking DLL children tend to have fewer words in their vocabularies than do English-speaking monolingual children. Here the focus tends to be on what children are lacking, leading to misinterpretations and biased conclusions about these populations (Cabrera et al. 2013; Castro et al. 2013). However, by focusing on strengths and examining Latino DLL's vocabulary in both languages combined, their vocabularies are at level-with, if not greater than, their monolingual peers (e.g., Oller and Jarmulowicz 2007; Oller et al. 2007), and although the variability in language development is large, it makes it possible for DLL children to "lag" behind monolinguals yet still fall within the normal range (Bialystok and Feng 2011). In effect, the positive development of U.S. Latino DLL children is often masked by inferences made for Latinos as a group. Research should thus attend to the variability that might not have been examined or identified when comparing children to monolingual, mainstream counterparts. Understanding variability in the language development of Latino DLL children will help researchers and practitioners better support young DLLs by considering a wide range of features that uniquely characterize their development (Castro et al. 2013).

Moreover, understanding the variability and positive development of Latino DLLs will highlight unique skills and advantages beyond the domain of language development. For example,

DLL children vary significantly in the extent to which they are exposed to and use both Spanish (L1) and English (L2). Consistent dual-language exposure and usage trains the brain in a way that heightens the EF system, and thus Latino DLLs are likely to develop more efficient attentional and inhibitory skills as their proficiency in both languages increases (Kroll et al. 2014). In effect, increased multilingual experience leads to a cognitive advantage (Barac et al. 2014), and this advantage serves as a developmental asset that might explain help DLL children's academic success (Galindo and Fuller 2010).

Accordingly, there is need for research on U.S. Latino DLLs from immigrant families during the *early* years, as DLL children are exposed to varying degrees of each language from birth, and their dual language experiences are associated with the development of various academic, cognitive, and socio-emotional skills (e.g., Barac et al. 2014; Bialystok and Feng 2011). This gap in the knowledge base has created challenges for schools and communities, leaving teachers and policy makers ill-equipped to meet the needs of U.S. Latino DLL children by the time they reach the early school years (Castro et al. 2013). In this chapter, we focus on the language development of U.S. Latino DLLs during infancy, with attention to the variability of children's language experiences, and how variability shapes children's language development.

Theoretical Perspectives

Research on the language development of U.S. Latino DLLs requires an ecocultural approach (Bronfenbrenner 1989; Weisner 2002), which focuses on the intersecting, multiple systems in which children are embedded, and the ways children relate to and interact within those systems. We focus on the microsystem of the home setting because the early experiences of Latino DLLs begin in the home and comprise the core social influences within young children's zone of proximal development (Vygotsky 1978). This approach attends to the values and goals that underlie parenting practices. Immigrant and

Latino parents have high hopes that their children will do well in school, master English, and excel in the future labor market (Ng et al. 2012; Yoshikawa 2011). When asked about the qualities they hope to see in their children, mothers of Dominican and Mexican descent uniformly highlighted the importance of children's learning, achievement, and personal growth (Ng et al. 2012). Many Latino immigrant parents faced extreme hardships to migrate to the United States, and given their low socioeconomic status and levels of formal schooling, educating their children is viewed as a path to children's social and economic mobility (Ng et al. 2012).

The theoretical framework of *developmental cascades* highlights the cumulative effects of early disparities and motivates our focus on language development during the first years of life (Bornstein et al. 2006; Marchman and Fernald 2008; Masten and Cicchetti 2010; Smith and Thelen 2003). According to this theory, emerging skills and experiences during infancy have cascading influences on development across domains and at later points in time. For example, children growing up in a language-rich home environment excel in their vocabulary and language development (e.g., Hart and Risley 1995), which in turn has consequences for language and literacy development years later (e.g., Marchman and Fernald 2008; Snow et al. 1998). Thus, understanding language development from birth through age 4 years is of paramount importance, as children's early skills are rapidly emerging through interactions in their daily settings, allowing them to acquire foundational competencies that will prepare them for later school experiences.

Young children who enter school with the requisite developmental abilities are at an advantage in their ability to learn language-based skills, such as reading, writing, and communicating appropriately, for two main reasons. First, "skills build on skills" such that later achievements rest on foundations that were laid down earlier (e.g., early oral language supports later storytelling; Smith and Thelen 2003). Second, young children "co-construct" their social experiences, such that their skills shape other people's

interactions with them (Sameroff and Fiese 2000). For example, children who display strong language skills elicit responsiveness and stimulation from their parents and teachers, which in turn facilitate the acquisition of new skills (Hoff 2006; Pearson 2007; Tamis-LeMonda et al. 2001). In this regard, young children's social experiences, including their own contributions to interactions with other people, provide a springboard for later learning and school success.

Current Research Questions

Children experience a great deal of variability during early language development (Hoff 2009). Although variability in monolingual children is reasonably well documented, variability in multilingual children is not. Multilingual children display greater variability than do their monolingual counterparts because they typically experience each language in different contexts and with different people throughout the life course (Conboy and Mills 2006; Marchman et al. 2010). Accordingly, two questions frame the current chapter: What does the early language variability of young U.S. Latino DLLs look like? What factors contribute to this variability? To date, these questions remain largely unanswered.

Conceptualizing Variability

Variability of language development in DLL Latino children can be conceptualized in several ways, just as is the case for the language development of children more broadly. First, we consider variability within time, that is, at a specific child age. At the *group level*, substantial differences exist in both the language development and experiences that support skill development of U.S. Latino children from different backgrounds. The adult Latino population varies on income, education, language preference, English proficiency, literacy practices, generational status, and acculturation, thereby creating vastly different home environments for children

(Zong and Batalova 2015). However, focus is typically on low-income, at-risk Latino families, which overlooks the unique cultural factors that may affect the language development of Latino children from more advantaged backgrounds. Information on Latino populations from relatively higher socio-economic strata is lacking, perhaps because they comprise a smaller proportion of the Latino population in the United States. Nonetheless, this omission paints a narrow picture of language development in the population of U.S. Latino DLLs, and also confounds socio-economic status with culture.

We also consider variability within time at the *individual level*. Children vary at any given age in their language skills (Song et al. 2012). For instance, although there tend to be mean level differences favoring high-income children, there exist substantial within-group variations. Even when researchers focus on what is considered to be a "homogenous" group of low-income, first-generation Latino children, such as infants of Mexican immigrants, they find that children's skills span the full range seen in any other sample.

Third, we consider variability across *developmental time*, including rates of change in children's language skill growth. For instance, children vary in how many new words they add to their lexicons each month. Rate of language growth is certainly relevant to the U.S. Latino DLLs. In one study, the vocabulary development of low-income Dominican and Mexican children showed substantial variation from 14 months to 2 years (Song et al. 2012), a finding previously observed in children from other ethnic groups (Jackson-Maldonado et al. 2003).

Notably for DLLs, the three forms of heterogeneity—between groups, across individuals, and across developmental time—must be examined in *multiple languages*. That is, Latino DLLs vary in the relative sizes of their Spanish *and* English vocabularies at any given age. Moreover, Latino DLLs vary in the growth of their English and Spanish across developmental time. Examples of these different forms of variability are presented later in the chapter.

What Factors Contribute to Variability?

Identifying the determinants of language variability is critical to supporting the future academic success of diverse children in the United States. We consider three parent-level variables that might influence variability: (1) parental dual-language input, (2) parents' generational status and time in the United States, and (3) socioeconomic status. Although there are many more broad contextual factors that influence children's dual-language development (e.g., experiences with other caregivers), we focus on these three contextual factors to highlight the prevalence of parent-level influences during the first years of life.

Research Measurement and Methodology

In general, it is difficult to directly assess children's language skills in the laboratory during the first 2 years of life, and thus a variety of methods have been employed by researchers to measure language development in children, including direct assessments of child language as well as information gathered from parents (predominantly mothers). Some researchers have used preferential looking tasks in the laboratory to capture estimates of children's early language processing and receptive language skills (e.g., Fernald et al. 2008; Hurtado et al. 2014), whereas others often rely on parent-report measures acquire or list of words that children currently use and understand (such as the MacArthur CDI; Fenson et al. 2004). Other types of methods include naturalistic observations of caregiver-child interactions, which provide researchers the opportunity to examine parent and child language use, as well as the temporal features of language inputs and the non-verbal exchanges between children and caregivers. These naturalistic methods are particularly valuable in studies of early child language in social context (Pan et al. 2004), especially when trying to consider sources of variability in children's language development. As children increase in their language skills, researchers might turn to standardized assessments to measure children's receptive and expressive skills (Duursma et al. 2008).

However, there are several factors that need to be taken into consideration when assessing the language skills of DLL children. Latino children who speak Spanish and English might not be equally proficient in both languages, and often researchers consider assessing children in their dominant language. In doing so, researchers might miss the full spectrum of children's lexical and grammatical knowledge, and thus many assessments have been translated from English to Spanish, such as the TVIP (Spanish version of the PPVT) and the IDHC (Spanish version of the MacArthur CDI). However, many translated assessments do not show as strong validity reliability as their English counterparts when used with culturally and linguistically diverse samples (Vogel et al. 2008), creating opportunities for measurement error. For this reason, researchers might consider assessments normed with Spanish–English bilingual children, such as the PLS-5 (Zimmerman et al. 2012), which aim to capture children's conceptual language skills rather than the individual lexical and grammatical skills in Spanish and in English. Decisions about language administration should depend on whether researchers want to capture children's lexical and grammatical skills in each language individually, or whether they want to capture children's total conceptual knowledge as a combination of both languages (Barrueco et al. 2012). Nevertheless, the variety of available methods provide valuable information on children's language skills and experiences.

Empirical Findings

We address the first research question by describing what is currently known about the variability in Latino DLL's early language development. Then we turn to a review of the factors found to contribute to these various forms of variability to answer the second research question.

Characterizing Variability in Language Development

As previously discussed, variability in language development for Latino children can be conceptualized in three ways: (1) within time (at the group level and individual level); (2) over developmental time; and (3) across two languages (Spanish and English).

Variability Within Time

Considering variability at one point in time, there exist meaningful between-group differences in children's language skills. Data from our lab show that 2-year old children from low-income Dominican immigrant backgrounds produced more words in both L1 and L2 combined than did children from Mexican immigrant backgrounds. Specifically, the average productive vocabulary size of Dominican children was 178.79 words and the productive vocabulary size of Mexican children was 137.89 words (Fig. 1).

However, a sole emphasis on between-group differences overlooks the enormous within-group heterogeneity that exists. Infants of any given group vary in language skill, such as how many words they can produce or understand. For instance, the vocabularies of the Dominican- and Mexican-heritage 2-year olds were characterized by enormous standard deviations (SD = 115.70 and 106.43, respectively). Thus, Dominican 2-year old children had productive vocabularies that ranged from 2 words to 527 total words (L1 and L2 combined), and Mexican children's productive vocabularies ranged from 15 to 446 words. Data such as these indicate the need to consider Latino DLL children's language development at the individual level. By focusing only on between-group differences, researchers emphasize language disparities but fail to recognize subgroups of children within each population who demonstrate relatively strong or weak language skills.

This large within-group, within-time variability has been documented by others (Hurtado et al. 2014). A study measuring vocabulary in Spanish and in English separately found that U.S.

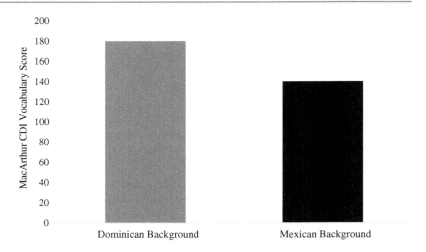

Fig. 1 Expressive vocabulary scores for Dominican and Mexican children at 24 months as measured by the MacArthur MCDI

Latino children's expressive Spanish vocabulary at 30 months ranged from 4 words to 676 words, and their receptive vocabulary in Spanish ranged from 87 words to 120 words. Large variability was also observed in their English vocabularies, such that expressive vocabulary ranged from 47 to 131 words and receptive vocabulary ranged from 17 to 667 words (Hurtado et al. 2014). These findings also show the importance of considering what language looks like in each of the two languages—L1 and L2—a point we return to in sections following.

Variability Over Time

Young children—monolingual and bilingual alike—also demonstrate considerable individual differences in their growth of language as they get older (Huttenlocher et al. 2010). These findings on varying rates of change generalize to the growth trajectories of Spanish–English speaking children as well. For example, in our lab, we followed U.S.-born Latino children yearly from ages 2 to 5, and examined their growth in both L1 and L2 word usage (Tamis-LeMonda et al. 2014a, b). For each language, children varied immensely in their rates of change across the three year period in terms of how many different words they used (word types) and how many words they used (word tokens) during a book-sharing interaction with their mothers. To illustrate, consider the variability that characterizes changes in Spanish word types of children from

Dominican immigrant backgrounds (Fig. 2). Each line represents an individual child, and shows that children show growth as well as decline in the L1 usage, and rates of change, represented by the different slopes of lines, vary considerably among the sample. These results highlight the importance of moving beyond group averages to documenting individual variability in Latino children's growth in language over time.

Variability Over Time in Two Languages

The across-age findings reported above are based on changes in children's use of Spanish. However, it is important to consider profiles of developmental change over time in both L1 and L2. These over-time-two- language profiles can be presented at either the group or individual level. To illustrate, Fig. 3 shows the group function of low-income Dominican children in the sample, indicating that although as a group children averaged equal numbers of word types per minute in L1 and L2 at 2 years of age, their L2 skills continued to grow while their L1 skills began to level off, likely reflecting children's increased exposure to English during preschool and kindergarten. The growth in English vocabulary over time is similar to what is seen in monolingual children, who also expand their vocabularies over the childhood years with exposure to new words and concepts at school.

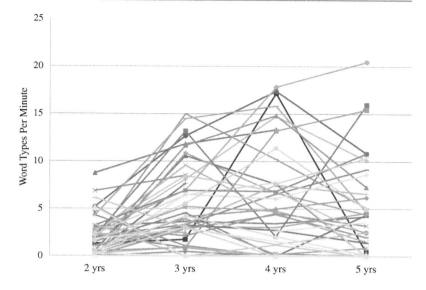

Fig. 2 Individual differences in Spanish language trajectories of Dominican children from ages 2 to 5, as measured by average number of word types produced per minute

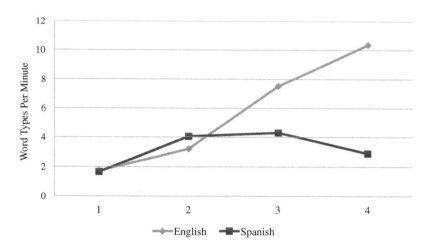

Fig. 3 Average language trajectory of Dominican heritage children from ages 2 to 5 as measured by average number of word types produced per minute

Considering variability by language in individual children, different profiles of changing language use can be identified. Some children display growth in *both* L1 and L2, perhaps reflecting emphases by families on the importance of children learning English at school while maintaining the Spanish language and culture in their homes (Worthy and Rodríguez-Galindo 2006). Strong support for each language creates a language profile that shows simultaneous growth in vocabulary and language skills in English and Spanish. Some Latino children switch from predominantly L1 to predominantly L2 usage over time. As family members become increasingly acculturated and children enter childcare and preschool settings, there is often increased exposure to English that will prevail over the current knowledge of Spanish. Under such circumstances, if Spanish is not strongly supported in the home or school, children will begin to reduce in their Spanish use while concurrently showing growth in their English language skills.

In our own research we identified four profiles of changes in children's English and Spanish

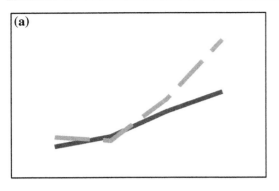

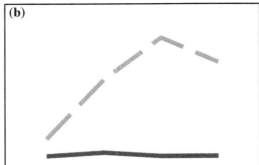

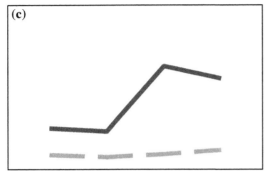

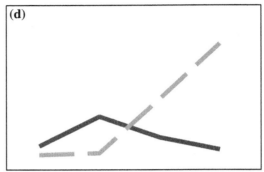

Fig. 4 Observed profiles of Latino children's language trajectories. *Solid lines* represent expressed word types per minute in English; *dashed lines* represent expressed word types per minute in Spanish. Profiles include: **a** Dual-language growth; **b** Growth in English; **c** Growth in Spanish; and **d** Change from Spanish to English dominance

language use across the ages of 2–5 years. Some children showed concomitant gains in both languages (Fig. 4a), likely reflecting strong support for the use of English and Spanish in their home environments. Some children were consistent in their English-dominance across time, likely reflecting predominantly English inputs at home, despite the immigrant status of their parents (Fig. 4b). Still others were consistently Spanish-dominant and used more Spanish than English from ages 2 to 5 (Fig. 4c), most likely representing the types of language development seen in children of recently immigrated parents. Conversely, some children were initially more Spanish-dominant, and over time shifted to become more English-dominant (Fig. 4d). This profile of change is likely to be most common for many children of immigrant parents as they are increasingly exposed to English in the host country, particularly at school. Notably, we did not

observe a shift in language dominance from English to Spanish. This is not surprising, since Latino children in the United States increasingly use English as they are exposed to the host language.

Explaining Variability in Language Development

Above we presented different ways that variability can be conceptualized in the study of young Latino children's language development. A question that naturally arises is: What might explain these individual differences? Here, we consider two main contributors to individual differences in young children's language development: (1) the nature of input from parents, and (2) broader contextual factors that influence parents' child-directed language use. Children's language development is also affected by inputs from caregivers outside the home as well as siblings and peers; however, parents tend to be the primary influences on language development in the first years of life. Moreover, U.S. Latino children, particularly those of recent immigrants, are less likely to attend nursery or preschool in the early years than are their monolingual English-speaking peers (Yoshikawa 2011). Older siblings often provide young Latino DLLs with opportunities to be exposed to and use English (Anderson 2012; Iglesias and Rojas 2012). As such, Latino DLL children with older siblings tend to become proficient in English at an earlier age than those without older siblings. However, siblings are rather understudied in any cultural group, compared to the vast majority of work done on mother-child relationships and the effect of peers and teachers on children (Barron-Hauwaert 2011). As a result, we focus on parent-level contextual factors, which only touch the surface of variability within Latino families, but can serve as a framework for thinking about variability more explicitly.

Nature of the Input

During the early years, mothers and fathers are main contributors to infants' language experiences. A recent study on Latino bilingual infants showed that parent–child interactions accounted for 77 % of the total time spent in conversations with others in the environment (Place and Hoff 2011), meaning that the majority of the time children are exposed to language, they are in the presence of their primary caregivers. Three features of parental language input largely affect the language development of DLL's: (1) amount and quality of language, (2) proficiency of language, and (3) relative use of Spanish and English. Moreover, all three features are influenced by broader contextual factors, including parent SES, which are reviewed later in the chapter.

Amount and quality of parent language are two of the strongest predictors of children's language skill. Children can only learn the words to which they are exposed, and adult caregivers offer children a multitude of language experiences during interactions that support children's growth in vocabulary. Specifically, the complexity, diversity, and frequency of parent-language use

with children predict children's vocabulary development (e.g., Hart and Risley 1995; Hoff 2003, 2006; Tamis-Lemonda et al. 2012a). In a study of children of Mexican and Dominican descent, changes in parents' language use over time predicted children's vocabulary growth in the respective language (Tamis-Lemonda et al. 2014a). In another study, Latina mothers of Spanish-learning infants were highly variable in their input to children, and these differences related to children's vocabulary size at age 2 (Hurtado et al. 2008). Specifically, infants of relatively talkative mothers heard seven times more words on average, three times more different words, and more complex sentences than those heard by infants of less talkative mothers. Additionally, positive associations were found between the percentages of words children produced in Spanish and English and estimates of input in each language (Hoff et al. 2012), such that substantial parental language input fosters a supportive environment for children to acquire any given language (Place and Hoff 2011).

Parents' proficiency of language input is also central to the development of children's language skills, such that children acquire language best when parents speak with them in the language in which parents are most comfortable (McCabe et al. 2013). Nearly ¾ (71 %) of Latino DLLs have at least one parent with limited English proficiency (LEP; Hernandez et al. 2007), and children of Mexican, Dominican, and Central American descent in particular are less likely to have parents who are proficient in English relative to other Latino children (Hernandez 2006). When parents with LEP speak English with their children, they are not necessarily improving children's skills in English, but might be sacrificing children's skills in Spanish (Hammer et al. 2009; Paradis et al. 2011).

However, exposure to fluent and native Spanish from early on can support children's development of their L2 (Brisk and Harrington 2007; Rinaldi and Páez 2008). Rich, high quality language exposure during early language development results in enhanced skills for children in the languages they are learning (McCabe et al. 2013). Children who are exposed to Spanish and

English from infancy start to learn both languages simultaneously, and their language trajectories in each language seem to follow the patterns observed for monolingual children (Conboy and Thal 2006; Parra et al. 2011). DLL children whose caregivers expose them to consistent, high quality, and proficient language input in both languages (to any degree of use in each language) before the age of 3 outperform other bilinguals who are exposed to the second language later (age 3 and on) on reading, phonological and syntactical awareness and overall language competence (Kovelman et al. 2008a, b). Children who are given opportunities to learn both languages from fluent speakers starting in infancy are unlikely to be hindered in their language development.

Parents' distribution of English and Spanish usage within and over time affects children's emerging skills in each of the two languages. Just as was observed for Latino children's language trajectories in English and Spanish, individual profiles of maternal language trajectories varied for both Mexican and Dominican mothers: Some mothers use English more than Spanish, whereas others use Spanish more than English, usually related to how long the mother has resided in the United States and how comfortable the mother is in each language. Moreover, mothers often switch their language use over time, such as by increasing the use of English and decreasing the use of Spanish. Findings from our work, however, did not show a profile of change in which mothers decreased English and increased Spanish, mirroring what was found for children's changing language use.

The profiles of parents' L1 and L2 use highlight variability in the *timing of children's exposure to different languages*. Some DLL children are referred to as simultaneous bilinguals, since they have been exposed to both languages early in life before L1 is solidified (Genesee 1989). Although their exposure to both languages is present very early on, their experiences with each of the two languages may be quantitatively and qualitatively distinct at any given time (Genesee et al. 1995). As a result, their comprehension and performance in each of

these languages will vary as a function of age of exposure and quantity and quality of the input. Sequential bilinguals, in contrast, are those who are exposed to one language (L1) in infancy and a second language (L2) a few years later, with significant variation existing in the timing and conditions under which the second language is introduced (Iglesias and Rojas 2012).

Broader Contextual Factors

As reviewed thus far, Latino parents provide dramatically different language environments to their children, and these differences powerfully influence the rates and profiles of children's vocabulary growth. However, parenting does not occur in a vacuum. Rather, several factors influence the amount of parent talk to children, the richness of their talk, and the language they use with their children on a daily basis. We discuss three characteristics that have been found to be of importance: generational status, parents' education, and family economic circumstances.

Parents' generational status and time spent in the United States are associated with parents' skills in the host language, and in turn the language development of their children. For example, the use of L2 within immigrant families increases over successive generations, such that the first generation tends to maintain the native language (Silva-Corvalan 2003; Veltman 2003), whereas subsequent generations begin to integrate L2 into their daily conversations and use L1 to varying degrees (Hurtado and Vega 2004). By the third generation, the native language is almost lost, leaving L2 as the primary spoken language used at home (Arriagada 2005). Generational status predicts DLL's vocabulary above parents' education, such that children of more educated parents have higher English vocabulary skills, but education did not play a role in children's Spanish vocabulary; rather, children's Spanish vocabularies were larger for those children whose mothers were immigrants (Hammer et al. 2012).

Consequently, it is important to consider the amount of time that family has resided in the United States rather than categorizing Latino immigrants into a homogenous group. Latino children from immigrant families (approximately

2/3 of the Latino population; Hernandez 2006) will encounter dramatically different experiences than will children whose parents are U.S. born. Latinos of different ethnicities, such as Mexican, Puerto Rican, or Peruvian, vary in nuanced aspects of culture, generation and legal status, years spent in the United States, and the degree of acculturation, which shape the daily contexts and experiences of children.

Drawing from the examples in our laboratory, low-income U.S.-born Dominican mothers showed greater increases in English language use over children's first 5 years of life than did low-income, immigrant Mexican mothers, an ethnic difference that reflects differences in mothers' time in the United States and skills with English (Tamis-LeMonda et al. 2014a, b). Specifically Dominican mothers had resided in the United States longer and were more educated than Mexican mothers.

Parents' socioeconomic status strongly relates to children's language outcomes (e.g. Fernald et al. 2013). Parent education levels are typically much lower in immigrant Latino families than they are for native-born Latinos and the U.S. adult population at large (Hernandez et al. 2007), and children from immigrant families originating in Mexico, Central America, and the Dominican Republic are likely to be among those whose parents have completed the fewest years of school (Hernandez et al. 2008). More years of schooling for immigrant parents is associated with higher levels of English proficiency, which affects children's English language skills by kindergarten (Bohman et al. 2010). Moreover, SES differences have implications for the quality and quantity of parents' language spoken to children (Hoff 2003, 2006). There exists a 6 month gap in language ability in DLL Latinos compared to monolinguals as early as 18 months (Fernald et al. 2013). Compared to low-responsive mothers, more responsive Latina mothers who talk more to their children at 18 months have children with larger vocabularies and faster language processing at 24 months (Hurtado et al. 2008).

Universal Versus Culture-Specific Mechanisms

We have provided a review of some of the contextual factors that contribute to the language development of U.S. Latino DLLs from immigrant backgrounds. Although we highlighted specific challenges and opportunities that come with learning two languages, several fundamental, universal principles of early language development based on research with monolingual children readily apply to the development of all DLL children. Consequently, many lessons learned in the language field more broadly are relevant to the language development of Latino DLL children (for a review, see McCabe et al. 2013).

First, the languages children learn, the rate at which they learn them, and thus the skill levels children display at every age reflect their everyday language experiences. Decades of research with monolingual children and more recent research with DLLs have identified properties of language experience that support children's language learning including the quantity and quality of caregiver speech, as described in this chapter.

Second, parents provide children the words of their language through both verbal and nonverbal behaviors. For example, parents' use of gestures facilitates matching words to referent objects by "narrowing the search space" and offering children a unitary language experience that allows them to perceive the word and the stimulus as "belonging together" (Rader and Zukow-Goldring 2010). Individuals from some cultural communities use gestures to a greater extent in communication than do others. Two-year old children from these cultural groups (e.g., Mexican children) display more gesture use and higher skills at sequencing and imitating actions and following commands that incorporate gestures despite lower expressive language than do children from other minority backgrounds (Tamis-LeMonda et al. 2012a, b). Moreover, language experiences that are prompt, contingent, and appropriate consistently predicts children's gains in language, especially during the first 2 years of life (e.g., Bornstein et al. 2008;

Goldstein and Schwade 2010). Contingent responses to infant behaviors promotes word learning by increasing the likelihood that infants will hear words that are the focus of their attention, thereby easing the referent-mapping task (Tamis-LeMonda et al. 2014a, b). Using both verbal and nonverbal language in integrated and meaningful contexts deepens children's conceptual knowledge and lexicons (Hirsh-Pasek et al. 2009). For example, an adult who talks about hammers, hard hats, screw drivers, and tool belts while building something with a child or reading a book about building things is providing an optimal type of context for acquiring extensive, connected vocabulary and concepts.

In the context of these universal principles, there exist several unique features of language experiences and development that are important to consider when investigating the development of DLLs. First, age of exposure to different languages is a topic of specific relevance. Children who hear two languages from infancy start to learn both languages simultaneously and the course of development in each language looks similar to that of monolingual children (Parra et al. 2011). Moreover, children who are exposed to proficient speakers in native and host languages before the age of 3 years outperform children with L2 exposure later than age 3 in language organization, such as morphology and phonology in both languages (Weber-Fox and Neville 1996, 2001; Kovelman et al. 2008a, b). Thus, if opportunities to learning more than one language from native speakers are available early on, the language development of DLL children will not be hindered.

Second, children exposed to more than one language differ in the strategies they use to map words to their referents when compared to monolingual children. Children learning multiple languages are more likely than are monolingual children to accept an additional, second label for a previously known object or action (Kovács and Mehler 2009; Yoshida 2008; but see Mervis et al. 1994). This makes sense since they soon learn that things in the world can have at least two names, one label for each language. In contrast, monolingual children assume that novel words refer to objects or events that do not yet have a label, since most things typically have a single name. Perhaps unsurprisingly, because dual language learning infants must navigate a world of multiple labels for the same object or event, growth in the individual vocabularies in each of the DLL's languages is slower compared to children learning one language (Carlo et al. 2004; McCabe et al. 2013). However, when the total language of DLL children is considered inclusive of L1 and L2, the overall rate of lexical growth and conceptual knowledge is at least equal to, if not greater than, the rates of growth seen in monolingual children (Hoff et al. 2012).

Finally, the cognitive advantage seen in executive functioning and attentional control in children who become fluent in two or more languages (e.g. Akhtar and Menjivar 2012; Bialystok 2015; Carlson and Meltzoff 2008; Poulin-Dubois et al. 2011) is particularly relevant to U.S. Latino DLL children. Multilinguals must constantly hold in mind the relevant language and inhibit the non-relevant language depending on the environment, and thus must pay attention to abstract dimensions of language and engage executive functions that monolinguals do not regularly have to do (Bialystok 2015). Preschoolers who are able to apply these regulatory skills to general classroom learning tasks and goals show higher levels of academic achievement than do their less regulated peers in later years (Denham et al. 2011), and thus multilingual children might have opportunities to develop and employ advanced regulatory skills. Consistent activation of these executive function areas affects and restructures neural pathways and brain structures (Costa and Sebastián-Gallés 2014), which might possibly slow the decline of executive functions during adulthood (e.g. Luk et al. 2011), suggesting that multilingual use and exposure throughout the lifespan could slow down the effects of aging.

Policy Implications and Future Directions

Research and practice at the level of the family should emphasize the ways that Latino parents can promote their children's development of early foundational skills. From a strengths-based perspective, Latino parents provide their children with emotional support, place high value on children's academic achievement and also put much effort into preparing their children for school (Cabrera et al. 2013). Thus, Latino parents' goals for children can serve as a starting point for designing strategies to effectively support children's development. These strategies might include highlighting practices that foster the development of language and literacy skills, such as book-reading (Raikes et al. 2006), reciting nursery rhymes and playing rhyming games (Baker et al. 1995), and sharing oral stories (Schick and Melzi 2010; Snow and Dickinson 1990). Additionally, practitioners should work with parents to identify family routines that present meaningful opportunities for children's everyday learning. For instance, we found that the emphasis on family solidarity in Mexican families means that most Mexican children eat meals with both their mothers and fathers on a daily basis (Tamis-LeMonda et al. 2009). Conversations during mealtime or other everyday routines provide young children with opportunities to practice and build oral language skills with different partners (e.g. Pan 1995; Ochs and Capps 2001; Reese 2012; Snow and Beals 2006). In order to effectively incorporate language and literacy into children's daily lives, some researchers are calling for two-generation literacy programs in which children and their parents can learn English together without losing their home language. Interventions must target parents and young children, keeping in mind that unauthorized immigrants are often excluded from programs (Crosnoe 2009).

Notably, parents' practices to promote their children's language development would be best when using the language with which the parent is most comfortable. Often, immigrant Latino parents with limited English proficiency believe that their children will not enter school with sufficient English skills if they do not speak English with them at home, resulting in the child being exposed to poor English that may impede development. The use of the host language in the homes of young immigrants only predicts positive development once parents have reached a certain level of proficiency in the L2 (Paradis et al. 2011). Early exposure to proficient language promotes fluent acquisition of that language (Kovelman et al. 2008a, b), which in turn has implications for the children's school readiness.

Because language experiences in the first years of life are critical to children's language development, it is important to educate and engage parents in children's language development early on, rather than wait until children are in school. One effective platform for such outreach is through pediatricians. Young children visit the doctor about fifteen times before the age of five (Hagan et al. 2008), thus the use of pediatric visits is an efficient way to reach difficult-to-reach populations, especially low-income and multilingual Latino families. The Video Interaction Project (VIP; Mendelsohn et al. 2005) is one example of a program that reached out to Latino families during child well visits. In the intervention group, mothers and newborns participated in one-on-one sessions with child development specialists who facilitated interactions during play and reading, using previously videotaped interactions from primary care visit days as guides for areas to work on. Studies of the VIP program found increased parent- child interactions from the intervention group, indicating effective engagement from multilingual families during early infancy (Mendelsohn et al. 2011).

Center-based programs provide the added opportunity to engage with caregivers from at-risk families with DLL children (McCabe et al. 2013). For example, federally funded programs such as Early Head Start work with parents directly (on site or through home visitation) to facilitate parent–child interactions. Although historically, DLL's have been underrepresented in all forms of early childhood education (García and García 2012), several federal programs have recently begun to establish learning principles specifically for children who are DLLs (Castro et al. 2013), requiring programs to address the needs of DLLs and their families across multiple development and service areas.

As is evident from this chapter, there is a need to identify ways to support and promote Latino DLLs' skills in both Spanish and English so that they become proficient speakers of the two languages and maintain proficiency over time. For many young U.S. Latino DLLs, school is the first setting that introduces them to English, which might lead to a considerable disadvantage at the start of school (Magnuson et al. 2006). Not all Latino children develop proficiency in both English and Spanish and some children develop English at the expense of competence in Spanish (García and Jensen 2009). For many such children these early disadvantages persist into adolescence, indicating the need for continued language support.

However, U.S. Latino children who develop solid bilingual skills can reap the benefits of bilingualism with regard to both language development and executive function. Thus researchers and practitioners must work to promote the development of both languages throughout the early years. Latino children with a strong bilingual skill set may ultimately perform at level with, if not better, than their monolingual counterparts upon entrance to formal schooling. These skills can be developed in the context of the family, and continue to be supported as needed by schools or programs that are equipped to work effectively with Spanish speakers (Hernandez et al. 2007). By understanding the variability the exists within the population of U.S. Latino children, researchers and policymakers can build on the strengths of children's language abilities and develop interventions to effectively improve Latino children's academic outcomes.

References

Akhtar, N., & Menjivar, J. A. (2012). Cognitive and linguistic correlates of early exposure to more than one language. In J. B. Benson (Ed.), *Advances in child development and behavior* (Vol. 42, pp. 41–78). Amsterdam: Elsevier.

Anderson, R. T. (2012). First language loss in Spanish-speaking children: Patterns of loss and implications for clinical practice. In B. A. Goldstein (Ed.), *Bilingual language development & disorders in Spanish–English speakers* (pp. 193–212). Baltimore, MD: Paul H. Brookes Publishing Co.

Arriagada, P. A. (2005). Family context and Spanish-language use: A study of Latino children in the United States. *Social Science Quarterly, 86,* 599–619.

Baker, L., Serpell, R., & Sonnenschein, S. (1995). Opportunities for literacy learning in the homes of urban preschoolers. In L. Morrow (Ed.), *Family literacy: Connections in schools and communities.* Newark: International Reading Association.

Barac, R., Bialystok, E., Castro, D. C., & Sanchez, M. (2014). The cognitive development of young dual language learners: A critical review. *Early Childhood Research Quarterly, 29,* 159–163.

Barron-Hauwaert, S. (2011). *Bilingual siblings: Language use in families.* Clevedon: Multilingual Matters.

Barrueco, S., López, M. L., Ong, C. A., & Lozano, P. (2012). *Assessing Spanish–English bilingual preschoolers: A guide to best measures and approaches.* Baltimore, MD: Brookes Publishing.

Bialystok, E. (2015). Bilingualism and the development of executive function: The role of attention. *Child Development Perspectives, 9,* 117–121.

Bialystok, E., & Feng, X. (2011). Language proficiency and its implications for monolingual and bilingual children. In A. Y. Durgunoğlu & C. Goldenberg (Eds.), *Language and literacy development in bilingual settings* (pp. 121–138). New York, NY: Guilford Press.

Bohman, T. M., Bedore, L. M., Peña, E. D., Mendez-Perez, A., & Gillam, R. B. (2010). What you hear and what you say: Language performance in Spanish–English bilinguals. *International Journal of Bilingual Education and Bilingualism, 13,* 325–344.

Bornstein, M. H., Hahn, C., Bell, C., Haynes, O. M., Slater, A., Golding, J., et al. (2006). Stability in cognition across early childhood: A developmental cascade. *Psychological Science, 17,* 151–158. doi:10.1111/j.1467-280.2006.01678.x

Bornstein, M. H., Tamis-LeMonda, C. S., Hahn, C., & Haynes, O. M. (2008). Maternal responsiveness to young children at three ages: Longitudinal analysis of a multidimensional, modular, and specific parenting construct. *Developmental Psychology, 44,* 867–874. doi:10.1037/0012-1649.44.3.867

Brisk, M. E., & Harrington, M. M. (2007). *Literacy and multilingualism: A handbook for all teachers* (2nd ed.). Mahwah, NJ: Erlbaum.

Bronfenbrenner, U. (1989). Ecological systems theory. *Annals of Child Development, 6,* 187–249.

Cabrera, N. J., Ethnic, The. S. C. R. D., & Committee, Racial Issues. (2013). Positive development of minority children. *Social Policy Report, 27,* 3–22.

Carlo, M. S., August, D., McLaughlin, B., Snow, C. E., Dressler, C., Lippman, D., et al. (2004). Closing the gap: Addressing the vocabulary needs for English language learners in multilingual and mainstream classrooms. *Reading Research Quarterly, 39*, 188–215. doi:10.1598/RRQ.39.2.3

Carlson, S. M., & Meltzoff, A. N. (2008). Bilingual experience and executive functioning in young children. *Developmental Science, 11*, 282–298.

Castro, D. C., García, E. E., & Markos, A. M. (2013). *Dual language learners: Research informing policy.* Chapel Hill, NC: The University of North Carolina, Frank Porter Graham Child Development Institute.

Collins, B. A., O'Connor, E. E., Suarez-Orozco, C., Nieto-Castanon, A., & Toppelberg, C. O. (2014). Dual language profiles of Latino children of immigrants: Stability and change over the early school years. *Applied Psycholinguistics, 35*, 581–620.

Conboy, B. T., & Mills, D. L. (2006). Two languages, one developing brain: Event-related potentials to words in bilingual toddlers. *Developmental Science, 9*, F1–F12.

Conboy, B. T., & Thal, D. J. (2006). Ties between the lexicon and grammar: Cross-sectional and longitudinal studies of bilingual toddlers. *Child Development, 77*, 712–735.

Costa, A., & Sebastián-Gallés, N. (2014). How does the bilingual experience sculpt the brain? *Nature Reviews Neuroscience, 15*, 336–345.

Crosnoe, R. (2009). Low-income students and the socioeconomic composition of public high schools. *American Sociological Review, 74*, 709–730.

Denham, S. A., Brown, C., & Domitrovich, C. E. (2011). Plays nice with others': Social emotional learning and academic success. *Corrigendum. Early Education and Development, 22*, 180.

Duursma, E., Pan, B. A., & Raikes, H. (2008). Predictors and outcomes of low-income fathers' reading with their toddlers. *Early Childhood Research Quarterly, 23*, 351–365.

Fenson, L., Dale, P. S., Reznick, J. S., Thal, D., Bates, E., Hartung, J. P., et al. (2004). *Macarthur communicative development inventories: User's guide and technical manual.* Baltimore, MD: Brookes.

Fernald, A., Marchman, V. A., & Weisleder, A. (2013). SES differences in language processing skill and vocabulary are evident at 18 months. *Developmental Science, 16*, 234–248.

Fernald, A., Zangl, R., Portillo, A. L., & Marchman, V. A. (2008). Looking while listening: Using eye movements to monitor spoken language comprehension by infants and Young children. In I. Sekerina, E. M. Fernández, & H. Clahsen (Eds.), *Developmental psycholinguistics: On-line methods in children's language processing* (pp. 97–135). Amsterdam: John Benjamins.

Galindo, C., & Fuller, B. (2010). The social competence of Latino kindergartners and growth in mathematical understanding. *Developmental Psychology, 46*, 579–592.

García, E., & García, E. (2012). *Understanding the language development and early education of Hispanic children.* New York: Teachers College Press.

García, E., & Jensen, B. (2009). Early educational opportunities for children of Hispanic origins. *Social Policy Report, 23*, 1–20.

Genesee, F. (1989). Early bilingual development: One language or two? *Journal of Child Language, 16*, 161–179.

Genesee, F., Nicoladis, E., & Paradis, J. (1995). Language differentiation in early bilingual development. *Journal of child language, 22*, 611–632.

Goldstein, M. H., & Schwade, J. (2010). From birds to words: Perception of structure in social interactions guides vocal development and language learning. In M. S. Blumberg, J. H. Freeman, & S. R. Robinson (Eds.), *The Oxford handbook of developmental behavioral neuroscience* (pp. 708–729). Oxford: Oxford University Press.

Gutiérrez, K. D., Zepeda, M., & Castro, D. C. (2010). Advancing early literacy learning for all children implications of the NELP report for dual-language learners. *Educational Researcher, 39*, 334–339.

Hagan, J. F., Shaw, J. S., & Duncan, P. M. (2008). AAP bright futures: Guidelines for health supervision of infants, children, and adolescents. *Pediatrics.*

Hammer, C. S., Davison, M. D., Lawrence, F. R., & Miccio, A. W. (2009). The effect of maternal language on bilingual children's vocabulary and emergent literacy development during head start and kindergarten. *Scientific Studies of Reading, 13*, 99–121.

Hammer, C. S., Hoff, E., Uchikoshi, Y., Gillanders, C., Castro, D. C., & Sandilos, L. E. (2014). The language and literacy development of young dual language learners: A critical review. *Early Childhood Research Quarterly, 29*, 715–733.

Hammer, C. S., Komaroff, E., Rodriguez, B. L., Lopez, L. M., Scarpino, S. E., & Goldstein, B. (2012). Predicting Spanish–English bilingual children's language abilities. *Journal of Speech, Language, and Hearing Research, 55*, 1251–1264.

Hart, B., & Risley, T. R. (1995). *Meaningful differences in the everyday experiences of young American children.* Baltimore, MD: Brookes.

Hernandez, D. (2006). Young Hispanic children in the US: A demographic portrait based on Census 2000. *Report to the National Task Force on Early Childhood Education for Hispanics.* Tempe, AZ: Arizona State University.

Hernandez, D. J., Denton, N. A., & Macartney, S. E. (2007). Demographic trends and the transition years. In R. C. Pianta, M. J. Cox, & K. L. Snow (Eds.), *School readiness and the transition to kindergarten in the era of accountability* (pp. 217–282). Baltimore, MD: Brookes.

Hernandez, D. J., Denton, N. A., & Macartney, S. E. (2008). Children in immigrant families: Looking to America's future. *Social Policy Report, 21*, 3–22.

Hirsh-Pasek, K., Golinkoff, R. M., Berk, L. E., & Singer, D. (2009). *A mandate for playful learning in preschool: Presenting the evidence*. New York, NY: Oxford University Press.

Hoff, E. (2003). The specificity of environmental influence: Socioeconomic status affects early language vocabulary development via maternal speech. *Child Development, 74*, 1368–1378.

Hoff, E. (2006). How social contexts support and shape language development. *Developmental Review, 26*, 55–88. doi:10.1016/j.dr.2005.11.002.

Hoff, E. (2009). Language development at an early age: Learning mechanisms and outcomes from birth to five years. *Encyclopedia on early childhood development*, pp. 1–5.

Hoff, E., Core, C., Place, S., Rumiche, R., Señor, M., & Parra, M. (2012). Dual language exposure and early bilingual development. *Journal of Child Language, 39*, 1–27.

Hurtado, N., Grüter, T., Marchman, V. A., & Fernald, A. (2014). Relative language exposure, processing efficiency and vocabulary in Spanish–English bilingual toddlers. *Bilingualism: Language and Cognition, 17*, 189–202. doi:10.1017/S136672891300014X.

Hurtado, N., Marchman, V. A., & Fernald, A. (2008). Does input influence uptake? Links between maternal talk, processing speed and vocabulary size in Spanish-learning children. *Developmental Science, 11*, F31–D39. doi:10.1111/j.1467-7687.2008.00768.x.

Hurtado, A., & Vega, L. A. (2004). Shift happens: Spanish and English transmission between parents and their children. *Journal of Social Issues, 60*, 137–155.

Huttenlocher, J., Waterfall, H., Vasilyeva, M., Vevea, J., & Hedges, L. (2010). Sources of variability in children's language growth. *Cognitive Psychology, 61*, 343–365.

Iglesias, A., & Rojas, R. (2012). Bilingual language development of English language learners: Modeling the growth of two languages. In B. A. Goldstein (Ed.), *Bilingual language development & disorders in Spanish–English speakers* (2nd ed., pp. 1–30). Baltimore, MD: Brooke.

Jackson-Maldonado, D., Thal, D. J., Fenson, L., Marchman, V. A., Newton, T., & Conboy, B. (2003). *MacArthur Inventarios del Desarrollo de Habilidades Comunicativas: User's guide and technical manual [MacArthur Communicative Development Inventory: User's guide and technical manual]*. Baltimore, MD: Brookes.

Kovács, Á. M., & Mehler, J. (2009). Cognitive gains in 7-month-old bilingual infants. *Proceedings of the National Academy of Sciences, 106*, 6556–6560.

Kovelman, I., Baker, S. A., & Petitto, L. A. (2008a). Age of first bilingual language exposure as a new window into bilingual reading development. *Bilingualism: Language and Cognition, 11*, 203–223.

Kovelman, I., Baker, S. A., & Petitto, L. A. (2008b). Bilingual and monolingual brains compared: A functional magnetic resonance imaging investigation of syntactic processing and a possible "neural signature" of bilingualism. *Journal of Cognitive Neuroscience, 20*, 153–169.

Kroll, J. F., Bobb, S. C., & Hoshino, N. (2014). Two languages in mind: Bilingualism as a tool to investigate language, cognition, and the brain. *Current Directions in Psychological Science, 23*, 159–163.

Luk, G., Bialystok, E., Craik, F. I. M., & Grady, C. L. (2011). Lifelong bilingualism maintains white matter integrity in older adults. *The Journal of Neuroscience, 31*, 16707–16813.

Magnuson, K., Lahaie, C., & Waldfogel, J. (2006). Preschool and school readiness of children of immigrants. *Social Science Quarterly, 87*(1241), 1262.

Marchman, V. A., & Fernald, A. (2008). Speed of word recognition and vocabulary knowledge in infancy predict cognitive and language outcomes in later childhood. *Developmental Science, 11*, F9–F16.

Marchman, V. A., Fernald, A., & Hurtado, N. (2010). How vocabulary size in two languages relates to efficiency in spoken word recognition by young Spanish–English bilinguals. *Journal of Child Language, 37*(4), 817–840.

Masten, A. S., & Cicchetti, D. (2010). Developmental cascades. *Development and Psychopathology, 22*, 491–495.

Mendelsohn, A. L., Dreyer, B. P., Flynn, V., Tomopoulos, S., Rovira, I., Tineo, W., et al. (2005). Use of videotaped interactions during pediatric well-child care to promote child development: A randomized, controlled trial. *Journal of Developmental and Behavioral Pediatrics, 26*, 34–41.

Mendelsohn, A. L., Huberman, H. S., Berkule, S. B., Brockmeyer, C. A., Morrow, L. M., & Dreyer, B. P. (2011). Primary care strategies for promoting parent–child interactions and school readiness in at-risk families: The Bellevue project for early language, literacy, and education success. *Archives of Pediatrics and Adolescent Medicine, 165*, 33–41.

Mervis, C. B., Golinkoff, R. M., & Bertrand, J. (1994). Two-year-olds readily learn multiple labels for the same basic-level category. *Child Development, 65*, 1163–1177.

McCabe, A., Tamis-LeMonda, C. S., Bornstein, M. H., Cates, C. B., Golinkoff, R., Guerra, A. W., et al. (2013). Multilingual children. *Social Policy Report, 27*, 1–21.

Ng, F. F. Y., Tamis-LeMonda, C. S., Godfrey, E. B., Hunter, C. J., & Yoshikawa, H. (2012). Dynamics of mothers' goals for children in ethnically diverse populations across the first three years of life. *Social Development, 21*, 821–848.

Ochs, E., & Capps, L. (2001). *Living narrative: Creating lives in everyday storytelling*. Cambridge, MA: Harvard University Press.

Oller, D. K., & Jarmulowicz, L. (2007). Language and literacy in bilingual children in the early school years. In E. Hoff & M. Shatz (Eds.), *Blackwell handbook of language development* (pp. 368–386). Malden, MA: Blackwell.

Oller, D. K., Pearson, B. Z., & Cobo-Lewis, A. B. (2007). Profile effects in early bilingual language and literacy. *Applied Psycholinguistics, 28,* 191–230.

Pan, B. A. (1995). Code negotiation in bilingual families: "My body starts speaking English". *Journal of Multilingual and Multicultural Development, 16,* 315–327.

Pan, B., Rowe, M., Spier, E., & Tamis-LeMonda, C. S. (2004). Measuring productive vocabulary of toddlers in low-income families: Concurrent and predictive validity of three sources of data. *Journal of Child Language, 31,* 587–608.

Paradis, J., Genesee, F., & Crago, M. B. (2011). *Dual language development and disorders: A handbook on bilingualism and second language learning* (2nd ed.). Baltimore, MD: Brookes.

Parra, M., Hoff, E., & Core, C. (2011). Relations among language exposure, phonological memory, and language development in Spanish–English bilingually developing 2-year- olds. *Journal of Experimental Child Psychology, 108,* 113–125.

Pearson, B. Z. (2007). Social factors in childhood bilingualism in the United States. *Applied Psycholinguistics, 28,* 399–410.

Place, S., & Hoff, E. (2011). Properties of dual language exposure that influence 2-year-olds' bilingual proficiency. *Child Development, 82,* 1834–1849.

Poulin-Dubois, D., Blaye, A., Coutya, J., & Bialystok, E. (2011). The effects of bilingualism on toddlers' executive functioning. *Journal of Experimental Child Psychology, 108,* 567–579.

Rader, N. D. V., & Zukow-Goldring, P. (2010). How the hands control attention during early word learning. *Gesture, 10,* 202–221.

Raikes, H., Alexander Pan, B., Luze, G., Tamis-LeMonda, C. S., Brooks-Gunn, J., Constantine, J., et al. (2006). Mother–child bookreading in low-income families: Correlates and outcomes during the first three years of life. *Child Development, 77,* 924–953.

Reese, L. (2012). Storytelling in Mexican homes: Connections between oral and literacy practices. *Bilingual Research Journal, 35,* 277–293.

Rinaldi, C., & Páez, M. (2008). Preschool matters: Predicting reading difficulties for Spanish—Speaking bilingual students in first grade. *Learning Disabilities: A Contemporary Journal, 6,* 71–84.

Sameroff, A. J., & Fiese, B. H. (2000). Transactional regulation: The developmental ecology of early intervention. *Handbook of Early Childhood Intervention, 2,* 135–159.

Schick, A., & Melzi, G. (2010). The development of children's oral narratives across contexts. *Early Education and Development, 21,* 293–317.

Silva-Corvalan, C. (2003). *Language contact and change. Spanish in Los Angeles.* Oxford, UK: Oxford University Press.

Smith, L. B., & Thelen, E. (2003). Development as a dynamic system. *Trends in Cognitive Sciences, 7,* 343–348.

Snow, C. E., & Beals, D. E. (2006). Mealtime talk that supports literacy development. In *New directions for child and adolescent development: family meals as contexts of development and socialization.* No. 111 (pp. 51–66). San Francisco: Jossey-Bass.

Snow, C. E., Burns, M. S., & Griffin, P. (1998). *Preventing reading difficulties in young children committee on the prevention of reading difficulties in young children.* Washington, DC: National Research Council.

Snow, C. E., & Dickinson, D. K. (1990). Social sources of narrative skills at home and at school. *First Language, 10,* 87–103.

Song, L., Tamis-LeMonda, C. S., Yoshikawa, H., Kahana-Kalman, R., & Wu, I. (2012). Language experiences and vocabulary development in Dominican and Mexican infants across the first 2 years. *Developmental Psychology, 48,* 1106–1123.

Tamis-LeMonda, C. S., Baumwell, L., & Cristofaro, T. (2012a). Parent–child conversations during play. *First Language, 32,* 413–438.

Tamis-LeMonda, C. S., Song, L., Leavell, A. S., Kahana-Kalman, R., & Yoshikawa, H. (2012b). Ethnic differences in mother-infant language and gestural communications are associated with specific skills in infants. *Developmental Science, 15,* 384–397. doi:10.1111/j.1467-7687.2012.00136.x.

Tamis-LeMonda, C. S., Bornstein, M. H., & Baumwell, L. (2001). Maternal responsiveness and children's achievement of language milestones. *Child Development, 72,* 748–767.

Tamis-LeMonda, C. S., Kahana-Kalman, R., & Yoshikawa, H. (2009). Father involvement in immigrant and ethnically diverse families from the prenatal period to the second year: Prediction and mediating mechanisms. *Sex roles, 60,* 496–509.

Tamis-LeMonda, C. S., Kuchirko, Y., & Song, L. (2014a). Why is infant language learning facilitated by parental responsiveness? *Current Directions in Psychological Science, 23,* 121–126.

Tamis-Lemonda, C. S., Song, L., Luo, R., Kurchirko, Y., Kahana-Kalman, R., Yoshikawa, H., et al. (2014b). Children's vocabulary growth in English and Spanish across early development and associations with school readiness skills. *Developmental Neuropsychology, 39,* 69–87.

Tienda, M., & Haskins, R. (2011). Immigrant children: Introducing the issue. *The Future of Children, 21,* 3–18.

Veltman, C. (2003). The American linguistics mosaic: Understanding language shift in the United States. In S. L. Mckay & S. C. Wong (Eds.), *New immigrants in the United States* (pp. 58–93). Cambridge, UK: Cambridge University Press.

Vogel, C., Aikens, N., Atkins-Burnett, S., Martin, E.S., Caspe, M., Sprachman, S., & Love, J. M. (2008). Reliability and validity of child outcome measures with culturally and linguistically diverse preschoolers: The first 5 LA Universal Preschool child outcomes study Spring 2007 Pilot study.

Vygotsky, L. (1978). *Mind in society*. Cambridge, MA: Harvard University Press.

Weber-Fox, C. M., & Neville, H. J. (1996). Maturational constraints on functional specializations for language processing: ERP and behavioral evidence in bilingual speakers. *Journal of Cognitive Neuroscience, 8*, 231–256.

Weber-Fox, C., & Neville, H. J. (2001). Sensitive periods differentiate rrocessing of open-and closed-class words: An ERP study of bilinguals. *Journal of Speech, Language, and Hearing Research, 44*(6), 1338–1353.

Weisner, T. S. (2002). Ecocultural understanding of children's developmental pathways. *Human Development, 45*, 275–281.

Winsler, A., Burchinal, M. R., Tien, H. C., Peisner-Feinberg, E., Espinosa, L., Castro, D. C., et al. (2014). Early development among dual language learners: The roles of language use at home, maternal immigration, country of origin, and socio-demographic variables. *Early Childhood Research Quarterly, 29*, 750–764.

Worthy, J., & Rodríguez-Galindo, A. (2006). "Mi hija vale dos personas": Latino immigrant parents' perspectives about their children's bilingualism. *Bilingual Research Journal, 30*, 579–601.

Yoshida, H. (2008). The cognitive benefits of early multilingualism. *Zero to Three, 2*, 26–30.

Yoshikawa, H. (2011). *Immigrants raising citizens: Undocumented parents and their young children*. New York: Russell Sage Foundation.

Zimmerman, I. L., Steiner, V. G., & Pond, R. E. (2012). *Preschool language scales Spanish* (5th ed.). San Antonio: Person.

Zong, J., & Batalova, J. (2015). *Frequently requested statistics on immigrants and immigration in the United States*. Retrieved from: http://www.migrationpolicy.org/article/frequently-requested-statistics-immigrants-and-immigration-united-states#Demographic,Educational,andLinguistic

An International Perspective on Parenting and Children's Adjustment

Jennifer E. Lansford

Abstract

This chapter provides an international perspective on parenting and children's adjustment, which can inform understanding of the development of minority children. It begins with an historical overview of this area of inquiry, which has been conducted primarily with North American and Western European samples, and presents two of the main theories that have guided research attempting to understand children's development in cultural contexts. The chapter then describes current key research questions as well as measurement and methodological issues in adopting an international perspective. The bulk of the chapter reviews empirical research on links between parenting and children's adjustment in a variety of domains (socioemotional adjustment, behavioral adjustment, academic achievement, moral development, social relationships) around the world. The chapter then highlights universal versus culture-specific mechanisms through which parenting has been found to relate to children's adjustment. Finally, the chapter suggests policy implications and directions for future research. Throughout, the review of theories and empirical research is not comprehensive but rather illustrative, attempting to provide an international framework in which to conceptualize parenting and children's adjustment.

Historical Overview and Theoretical Perspectives

Historically, the majority of research on parenting and children's adjustment has been conducted in the United States, Canada, and Western Europe. Arnett's (2008) analysis of the research participants in the most influential journals in six sub-disciplines of psychology from 2003 to 2007 revealed that 96 % of the participants were from

J.E. Lansford (✉)
Duke University, Durham, NC, USA
e-mail: Lansford@duke.edu

© The Editor(s) 2017
N.J. Cabrera and B. Leyendecker (eds.), *Handbook on Positive Development of Minority Children and Youth*, DOI 10.1007/978-3-319-43645-6_7

Western industrialized countries, with 68 % from the United States alone. Thus, 96 % of the research participants in these studies were from countries with only 12 % of the world's population (Henrich et al. 2010). These findings are corroborated by analyses of other journals conducted in different ways. For example, in a review of developmental studies published between 1986 and 2005, only 1.8 % involved Central or South American countries (Ribas 2010). This historical underrepresentation in the research literature of populations from most of the world's countries is concerning because findings from Western, educated, industrialized, rich, and democratic (WEIRD) societies may not generalize to the majority of the world's population, which does not live in such countries (Henrich et al. 2010). Despite this historical underrepresentation, recent efforts by professional organizations, universities, and bodies such as the United States National Academy of Sciences have focused on promoting international collaborative research and increasing international representativeness of study samples and researchers in the social sciences.

In the past, studies that included samples from underrepresented countries tended to take a deficit approach in which findings from the minority world of WEIRD countries were used as the gold standard against which findings from the majority world were compared and often interpreted as lacking (particularly in psychology, not as much in anthropology). For example, parent and child behaviors observed in low- and middle-income countries were often compared unfavorably to parenting in high-income countries. This has posed a lasting weakness in the developmental research base because indigenous childrearing practices and aspects of child adjustment historically were treated not as crucial to scientific knowledge in their own right but instead as confirming or failing to confirm theories that had been developed primarily using middle-class European American norms (Nsamenang and Lo-Oh 2010). Scholars have increasingly recognized the importance not only of including individuals from many countries as participants in research studies, but also of having native researchers lead scientific

study of parenting and children's adjustment to be able to bring an emic perspective to the research questions, methods, and interpretation of results.

Two particularly notable theories have guided research on children's development as situated in broad cultural contexts: Bronfenbrenner's (2005) bioecological model and Super and Harkness's (1986) developmental niche model. First, Bronfenbrenner's theory places child development within a set of systems ranging from proximal processes (e.g., direct parent–child interactions) to more distal processes (e.g., sociopolitical contexts and cultural beliefs), which are situated within chronosystems that acknowledge the importance of historical time and cohort effects. One of the primary contributions of Bronfenbrenner's theory is the idea that parent–child interactions are embedded in larger ecological and cultural contexts that can have a profound effect on parents, children, and their ways of interacting together.

Second, Super and Harkness's (1986) developmental niche model emphasizes how culture shapes children's development through physical and social environments, childrearing customs and practices, and culturally-influenced beliefs, attitudes, and values about parenting and children's development. This framework is built from the understanding that different parts of cultural systems influence one another such that modes of childrearing stem from opportunities and constraints in the larger society. For example, in agrarian societies, children tend to be taught responsibility and obedience from an early age so that they can contribute to the family's livelihood through household chores. Their framework also acknowledges similarities in human development across the widely varied contexts in which children are reared; for example, children everywhere must learn to walk, to get along with their peers, and to contribute in meaningful ways to their communities.

Current Research Questions

Individuals in different countries conceptualize positive parenting and child adjustment in ways that vary in some respects by cultural context.

Parents in all countries share goals of rearing their children to be successful, competent members of their respective societies, but what parents believe is necessary to achieve these goals and what defines success and competence varies around the world. Current research questions center on between-country differences in parenting and children's adjustment, mechanisms linking parenting with children's adjustment in different countries, and understanding universality versus cultural specificity in developmental processes.

Research Measurement and Methodology

Many measurement and methodology issues in international research on parenting and children's adjustment are the same as in other areas of psychological and developmental inquiry. For example, researchers must attend to questions about how samples should be drawn such as whether it is possible to recruit a nationally representative sample and, if time and budget constraints make national representativeness unfeasible, how a convenience sample can be constructed to be as generalizable as possible. Issues of measurement reliability and validity are important to all research, particularly if measures are being used for the first time with new populations. Decisions must be made about the mode of data collection (e.g., whether to use observations, parent reports, or direct assessments of children).

Despite these similarities, international research on parenting and children's adjustment faces several measurement and methodology issues that differ from issues in research with just a single population in one locale (Bornstein and Lansford 2013). One of the most pressing issues is whether to import into one country measures that have been developed in another or to develop new measures in the new country. Each approach has advantages and disadvantages. Adopting measures developed elsewhere has the advantage of building on previous research and making it easier to compare findings from the

new population with findings from previous populations, perhaps identifying universal aspects of parenting. However, taking an emic approach and developing new measures instead of importing already existing ones has the advantage of being able to capture aspects of parenting and children's adjustment that may be unique to the new context and therefore not covered on measures imported from elsewhere. If measures are imported from a different country, then translation from the original language to the target language, back-translation from the target language to the original language to identify problems in the translation, and a process of cultural adaptation to check for inappropriate items are necessary (Erkut 2010). Hambleton and Zenisky (2010) described 25 criteria useful in evaluating the quality of translated and adapted measures. For example, does a particular item have the same or highly similar meaning in the two languages? Are there differences between the two versions in the use of metaphors, idioms, or colloquialisms? Are the format of the items and required tasks equally familiar in the two languages? Using these methods, one might be able to tap into universal constructs using measures that are culturally-tailored.

A second issue involves establishing measurement equivalence or invariance across countries, a process meant to assure that constructs are being measured in the same way in different groups. Vandenberg and Lance (2000) outline a series of steps through which measurement invariance should be established, ranging from whether items load on the same factors across groups to whether intercepts of indicators are equal across groups. In practice, it can be very difficult to establish strict measurement invariance, particularly when working with a large number of groups. Therefore, a challenge for the field lies in determining when measures have captured a construct similarly enough across countries to produce confidence in the comparability of the findings.

Finally, socioeconomic factors pose a number of methodological challenges in conducting international research because such factors within countries can play as meaningful a role in shaping parenting and children's adjustment as differences between countries. For example, less educated parents and parents with less household income are less likely to provide cognitive stimulation and more likely to behave harshly toward their children (Hoff et al. 2002). Countries differ widely in the socioeconomic conditions of daily life. Many countries in sub-Saharan Africa and Asia, for example, have large proportions of their populations (as high as 88 % in Madagascar, World Bank 2014) living below the international poverty line of less than US$1.25 per day, but this standard of poverty is seldom found in North America and Western Europe. Socioeconomic factors are reflected in large differences in infant and child mortality rates, life expectancy, literacy rates, and numerous other indicators. For example, in sub-Saharan Africa, the infant mortality rate is 10 %, and of children who live to be age 6 years, one-third are chronically malnourished; life expectancy is just 36 years in Zimbabwe and 38 years in Zambia, in contrast to life expectancy of 82 years in Japan and 80 years in Iceland and Switzerland (Nsamenang and Lo-Oh 2010). Therefore, any international comparison of research findings must attend carefully to socioeconomic differences to avoid confounding country differences with SES differences.

Yet, cultural contexts are varied above and beyond differences between countries in poverty. For example, Durbrow et al. (2001) collected data from mothers of 5–18-year-old children in a poor village in the Philippines, in a poor village in St. Vincent in the Caribbean, and in an inner-city African American homeless shelter. In all three samples, mothers believed that children's competence was promoted by encouragement, attention, and discipline, but American mothers also stressed the importance of physical affection, praise, and minimizing the impact of dangerous neighborhoods whereas mothers in the Philippines and St. Vincent were more likely to emphasize the importance of health and nutrition. Attempts to understand parenting and children's adjustment in different countries should attend carefully to socioeconomic in addition to cultural factors.

Empirical Findings

The following sections provide illustrative empirical findings regarding ways that parenting is related to children's adjustment in socioemotional, behavioral, academic, moral, and social relationship domains. Taken together, the empirical literature suggests both similarities and differences across countries in associations between parenting and children's adjustment.

Socioemotional Adjustment

Attachment theory has been one of the leading frameworks through which developmentalists have sought to understand children's socioemotional adjustment, but the basic tenets of attachment theory are biased toward Western ways of thinking (Rothbaum et al. 2000). A large body of research using samples primarily from the United States, Canada, and Western Europe supports links between maternal sensitivity and secure attachment (De Wolff and van IJzendoorn 1997), between secure attachment and the development of children's social competence (Groh et al. 2014), and between secure attachment and exploration (Grossmann et al. 2008). However, each of those links is called into question using data from Japan (Rothbaum et al. 2000). For example, Japanese mothers anticipate their infants' needs and behave proactively to minimize infants' distress (e.g., avoiding situations that are stressful to their infants), whereas primarily middle-class European American mothers tend to wait until their infants communicate needs (e.g., by crying to show distress) and then respond to those needs. Thus, a review of research drawing from several samples suggests that, on average, Japanese and American mothers construe sensitive caregiving differently; when American mothers behave in ways that would appear to be sensitive caregiving in Japan, American mothers have been described as insensitive and their infants as insecurely attached (George and Solomon 1999). Likewise, social competence in children is regarded differently in Japan and the United States. In Japan, social competence is demonstrated by a child who works well in a group and is interdependent with others, whereas in the United States social competence is demonstrated by autonomy, open expression of emotions, and independently exploring the environment. Different types of parenting promote these different kinds of social competence. For example, Japanese mothers orient infants' attention to themselves, whereas American mothers orient infants' attention to objects in the environment (Rothbaum et al. 2000). American parents act as a secure base from which infants can explore the environment, whereas Japanese parents promote interdependence instead of exploration.

Chao (1994) described a conception of control in China called *guan*, meaning "to govern," which has been related to upper middle class American Chinese children's socioemotional adjustment. *Guan* involves firm control and training but also love and caring (with some similarities to authoritative parenting); without *guan*, parents of Chinese origin would be regarded as neglectful. This research suggests that the meanings and manifestations of parental control differ in different cultural contexts. Indeed, the association between warmth and control differed across 13 cultural groups in nine countries, with correlations that averaged from a low of −0.35 for European Americans in the United States to a high of 0.85 for Luos in Kenya (Deater-Deckard et al. 2011). Thus, the association between control and children's adjustment may depend on the meaning conveyed by parental control within a specific cultural context.

Differences across countries in aspects of parenting that promote socioemotional adjustment also are found during adolescence. For example, increases in autonomy over decision-making in grades 7–8 are more predictive of working- and middle-class adolescents' emotional functioning (operationalized as a combination of life satisfaction, experience of positive emotions, self-esteem, experience of negative emotions, and anxiety) in the United States (with a sample that was 88 % European American, 9 % Hispanic American, 2 % African American, and 1 % Asian American) than in China, in part because decision-making autonomy is more normative during adolescence in the United States than in China (Qin et al. 2009).

Different environmental conditions in different countries sometimes lead to different forms of parenting. For example, among the Yoruba in Nigeria, interactions involving food are used by parents to teach their children key life lessons to socialize them to be well-functioning members of their society (Babatunde and Setiloane 2014). This part of West Africa has a rainy season and a dry season, which results in fluctuations in the availability of food during different parts of the year. Parents teach children to wait patiently for food, not to visit other families during mealtimes, and to leave meat and fish (which are rare and valuable) untouched until the end of the meal. In this way, parents use food as a way of instilling the importance of delaying gratification, being thrifty, and showing proper etiquette, which will contribute to success later in life (Babatunde and Setiloane 2014).

Behavioral Adjustment

Perceptions of what constitutes desirable and undesirable child behaviors differ across countries. For example, adults in the United States are more likely to tolerate undercontrolled behavior than are adults in Thailand, who are more likely to emphasize the importance of respect toward others and nonaggression compatible with Buddhist teachings, which can manifest as overcontrolled behavior (Weisz et al. 1995). Similarly, in a review of several studies comparing samples in the United States and Canada with samples in China, Chen and French (2008) concluded that shyness and behavioral inhibition are perceived by American and Canadian mothers as being undesirable characteristics; shy children are less accepted by their mothers and less well liked by their peers than children who are not shy, and shyness is associated with the development of maladaptive behaviors such as poor academic achievement (Chen and French 2008). In contrast, behavioral inhibition and shyness are perceived by Chinese children and adults as being desirable; accordingly, shy children are treated with warmth and favor by their mothers and are perceived positively by their teachers and peers (Chen and French 2008).

Discipline is one of the primary means parents use to shape children's behaviors, by punishing undesired behaviors and rewarding desired behaviors. Parents' use of different forms of discipline varies dramatically across countries. For example, as of 2016, 50 countries have outlawed all forms of corporal punishment (www.endcorporalpunishment.org), a number that is increasing steadily as countries attempt to comply with standards related to protecting children from abuse and exploitation as set forth in the United Nations Convention on the Rights of the Child (CRC). Yet, in other countries (including the United States), the use of corporal punishment remains widespread. In a comparison of rates of corporal punishment of 2–4-year-old children in 24 low- and middle-income countries, Lansford and Deater-Deckard (2012) found that 27–38 % of the variance in whether corporal punishment was deemed necessary to rear a child properly was accounted for by country of residence. Use of psychological aggression and nonaggressive forms of discipline (such as offering explanations) also varied widely across countries.

Despite these differences in rates of different forms of discipline in different countries, there are many similarities in links between different forms of discipline and children's adjustment. For example, although the strength of the relation between corporal punishment and children's adjustment (aggression and anxiety) is moderated by the cultural normativeness of corporal punishment, more frequent corporal punishment is related to more child aggression and anxiety in China, India, Italy, the Philippines Thailand, and the United States (Lansford et al. 2005). A review of studies primarily with different ethnic groups in the United States concluded that corporal punishment is harmful to children regardless of its intended purpose or cultural context (Gershoff 2013).

Of course, behavioral adjustment involves not just avoiding problem behaviors but also engaging in prosocial behaviors. In a study of Ngecha children in Gikuyu, Kenya, de Guzman et al. (2005) found that contexts in which children spent time elicited different types and amounts of prosocial behavior. For example, in this subsistence economy, infants and toddlers are often cared for by older siblings; in the context of caring for younger siblings, older siblings were likely to display nurturant prosocial behavior. Likewise, children are expected to contribute to the family's sustenance through household chores, taking care of livestock, and engaging in other types of labor for the benefit of the family, all of which elicited responsible prosocial behavior. Playing with other children and taking care of oneself were the contexts least likely to elicit prosocial behavior. Many industrialized countries provide few opportunities for children to engage in meaningful work to benefit their families and communities, thereby limiting their access to contexts that elicit prosocial behavior. An important implication of these findings is that parents in such countries or communities may need to be especially mindful about how to promote children's prosocial behaviors when children are not often able to see the direct benefits of their actions on others.

Academic Achievement

Since Stevenson's seminal studies of academic achievement in China, Japan, and the United States (e.g., Stevenson et al. 1986), comparisons of what parents in different countries do to promote their children's academic achievement have been a major focus of international research on parenting and children's adjustment. In a review of studies using several economically diverse samples, on average, compared to parents in the United States, parents in China spend more time working on homework with their children, extend learning opportunities beyond assigned homework, and are more controlling in their teaching-related interactions with their children (Pomerantz et al. 2014). In working- and middle-class families, when parents in the United States are involved with their children's learning, they tend to promote autonomy, whereas parents in China are more controlling (Cheung and Pomerantz 2011). Chinese and American parents also respond differently to children's successes and failures, with Chinese parents reflecting on children's mistakes and minimizing their successes more than American parents (Ng et al. 2007). These aspects of parenting are related to children's academic achievement (Ng et al. 2007), with Chinese children consistently outperforming American children academically, particularly in math and science. Despite the academic advantages conferred by Chinese parenting, emphasis on mistakes and controlling behaviors also appear to take an emotional toll, with Chinese children feeling less happy and having lower perceptions of their own worth (Pomerantz et al. 2014). Pomerantz et al. suggested that optimizing children's academic achievement and emotional well-being could be promoted by parents' greater involvement in their children's education (as in traditional Chinese parenting) while at the same time using strategies that are more autonomy-promoting than controlling (as in traditional American parenting, which has been found to promote emotional well-being in both the United States and China; Pomerantz and Wang 2009).

Moral Development

Historically, researchers focused on whether children's moral development proceeded through a universal set of stages such as Kohlberg's (1984) progression from an obedience and punishment orientation to a stage defined by universal ethical principles. As in other areas of child development, this approach took a theory developed primarily from studying middle-class European Americans (in this case, just males) and used it as a gold standard against which to compare the moral development of females and children in many other countries and cultural contexts. This set of research sometimes concluded that children from certain countries were less morally advanced compared to children from other countries, a perspective that has been

criticized as being biased because Kohlberg's stages place more emphasis on individual rights and social justice than is common in many places. For example, individuals from India emphasize the importance of social relationships and fulfilling one's obligations to others and meeting others' needs, whereas individuals from the United States are more likely to emphasize what is fair or just as the basis for morality (Miller and Bersoff 1992). In their work with Black and White adolescents in South Africa, Ferns and Thom (2001) have described how these differences in cultural orientation can lead to different end points in moral development.

More contemporary research has focused less on stages of moral development and more on different social cognitive domains (e.g., social conventions versus morality; Smetana 2006; Turiel 2002) and factors that affect children's moral judgments in different contexts (Lapsley and Carlo 2014). In some cases, these factors have been found to differ across countries. In a comparison of primarily middle-class Japanese and American (82 % European American, 8 % Asian American, 6 % Hispanic American, 1 % African American, and 3 % multiethnic) 7-, 9-, and 11-year-old children, younger children in both countries were more likely than older children to indicate that they would report their peers' minor transgressions to authority figures; however in Japan, participants of all ages reported thinking it was more appropriate to report minor transgressions than did American participants (Loke et al. 2014). Compared to middle-class Japanese mothers, middle-class Israeli mothers are more likely to find children's disobedience acceptable when such disobedience results from an expression of the child's individuality (Osterweil and Nagano 1991). Prosocial behavior may be fostered in different ways in different societies. For example, in societies in which children are responsible for meeting others' needs (e.g., by taking care of younger siblings or doing housework for the good of the family), parents may not feel the need to specifically socialize prosocial behavior because such behavior is encouraged implicitly as children contribute to their families' well-being (de Guzman et al. 2005). In societies in which children have fewer opportunities to contribute to the welfare of the family through daily responsibilities, parents may try to socialize prosocial behavior through inductive reasoning and authoritative parenting (e.g., Hastings et al. 2007). Burr (2014) describes how morality and conceptions of what it means to be a "good child" are entwined with a web of cultural values in Vietnam. For example, knowing one's place in the social hierarchy is highly valued, and children are expected to behave in ways consistent with their position in this hierarchy. A child might be expected to work on the streets to earn money to support a brother's education or to live in an orphanage to give the family the opportunity to try for more sons (Burr 2014). Zucker and Howes (2009) found similar goals of Mexican mothers in the United States for their children to relate to other people by meeting their needs and expectations.

Social Relationships

Different beliefs about the importance of social relationships shape parent–child interactions in a variety of ways. For example, many parents in Bangladesh believe that showing children too much affection will spoil them and that speaking to infants is not important because infants cannot understand language (Hamadani and Tofail 2014). A classic ethnographic study of a rural, poor sample of the Gusii in Kenya revealed that co-sleeping, breastfeeding on demand, frequent physical contact, and immediate consoling of infants are expected features of mother–infant relationships (LeVine et al. 1994). Gusii mothers expressed shock when they were told that American parents rarely sleep with their infants, and when shown videotapes of American families, Gusii mothers were distressed by how long it took American mothers to respond to infant crying (LeVine et al. 1994). Gusii mothers do not believe that infants are capable of understanding language so do not speak with them in face-to-face interactions that are common in American mother–infant interactions. Gusii mothers spend more time soothing their infants, whereas American mothers spend more time stimulating their infants (LeVine et al. 1994). With older children Gusii mothers stress obedience and respect and would not praise their child for fear that praise would lead to conceit and rudeness (LeVine et al. 1994). More contemporary research with socioeconomically diverse and more urban Kenyan samples from different ethnic groups shows diversity in parenting attitudes and behaviors (see Oburu 2011).

Socialization in many countries focuses on promoting social relationships more than any other aspect of development. For example, in South Africa, the Zulu nurture *umuntu umuntu ngabantu*, which means that a person is only a person with other people (Zimba 2002). Likewise, the Yoruba people of Nigeria rear children using the concept of *omoluwabi*, which involves a holistic approach emphasizing loyalty to family obligations and traditions in interpersonal interactions (Akinsola 2011). Family obligations are emphasized in socialization in many countries, as exemplified in the Filipino notion of *utang na loob*, which involves a deep sense of gratitude and respect that children feel toward their parents and honor by carrying out their family obligations (Alampay 2014).

Developmental and Gender Considerations

Differences across countries have been reported in what is considered developmentally appropriate and desirable at a given age. For example, the timing of motor skill acquisition during infancy and early childhood varies across countries, in large part because of differences in parent–child interactions related to the development of these skills (Karasik et al. 2010). During adolescence, increasing autonomy is expected in the United States, but a large increase in autonomy is not expected in China (Qin et al. 2009). Countries differ even in how much influence parents are expected to have on their adult children's lives (e.g., Alampay 2014).

Cultural differences exist not only in parenting and child behaviors at different ages but also in how much parents believe they can shape children's development at all. For example, rural, poor Yucatec Mayan parents in Mexico believe that children's development unfolds over time in a steady progression regardless of what parents might do; therefore, they do not attempt to improve or hasten children's development (Gaskins 2000). In contrast, Luo parents in Kenya believe that parents have the ability to mold children's development deliberately toward desired outcomes, as illustrated in the Luo saying, "A tree is shaped while young, or when it is grown up it breaks" (Oburu 2011, p. 155). In some countries, parents believe that they begin influencing children even before they are born (e.g., Shwalb et al. 2010). Similarly, socioeconomically diverse mothers and fathers in primarily urban areas of China, Colombia, Italy, Jordan, Kenya, the Philippines, Sweden, Thailand, and the United States differ in the extent to which they believe they have control over successes and failures in caregiving situations (Bornstein et al. 2011).

Gender warrants consideration, both in terms of differences in mothers' and fathers' parenting and in terms of how daughters and sons are parented by both parents. Countries vary in societal-level goals, expectations, and behaviors related to gender such as girls' versus boys' access to education, women's and men's participation in the paid labor force, and gender equality or disparities in rights within the family and broader communities. In international rankings of countries by gender equality in health, education, economy, and politics, Iceland, Finland, Norway, Sweden, and Denmark are the most gender equitable countries; Mali, Syria, Chad, Pakistan, and Yemen are the least equitable (World Economic Forum 2014). Societal factors related to gender have implications for the ways parents rear sons and daughters, particularly with respect to gender-typed activities such as toy choices and household chores (Lytton and Romney 1991). Nevertheless, effect sizes for

differences in how boys and girls are parented are small when examined across a large number of low- and middle-income countries (Bornstein et al. 2016). Gender differences in how children are parented may depend on developmental stage, with infants and young children treated more similarly than adolescents, particularly in countries in North Africa and the Middle East where girls' mobility is more restricted after puberty in contrast to boys' mobility, which increases to include more community involvement and work outside the home (Ahmed 2010).

In a study of nationally representative samples of more than 170,000 families in 39 low- and middle-income countries, mothers were more likely to spend time with children under 5 years of age in primary caregiver roles than fathers (Bornstein and Putnick 2016). In some countries (e.g., Australia, Canada, the United States), the proportion of caregiving done by fathers has increased over time (Bianchi and Milkie 2010). Differences in caregiving between mothers and fathers are minimized in countries that have paternal as well as maternal leave policies following the birth or adoption of a child (International Labour Organization 2014). Factors such as family structure, socioeconomic status, and the age of children also affect the relative contributions of fathers and mothers to caregiving (Bianchi and Milkie 2010). Although fatherhood has been going through a reshaping toward more involvement by fathers in roles previously assumed primarily by mothers, historically, in many countries, fathers have served as playmates (Parke 2002) and as disciplinarians (Li and Lamb 2013), as embodied in the Chinese adage, "Kind mother, strict father," a Confucian-based distinction also common in other Asian countries (Shwalb et al. 2010). However, recent research shows that fathers are more than just playmates and take on as many different roles as mothers in childrearing (Cabrera et al. 2007, 2011, 2014). Overall, attention to gender is warranted when considering how mothers and fathers parent their daughters and sons in different countries.

Universal Versus Culture-Specific Mechanisms

Norenzayan and Heine (2005, p. 763) assert that "The existence of cultural diversity poses a great challenge to psychology: The discovery of genuine psychological universals entails the generalization of psychological findings across disparate populations having different ecologies, languages, belief systems, and social practices." Both theoretical and empirical approaches have attempted to elucidate universal versus culture-specific mechanisms through which parenting affects children's adjustment. Rohner's parental acceptance-rejection theory represents one example of an account of universal mechanisms. Children's perceptions of their parents' rejection appear to be a universal mediator of the link between parenting behaviors and children's maladjustment, whereas children's perceptions of their parents' acceptance appear to be a universal mediator of the link between parenting behaviors and children's positive adjustment (Rohner 2004; Rohner and Britner 2002). For example, children's perception of their parents as being rejecting mediates the link between parents' use of corporal punishment and children's psychological adjustment (Rohner et al. 1996). There is also some evidence for universality in social cognitive mechanisms as predictors of parents' behaviors and in the relation between parents' behaviors and children's adjustment. For example, Lansford et al. (2014) found in nine countries that mothers and fathers who endorsed aggressive forms of discipline in hypothetical situations were more likely to report using such forms of discipline with their own children. Finally, several studies suggest universality in how SES influences children's well-being through qualities of the home, including parent–child interactions such as cognitive stimulation and maternal supportiveness (Guo and Harris 2000; Mistry et al. 2008).

In contrast, some mechanisms appear to be culture-specific. Bornstein (1995) distinguished between the form and function of caregiving. Form encompasses parents' behaviors; function encompasses the purpose served for the child by parents' behavior. The form and function of parenting can be either the same or different across countries. In all countries, caregivers (including parents and other adults) need to fill the function of making their children feel loved and accepted (Rohner 2004), but the form of caregiving they use to fill this function may differ (e.g., physical affection, including its intensity and where affection is displayed, and verbal expressions of love in some countries but indirect actions such as preparing special foods in others). In contrast, a particular form of parenting (e.g., making direct eye contact with a child) may serve different functions depending on the broader context in which it is used (e.g., establishing open communication with the child in some countries but signaling aggression and disrespect in other countries).

One consistency across both the apparently universal versus culture-specific mechanisms is that the meaning delivered by parents' behavior is more strongly related to children's adjustment than the behavior itself. If parents behave in a manner that is accepted and endorsed by their cultural group, on average, their behavior will be more likely to have intended effects on children's adjustment than if parents behave in a way that is at odds with the larger cultural group. Children interpret their parents' behavior from a perspective that involves social norms gathered from observing others in the community.

Policy Implications

In the large majority of cases, one type of parenting strategy or behavior is neither better nor worse than a different kind of parenting, but caution is needed in not adopting a strict position on cultural relativism because there are some instances in which the international community has reached consensus that a particular practice is harmful to children and should not be implemented regardless of how culturally normative it is (see Coleman 1998). Female circumcision is one example of such a practice. Corporal punishment is increasingly regarded as another example. The United Nations (1989) has included mild corporal punishment as a human rights violation in several official documents since the time of the ratification of the CRC. For example, the United Nations Committee on the Rights of the Child, which is the body assigned to monitor implementation of the CRC, defines corporal punishment as "any punishment in which physical force is used and intended to cause some degree of pain or discomfort, however light. Most involves hitting ('smacking', 'slapping', 'spanking') children, with the hand or with an implement—whip, stick, belt, shoe, wooden spoon, etc." (paragraph 11, United Nations 2007). The Committee has specifically targeted legislation in some countries that allows corporal punishment as "reasonable chastisement," "moderate correction," and so forth. In referring to Article 19 of the CRC, which requires protecting children "from all forms of physical or mental violence," the Committee states (paragraph 18, United Nations 2007): "There is no ambiguity: 'all forms of physical or mental violence' does not leave room for any level of legalized violence against children. Corporal punishment and other cruel or degrading forms of punishment are forms of violence and the State must take all appropriate legislative, administrative, social and educational measures to eliminate them." The Committee goes on to explain, "In the light of the traditional acceptance of violent and humiliating forms of punishment of children, a growing number of States have recognized that simply repealing authorization of corporal punishment and any existing defences is not enough. In addition, explicit prohibition of corporal punishment and other cruel or degrading forms of punishment, in their civil or criminal legislation, is required in order to make it absolutely clear that it is as unlawful to hit or 'smack' or 'spank' a child as to do so to an adult, and that the criminal law on assault does apply equally to such violence, regardless whether it is termed discipline or 'reasonable correction'" (paragraph 34, United Nations 2007). In outlawing all forms of corporal punishment against children, countries are trying to change what is considered normative and acceptable parenting behavior in the interest of protecting

children from abuse and promoting their positive development.

In addition to broad policy implications, international research on parenting and children's adjustment also has implications for parenting interventions designed to improve parenting and, thereby, child outcomes. In low-income countries, parenting programs tend to focus on improving parents' knowledge about topics that increase child survival (e.g., how to prevent mother to child transmission in countries where HIV/AIDS is endemic, the importance of having children sleep under insecticide-treated nets in countries where malaria is a risk). Yet even in countries with high infant and early childhood mortality rates, most children survive, making it important for parenting programs to include socioemotional and cognitive caregiving components to optimize children's development, not just survival. In a review of interventions designed to increase maternal responsiveness, such interventions were found to be especially effective in developing countries, leading the authors to recommend that interventions to promote child survival should also include responsiveness training (Eshel et al. 2006). Although some parenting programs specifically target fathers, the majority of programs either target only mothers [e.g., the responsiveness interventions reviewed by Eshel et al. (2006)] or are open to either parent, which usually ends up drawing more mothers than fathers (Lansford and Bornstein 2007). Evaluating interventions directed toward fathers is an important direction for future research.

In a meta-analysis of 76 studies, mental health interventions that were adapted for use in particular cultures were four times more effective than interventions not targeted to a specific cultural group (Griner and Smith 2006). An important implication of findings about the role of culture in parenting and children's adjustment is that parenting interventions that are tailored to particular cultural contexts are preferable to implementing one-size-fits all programs. In practice, the process of cultural adaptation can occur in both content and mode of delivery. For example, one goal of the Better Parenting

Program in Jordan was to increase fathers' time with their children and knowledge about ways they could positively interact with their children, but the program initially had a difficult time reaching fathers because they perceived child-rearing as the responsibility of mothers and were unmotivated to spend time participating in a parenting program (Al-Hassan 2009). Using a culturally-grounded approach, the implementers adapted the program so that it could be delivered to fathers by Imams in mosques when fathers were there for Friday night prayers; in this way, fathers received the program's messages from highly respected authority figures who stressed fathers' roles within the family.

Future Directions

Adopting an international perspective offers several lessons that can be applied to understanding the development of minority children within a particular country. For example, research questions centering on between-country differences in parenting and children's adjustment, mechanisms linking parenting with children's adjustment in different countries, and understanding universality versus cultural specificity in developmental processes apply not just to international comparisons but also to understanding minority children within a society. In addition, methodological challenges such as establishing measurement equivalence and handling socioeconomic factors are important in research on minority children within a country as well as in international research. Because international research often grapples with issues related to studying populations other than the middle-class Western samples that comprise the majority of psychological research (Henrich et al. 2010), international research is well positioned to inform the study of minority children.

Future studies can advance understanding and promote minority children's positive development in diverse international contexts in at least four ways. First, future research should sample minority and majority children from countries that have been historically underrepresented in the research literature and should involve scholars from those countries who can bring an emic approach to understanding parenting and child development in particular locales. This will advance developmental science by illuminating processes that are culture-specific versus more universal. In some countries, researchers publish their findings almost exclusively in country-specific journals in the local language, making the research inaccessible to readers outside of that country. As part of an attempt to broaden the international knowledge base, researchers should be mindful to present their findings at conferences that draw international audiences and to publish their findings in international journals.

Second, future research should attend to within- as well as between-country differences. Within-country differences may reflect ethnicity, socioeconomic status, rural versus urban distinctions, and other factors that differentiate individuals within countries. Within-country differences also may reflect changes over historical time. In some countries political, economic, or other sociohistorical factors have shaped the extent to which developmental science is even an academic discipline. For example, Soviet repression of the social sciences hampered the fields of developmental psychology and family studies until perestroika, and it has taken some time since then to build a developmental research base in Russia (Nelson et al. 2010). Just as children develop over time, so do countries. Traditional values and parenting practices evolve over time, especially during times of economic growth and modernization (Chang et al. 2011), so parenting and child development in a particular country should be situated in broader historical contexts. The circumstances of minority children within a society can change in tandem with forces such as immigration policies and demographic shifts in the full population.

Third, studies of parenting and children's development would benefit from including not just mothers and fathers but other caregivers as well. In some countries and in some ethnic groups within countries, parents are children's primary caregivers, whereas in other groups, parents, grandparents, siblings, and other extended family members share the caregiving role. For example, in India the majority of households include extended family members who actively participate in childrearing (Saraswathi and Dutta 2010). Including other caregivers will broaden the definition of family and advance the field beyond the study of traditionally middle-class Western nuclear families and contribute to understanding of child development in broader family systems with complex configurations and multiple caregivers that are common in many parts of the world.

Finally, future research should try to determine which parenting programs work well in which contexts and with which children. Especially in low- and middle-income countries, there is a strong desire by researchers and practitioners not just to gain knowledge for its own sake but also to use this knowledge to improve the lives of children and their families. By using knowledge about parenting and child development in a particular country or with a particular ethnic group to tailor interventions to be culturally appropriate, it will be possible to maximize the potential effectiveness of such interventions. Rigorous evaluation studies will then be needed to determine whether the interventions are working as intended.

Adopting an international, cross-cultural framework in understanding parenting and children's adjustment offers several advantages over using a monocultural approach. Such a framework reduces the bias toward universality and overgeneralization that comes from adopting a monocultural approach and also adds important cultural variation. Although the ideas and findings discussed in this chapter reflect primarily a between-country perspective, they likely apply within countries as well. That is, they are relevant for understanding factors that improve development in ethnic, religious, socioeconomic, and other minority groups. An international approach advances understanding of the diverse ways that competence and adaptation can be defined and promoted around the world.

References

Ahmed, R. A. (2010). North Africa and the Middle East. In M. H. Bornstein (Ed.), *Handbook of cultural developmental science* (pp. 359–381). New York, NY: Taylor and Francis.

Akinsola, E. F. (2011). "Omoluwabi's approach" to educating the African child. In A. B. Nsamenang & T. M. S. Tchombe (Eds.), *Handbook of African educational theories and practices: A generative teacher education curriculum* (pp. 221–232). Bamenda, Cameroon: Human Development Resource Centre.

Alampay, L. P. (2014). Parenting in the Philippines. In H. Selin (Ed.), *Parenting across cultures: Childrearing, motherhood and fatherhood in non-western cultures* (pp. 105–121). New York, NY: Springer.

Al-Hassan, S. (2009). *Evaluation of the Better Parenting Program: A study conducted for UNICEF*. Amman: UNICEF.

Arnett, J. J. (2008). The neglected 95 %: Why American psychology needs to become less American. *American Psychologist, 63*, 602–614.

Babatunde, E. D., & Setiloane, K. (2014). Changing patterns of Yoruba parenting in Nigeria. In H. Selin (Ed.), *Parenting across cultures: Childrearing, motherhood and fatherhood in non-western cultures* (pp. 241–252). New York, NY: Springer.

Bianchi, S. M., & Milkie, M. A. (2010). Work and family research in the first decade of the 21st century. *Journal of Marriage and Family, 72*, 705–725.

Bornstein, M. H. (1995). Form and function: Implications for studies of culture and human development. *Culture & Psychology, 1*, 123–137.

Bornstein, M. H., & Lansford, J. E. (2013). Assessing early childhood development. In P. R. Britto, P. L. Engle, & C. M. Super (Eds.), *Early childhood development research and its impact on global policy* (pp. 351–370). New York, NY: Oxford University Press.

Bornstein, M. H., & Putnick, D. L. (2016). Mothering and fathering daughters and sons in low- and middle-income countries. *Monographs of the Society for Research in Child Development, 81*(1), 60–77.

Bornstein, M. H., Putnick, D. L., Bradley, R. H., Deater-Deckard, K., & Lansford, J. E. (2016). Gender across the developing world: Reflections, limitations, directions, and implications. *Monographs of the Society for Research in Child Development, 81*(1).

Bornstein, M. H., Putnick, D. L., & Lansford, J. E. (2011). Parenting attributions and attitudes in cross-cultural perspective. *Parenting: Science and Practice, 11*, 214–237.

Bronfenbrenner, U. (2005). *Making human beings human*. Thousand Oaks, CA: Sage.

Burr, R. (2014). The complexity of morality: Being a 'good child' in Vietnam? *Journal of Moral Education, 43*, 156–168.

Cabrera, N. J., Fitzgerald, H. E., Bradley, R. H., & Roggman, L. (2007). Modeling the dynamics of paternal influences on children over the life course. *Applied Development Science, 11*, 185–189.

Cabrera, N. J., Fitzgerald, H. E., Bradley, R. H., & Roggman, L. (2014). The ecology of father–child relationships: An expanded model. *Journal of Family Theory & Review, 6*, 336–354.

Cabrera, N. J., Hofferth, S. L., & Chae, S. (2011). Patterns and predictors of father–infant engagement across race/ethnic groups. *Early Childhood Research Quarterly, 26*, 365–375.

Chang, L., Chen, B.-B., & Ji, L. Q. (2011). Parenting attributions and attitudes of mothers and fathers in China. *Parenting: Science and Practice, 11*, 102–115.

Chao, R. K. (1994). Beyond parental control and authoritarian parenting style: Understanding Chinese parenting through the cultural notion of training. *Child Development, 65*, 1111–1119.

Chen, X., & French, D. C. (2008). Children's social competence in cultural context. *Annual Review of Psychology, 29*, 591–616.

Cheung, C. S., & Pomerantz, E. M. (2011). Parents' involvement in children's academic lives in the US and China: Implications for children's academic and emotional adjustment. *Child Development, 82*, 932–950.

Coleman, D. L. (1998). The Seattle compromise: Multicultural sensitivity and Americanization. *Duke Law Journal, 47*, 717–783.

de Guzman, M. R. T., Edwards, C. P., & Carlo, G. (2005). Prosocial behaviors in context: A study of Gikuyu children of Ngecha, Kenya. *Journal of Applied Developmental Psychology, 26*, 542–558.

De Wolff, M. S., & van IJzendoorn, M. H. (1997). Sensitivity and attachment: A meta-analysis on parental antecedents of infant attachment. *Child Development, 68*, 571–591.

Deater-Deckard, K., Lansford, J. E., Malone, P. S., Alampay, L. P., Sorbring, E., Bacchini, D., et al. (2011). The association between parental warmth and control in thirteen cultural groups. *Journal of Family Psychology, 25*, 790–794.

Durbrow, E. H., Peña, L. F., Masten, A., Sesma, A., & Williamson, I. (2001). Mothers' conceptions of child competence in contexts of poverty: The Philippines, St. Vincent, and the United States. *International Journal of Behavioral Development, 25*, 438–443.

Erkut, S. (2010). Developing multiple language versions of instruments for intercultural research. *Child Development Perspectives, 4*, 19–24.

Eshel, N., Daelmans, B., de Mello, M. C., & Martines, J. (2006). Responsive parenting: Interventions and outcomes. *Bulletin of the World Health Organization, 84*, 991–998.

Ferns, I., & Thom, D. P. (2001). Moral development of Black and White South African adolescents: Evidence against cultural universality in Kohlberg's theory. *South African Journal of Psychology, 31*, 38–47.

Gaskins, S. (2000). Children's daily activities in a Mayan village: A culturally grounded description. *Cross-Cultural Research, 34*, 375–389.

George, C., & Solomon, L. (1999). The caregiving behavioral system. In J. Cassidy & P. R. Shaver (Eds.), *Handbook of attachment: Theory, research, and clinical applications* (pp. 649–670). New York, NY: Guilford Press.

Gershoff, E. T. (2013). Spanking and child development: We know enough now to stop hitting our children. *Child Development Perspectives, 7*, 133–137.

Griner, D., & Smith, T. B. (2006). Culturally adapted mental health interventions: A meta-analytic review. *Psychotherapy: Theory, Research, Practice, Training, 43*, 531–548.

Groh, A. M., Fearon, R. P., Bakermans-Kranenburg, M. J., van IJzendoorn, M. H., Steele, R., & Roisman, G. I. (2014). The significance of attachment security for children's social competence with peers: A meta-analytic study. *Attachment and Human Development, 16*, 103–136.

Grossmann, K., Grossmann, K. E., Kindler, H., & Zimmermann, P. (2008). A wider view of attachment and exploration: The influence of mothers and fathers on the development of psychological security from infancy to young adulthood. In J. Cassidy & P. R. Shaver (Eds.), *Handbook of attachment: Theory, research, and clinical applications* (2nd ed., pp. 857–879). New York, NY: Guilford Press.

Guo, G., & Harris, K. M. (2000). The mechanisms mediating the effects of poverty on children's intellectual development. *Demography, 37*, 431–447.

Hamadani, J. D., & Tofail, F. (2014). Childrearing, motherhood and fatherhood in Bangladeshi culture. In H. Selin (Ed.), *Parenting across cultures: Childrearing, motherhood and fatherhood in non-western cultures* (pp. 123–144). New York, NY: Springer.

Hambleton, R. K., & Zenisky, A. L. (2010). Translating and adapting tests for cross-cultural assessments. In D. Matsumoto & F. J. R. van de Vijver (Eds.), *Cross-cultural research methods in psychology* (pp. 46–74). New York, NY: Cambridge University Press.

Hastings, P. D., Utendale, W. T., & Sullivan, C. (2007). The socialization of prosocial development. In J. E. Grusec & P. D. Hastings (Eds.), *Handbook of socialization: Theory and research* (pp. 638–664). New York, NY: Guilford.

Henrich, J., Heine, S. J., & Norenzayan, A. (2010). The weirdest people in the world? *Behavioral and Brain Sciences, 33*, 1–75.

Hoff, E., Laursen, B., & Tardif, T. (2002). Socioeconomic status and parenting. In M. H. Bornstein (Ed.), *Handbook of parenting: Biology and ecology of parenting* (2nd ed., Vol. 2, pp. 231–252). Mahwah, NJ: Erlbaum.

International Labour Organization. (2014). *Maternity and paternity at work: Law and practice across the world.* Geneva: International Labour Organization.

Karasik, L. B., Adolph, K. E., Tamis-LeMonda, C. S., & Bornstein, M. H. (2010). WEIRD walking: Cross-cultural research on motor development. *Behavioral and Brain Sciences, 33,* 95–96.

Kohlberg, L. (1984). *Essays on moral development: The psychology of moral development: Moral stages, their nature and validity* (Vol. 2). San Francisco, CA: Harper & Row.

Lansford, J. E., & Bornstein, M. H. (2007). *Review of parenting programs in developing countries.* New York, NY: UNICEF.

Lansford, J. E., Chang, L., Dodge, K. A., Malone, P. S., Oburu, P., Palmérus, K., et al. (2005). Physical discipline and children's adjustment: Cultural normativeness as a moderator. *Child Development, 76,* 1234–1246.

Lansford, J. E., & Deater-Deckard, K. (2012). Childrearing discipline and violence in developing countries. *Child Development, 83,* 62–75.

Lansford, J. E., Woodlief, D., Malone, P. S., Oburu, P., Pastorelli, C., Skinner, A. T., et al. (2014). A longitudinal examination of mothers' and fathers' social information processing biases and harsh discipline in nine countries. *Development and Psychopathology, 26,* 561–573.

Lapsley, D., & Carlo, G. (2014). Moral development at the crossroads: New trends and possible futures. *Developmental Psychology, 50,* 1–7.

LeVine, R. A., Dixon, S., LeVine, S., Richman, A., Leiderman, P. H., Keefer, C. H., et al. (1994). *Child care and culture: Lessons from Africa.* New York, NY: Cambridge University Press.

Li, X., & Lamb, M. E. (2013). Fathers in Chinese culture: From stern disciplinarians to involved parents. In D. W. Shwalb, B. J. Shwalb, & M. E. Lamb (Eds.), *Fathers in cultural context* (pp. 15–41). New York, NY: Routledge/Taylor & Francis Group.

Loke, I. C., Heyman, G. D., Itakura, S., Toriyama, R., & Lee, K. (2014). Japanese and American children's moral evaluations of reporting on transgressions. *Developmental Psychology, 50,* 1520–1531.

Lytton, H., & Romney, D. M. (1991). Parents' differential socialization of boys and girls: A meta-analysis. *Psychological Bulletin, 109,* 267–296.

Miller, J. G., & Bersoff, D. M. (1992). Culture and moral judgment: How are conflicts between justice and interpersonal responsibilities resolved? *Journal of Personality and Social Psychology, 62,* 541–554.

Mistry, R. S., Biesanz, J. C., Chien, N., Howes, C., & Benner, A. D. (2008). Socioeconomic status, parental investments, and the cognitive and behavioral outcomes of low-income children from immigrant and native households. *Early Childhood Research Quarterly, 23,* 193–212.

Nelson, D. A., Hart, C. H., Keister, E. K., & Piassetskaia, K. (2010). Russia. In M. H. Bornstein (Ed.), *Handbook of cultural developmental science* (pp. 409–428). New York, NY: Taylor and Francis.

Ng, F. F., Pomerantz, E. M., & Lam, S. F. (2007). European American and Chinese parents' responses to children's success and failure: Implications for children's responses. *Developmental Psychology, 43,* 1239–1255.

Norenzayan, A., & Heine, S. J. (2005). Psychological universals: What are they and how can we know? *Psychological Bulletin, 131,* 763–784.

Nsamenang, A. B., & Lo-Oh, J. L. (2010). Afrique Noire. In M. H. Bornstein (Ed.), *Handbook of cultural developmental science* (pp. 383–407). New York, NY: Taylor and Francis.

Oburu, P. O. (2011). Attributions and attitudes of mothers and fathers in Kenya. *Parenting: Science and Practice, 11,* 152–162.

Osterweil, Z., & Nagano, K. N. (1991). Maternal views on autonomy: Japan and Israel. *Journal of Cross-Cultural Psychology, 22,* 362–375.

Parke, R. D. (2002). Fathers and families. In M. H. Bornstein (Ed.), *Handbook of parenting status and social conditions of parenting* (2nd ed., Vol. 3, pp. 27–73). Mahwah, NJ: Erlbaum.

Pomerantz, E. M., Ng, F., Cheung, C. S.-S., & Qu, Y. (2014). Raising happy children who succeed in school: Lessons from China and the United States. *Child Development Perspectives, 8,* 71–76.

Pomerantz, E. M., & Wang, Q. (2009). The role of parental control in children's development in Western and East Asian countries. *Current Directions in Psychological Science, 18,* 285–289.

Qin, L., Pomerantz, E. M., & Wang, Q. (2009). Are gains in decision-making autonomy during early adolescence beneficial for emotional functioning? The case of the United States and China. *Child Development, 80,* 1705–1721.

Ribas, R. C., Jr. (2010). Central and South America. In M. H. Bornstein (Ed.), *Handbook of cultural developmental science* (pp. 323–339). New York, NY: Taylor and Francis.

Rohner, R. P. (2004). The parental "acceptance-rejection syndrome": Universal correlates of perceived rejection. *American Psychologist, 59,* 830–840.

Rohner, R. P., Bourque, S. L., & Elordi, C. A. (1996). Children's perceptions of corporal punishment, caretaker acceptance, and psychological adjustment in a poor, biracial southern community. *Journal of Marriage and the Family, 58,* 842–852.

Rohner, R. P., & Britner, P. A. (2002). Worldwide mental health correlates of parental acceptance-rejection: Review of cross-cultural and intracultural evidence. *Cross-Cultural Research, 36,* 16–47.

Rothbaum, F., Weisz, J., Pott, M., Miyake, K., & Morelli, G. (2000). Attachment and culture: Security in the United States and Japan. *American Psychologist, 55,* 1093–1104.

Saraswathi, T. S., & Dutta, R. (2010). India. In M. H. Bornstein (Ed.), *Handbook of cultural developmental science* (pp. 465–483). New York, NY: Taylor and Francis.

Shwalb, D. W., Shwalb, B. J., Nakazawa, J., Hyun, J.-H., Le, H. V., & Satiadarma, M. P. (2010). East and Southeast Asia: Japan, South Korea, Vietnam, and Indonesia. In M. H. Bornstein (Ed.), *Handbook of* cultural developmental science (pp. 445–464). New York, NY: Taylor and Francis.

Smetana, J. G. (2006). Social domain theory: Consistencies and variations in children's moral and social judgments. In M. Killen & J. G. Smetana (Eds.), Handbook of moral development (pp. 119–154). Mahwah, NJ: Erlbaum.

Stevenson, H. W., Lee, S.-Y., & Stigler, J. W. (1986). Mathematics achievement of Chinese, Japanese, and American children. Science, 231, 693–699.

Super, C. M., & Harkness, S. (1986). The developmental niche: A conceptualization at the interface of child and culture. International Journal of Behavioral Development, 9, 545–569.

Turiel, E. (2002). The culture of morality: Social development, context, and conflict. Cambridge, England: Cambridge University Press.

United Nations. (1989). United Nations Convention on the Rights of the Child, Geneva. Washington, DC: Office of the United Nations High Commissioner for Human Rights. www.unhchr.ch/html/menu3/b/k2crc.htm

United Nations Committee on the Rights of the Child. (2007). General comment number 8: The right of the child to protection from corporal punishment and other cruel or degrading forms of punishment. http://daccess-dds-ny.un.org/doc/UNDOC/GEN/G07/407/71/PDF/G0740771.pdf?OpenElement

Vandenberg, R. J., & Lance, C. E. (2000). A review and synthesis of the measurement invariance literature: Suggestions, practices, and recommendations for organizational research. Organizational Research Methods, 3, 4–70.

Weisz, J. R., Chaiyasit, W., Weiss, B., Eastman, K. L., & Jackson, E. W. (1995). A multimethod study of problem behavior among Thai and American children in school: Teacher reports versus direct observations. Child Development, 66, 402–415.

World Bank. (2014). Poverty headcount ratio at $1.25 a day (PPP) (% of population). Retrieved December 9, 2014 from http://data.worldbank.org/indicator/SI.POV.DDAY

World Economic Forum. (2014). The global gender gap report 2014. Geneva: World Economic Forum.

Zimba, R. F. (2002). Indigenous conceptions of childhood development and social realities in southern Africa. In H. Keller, Y. P. Poortinga, & A. Scholmerish (Eds.), Between cultures and biology: Perspectives on ontogenetic development (pp. 89–115). Cambridge: Cambridge University Press.

Zucker, E., & Howes, C. (2009). Respectful relationships: Socialization goals and practices among Mexican mothers. Infant Mental Health Journal, 30, 501–522.

Cultural Identity Development as a Developmental Resource

Paul Vedder and Mitch van Geel

Abstract

Cultural identities can have a positive role in youths' lives. Cultural identity refers to cognitive and affective appreciation of group membership. Depending personal and social circumstances, cultural identity can either be an asset or a danger. Efforts to help youth achieve a positive cultural identity should seek to create contexts in which they can safely explore their identities.

Historical Overview and Theoretical Perspectives

In 1968, in the preface of his book entitled "Identity: Youth and Crisis", Erikson contended that to understand the concept of identity one should analyze what and how people experience its absence or incompleteness and what this does to a person's functioning in a variety of contexts. This view suggests that identity depends on the contexts in which a person functions and that much can be written or said about it. And, indeed, much has been written about it, reflecting that there is neither consensus about the definition of cultural identity nor on adequate methodological approaches to studying identity

formation. Actually, the concept of identity is used in many different ways, often without a clear definition, resulting in misunderstanding and vagueness (Verkuyten 2005). Nevertheless identity is an inspiring notion in psychology. To avoid adding to the confusion, in this chapter we use a definition of identity presented earlier by Vedder and Phinney (2014). They describe identity as a sense of self that is formed over time, and that resolves doubt about personal purpose and goals in life. The doubt as well as the purpose and goals are linked to particular activities that a person is engaged in. The sense of goal and purpose a person is aspiring to is linked to a particular time and situation. At the same time this bond with time and place is transcended because a secure sense of purpose and goals not only guides current behavior, but also future behaviors and activities. Erikson (1968) refers to this quality of identity as "self-sameness": a personal sense of constancy and continuity beyond time and situations. He

P. Vedder (✉) · M. van Geel
Institute of Clinical Child and Adolescent Studies,
Leiden University, Leiden, The Netherlands
e-mail: vedder@fsw.leidenuniv.nl

© The Editor(s) 2017
N.J. Cabrera and B. Leyendecker (eds.), *Handbook on Positive
Development of Minority Children and Youth*, DOI 10.1007/978-3-319-43645-6_8

stresses its social nature by emphasizing that not only the person recognizes this selfsameness, but others do as well. Identity has to do with personal agency that is used to connect with the social world to access resources that increase personal well-being or that signifies the right thing to do in a social setting.

In the remainder of this chapter we limit our scope in that we focus on cultural identity. We define cultural identity, a component of identity, in the tradition of social identity theory (Tajfel and Turner 1979) as a cognitive appreciation of group membership together with an affective appreciation of the group (Tajfel 1981). We use the adjective "cultural" to refer to a group or groups defined by ethnicity (e.g., the Frisians in the Netherlands and Germany), phenotypical characteristics (e.g., black versus white South Africans), country of origin (e.g., immigrants from Morocco) or of residence (e.g., nationals in the Netherlands), or some combination of the four. Strictly speaking these substantiations may each refer to a different reality. Ethnic identity, for instance primarily deals with the exploration and confirmation of one's cultural heritage and ancestral roots, including beliefs and practices that are transmitted from generation to generation. In contrast, cultural identity primarily referring to one's phenotype and which is shaped by experiences akin to the phenotype, is likely linked to experiences of prejudice and discrimination or of dominance and privilege. Indeed, all these substantiations or qualifications of cultural identity in terms of ethnicity, phenotype, country of origin, etc. may refer to quite distinct entities (Navarrete and Jenkins 2011; Williams et al. 2012). Still, they are frequently used as overlapping or interchangeable (Berry et al. 2006; Vedder and Phinney 2014). All refer to socially constructed labels used for ascribing and claiming cultural group membership.

This chapter is predominantly about ethnic or cultural minority children who, almost by definition, grow up developing more than a single cultural identity. They are commonly exposed to and engaged with their own ethnic culture and the culture of the surrounding society or their society of settlement. The two cultures and accompanying identities influence each other, with the surrounding culture often having a strong impact (Horenczyk et al. 2013). Indeed, people acquire multiple identities and use different identities or combinations of identities depending on the situation or context in which they engage. In a sense, people act like chameleons. To feel safe and secure and accepted by their social entourage, or to reconfirm a personally appreciated ideological stance, people may decide to use the identity that best serves their purposes in a particular situation. Liebkind (2001), working within the social identity framework, contends that the notion of multiple identities is better understood in terms of partial identities, each referring to a different social category (e.g., girl, Muslim, head scarf wearer, sister, oldest daughter, good swimmer, white, etc.). More so than adults, children want to select situation or activity adapted identities and manifest the accompanying behaviors to have access to and to enjoy activity contexts and corresponding activities. Young people make sure that they fit into a variety of "activity cultures" (Liebkind 2001; Verkuyten 2005). Most of the literature we discuss in this chapter has focused on adolescents or young adults. It is not surprising that this developmental stage has received so much attention, for it is during adolescence that identity undergoes a major developmental spurt (Erikson 1968) in which processes such as exploration and commitment are used to create a cultural identity. Even though many of the spectacular processes connected to identity formation may happen during adolescence, it is important to realize that the development of identity starts much earlier in life. Between the ages of three and five most children develop the ability to correctly label themselves in terms of an ethnic or cultural group, though it is unclear whether this label carries any meaning, let alone functions as a developmental resource. Between the ages of six and ten, children start to connect 'their group' to concrete cultural practices such as food consumption or language use. Between

10 and 14 children may become aware of the social status and stereotypes associated with their group. Later in adolescence, they develop an increasingly clear sense of cultural identity, and their cultural identity may become a source of pride and inspiration for affecting and supporting persons in one's social network and feel cared for by these same persons (Ruble et al. 2004). The resulting sense of connection, direction, and fulfillment not only has an energizing function for engaging in activities with peers, but also protects against confusion and feelings of fear and threat linked with experiences of discrimination Indeed, ample studies show the positive consequences and correlates of cultural identity (Alvarado and Ricard 2013; Neblett and Carter 2012; Umaña-Taylor et al. 2014).

The positive, protective quality of cultural identity is also available from so-called multicultural identities. Particularly in contexts in which different cultural groups come in first hand contact, for instance through immigration, it is important for children to develop multicultural identities that allow them to adapt their mode of behaviors to requirements or preferences typical of people and situations whom they want to engage with in activities, either for enjoying a good time or for achieving access to desired resources (knowledge, company, help, material goods). Liebkind (2001) mentions challenges and resources that people encounter in their different cultural "worlds". She stresses that this corresponds to a so-called additive model of cultural acquisition; additive because multiple identities have the potential to enrich a person's world. The alternative is subtractive in which a second identity is developed at the expense of identities acquired earlier. Indeed, studies show that in adolescence the development of a cultural identity goes hand in hand with learning the language, values, beliefs, behaviors and customs typical of the cultural group that is the referent to the acquired identity. Together these are conducive to positive developmental outcomes and psychological wellbeing (Berry et al. 2006; Phinney et al. 2001).

Growth conducive for realizing an additive function of cultural or multicultural identity is not achieved automatically and without specific effort. To clarify this we refer to the work of Marcia (1966). She presented two concepts that are important for identity development: commitment and exploration. Commitment refers to the affective appreciation and exploration to the cognitive appreciation. These concepts are used to describe four identity statuses: foreclosure, identity diffusion, moratorium, and identity achievement. Foreclosure refers to commitments without exploring alternatives. This is typical of children who do as their parents and other influential people do (Wong et al. 2010). Identity diffusion is typical of young people who do not commit themselves and do not explore opportunities for, or the desirability of commitment. This status seems to resemble the notion of marginalized or isolated people (Berry et al. 2006) and it is hard to imagine that it can be an element in realizing an additive function of cultural identity. Moratorium refers to a state of intensive exploration of opportunities for commitment without commitment. And finally, identity achievement is the state that follows after a profound exploration and starts with the choice of a particular commitment. Identity diffusion is considered the least adaptive status and achievement the most adaptive (Kroger et al. 2010). Lichtwarck-Aschoff et al. (2008) contend that Marcia's model is incomplete because it insufficiently recognizes that exploration does not necessarily lead to questioning commitment, and consequently to status change. They, as well as Crocetti et al. (2008), add a third process, reconsideration. This third process means that the outcomes that emerge from one's explorations may lead to a reconsideration of one's commitments. This can even happen when a person has reached the stage of identity achievement but then encounters new circumstances that promote further consideration. Although no direct empirical evidence is available, it is likely that an additive function of multiple cultural identities can only be achieved when the level of commitment is such that the commitment is converted into or goes hand in hand with support and engagement in one's social networks (cf. Fleischman and Verkuyten 2016), hence, when the stage of moratorium or achievement has been reached.

Umaña-Taylor et al. (2014) followed a more empirical approach to find out about conditions that impact how strongly cultural identity serves positive functions. They provide evidence that the relationship between ethnic identity and youths' confidence in their capacities to learn (academic self-efficacy) varies in strength depending the school's ethnic composition. Participants were Mexican-American 5th grade children living in Phoenix, Arizona, diverse on socio-economic indicators, generational status and language preference. The researchers compared children from schools in which they were a numerical minority to children from schools in which the Mexican-American children were a numerical majority. In the first group the relationship between ethnic identity and academic self-efficacy was stronger than in the second group. The researchers argue that this is likely to be caused by the higher salience of being Mexican-American in schools in which the Mexican-American children formed a numerical minority. In this context the sense of security and resourcefulness attached to ethnic identity is likely to be experienced as more important, and consequently activated more. Possible interactions with other contextual variables (e.g., SES make-up of schools and neighborhoods) were not analyzed. Later in this chapter, in the section on empirical findings, we return to the positive and protective function of cultural identity, providing examples of how it works as well as further qualifications.

Current Research Questions

In this section we discuss a variety of research questions, ranging from questions like what a normative course of cultural identity development looks like and what challenges the development of such a normative model, to what the nature is of the relationship between social contacts and cultural identity development; is one of them leading and the other following or is the relationship rather reciprocal? This latter question is one of a series of questions that are all variations on the notion that cultural identity is context dependent.

In their editorial to a special issue for Child Development about research on race, ethnicity, and culture in child development Quintana et al. (2006) suggest that we need more studies on the normative development of ethnic minority children and adolescents. Models of normative development are important because they form a referent or standard for evaluating the quality of a young persons' cultural identity development. As such they lead to a better view on how to support this development and how to overcome challenges when the development takes an unhealthy, undesirable course. Creating such models is a challenge that has not yet been resolved in the domain of cultural and multicultural identity. One of the reasons is that there is a multitude of groups that vary in definition and size, making feasibility and prioritization cumbersome hurdles. Another challenge is that group membership has to be defined and ascribed or claimed. Ascription, however, may be problematic. An approach like the one represented in the "one drop rule", which states that anyone with a Black ancestor is to be considered Black (Hickman 1997), does not square with how many individuals identify themselves. Science does not and cannot clarify how many generations should pass before scholars quit categorizing people with a heritage that includes ancestors of a given background as a member of a particular minority or immigrant group. Does this vary by group or is self-labeling the way to go? In many cases, particularly when it involves people with mixed backgrounds, it is likely that self-labeling plays a role; who else would know? If, however, the issue is surrounded by fierce competition about access to scarce resources (e.g., for getting refugee status in the US or returnee status in Germany), then self-labeling will not suffice. The same editors warn that normative theories that were constructed and validated with a particular cultural group should not be applied uncritically to other groups. Generalizability and applicability should not be assumed, but explored time and again.

Vedder and Phinney (2014) state that dynamic times ask for dynamic notions of cultural identity. They clarified that culture as the referent for identity is increasingly conceptualized as something that constantly changes. Culture is created and renovated, but as important, or perhaps even more important, is that inter- and intra-generational processes of cultural transmission do not result in a simple multiplier effect leading to endless copies of cultural elements or building blocks that are transmitted; they lead to changes in culture. And cultural changes result in changes in the input for the manifestations and emergence of cultural identity. New variations show up with changing times and places. The experience and recognition of this dynamism have led researchers to try to understand and model a dynamic, developmental view of (multi)cultural identities. In studies focusing on this dynamic nature of cultural identity development, contexts receive ample attention.

Studies on identity development, although recognizing the importance of a social context, traditionally focus on the development of the self as a primarily individually self-contained process. In the last few decades, frameworks have been developed that present identity development as a contextualized transactional process in which social interactions are not just manifestations of developmental processes, but also processes that determine the course of the development. In the introduction we referred to studies typical of this latter understanding, viz., studies showing that multicultural youth adapts their mode of behaviors to requirements or preferences typical of persons and situations whom they want to engage with in activities (Liebkind 2001). Padilla (2006) refers to this phenomenon when explaining what bi- or multi-culturalism entails. He refers to the completely bicultural person as one who has acquired cultural competencies to a high degree and who, when the situation demands, easily switches or alternates between the competencies required in the different cultural communities. This alternating facility makes it easier to interact with members of a broad variety of cultures. This capability is linked to the acquisition and use of different sets of knowledge, each linked to particular cultural contexts or frames. Studies (Mok and Morris 2012; Verkuyten and Pouliasi 2002) show that by priming a particular cultural frame, or by manipulating the salience of particular characteristics relevant to a particular identity (e.g., by introducing persons representing a particular ethnic group by appearance or outfit), a bicultural person makes sense of a presented situation in a way quite distinct from the way the same situation would have made sense if the situation would not have changed. This comes close to what we know about multilingualism and language shifting (Diamond 2010).

Studies of the context dependency of identity development also clarify that skills, and knowledge are closely linked to persons' identity development (Hong et al. 2000; Luna et al. 2008). Kim and Chao (2009), working with 207 Chinese (1st and 2nd generation) and 354 Mexican (1st, 2nd and 3rd generation) 14–18 years old adolescents living in Los Angeles, California, showed that ethnic language proficiency and use is an important component of 2nd generation Mexican adolescents' identity, but not of 2nd generation Chinese youth. Between generations in the Chinese community in Los Angeles this proficiency and use of the heritage language drastically declines, due to limited exposure to the language and due to the difficulty to learn the heritage language. For the Mexican adolescents' heritage language this is different: exposure and possibilities for use are ample and the language, Spanish, is structurally more similar to English, hence less difficult to learn. The study further clarifies that language may be, but not necessarily is, an important facilitator of identity development. Kiang and Fuligni (2009), stress the importance of the ethnic background of the peers whose company one keeps. If peers share their ethnic background, ethnic identity tends to be stronger than when peers have a different ethnic background. Kiang and Fuligni (2009) suggest that we are in need of studies that show the extent to which the strength of ethnic identity affects the social contacts that young people establish and try to maintain. In effect, they ask do contacts follow from identity, does identity follow contacts, or is the relation reciprocal? And if the two are closely interrelated could relational variation in ethnic identity correspond to fluctuating levels of well-being over shorter and longer stretches of time?

A final research question to be dealt with in this section is "What causes radicalization?" In the preceding section we stated that moratorium refers to a state of intensive exploration of opportunities for commitment, but without having committed yet. Adolescence is a stage in life during which individuals seem most susceptible to radicalization. Radicalization is a concept that refers to a process that combines a lower sympathy for the commonly accepted value climate, and a growing sympathy for or identification with values, opinions and behaviors which conflict with the dominant value climate. It is the expression of a strong urge to no longer abide by the rules of common organizations, and a loss of respect for earlier relations, attitudes and life styles; in short, de-identification (Becker et al. 2011). At the same time radicalization is characterized by efforts to seek and find a community of like-minded people who share similar radical opinions and behaviors. In terms of social belongingness, as already described by Erikson (1968), identity develops in such a way that the social ties to the dominant majority are not only severed, but there is actually an aversion to this identity and the values it stands for, while at the same time a very strong social belongingness is felt towards the ethnic, religious or cultural minority group to which a person belongs. In short, there is a widening gap between "us and them". In the last decade it has been studied mostly with respect to Muslim youth living in the western world (Stevens 2011; Vedder and Van Geel 2013). Though the focus is not explicitly on radicalization, the Rejection Identification Model (RIM) suggests that experiences of discrimination can lead to feelings of anger, and an increased identification with the ethnic identity, as well as rejection of the majority identity (Branscombe et al. 1999). The RIM focuses on personal experiences of discrimination and rejection, but theories on radicalization stress that feelings of discrimination, rejection, and deprivation towards the group one identifies with are the primary catalysts in the radicalization process (Borum 2011); these theories suggest that the way in which immigrants and minorities are received and treated in the receiving countries may contribute to the development of radicalization. However, empirical research on radicalization processes is scarce, thus we cannot be fully sure of what the push and pull factors pertaining to radicalization are. More empirical research is needed, because the personal and societal consequences of this type of identification processes are so grave, while we know so little about how to prevent or cure it.

Research Measurement and Methodology

For studying the questions identified in the preceding section we need a broad variety of research approaches. Specifically, we need methodologies that unravel the processes that constitute the growth in youth's balancing between personal developmental needs of belonging, purpose and accomplishment and the contextual forces that define developmental tasks and social participation to achieve those tasks. We also need surveys to identify normative processes of cultural identity development in a variety of cultural groups and social contexts and settings (Umaña-Taylor et al.

2014). Such studies provide a basis for monitoring youth cultural identity development and its protective, motivating, health enhancing qualities, while allowing us to timely signal circumstances and developmental courses jeopardizing these positive qualities. We need more longitudinal studies to learn more about the dynamics of the development of cultural identities; not just to know more about the order in which particular aspects and manifestations of the development of cultural identities follow each other, if at all, but also to identify causes, consequences and transactional processes linking these aspects.

When it comes to causes and consequences, longitudinal studies are important, but not sufficient. One of the challenges with longitudinal studies is the risk of attribution errors that are due to the infeasibility to control for the effects of confounders. A type of design that allows for more control and better exclusion of confounders is an experimental design. Experimental designs can, for instance, clarify how contextual cues raise the salience of a particular cultural orientation and activate particular identity relevant cognitions in bicultural youths. The change of contextual cues leads to cultural frame switching and triggers particular knowledge structures that play a role in identity development (cf. Luna et al. 2008). Earlier in the chapter we referred to Mok and Morris (2012) who showed that by priming a particular cultural frame in a given situation (e.g., by changing the use of the language primarily linked to a particular culture) a multicultural person appreciates the situation different depending on the primed cultural frame. This type of research may eventually clarify how and why people experience and label particular information and social interactions differently from other persons (e.g., as culturally biased, as abusive).

One might wonder about the impact of policy and events on the development of cultural identity. It is not difficult to think of both policies (e.g., legislation against headscarves), and events (the Arab Spring, the terrorist attacks of the 11th of

September 2001) that may be sources of pride, shame or anger, and lead an individual to reaffirm, question or even alter that individual's cultural identities. Sirin and Fine (2007) used a mixed method design to demonstrate how the terrorist attacks of the 11th of September 2001 affected the identity formation of Arab American youth, and this study serves to demonstrate that major events can indeed influence identity development among minority youth. Another potentially powerful technique to understand processes connected with identity development are natural experiments. Specifically, scholars can document the development of identity amongst cultural minority youth before and after a major event or policy change. Such events or policy changes would serve to define the "natural experimental condition". Since these grave events and policy changes are mostly not foreseen or planned by researchers interested in such natural experiments, such experiment are largely lacking. Thus though we know that policies and events may have an influence, data to study such general tendencies are lacking.

We wrote about the embeddedness of cultural identity development in social contexts. In terms of designs this almost automatically calls for the use of multilevel designs. They are not just relevant for studying the connection between changes in social contexts and changes at the individual plane (Christ et al. 2013; Fasel et al. 2013), they also may be applied to repeated measures for modeling individual trajectories (Hox and Stoel 2005).

True experiments, natural experiments, and multi-level methods are all valuable in the study of cultural identity formation, but each by itself is too limited given the complex nature of the processes involving the interaction of multiple individual and contextual factors occurring over time. Unfortunately, most studies of identity that explore changes in cultural identity use single wave measures; typically surveys that require individuals to reflect on their attitudes. This may result in an indication of a current position in an adolescent cultural identity development, but it provides no information of how the youth came to this position. Lichtwarck-Aschoff et al. (2008) even contend that when surveys are used repeatedly in a longitudinal design, it is likely to result in just "snapshots" of development. Survey data do not consistently provide accurate and comprehensive pictures of how relevant processes take shape and what triggers the processes to change or adapt to changing circumstances. To overcome this limitation they propose to conduct micro-level research focusing on concrete experiences where actions and interactions take place in minutes or hours. Micro level research, such as case studies, interviews, narratives, and vignettes, can reveal moments in which individuals are faced with identity challenges and make decisions that shape identity development. These identity challenges can be triggered by others such as parents who try to regulate a person's identity choice and accompanying identity manifestations. Examination of a series of such moments could trace progress of identity development. As clarified by Vedder and Phinney (2014) these types of designs are challenging because they are extremely intensive and time consuming, hence feasibility is under constant pressure. Moreover, due to the scale and specificity, such studies are likely to produce results of limited generalizability. Nevertheless the promise to come closer to a good representation of the emergence of cultural identity is a tempting perspective.

Empirical Findings

In this section we focus on how cultural identity leads or corresponds to protection against negative influences and positive developmental adaptations. We present research showing that a sense of cultural identity often has these positive correlates or consequences. Yet, not in all situations and with respect to all manifestations of development and personal appreciations this is always experienced as something positive.

We return to the notion that cultural identity in modern western societies often entails multicultural identity. We contend that cultural identity is often experienced as a resource. The feeling of connectedness with a community of like-minded people and the accompanying perception of the availability of support from these people imbues a sense of resourcefulness. Another instantiation is found in the skills and knowledge accompanying a particular identity (i.e., language competence, commonalities of style, social participation and culture specific as well as intercultural competences). And finally, the capacity to shift between different cultural frames and move with confidence in a variety of cultural contexts testifies to a person's cultural identity as a resource. These capacities all facilitate a person's connection to and engagement with multiple cultural groups.

This being said, it is important to note that youth growing up with more than one cultural frame of reference do not necessarily grow up with a positive and strong sense of belonging, good availability of, and access to social resources. The different cultural frames of reference may be all linked to some minority group. The status and sense of identity derived from belonging to multiple minority groups depends on how each is viewed within the larger society, the distribution of power and wealth in society as well as how members of each of the minority groups perceives the other. This is, for instance, the case for children growing up in the Netherlands with a mother who has an Indo-Caribbean background and a father from Morocco. Neither the Indo-Caribbean frame, with its Hindu cultural connections, nor the Muslim-Moroccan frame is commonly seen as an asset by members of the majority group; in this case, white European Dutch. Such children will grow up in a culturally diversified and rich environment but frequently experience that neither minority cultural group is appreciated by the majority group. They may grow up as a member of multiple minority groups, experiencing harassment, disappointments and rejection whatever cultural frame of reference they use in a given situation. Navarrete and Jenkins (2011), referring to multi-racial emergent adult, undergraduate students living in the USA show that such youth runs a higher risk of feeling lost. In effect, they experience a kind of cultural homelessness. This study shows that the contextualized nature of cultural identity in practice deals with multiple and hierarchically structured contexts that are connected by particular power relationships. The young adults in the study of Navarrete and Jenkins (2011) deal with social contexts substantiated by members of two minority cultures to which the students are linked through their father and mother. These two culture specific social contexts are overshadowed by the American majority culture that at the level of personal and institutional contacts not always provides equal rights to all its inhabitants. Such circumstances are not uncommon throughout the Western world (cf. Berry and Vedder 2016).

A further qualification of the notion of cultural identity as a resource can be found in studies on radicalization. Radicalization in a sense is a process of re-identification. Skrobanek (2009) studied this phenomenon in Germany with Turkish immigrants of first and second generation. Results showed that when Turkish immigrants felt that members of their own group were victims of discrimination, such a perception enhanced the distance between Turks and Germans as well as a reorientation of Turks towards their fellow Turks. To replenish the feelings of loss and frustration, people look for improved access to and intensified social bonds with their own group. As a result of these processes, Turks become increasingly more conservative, more radical and less open to the German society (Ramm 2010). This process does not take shape in all Turks and when it does it is not equally intensive between Turks. Whether it takes shape and how intensively depends on concrete living conditions in the country of settlement (Berry et al. 2006; Ersanilli and Koopmans 2010). Vedder and Van Geel (2013) define

this process as basic to radicalization processes and add that feelings of discrimination and depreciation preceding radicalization may be relieved by seeking revenge (e.g., demolishing public property). When it is combined with identification processes, seeking connections and having discussions with like-minded youth, opinions tend to become more extreme (Thompson et al. 2000). In such situations, youth may voice support for acts of terrorism or argue the justification of terrorist acts. In rare cases this may eventually be followed by actual involvement in terrorism.

The process of identity exploration and mutual commitment that often occurs when youth feel alienated from the larger society is nicely depicted in a study by Adraoui (2009). Referring to Muslim youth in France, Adraoui shows how group consensus on the correct interpretation of particular parts of the scripture helps Muslim youth to cope with the situation of depreciation that they experience. From being judged and rejected by others, they move to a situation that allows them to see themselves as safeguards of truth and the just. From victims or losers they change into the imposers of the standard of right and wrong. In short, they gain control of their lives. We refer to this process as akin to cultural identity, but in the end it is probably better to refer to it as a religious identity. Note that also for these adolescents cultural identity is experienced as a resource. It adds to a feeling of fulfillment and direction in life that is connected with feelings of happiness and inner strength. It concurs to the notions and expectations entailed in the RIM put forward by Branscombe et al. (1999).

Findings by Knight et al. (2012) demonstrate how the value of ethnic identity as a resource depends on the social context. The researchers followed 300 14–17 years old Mexican American juvenile offenders over a period of 7 years analyzing relationships between changes in ethnic identity, gang membership and offending. Most of these adolescents came from single parent homes (67 %) and 42 % had parents who had not complete high school. They suspected that adolescents who actively and intensively seek to know more about their ethnic background have a higher chance of becoming a gang member of an ethnically homogeneous gang, and then find opportunities to explore their ethnic identity, but are simultaneously modeled and enticed to engagement in serious offending. Their findings suggest a more subtle story. They distinguished four groups: the first two were youth low on offending but one was high on ethnic identity, whereas the other was moderate. The other two groups were moderate on ethnic identity, and one was moderate on offending and the other was high on offending. These results clarify that there is no simple relation between ethnic identity and offending. Gang membership was most prevalent in the two groups moderate on ethnic identity, of which one was moderate on offending and the other high on offending. In comparison to the group with adolescents who scored low on ethnic identity and low on offending the group combining high ethnic identity scores and low offending scores were predominantly 1st and 2nd generation immigrant adolescents whose mothers predominantly spoke Spanish and who more often were gang members, whereas in the first group the adolescents were predominantly 3rd and 4th generation immigrants, far less had a Spanish speaking mother and they were far less often gang members. The researchers suggest that for the latter group ethnic exploration was likely less important than it was for those high on ethnic identity and with this came a lower chance of getting involved in a gang. A final interesting finding was that youth in the moderate ethnic identity and high offending group, not only had the highest chance of being involved in a gang, but also showed the lowest stability over time in ethnic identity. They started relatively low in ethnic identity, but increased considerably over time, which corresponds with increases in time spent with ethnically homogeneous gang members. The authors conclude that the quality of ethnic identity as a protective or risk factor depends to a large extent on such circumstances or opportunities available through peer relationships, accessibility of cultural resources and probably many more. Nevertheless, even given the context dependence of the resourcefulness of cultural identity, it is tempting to use a telling title of an article by Elmore and Oyserman (2012) as a general rule that stresses contextuality but also shows that it can transcend particular contexts or situations: "If 'we' can succeed, 'I' can too!"

Universal Versus Culture-Specific Mechanisms

More than a decade ago Phinney et al. (2001) argued that there is no common global process of multicultural identity development in immigrant youth. Rather, data and the literature indicate that the most positive outcomes of this process result when societies provide real opportunities for immigrants to make choices as to the way and the extent to which they retain their ethnic identity. Hence, supportive societies or communities make for resourceful cultural identities (Shweder et al. 2006). This expresses what is likely a very broadly applicable rule: a sense of alignment between personal and group purposes with respect to personal as well as social challenges makes for inner personal as well as group based strength to invest effort and time in changing one's life and community in a desired direction.

Such basic processes as exploration, commitment and reconsideration are the cognitive tools for developing a notion about "who I am". They also help in the formulation of ideas of how I am perceived by others and what these others want of me (Phinney and Baldelomar 2011). These processes shape the building blocks of any cultural identity and are, in that sense, universal. The outcomes, however, always will be person, time and situation specific. Even when the goal is, as suggested by Erikson (1968), to transcend particular situations and particular times and sometimes even particular cultural or group related appreciations, identity development and cultural context are interdependent (Hammack 2008; Schachter 2005; Vedder and Phinney 2014). Moreover, arguing that the processes of exploration, commitment, and reconsideration are universal does not mean that the outcomes in terms of identity status are universal. What is evaluated or presented as the status that normatively represents the most advanced level of identity development depends on the dominant view on desirable relationships between dependent persons and on preferences for types of interactions and interpersonal restraint between these people (Phinney and Baldelomar 2011). For instance, the achieved status, may be seen as the most preferred status from an American or western perspective. In communities that are characterized by more and strong interdependent relationships, or even dependent relationships between children and adults, foreclosure may be the preferred status. There is no universal goal or standard in identity development (Vedder and Phinney 2014).

Johnson et al. (2012) provide a nice example in a study employing the Multigroup Ethnic Identity Measure (Phinney 1992) to compare the ethnic identity between 11 and 27 years old students living in Uganda (242), Tanzania (231), and the USA (81). Students in Uganda and Tanzania came from lower SES backgrounds than students in the USA. About 40 % of the students in Uganda and Tanzania lived under harsh economic conditions, often lacking basic needs such as food and shelter. None of the American students lived under such circumstances. Most US-students were Caucasian, while the East-African students came from a wide variety of self-reported groups, predominantly

with tribal references or reference to linguistic communities. A remarkable finding was that the East-African students had extremely low scores on the exploration part of the MEIM. This is not to say that they do not explore their cultural roots, but it is likely to reflect that no one in their community questions it. They live in highly culturally diverse communities and it is taken for granted that adolescents belong to and represent a particular tribal or linguistic segment. Most of these youth communicate in a variety of languages allowing them to understand each other and blend whenever needed. They are likely to feel like a fish in water that accommodates a fish's needs. This is different with the US students. They grow up with the experience that cultural distinctions do matter in terms of social mobility and access to desirable places and commodities. They have to explore, find, establish, deny or reconfirm their cultural identity on their way to adulthood, particularly if they belong to a visible minority. In their study Johnson et al. (2012) clarify that for the American Caucasian youth this is less a challenge at the moment, but they predict that this will change by 2050 when the Caucasian Americans will likely be an ethnic minority in the USA.

Policy Implications

Throughout this chapter we mentioned studies that have repeatedly demonstrated that identity is related to both feeling well and doing well for youth. Youth may derive a sense of pride and a sense of belonging from their cultural identity, which may make them feel good about themselves, and that may urge them to do their best in school, and help out in the family and the wider community. Furthermore, a strong cultural identity may buffer against experiences of discrimination, as youth who feel certain about their cultural identity may see discrimination as an act of the perpetrator and not blame themselves or internalize the experience. Allowing youth to explore and form their own identities is also a cornerstone of a truly multicultural society, in which youth can learn about different cultures and prepare for participation in a culturally diverse world.

Yet the identity formation process also comes with risks and challenges both to youth personally and to the larger community in the instance of radicalization. A common denominator for both these problems appears to be that youth can feel that the larger community may not value, or may even derogate, the cultural group(s) that they belong to. Feelings of alienation, derogation and discrimination may frustrate a healthy exploration of identity and lead youth to unhappiness, marginalization or radicalization rather than transcendence. We may than conclude that policy regarding cultural identity should stimulate the healthy exploration and development of cultural identity, but prevent the pitfalls of marginalization and radicalization. This is not an easy task, but in democratic societies certainly one that should be taken up by schools. And yet, because longitudinal studies are largely lacking, and results are difficult to generalize across contexts and ethnic groups it is difficult to provide a one-size-fits-all advice. Yes, schools are likely to play an important role, but how and what about other people or institutions? We miss important information. For instance, we need to know what support is needed and acceptable to adolescents. Would peers make for good coaches and do they need training? Would kin be a better option, or is a self-help app a preferred one? We don't have the answers. Given what we know, however, it seems safe to say that we should allow youth to explore and discuss their identity in freedom, provide them with the resources necessary for exploration, provide advice and support where needed, and create a safe environment free of discrimination and ostracism in which youth can explore.

Future Directions

At the end of a paper emphasizing the complex and dynamic nature of cultural identity, it is tempting to suggest that this complexity and dynamism are the precise reasons for returning to a more simple approach of cultural identity in research. And indeed, we do need better-validated instruments that more accurately represent the contextualized nature of cultural identity development (Johnson et al. 2012). To be able to do this we need to stick to the notion of self-sameness as an important constituent element or process of identity development. It is at the same time the representation that allows scholars to distinguish the object of their study that is constantly changing and adapting to constraints and requirements that differ over time and between situations. It should allow us to keep track of the essence of what we are studying. We need better instruments to capture the complexities and developments in identity, and future research should focus on developing and validating such instruments.

Cultural identity is not a static characteristic. Like many risk factors and processes of adaptation, identity is always under construction, even when a mature sense of identity has been largely achieved (Masten 2014). There is ongoing interplay between context, a person's competencies and proclivities, and a person's sense of identity. It is, therefore, particularly interesting to examine their longitudinal interplay. This interplay is likely to reveal when and to what extent cultural identity is functioning as a resource that really supports a child or adolescents' development and health.

Earlier in the chapter we contended that there is a continued need for studies on normative cultural identity processes. These studies will likely be group or community specific. And yet the question remains whether it is possible to identify normative paths of cultural identity development that are effectively universal. Vedder and Phinney (2014) wondered whether we can develop relatively stable notions of ideal and optimal bicultural identities for youths from particular cultural groups, and if so, how? These scholars suggest that we need more research on the way developmental paths of cultural identity take shape. We need information on the relationship of cultural identity development to child and adolescent cognitive, linguistic and emotional development and on the influence of family, community, and societal contexts. In short, it makes sense to accept the challenge of the complex nature of cultural identity development in context as our study object.

References

Adraoui, M.-A. (2009). Salafism in France: Ideology, practices and contradictions. In R. Meijer (Ed.), *Global salafism: Islam's new religious movement* (pp. 364–379). New York: Columbia University Press.

Alvarado, M., & Ricard, R. J. (2013). Developmental assets and ethnic identity as predictors of thriving in Hispanic adolescents. *Hispanic Journal of Behavioral Sciences, 34,* 510–523.

Becker, J. C., Tausch, N., Spears, R., & Christ, O. (2011). Committed dis (s) idents: Participation in radical collective action fosters disidentification with the broader in-group but enhances political identification. *Personality and Social Psychology Bulletin, 37,* 1104–1116.

Berry, J. W., Phinney, J. S., Sam, D. L., & Vedder, P. (2006). *Immigrant youth in cultural transition: Acculturation, identity and adaptation across national contexts.* Mahwah: Lawrence Erlbaum Associates.

Berry, J. W., & Vedder, P. (2016). Adaptation of Immigrant Children, Adolescents and their Families. In U. P. Gielen & J. L. Roopnarine (Eds.), *Childhood and adolescence: Cross-cultural perspectives and applications* (2nd ed.) (pp. 321–346). Santa Barbara, CA: Praeger.

Borum, R. (2011). Radicalization into violent extremism I: A review of social science theories. *Journal of Strategic Security, 4,* 7–36.

Branscombe, N. R., Schmitt, M. T., & Harvey, R. D. (1999). Perceiving pervasive discrimination among African-Americans: Implications for group identification and well-being. *Journal of Personality and Social Psychology, 77,* 135–149.

Christ, O., Asbrock, F., Dhont, K., Pettigrew, T. F., & Wagner, U. (2013). The effects of intergroup climate on immigrants' acculturation preferences. *Zeitschrift für Psychologie, 221,* 252–257.

Crocetti, E., Rubini, M., & Meeus, W. (2008). Capturing the dynamics of identity formation in various ethnic groups: Development and validation of a three-dimensional model. *Journal of Adolescence, 31*(2), 207–222.

Diamond, J. (2010). The benefits of multilingualism. *Science, 330,* 332–333.

Elmore, K. C., & Oyserman, D. (2012). If 'we' can succeed, 'I' can too: Identity-based motivation and gender in the classroom. *Contemporary Educational Psychology, 37,* 176–185.

Erikson, E. (1968). *Identity: Youth and crisis.* New York: Norton.

Ersanilli, E., & Koopmans, R. (2010). Rewarding integration? Citizenship regulations and the socio-cultural integration of immigrants in the Netherlands, France and Germany. *Journal of Ethnic and Migration Studies, 36,* 773–791.

Fasel, N., Green, E. G. T., & Sarrasin, O. (2013). Unveiling naturalization: A multilevel study on minority proportion, conservative ideologies and attitudes towards the Muslim veil. *Zeitschrift für Psychologie, 221,* 242–251.

Fleischmann, F., & Verkuyten, M. (2016). Dual identity among immigrants: Comparing different conceptualizations, their measurement and implications. *Cultural Diversity and Ethnic Minority Psychology, 22,* 151–165.

Hammack, P. L. (2008). Narrative and the cultural psychology of identity. *Personality and Social Psychology Review, 12,* 222–247.

Hickman, C. B. (1997). The devil and the one drop rule: Racial categories, African Americans, and the US census. *Michigan Law Review, 95,* 1161–1265.

Hong, Y., Morris, M. W., Chiu, C., & Benet-Martinez, V. (2000). Multiple minds: A dynamic constructivist approach to culture and cognition. *American Psychologist, 55,* 709–720.

Horenczyk, G., Jasinskaja-Lahti, I., Sam, D. L., & Vedder, P. (2013). Mutuality in acculturation: Towards an integration. *Zeitschrift für Psychologie, 221,* 205–213.

Hox, J. J., & Stoel, R. D. (2005). Multilevel and SEM approaches to growth curve modelling. In B. S. Everitt & D. C. Howell (Eds.), *Encyclopedia in statistics in behavioral science* (pp. 1296–1305). Chichester: Wiley.

Johnson, L. R., Kim, E. A., Johnson-Pynn, J. S., Schulenberg, S. E., Balagaye, H., & Lugumya, D. (2012). Ethnic identity, self-efficacy, and intercultural attitudes in East African and U.S. youth. *Journal of Adolescent Research, 27,* 256–289.

Kiang, L., & Fuligni, A. J. (2009). Ethnic identity in context: Variations in ethnic exploration and belonging within parent, same-ethnic peer, and different-ethnic peer relationships. *Journal of Youth and Adolescence, 38,* 732–743.

Kim, S. Y., & Chao, R. K. (2009). Heritage language fluency, ethnic identity, and school effort of immigrant Chinese and Mexican adolescents. *Cultural Diversity and Ethnic Minority Psychology, 15*, 27–37.

Knight, G. P., Losoya, S. H., Cho, Y. I., Chassin, L., Williams, J. L., & Cota-Robles, S. (2012). Ethnic identity and offending trajectories among Mexican-American juvenile offenders: gang membership and psychosocial maturity. *Journal of Research on Adolescence, 22*, 782–796.

Kroger, J., Martinussen, M., & Marcia, J. E. (2010). Identity status change during adolescence and young adulthood: A meta-analysis. *Journal of Adolescence, 33*, 683–698.

Lichtwarck-Aschoff, A., Van Geert, P., Bosma, H., & Kunnen, S. (2008). Time and identity: A framework for research and theory formation. *Developmental Review, 28*, 370–400.

Liebkind, K. (2001). Acculturation. In R. Brown & S. Gaertner (Eds.), *Blackwell handbook of social psychology: Intergroup processes* (Vol. 4, pp. 386–406). Oxford: Basil Blackwell.

Luna, D., Ringberg, T., & Peracchio, L. A. (2008). One individual, two identities: Frame switching among biculturals. *Journal of Consumer Research, 35*, 279–293.

Marcia, J. E. (1966). Development and validation of ego identity status. *Journal of Personality and Social Psychology, 3*, 551–558.

Masten, A. S. (2014). Global perspectives on resilience in children and youth. *Child Development, 85*, 6–20.

Mok, A., & Morris, M. W. (2012). Managing two cultural identities the malleability of bicultural identity integration as a function of induced global or local processing. *Personality and Social Psychology Bulletin, 38*, 233–246.

Navarrete, V., & Jenkins, S. R. (2011). Cultural homelessness, multiminority status, ethnic identity development, and self-esteem. *International Journal of Intercultural Relations, 35*, 791–804.

Neblett, E. W., & Carter, S. E. (2012). The protective role of racial identity and Africentric worldview in the association between racial discrimination and blood pressure. *Psychosomatic Medicine, 74*, 509–516.

Padilla, A. M. (2006). Bicultural social development. *Hispanic Journal of Behavioral Sciences, 28*, 467–497.

Phinney, J. S. (1992). The multigroup ethnic identity measure a new scale for use with diverse groups. *Journal of Adolescent Research, 7*, 156–176.

Phinney, J. S., & Baldelomar, O. A. (2011). Identity development in multiple cultural contexts. In L. A. Jensen (Ed.), *Bridging cultural and developmental psychology: New syntheses for theory, research and policy* (pp. 161–186). New York: Oxford University Press.

Phinney, J. S., Horenczyk, G., Liebkind, K., & Vedder, P. (2001). Ethnic identity, immigration, and well-being: An interactional perspective. *Journal of Social Issues, 57*, 493–510.

Quintana, S. N., Aboud, F. E., Chao, R. K., Contreras-Grau, J., Cross, W. E., Hudley, C., et al. (2006). Race, ethnicity, and culture in child development: Contemporary research and future directions. *Child Development, 77*, 1129–1141.

Ramm, C. (2010). The Muslim-makers: How Germany 'Islamizes' Turkish immigrants. *Interventions: International Journal of Postcolonial Studies, 12*, 183–197.

Ruble, D., Alvarez, J., Bachman, M., Cameron, J., Fuligni, A., Garcia Coll, C., et al. (2004). The development of a sense of "we": The emergence and implications of children's collective identity. In M. Bennett & F. Sani (Eds.), *The development of the social self* (pp. 29–76). New York: Psychology Press.

Schachter, E. (2005). Context and identity formation: A theoretical analysis and a case study. *Journal of Adolescence Research, 20*, 375–396.

Shweder, R., Goodnow, J., Hatano, G., Levine, R., Markus, H., & Miller, P. (2006). The cultural psychology of development: One mind, many mentalities. In R. Lerner (Ed.), *Handbook of child psychology* (6th ed., Vol. 1, pp. 716–792). Hoboken, NJ: Wiley.

Sirin, S. R., & Fine, M. (2007). Hyphenated selves: Muslim American youth negotiating identities on the fault lines of global conflict. *Applied Development Science, 11*(3), 151–163.

Skrobanek, J. (2009). Perceived discrimination, ethnic identity and the (re-) ethnicisation of youth with a Turkish ethnic background in Germany. *Journal of Ethnic and Migration Studies, 35*, 535–554.

Stevens, D. (2011). Reasons to be fearful, one, two, three: The 'preventing violent extremism' agenda. *British Journal of Politics and International Relations, 13*, 165–188.

Tajfel, H. (1981). *Human groups and social categories*. Cambridge: Cambridge University Press.

Tajfel, H., & Turner, J. C. (1979). An integrative theory of intergroup conflict. In W. G. Austin & S. Worchel (Eds.), *The social psychology of intergroup relations* (pp. 33–47). Monterey, CA: Brookes-Cole.

Thompson, M. S., Judd, C. M., & Park, B. (2000). The consequences of communicating social stereotypes. *Journal of Experimental Social Psychology, 36*(6), 567–599.

Umaña-Taylor, A. J., O'Donnell, M., Knight, G. P., Roosa, M. W., Berkel, C., & Nair, R. (2014). Mexican-origin early adolescents' ethnic socialization, ethnic identity, and psychological functioning. *The Counseling Psychologist, 42*, 170–200.

Vedder, P., & Phinney, J. (2014). Identity formation in bicultural youth: A developmental perspective. In V. Benet-Martínez & Y.-Y. Hong (Eds.), *Handbook of multicultural identity* (pp. 335–354). Oxford: Oxford University Press.

Vedder, P., & Van Geel, M. (2013). Radicalizing Muslim youth; A conceptual analysis and consequences for interventions. In E. Tartakovsky (Ed.), *Immigration: Policies, challenges and impact* (pp. 395–414). Hauppauge, NY: Nova Science.

Verkuyten, M. (2005). *The social psychology of ethnic identity*. Hove: Psychology Press.

Verkuyten, M., & Pouliasi, K. (2002). Biculturalism among older children cultural frame switching, attributions, self-identification, and attitudes. *Journal of Cross-Cultural Psychology, 33*(6), 596–609.

Williams, J. L., Tolan, P. H., Durkee, M. I., Francois, A. G., & Anderson, R. E. (2012). Integrating racial and ethnic identity research into developmental understanding of adolescents. *Child Development Perspectives, 6,* 304–311.

Wong, T. M. L., Branje, S. J. T., VanderValk, I. E., Hawk, S. T., & Meeus, W. H. J. (2010). The role of siblings in identity development in adolescence and emerging adulthood. *Journal of Adolescence, 33,* 673–682.

Differential Susceptibility in Minority Children: Individual Differences in Environmental Sensitivity

Elham Assary and Michael Pluess

Abstract

In developmental psychology, individual differences in response to environmental influences have often been conceptualized from a perspective of diathesis-stress. According to this framework, adversity will lead to negative outcomes only in individuals that also carry some form of vulnerability (e.g. genetic, psychological traits). Children without such vulnerability, on the other hand, are likely to be resilient in the face of adversity. This model, however, does not lend itself to the examination of individual variability in response to effects of positive influences. Over the last decade, several new frameworks have been developed that describe individual differences in environmental sensitivity more generally, including differential susceptibility theory, biological sensitivity to context and sensory-processing sensitivity. These concepts are based on the notion that individual differences in response to environmental influences reflect an individual's general sensitivity to environmental influences. Importantly, such general sensitivity moderates the effects of negative as well as positive environmental influences. Empirical studies indicate that individual differences in environmental sensitivity may explain variation in the well-being of minority children when exposed to adverse environments, but also in response to supportive exposures (including intervention). Adopting a perspective of individual differences in general environmental sensitivity will benefit researchers, policy makers and practitioners alike in their efforts to better understand and promote positive development and well-being in minority children.

Overview and Theoretical Perspectives

Minority groups, in comparison to non-minority groups, are faced with more prejudice, discrimination and racism, which hinder their integration

E. Assary · M. Pluess (✉)
Department of Biological and Experimental Psychology, School of Biological and Chemical Sciences, Queen Mary University of London, Mile End Road, London E1 4NS, UK
e-mail: m.pluess@qmul.ac.uk

© The Editor(s) 2017
N.J. Cabrera and B. Leyendecker (eds.), *Handbook on Positive Development of Minority Children and Youth*, DOI 10.1007/978-3-319-43645-6_9

into society and, at times, lead to social exclusion, with adverse effects on the psychological health of minority children and families (Brody et al. 2006; Coll et al. 1996). For example, discrimination has been found to be associated with depressive symptoms and lower self-esteem (Pascoe and Smart Richman 2009). Furthermore, those with minority status are more likely than other groups to experience poverty and lower socio-economic status (SES) (Rogler 1994; Timberlake 2007), which means they are more likely to live in more dangerous neighborhoods and in more crowded conditions (Iceland and Bauman 2007). Not surprisingly, such living conditions are also associated with increased levels of stress and maladjustment (Dahl et al. 2010; Evans and Kim 2007; Schapkin et al. 2006).

Acknowledging the increased exposure of minority groups to environmental risk factors and the negative outcomes associated with these risks, much of the research with minority groups has concentrated on evaluating the detrimental effects of contextual adversities on a wide range of psychological and physical health outcomes. Findings from these studies with adult and child minority groups suggest that minority children, compared to non-minority children, are generally at increased risk of mental health problems such as anxiety, depression and conduct problems (Munroe-Blum et al. 1989; Rousseau et al. 1996). The psychological development and well-being of minority children can be directly or indirectly affected by discrimination, prejudice, poverty and lower levels of social support. For example, the child of an asylum-seeking family might develop depression or anxiety directly as a result of facing discrimination at school or, alternatively, may be affected indirectly, by parental conflict brought about by increased levels of stress due to parental unemployment and other migration related issues.

Given that this volume focuses on positive development of minority children, it must be noted that children's well-being and positive development can be conceptualized from two different perspectives: (1) positive development inferred by the absence of psychopathology

(i.e. resilience); or (2) positive development characterized by the presence of competence, ability and achievement (i.e. thriving), as is the position taken by the editors of this handbook. Considering the bias in much of psychological research to study the negative effects of adverse environments on individuals, positive development is often equated with the absence of psychopathology in the presence of adversity. However, though we acknowledge that positive development is fundamentally about more than being resilient to adversity, we will often discuss well-being from a perspective of resilience throughout this chapter, given that this is currently the perspective underlying much of the empirical research in the field (see Motti-Stefanidi and Masten, this volume). Despite this limitation in current research, the theoretical perspectives discussed in the forthcoming sections pertain to behavioral and psychological outcomes more broadly, including competence and well-being and not just maladaptive behaviors and mental health problems.

It is also important to note that the nature of environmental influences that minority children are exposed to depends on how they come to hold the minority position. Some children may be considered minority due to their ancestral ethnic background, even though they and previous generations were born in the same country as the majority ethnic population. Other children, born to a first generation economic migrant family or those settling in a new country as part of an asylum seeking family, can also be classified as minority. While these different types of minority groups may vary in respect to their SES, the majority are likely to be of lower SES, and children of asylum seekers may be exposed to additional challenges. Importantly, the specific cultural background of a minority group (e.g. moral values, social norms, parenting practices etc.) may account for further individual differences between minority groups in adjustment to the host context (Mohler 2001). Caution is thus required in taking a blanket approach in interpreting and applying the findings from studies with one type of minority group to others.

While, historically, research with minority groups have reported increased risk for mental health problems in minority children compared to non-minority children (Aronowitz 1984; Munroe-Blum et al. 1989), more recent research in the field suggest that this association may be exaggerated, or inflated by other factors, including SES. For example, a meta-analysis of studies with children of economic migrant families by Stevens and Vollebergh (2008) suggested that factors such as informant bias (e.g. differences in reports of problem behavior/depression depending on the information source) and cultural differences (e.g. teacher ratings of child behavior being influenced by cultural differences in behavioral standards between the minority and majority culture) complicates drawing firm conclusions as to whether minority children, in comparison to native children, are at genuinely increased risk of internalizing and externalizing problems. Interestingly, research suggests that in some cases, minority children, in comparison to non-minority children, do not differ or are actually at *lower risk* of developing externalizing and internalizing problems (Alati et al. 2003; Beiser et al. 2002; Harker 2001), possibly due to the presence of protective factors such as close relationships between family members and strong cultural identities (Harker 2001; Virta et al. 2004).

As alluded to earlier, holding a minority status is associated with higher risk of mental health problems, either directly as a result of minority group membership which exposes the individuals to more discrimination and racism, or more indirectly due to higher prevalence of poverty in minority groups. Notwithstanding the significant contribution of minority status to risk of developing mental health problems, there is a consensus for the existence of individual differences within minority groups, where environmental risk factors associated with minority status do not homogenously illicit the projected negative outcomes. Simply put, although poverty and discrimination are strongly implicated in increased risk of negative mental health outcomes, the risk does not materialize for all individuals exposed to them. The same observation tends to emerge

with regards to the effects of positive environmental influences on children's development. For example, in a recent study a school-based intervention program intended to prevent internalising problems, benefited some but not all children (Pluess and Boniwell 2015). Undeniably, researchers in the field of individual differences have long been attempting to explain how these individual differences emerge, and what factors contribute to this observed variation. To this end, resilience research has identified two main categories implicated in individual differences in well-being: one relates to individual characteristics (e.g. genetic, biological, and physiological factors or behavioural phenotypes such as temperament); and the other relates to contextual risk and protective factors (e.g. family, society). With regards to the latter, for example, while low SES is seen as an established risk factor for conduct problems and reduced cognitive abilities (Brooks-Gunn et al. 1996; Duncan et al. 1994), stimulating activities and maternal warmth have been reported to act as protective factors in low income families, ameliorating the adverse effects of low SES (Kim-Cohen et al. 2004).

The contribution of individual characteristics (such as genes or temperament) to variability in response to the effects of environmental influences across development has been the subject of extensive investigation. In the following sections, we will present different theoretical perspectives pertaining to individual differences in environmental sensitivity and consider how individual-level characteristics moderate the effects of environmental influences on behavioural outcomes including competence and psychological well-being.

Theoretical Perspectives of Individual Differences

Questions pertaining to individual differences in the development of competence and wellbeing can be investigated and interpreted from two similar but fundamentally different theoretical perspectives. The older and more widely embraced perspective supposes that variability in response to negative effects of environmental influences is due to inherent individual differences in *vulnerability* or *resilience*. The more recent, alternative perspective proposes that observed variation is due to individual differences in *general environmental sensitivity*.

The vulnerability/resilience view is best reflected in the *Dual-Risk* or *Diathesis-Stress* model (Monroe and Simons 1991; Zuckerman 1999). Based on this model, psychopathology emerges when environmental stressors interact with a vulnerability inherent in the individual (genetic, physiological, and psychological). From this perspective, individual differences in the development of mental health problems in response to contextual adversity emerge because these inherent vulnerability factors exist only in some individuals. The absence of psychopathology despite a history of environmental adversity is viewed as resilience and is usually a function of the absence of vulnerability factors or the presence of protective factors.

Historically, the focus of much research in psychology on the development of psychopathology led most researchers to adopt the diathesis-stress framework to explain individual differences in mental health outcomes (Gottesman and Shields 1967; Monroe and Simons 1991; Zuckerman 1999). The diathesis-stress perspective has been very helpful in conceptualizing the interactive effects of contextual risk (e.g. poverty), protective factors (e.g. sensitive parenting) and individual characteristics (e.g. temperament) to predict psychopathology (e.g. externalizing behaviors). However, while the diathesis-stress model aptly explains individual differences in response to adverse exposures, this model is not well suited to explain individual differences in response to positive/supportive environments. This is because diathesis-stress does not make any specific prediction about individual differences in the absence of adverse contextual influences, besides implying that in the absence of adversity, individual vulnerability factors would not necessarily result in any observable behavioral differences.

Over the last two decades, three related but different theoretical frameworks for individual differences in general environmental sensitivity have been developed as an alternative perspective to the vulnerability view embraced by the diathesis-stress model. Although these frameworks differ in important ways, including the hypothesized origins and specific mechanisms of environmental sensitivity, they are all rooted in evolutionary reasoning to explain why individual differences in environmental sensitivity should exist. Three theoretical frameworks that describe individual differences in environmental sensitivity more generally include: *biological sensitivity to context* (BSC; Boyce and Ellis 2005; Ellis et al. 2005), *sensory-processing sensitivity* (SPS; Aron 1996; Aron and Aron 1997) and *differential susceptibility theory* (DST; Belsky 1997, 2005; Belsky and Pluess 2009, 2013). All three frameworks build on the dynamic of the diathesis-stress model, where variation in well-being is the result of the interaction between environmental risk factors and individual characteristics. However, rather than considering these individual characteristics as vulnerability factors that increase vulnerability to the detrimental effects of adverse environments, they consider these factors to be sensitivity markers that predispose the individual to be more responsive to both negative and positive environmental influences. Consequently, this perspective proposes that individual variation in general environmental sensitivity may explain widely observed variability in the effects of both *negative and positive* environmental factors on psychological outcomes (both psychological problems and well-being).

To summarize, environmental sensitivity frameworks differ in important ways from the diathesis-stress model: (1) they all focus on variability in general sensitivity to environmental influences on the basis of evolutionary theory; and (2) they propose that individual differences in environmental sensitivity moderate the effects of both negative *and* positive environmental influences.

In what follows, we will discuss in more detail, the three dominant theoretical frameworks of environmental sensitivity and review selected empirical evidence. Importantly, although the aim of this chapter is to focus on individual differences in minority children, some of the reviewed research is conducted with non-minority populations, given the relative scarcity of research that examines these theories in minority groups.

Differential Susceptibility Theory

The *DST* (Belsky 1997, 2005; Belsky and Pluess 2009, 2013) postulates that individuals differ in the extent to which they are affected by environmental influences as a result of individual differences in general susceptibility—and not just vulnerability. Importantly, DST proposes that those individuals who are more susceptible to the effects of negative environments are also likely to be more susceptible to the effects of positive environmental exposures. The inherent general sensitivity thus functions in a "for better and for worse" manner (Belsky et al. 2007).

DST was initially proposed by Belsky (1997, 2005) on the basis of evolutionary theory, according to which the primary goal of all living beings is to pass on their genes to future generations. From that perspective, developmental strategies that enhance the chances of reproductive fitness are considered optimal even if they infer psychological maladjustment. For example, whereas heightened levels of aggression are considered maladaptive in most societies, an evolutionary-developmental view may suggest that aggression in a context of low resources may be an adaptive and optimal strategy that increases the chances of obtaining resources and, hence, promote reproductive fitness. Developmental plasticity, the ability to adapt the phenotype to environmental conditions, may increase reproductive fitness through optimal adaptation to the prevailing context. However, such plasticity also carries costs and includes risks due to a potential mismatch between the developing environment and the one in which the developed individual finds itself during the reproductive period. Thus, developmental plasticity is associated with both risks and opportunities. Consequently, DST proposes that there should be variation in such developmental plasticity. Drawing on

evolutionary theory, Belsky (1997, 2005) proposed that since the future is inherently unpredictable, high plasticity would not always prove to be adaptive—specifically in environments where the current environment is not predictive of what is to come. Hence, natural selection would have led to propagation of at least two plasticity types: high and low phenotypic plasticity. Following on from this line of reasoning, DST maintains that individual differences in environmental sensitivity are predominantly genetically determined, although more recently, it has been suggested that high susceptibility may also be shaped by early environmental influences (Belsky and Pluess 2009; Pluess and Belsky 2011).

Most importantly, DST suggests that individual susceptibility extends to the positive end of the quality of environment spectrum. While vulnerability, as captured in the diathesis-stress model, reflects the "dark side" of differential susceptibility, *Vantage Sensitivity* has been suggested more recently as a concept and terminology to describe the "bright side" of differential susceptibility (Pluess and Belsky 2013). The concept of Vantage Sensitivity is closely related to DST and characterizes the disproportionate advantage a highly susceptible individual may gain in the context of supportive environments, as opposed to the disproportionate disadvantage in response to adverse environments. Failure to benefit from positive environmental influences has been termed *Vantage Resistance* (Pluess and Belsky 2013). Vantage Sensitivity proposes that individual differences in response to positive environmental influences are a function of an individual's inherent environmental sensitivity. Importantly, although Vantage Sensitivity describes primarily the positive end of differential susceptibility, in some cases a sensitive individual might be especially responsive to the effects of positive environments but not necessarily to the effects of negative environments. Similarly, a vantage resistant individual may be resistant to the effects of positive environments but not necessarily resilient to the negative impact of adverse experiences. Hence, although

Vantage Sensitivity is part of DST, it is not the same as it.

Biological Sensitivity to Context

Similar to DST, *BSC* (Boyce and Ellis 2005; Ellis et al. 2005) is also concerned with development from an evolutionary perspective, but proposes that individuals adapt the degree of their environmental sensitivity to the conditions of the specific context. Notably, BSC suggests that individual differences in physiological reactivity—reflected in the stress response systems—contribute to individual difference in environmental sensitivity in response to both negative and positive environmental influences. According to this model, children in more positive environmental contexts, as well as more adverse conditions, will both develop higher physiological reactivity (Boyce and Ellis 2005; Ellis et al. 2005). In line with this reasoning, stressful childhood environments predispose a child to develop a heightened reactivity in order to detect and respond to environmental threats, whilst supportive early environments predispose a child to develop heightened reactivity in order to benefit from positive features of the environment. Environments that are not particularly adverse or supportive, on the other hand, lead to the development of physiological reactivity patterns that are less biased and less responsive to environmental influences. Although there are clear conceptual differences between DST and BSC, it is possible to integrate both by considering physiological reactivity as a marker of differential susceptibility reflecting environmental sensitivity at the physiological level (for a detailed comparison of both models, see Del Giudice et al. 2011).

Sensory-Processing Sensitivity

Though taking a slightly different approach than the aforementioned frameworks, *SPS* (Aron 1996; Aron and Aron 1997) is also concerned with individual differences in environmental sensitivity. However, in contrast to DST and BSC, SPS was originally less concerned with developmental processes and more focused on explaining individual differences in sensory sensitivity and depth of processing in adults (Aron 1996; Aron and Aron 1997). Most importantly, SPS theory approaches the notion of individual differences in environmental sensitivity from a personality perspective, suggesting that heightened environmental sensitivity is reflected in a highly sensitive personality type. SPS, similar to DST and BSC, proposes that individuals characterized as highly sensitive are more influenced by both negative and positive environmental influences. According to SPS, the highly sensitive personality trait is characterized by greater awareness of sensory stimulation, behavioral inhibition, higher emotional and physiological reactivity, and deeper cognitive processing of environmental stimuli (Aron et al. 2012). Although heightened SPS is hypothesized to have a genetic basis and to emerge in infancy, it is understood that this trait is further shaped by the specific environments that the individual is exposed to during development (Aron et al. 2005).

An Integrated Perspective

As noted earlier, although the three frameworks for individual differences in environmental sensitivity differ in several aspects, it has been suggested—in an attempt to integrate these different models—that heightened environmental sensitivity may be the function of a generally more sensitive central nervous system. This heightened sensitivity of the central nervous system may be reflected in various biological, physiological and psychological markers found to increase sensitivity to both negative and positive aspects of the environment (for review, see Pluess 2015). According to this hypothesis of "neurosensitivity", genetic and environmentally induced epigenetic factors influence physiological structures and functions of organs, including the central nervous system, which is hypothesized to result in a brain that is more sensitive to environmental influences. Indeed, a large number of gene–environment interaction studies provide empirical evidence that differences in environmental sensitivity are associated with specific genetic polymorphisms involved in brain function (Belsky et al. 2009; Belsky and Pluess 2009, 2013). For example, a genetic variation in the serotonin transporter gene (i.e. 5-HTTLPR) has been shown to moderate environmental influences in a differential susceptibility manner —for better and for worse (van IJzendoorn et al. 2012) and found to also predict amygdala reactivity (Munafo et al. 2009). Important to mention that, the same genetic factors that predict individual differences in environmental sensitivity are also associated with a range of other physiological outcomes besides brain functioning, including reactivity of the physiological stress system.

In summary, although these theoretical frameworks differ in some aspects, they share some important features regarding the notion of individual differences in environmental sensitivity: (1) they all adopt evolutionary reasoning—to some extent—for explaining why individual differences in environmental sensitivity should exist in the first place; (2) they propose that individual differences in environmental sensitivity would emerge in response to both negative as well as positive environmental influences; and (3) they suggest that individual differences in environmental sensitivity have a biological basis (i.e. are genetically influenced).

Current Research Questions

Whilst our knowledge of how risk and protective factors shape psychological development has greatly improved over the last 50 years, particularly as a result of extensive research related to resilience, our understanding of individual differences in more general environmental sensitivity is not as advanced yet. Since the publication of the first SPS, DST and BST papers in the late 1990s, most research inspired by these concepts has been aimed at investigating person–environment interactions in cross-sectional and longitudinal studies. The majority of these studies relied on simple visual comparisons or, in some cases statistical follow-up analyses, to test

whether emerging interaction patterns would fit better with diathesis-stress or general environmental sensitivity. In other words, researchers have been and still are examining the main assertion of DST, which posits that inherent general sensitivity to environmental influences functions in a *for better and for worse* manner, such that the sensitivity to the effects of environmental influences can be extended to positive as well as negative environments. Given the limitations of correlational designs, more recent research has focused on applying experimental designs to the investigation of individual differences in environmental sensitivity, including genetic moderation of intervention effects; some examples of which will be presented in this chapter.

In what follows, we will provide a brief overview of the methods and measurements currently used to address these questions and present selected empirical evidence for individual differences in environmental sensitivity.

Research Measurement and Methodology

The majority of research concerning individual differences in environmental sensitivity has been conducted from a DST- and BSC-influenced developmental perspective, which interprets environmental sensitivity as developmental plasticity—in contrast to SPS, which conceptualizes environmental sensitivity within a personality framework.

The developmental plasticity approach is mainly concerned with how environmental sensitivity is implicated in developmental processes, and the related studies tend to investigate the moderating effects of individual factors. These characteristics are hypothesized to reflect environmental sensitivity on the association between various environmental factors and psychological outcomes, usually in longitudinal prospective research designs. Depending on the research interests of the investigators, individual differences in environmental sensitivity can be studied using genetic (e.g. 5-HTTLPR), physiological (e.g. cortisol reactivity) or psychological (e.g. infant temperament) markers of environmental sensitivity. In molecular genetics studies, associations between a genetic variant, an environmental variable (e.g. life events) and a psychological outcome (depression) are examined in so-called gene-environment interaction studies. These studies usually test whether a given genetic marker moderates the association between the environmental variable and the psychological outcome. On the physiological level, skin conductance reactivity is used, for example, as a marker of environmental sensitivity which has been reported to moderate the relationship between marital conflict and child externalizing behavior consistent with DST (El-Sheikh et al. 2009). On the psychological/behavioral level, environmental sensitivity has been tested, for example, as a function of infant temperament, which has been found to moderate the effects of maternal discipline on child externalizing behavior in a Dutch non-minority sample, for better and for worse— consistent with DST (van Zeijl et al. 2007). Importantly, in all of these studies, and hence the majority of existing empirical evidence, individual differences in environmental sensitivity are being assessed indirectly, based on interaction patterns between individual characteristics and environmental factors, rather than direct measures of individual general environmental sensitivity.

A personality approach to individual differences in environmental sensitivity, as reflected in SPS, conceptualizes environmental sensitivity as a personality trait that is measurable, temporally stable and consistent across different contexts. To this end, the Highly Sensitive Person scale (HSP) has been developed as an index for an individual's self-reported propensity to be highly sensitive toward environmental influences (Aron and Aron 1997). This quantitative measure of environmental sensitivity allows direct examination of an individual's general environmental sensitivity, independent of the interaction between individual and environment.

It must be noted that whilst there are many longitudinal studies that have examined the various hypotheses of DST, BSC and SPS, the majority of these studies are correlational, meaning the findings cannot be interpreted causally. With regards to statistical analysis, much of the data have been analyzed using exploratory methods to test for hypothesized cross-over interactions, followed by visual inspection of interaction patterns to test whether observed interactions are more consistent with diathesis-stress or differential susceptibility. More recently, new statistical procedures have been developed and applied that allow for more advanced statistical testing of competing theoretical models, such as *Regions of Significance* analysis (Preacher et al. 2006; Roisman et al. 2012) and model fit comparison (Belsky et al. 2013; Widaman et al. 2012). Recent studies that applied these new statistical methods provide strong evidence that environmental sensitivity stretches indeed from the negative across the positive end of the spectrum of environmental quality (for a review see Belsky and Pluess 2013, 2016).

In the following section, we will review a selection of more recent empirical studies that applied the aforementioned advanced methodological approaches in investigating individual differences in environmental sensitivity.

Empirical Findings

A growing number of studies focus on the empirical investigation of individual differences in environmental sensitivity rather than vulnerability. In other words, they are concerned with testing a range of individual characteristics as potential susceptibility factors, investigating whether these characteristics moderate environmental effects in a 'for better and for worse manner' (i.e. differential susceptibility) rather than just 'for worse' (i.e. vulnerability). In other words, the investigation of diathesis-stress has been extended to include the moderation of effects of positive environmental influences (i.e. Vantage Sensitivity). Evidence in support of DST comes from two lines of research: (1) studies in which the DST was not directly examined, but results seemed supportive of differential susceptibility when interpreted post hoc (e.g. as reviewed in Belsky and Pluess 2009); and (2) studies that have specifically set out to test a hypothesis of differential susceptibility. Below, we review a selection of more recent studies that specifically focus on the a priori investigation of individual differences in environmental sensitivity from a perspective of differential susceptibility. We selected studies that include the kind of environmental influences that will be most relevant to minority children, even though the majority of these studies were not specifically conducted with minority children.

Empirical evidence for DST can be divided into three areas of investigation, which most likely reflect the same underlying mechanisms of environmental sensitivity but are measured at different levels of analysis: the genetic, the physiological and the behavioral level (Pluess 2015). Drawing on evidence from gene–environment interaction studies, findings suggest that certain variants of serotonergic and dopaminergic genes (e.g. 5-HLLTPR short allele and DRD4 7-repeat) act as markers of environmental sensitivity. For example, the short allele of the 5-HTTLPR has been shown to moderate the effects of maternal responsiveness on child's moral internalization (Kochanska et al. 2011), the influence of supportive parenting on child's positive affect (Hankin et al. 2011) and, among male African-American adolescents, the influence of perceived racial discrimination on conduct problems (Brody et al. 2011). In all three examples, those carrying the 5-HTTLPR short allele had the least adaptive outcome under less favorable conditions and the most adaptive outcome under more favorable conditions, compared to children with different gene variants.

On the behavioral level, some of the most consistent evidence in support of DST is found in developmental studies on parenting and infant temperament. Much of the research indicates that the negative emotional dimension of infant temperament moderates the effects of quality of care on various indices of children's psychosocial development (Dopkins Stright et al. 2008; Pitzer et al. 2011; Pluess and Belsky 2010; Poehlmann

et al. 2012). Generally, children with more negative emotionality in infancy have been found to be more adversely affected by unresponsive parenting as well as benefiting substantially more from responsive parenting, in comparison to those children with less negative emotionality (Obradovic et al. 2010; Pluess and Belsky 2009).

Because minority children in the US are more likely to be poor, poverty reflects an important component of the minority context. In a longitudinal study of 1259 poor White and African American children and their mothers, Raver et al. (2012) examined the effects of chronic poverty and poverty-related risks such as family financial strain and housing quality, and the moderating role of infant's temperament on variability in executive function. Controlling for demographic differences including ethnicity, geographic location, mother's age and educational level, the results supported DST. In children characterized with a high reactive temperament, chronic exposure to financial strain was associated with lower executive function at 4 years while lower exposure to financial strain was associated with higher executive functioning. For children with low-reactive temperament, however, financial strain was not related to differences in executive functioning. Hence, the more reactive children were more affected by both high and low levels of financial strain compared to children with a less reactive temperament.

Empirical investigation of the "bright side" of DST—individual differences in response to positive experiences (i.e. Vantage Sensitivity; Pluess and Belsky 2013)—is of particular relevance when focusing on positive development. Although research here is still relatively sparse, several recent studies (Cassidy et al. 2011; Eley et al. 2012; Pluess and Boniwell 2015; Scott and O'Connor 2012) have used randomized controlled trial designs to examine whether individual differences in environmental sensitivity moderate the positive effects of psychological intervention programs. For example, Eley et al. (2012) evaluated the moderating effects of 5-HTTLPR regarding the efficacy of cognitive behavioral therapy for anxiety in 6–13 year old children (N = 359). While all children followed up at 6 months post-treatment seemed to have improved from their baseline symptoms, those carrying the short allele had significantly lower scores, suggesting that they benefited more than the rest of the children from intervention. Similarly, testing the a priori hypothesis that children scoring high on a measure of SPS would be more responsive to psychological intervention, Pluess and Boniwell (2015) investigated variation in the anticipated positive effects of a school-based resilience-promoting program administered to a sample of more than 300 11-year old girls in one of the most deprived and multi-ethnic areas in London, United Kingdom. The intervention led to a significant decrease of depression symptoms, observable up to the 12 month follow-up assessment, but, consistent with Vantage Sensitivity, exclusively among children who scored high on the SPS measure. All other children failed to benefit from the intervention, at least regarding changes in depression symptoms.

Finally, it must be noted that although this selective set of empirical studies supports the notion of individual differences in environmental sensitivity, not all a priori studies of DST provide evidence consistent with its predictions, or find the same genetic markers to act in accordance with DST [see, e.g. for behavioral study: Kochanska and Kim (2012); for genetic studies: Cicchetti et al. (2012), Felmingham et al. (2013)]. Whether positive DST findings generalize to minority children is discussed in the following section.

Universal Versus Culture-Specific Mechanisms

Current findings from genetic and behavioral studies suggest that, in line with DST, the extent to which environmental risks (e.g. low SES, victimization) as well as promotive factors (i.e. sensitive parenting, psychological interventions) contribute to the development of psychological outcomes, including competence and well-being, may be a function of the individual's general sensitivity. Findings from intervention studies also indicate that individuals vary in the extent to which they

benefit from the well-being-promoting features of environmental factors. This variation in Vantage Sensitivity may be due to the same characteristics that drive more general individual differences in environmental sensitivity, including genetic factors. However, despite the fact that theoretical frameworks for individual differences in environmental sensitivity are rooted in evolutionary theory and, thus, imply some degree of universality, it is important to carefully consider whether current findings are likely to generalize across cultures and different contexts.

Most research on individual differences in environmental sensitivity has been conducted with European and American samples, and there are very few studies specifically testing variability in environmental sensitivity in minority groups (e.g. Brody et al. 2011). This is an important limitation of research in the field, since minority children as a group represent a special subpopulation within the general population, whose development is often shaped and influenced by more complex cultural and psychosocial dynamics (and environmental risks and opportunities). Notwithstanding this limitation, we suggest that findings from DST in the general population may generalize to minority children. This is because supportive parenting, as an example for a positive influence, can be considered beneficial independent of the cultural context (even though what constitutes good parenting is culturally defined), and poverty, as an example of adversity, can be universally considered a negative environmental influence (even though the extent of its negative impact on wellbeing may be culture-specific). Hence, while there are important cultural differences, the specific impact of contextual conditions will still be moderated by individual differences in environmental sensitivity. However, while the general principle of DST is applicable universally due to its root in evolutionary reasoning, the specific genetic markers of environmental sensitivity may differ across ethnicities. This is due to significant differences in the genetic architecture across different ethnicities, therefore limiting the generalizability of specific genetic findings from DST studies somewhat. For this reason, it is essential to replicate genetic findings in minority populations, before concluding that the same genetic factors that emerged in European and American non-minority children would predict individual differences in environmental sensitivity in minority groups.

In summary, although evolutionary considerations predict that individual differences in environmental sensitivity should be found in all populations, studies specifically targeting minority children will have to be conducted before concluding that these children are characterized by the same variability in environmental sensitivity as other children. This is especially important given that complex interactions between different aspects of the environment that minority children find themselves in may bring about different dynamics than in non-minority children.

Policy Implications

The notion of individual differences in environmental sensitivity suggests that environmental risks encountered by minority children will not affect all children to the same extent, and that those children most sensitive to the negative effects of adverse experiences may also benefit substantially more from positive features of the environment. While prevalent and pervasive contextual adversity may generally expose many minority children to greater risk for mental health problems or suboptimal development, individual differences in sensitivity to environments may indicate which children might be most likely to succumb to these negative exposures. On the other hand, individual differences in sensitivity to environments may also explain why some children seem to be more likely to benefit from well-being-promoting programs (Vantage Sensitivity). Acknowledging that variability in general environmental sensitivity may contribute to variations in psychological outcomes in response to both environmental risk and support, should encourage policy makers to focus on the provision of well-being promoting support rather than simply ameliorating risk, given that the children most negatively affected by risk may also be the

ones who would benefit most from improvements in their environments.

Furthermore, as current research suggests, provision of intervention efforts to individuals most likely to benefit given their heightened environmental sensitivity may produce the largest effects. In other words, the notion of individual differences in general environmental sensitivity calls for the provision of personalized programs that take this variation into account and argues against a "one-size fit all" approach, in order to promote optimal psychological functioning across all degrees of environmental sensitivity. Finally and importantly—as it relates to positive development—focusing intervention strategies specifically on those children who appear to be more environmentally sensitive may have the most significant impact given that these children are also the ones at greatest risk for the development of problems.

Future Directions

Despite growing empirical support for individual differences in general environmental sensitivity, there are important questions that future research in the field should prioritize (for a more detailed discussion, see Belsky and Pluess 2016; Pluess 2015). For example, while current evidence suggests both a genetic contribution as well as environmental programming of environmental sensitivity, the exact origins of environmental sensitivity remain largely unknown. Longitudinal research examining the contribution of genetic and environmental factors in the development of environmental sensitivity will be crucial in this respect. Additionally, one of the main propositions of environmental sensitivity theories is that the same individuals who are most negatively affected by adversity will also benefit most from positive aspects of the environment. However, due to the correlational nature of most differential susceptibility studies, it is difficult to test whether this is really the case. Future research will have to observe the same individuals in both adverse and supportive environments to test for consistency of environmental sensitivity across contexts. Particularly important for a better understanding of positive development is to investigate whether individual factors that contribute to increased vantage sensitivity are the same ones that predict vulnerability or whether there are some characteristics that are specific to increased sensitivity to supportive environments. Furthermore, it is important to investigate whether environmental sensitivity is limited to specific sensitive periods, during which individuals are more susceptible to environmental influences and whether environmental sensitivity changes over time. Investigation of these questions will require longitudinal prospective studies with repeated measures of environmental quality and environmental sensitivity. Finally, while there is substantial evidence for differential susceptibility in childhood, only a few studies have investigated individual differences in environmental sensitivity in adolescence and adulthood.

In conclusion, a growing number of studies provide empirical evidence for the proposition that children differ in the extent to which they are impacted by both positive and negative aspects of their environments as a function of their general environmental sensitivity. The more complex environmental settings of minority children warrants further research with these groups, in order to fully understand the genetic factors and environmental processes that may predispose them to developing high sensitivity. Researchers and policy makers, as well as practitioners, should consider that just as not all minority children will be affected by environmental risk to the same degree, not all minority children will benefit to the same degree from supportive components of the environment. Policies and services that take such differences into account are likely to be the most economic and effective ones.

References

Alati, R., Najman, J. M., Shuttlewood, G. J., Williams, G. M., & Bor, W. (2003). Changes in mental health status amongst children of migrants to Australia: A longitudinal study. *Sociology of Health & Illness, 25*(7), 866–888.

Aron, E. N. (1996). *The highly sensitive person: How to thrive when the world overwhelms you* (Rev ed.). New York: Broadway Books.

Aron, E. N., & Aron, A. (1997). Sensory-processing sensitivity and its relation to introversion and emotionality. *Journal of Personality and Social Psychology, 73*(2), 345–368.

Aron, E. N., Aron, A., & Davies, K. M. (2005). Adult shyness: The interaction of temperamental sensitivity and an adverse childhood environment. *Personality and Social Psychology Bulletin, 31*(2), 181–197.

Aron, E. N., Aron, A., & Jagiellowicz, J. (2012). Sensory processing sensitivity: A review in the light of the evolution of biological responsivity. *Personality and Social Psychology Review, 16*(3), 262–282. doi:10.1177/1088868311434213

Aronowitz, M. (1984). The social and emotional adjustment of immigrant children: A review of the literature. *International Migration Review, 18*(2), 237–257.

Beiser, M., Hou, F., Hyman, I., & Tousignant, M. (2002). Poverty, family process, and the mental health of immigrant children in Canada. *American Journal of Public Health, 92*(2), 220–227.

Belsky, J. (1997). Variation in susceptibility to rearing influences: An evolutionary argument. *Psychological Inquiry, 8*, 182–186.

Belsky, J. (2005). Differential susceptibility to rearing influences: An evolutionary hypothesis and some evidence. In B. Ellis & D. Bjorklund (Eds.), *Origins of the social mind: Evolutionary psychology and child development* (pp. 139–163). New York: Guildford.

Belsky, J., & Pluess, M. (2009). Beyond diathesis-stress: Differential susceptibility to environmental influences. *Psychological Bulletin, 135*(6), 885–908.

Belsky, J., & Pluess, M. (2013). Beyond risk, resilience, and dysregulation: Phenotypic plasticity and human development. *Development and Psychopathology, 25*(4 Pt 2), 1243–1261. doi:10.1017/S095457941300059X

Belsky, J., & Pluess, M. (2016). Differential susceptibility to environmental influences. In D. Cicchetti (Ed.), *Developmental Psychopathology* (3rd ed., Vol. 3, pp. 59). New York: Wiley.

Belsky, J., Bakermans-Kranenburg, M. J., & van IJzendoorn, M. H. (2007). For better and for worse: Differential susceptibility to environmental influences. *Current Directions in Psychological Science, 16*(6), 300–304.

Belsky, J., Pluess, M., & Widaman, K. F. (2013). Confirmatory and competitive evaluation of alternative gene–environment interaction hypotheses. *Journal of Child Psychology and Psychiatry and Allied Disciplines, 54*(10), 1135–1143. doi:10.1111/jcpp.12075

Belsky, J., Jonassaint, C., Pluess, M., Stanton, M., Brummett, B., & Williams, R. (2009). Vulnerability genes or plasticity genes? *Molecular Psychiatry, 14*, 746–754.

Boyce, W. T., & Ellis, B. J. (2005). Biological sensitivity to context: I. An evolutionary-developmental theory of the origins and functions of stress reactivity. *Development and Psychopathology, 17*(2), 271–301.

Brody, G. H., Beach, S. R. H., Chen, Y.-F., Obasi, E., Philibert, R. A., Kogan, S. M., et al. (2011). Perceived discrimination, serotonin transporter linked polymorphic region status, and the development of conduct problems. *Development and Psychopathology, 23*(2), 617–627. doi:10.1017/s0954579411000046

Brody, G. H., Chen, Y. F., Murry, V. M., Ge, X., Simons, R. L., Gibbons, F. X., et al. (2006). Perceived discrimination and the adjustment of African American youths: A five-year longitudinal analysis with contextual moderation effects. *Child Development, 77*(5), 1170–1189.

Brooks-Gunn, J., Klebanov, P. K., & Duncan, G. J. (1996). Ethnic differences in children's intelligence test scores: Role of economic deprivation, home environment, and maternal characteristics. *Child Development, 67*(2), 396–408.

Cassidy, J., Woodhouse, S. S., Sherman, L. J., Stupica, B., & Lejuez, C. W. (2011). Enhancing infant attachment security: An examination of treatment efficacy and differential susceptibility. *Development and Psychopathology, 23*(1), 131–148. doi:10.1017/s0954579410000696

Cicchetti, D., Rogosch, F. A., & Thibodeau, E. L. (2012). The effects of child maltreatment on early signs of antisocial behavior: Genetic moderation by tryptophan hydroxylase, serotonin transporter, and monoamine oxidase A genes. *Development and Psychopathology, 24*(3), 907–928.

Coll, C. G., Crnic, K., Lamberty, G., Wasik, B. H., Jenkins, R., Garcia, H. V., et al. (1996). An integrative model for the study of developmental competencies in minority children. *Child Development, 67*(5), 1891–1914.

Dahl, T., Ceballo, R., & Huerta, M. (2010). In the eye of the beholder: Mothers' perceptions of poor neighborhoods as places to raise children. *Journal of Community Psychology, 38*(4), 419–434.

Del Giudice, M., Ellis, B. J., & Shirtcliff, E. A. (2011). The adaptive calibration model of stress responsivity. *Neuroscience and Biobehavioral Reviews, 35*(7), 1562–1592. doi:10.1016/j.neubiorev.2010.11.007

Dopkins Stright, A., Cranley Gallagher, K., & Kelley, K. (2008). Infant temperament moderates relations between maternal parenting in early childhood and children's adjustment in first grade. *Child Development, 79*(1), 186–200.

Duncan, G. J., Brooks-Gunn, J., & Klebanov, P. K. (1994). Economic deprivation and early childhood development. *Child Development, 65*(2), 296–318.

El-Sheikh, M., Kouros, C. D., Erath, S., Cummings, E. M., Keller, P., & Staton, L. (2009). Marital conflict and children's externalizing behavior: Interactions between parasympathetic and sympathetic nervous system activity. *Monographs of the Society for Research in Child Development, 74*(1), vii, 1–79.

Eley, T. C., Hudson, J. L., Creswell, C., Tropeano, M., Lester, K. J., Cooper, P., et al. (2012). Therapygenetics: The 5HTTLPR and response to psychological therapy. *Molecular Psychiatry, 17*, 236–241. doi:10.1038/mp.2011.132

Ellis, B. J., Essex, M. J., & Boyce, W. T. (2005). Biological sensitivity to context: II. Empirical explorations of an evolutionary-developmental theory. *Development and Psychopathology, 17*(2), 303–328.

Evans, G. W., & Kim, P. (2007). Childhood poverty and health: Cumulative risk exposure and stress dysregulation. *Psychological Science, 18*(11), 953–957.

Felmingham, K. L., Dobson-Stone, C., Schofield, P. R., Quirk, G. J., & Bryant, R. A. (2013). The brain-derived neurotrophic factor Val66Met polymorphism predicts response to exposure therapy in posttraumatic stress disorder. *Biological Psychiatry,*. doi:10.1016/j.biopsych.2012.10.033

Gottesman, I. I., & Shields, J. (1967). A polygenic theory of schizophrenia. *Proceedings of the National Academy of Sciences of the United States of America, 58*(1), 199–205.

Hankin, B. L., Nederhof, E., Oppenheimer, C. W., Jenness, J., Young, J. F., Abela, J. R. Z., et al. (2011). Differential susceptibility in youth: Evidence that 5-HTTLPR × positive parenting is associated with positive affect 'for better and worse'. *Translational Psychiatry,*. doi:10.1038/tp.2011.44

Harker, K. (2001). Immigrant generation, assimilation, and adolescent psychological well-being. *Social Forces, 79*(3), 969–1004.

Iceland, J., & Bauman, K. J. (2007). Income poverty and material hardship: How strong is the association? *The Journal of Socio-Economics, 36*(3), 376–396.

Kim-Cohen, J., Moffitt, T. E., Caspi, A., & Taylor, A. (2004). Genetic and environmental processes in young children's resilience and vulnerability to socioeconomic deprivation. *Child Development, 75*(3), 651–668. doi:10.1111/j.1467-8624.2004.00699.x

Kochanska, G., & Kim, S. (2012). Difficult temperament moderates links between maternal responsiveness and children's compliance and behavior problems in low-income families. *Journal of Child Psychology and Psychiatry and Allied Disciplines,*. doi:10.1111/jcpp.12002

Kochanska, G., Kim, S., Barry, R. A., & Philibert, R. A. (2011). Children's genotypes interact with maternal responsive care in predicting children's competence: Diathesis-stress or differential susceptibility? *Development and Psychopathology, 23*, 605–616.

Mohler, B. (2001). Cross-cultural issues in research on child mental health. *Child and Adolescent Psychiatric Clinics of North America, 10*(4), 763–776.

Monroe, S. M., & Simons, A. D. (1991). Diathesis-stress theories in the context of life stress research: Implications for the depressive disorders. *Psychological Bulletin, 110*(3), 406–425. doi:10.1037/0033-2909.110.3.406

Munafo, M. R., Freimer, N. B., Ng, W., Ophoff, R., Veijola, J., Miettunen, J., et al. (2009). 5-HTTLPR genotype and anxiety-related personality traits: A meta-analysis and new data. *American Journal of*

Medical Genetics. Part B, Neuropsychiatric Genetics, 150B(2), 271–281.

Munroe-Blum, H., Boyle, M. H., Offord, D. R., & Kates, N. (1989). Immigrant children: Psychiatric disorder, school performance, and service utilization. *American Journal of Orthopsychiatry, 59*(4), 510.

Obradovic, J., Bush, N. R., Stamperdahl, J., Adler, N. E., & Boyce, W. T. (2010). Biological sensitivity to context: The interactive effects of stress reactivity and family adversity on socio-emotional behavior and school readiness. *Child Development, 81*(1), 270–289.

Pascoe, E. A., & Smart Richman, L. (2009). Perceived discrimination and health: A meta-analytic review. *Psychological Bulletin, 135*(4), 531.

Pitzer, M., Jennen-Steinmetz, C., Esser, G., Schmidt, M. H., & Laucht, M. (2011). Differential susceptibility to environmental influences: The role of early temperament and parenting in the development of externalizing problems. *Comprehensive Psychiatry, 52*(6), 650–658. doi:10.1016/j.comppsych.2010.10.017

Pluess, M. (2015). Individual differences in environmental sensitivity. *Child Development Perspectives, 9*(3), 138–143.

Pluess, M., & Belsky, J. (2009). Differential susceptibility to rearing experience: The case of childcare. *Journal of Child Psychology and Psychiatry, 50*(4), 396–404.

Pluess, M., & Belsky, J. (2010). Children's differential susceptibility to effects of parenting. *Family Science, 1*(1), 14–25.

Pluess, M., & Belsky, J. (2011). Prenatal programming of postnatal plasticity? *Development and Psychopathology, 23*(1), 29–38.

Pluess, M., & Belsky, J. (2013). Vantage sensitivity: Individual differences in response to positive experiences. *Psychological Bulletin, 139*(4), 901–916. doi:10.1037/a0030196

Pluess, M., & Boniwell, I. (2015). Sensory-processing sensitivity predicts treatment response to a school-based depression prevention program: Evidence of vantage sensitivity. *Personality and Individual Differences, 82*, 40–45.

Poehlmann, J., Hane, A., Burnson, C., Maleck, S., Hamburger, E., & Shah, P. E. (2012). Preterm infants who are prone to distress: Differential effects of parenting on 36-month behavioral and cognitive outcomes. *Journal of Child Psychology and Psychiatry and Allied Disciplines,*. doi:10.1111/j.1469-7610.2012.02564.x

Preacher, K. J., Curran, P. J., & Bauer, D. J. (2006). Computational tools for probing interactions in multiple linear regressions, multilevel modeling, and latent curve analysis. *Journal of Educational and Behavioral Statistics, 31*(4), 437–448.

Raver, C. C., Blair, C., & Willoughby, M. (2012). Poverty as a predictor of 4-year-olds' executive function: New perspectives on models of differential susceptibility. *Developmental Psychology,*. doi:10.1037/a0028343

Rogler, L. H. (1994). International migrations. A framework for directing research. *American Psychologist, 49*(8), 701–708.

Roisman, G. I., Newman, D. A., Fraley, R. C., Haltigan, J. D., Groh, A. M., & Haydon, K. C. (2012). Distinguishing differential susceptibility from diathesis-stress: Recommendations for evaluating interaction effects. *Development and Psychopathology, 24*(2), 389–409. doi:10.1017/S0954579412000065

Rousseau, C., Drapeau, A., & Corin, E. (1996). School performance and emotional problems in refugee children. *American Journal of Orthopsychiatry, 66*(2), 239–251.

Schapkin, S. A., Falkenstein, M., Marks, A., & Griefahn, B. (2006). Executive brain functions after exposure to nocturnal traffic noise: Effects of task difficulty and sleep quality. *European Journal of Applied Physiology, 96*(6), 693–702.

Scott, S., & O'Connor, T. G. (2012). An experimental test of differential susceptibility to parenting among emotionally-dysregulated children in a randomized controlled trial for oppositional behavior. *Journal of Child Psychology and Psychiatry and Allied Disciplines,*. doi:10.1111/j.1469-7610.2012.02586.x

Stevens, G. W., & Vollebergh, W. A. (2008). Mental health in migrant children. *Journal of Child Psychology and Psychiatry, 49*(3), 276–294. doi:10.1111/j.1469-7610.2007.01848.x

Timberlake, J. (2007). Racial and ethnic inequality in the duration of children's exposure to neighborhood poverty and affluence. *Social Problems, 54*(3), 319–342.

van Ijzendoorn, M. H., Belsky, J., & Bakermans-Kranenburg, M. J. (2012). Serotonin transporter genotype 5HTTLPR as a marker of differential susceptibility? A meta-analysis of child and adolescent gene-by-environment studies. *Translational Psychiatry, 2*, e147. doi:10.1038/tp.2012.73

van Zeijl, J., Mesman, J., Stolk, M. N., Alink, L. R., van Ijzendoorn, M. H., Bakermans-Kranenburg, M. J., et al. (2007). Differential susceptibility to discipline: The moderating effect of child temperament on the association between maternal discipline and early childhood externalizing problems. *Journal of Family Psychology, 21*(4), 626–636.

Virta, E., Sam, D. L., & Westin, C. (2004). Adolescents with Turkish background in Norway and Sweden: A comparative study of their psychological adaptation. *Scandinavian Journal of Psychology, 45*(1), 15–25.

Widaman, K. F., Helm, J. L., Castro-Schilo, L., Pluess, M., Stallings, M. C., & Belsky, J. (2012). Distinguishing ordinal and disordinal interactions. *Psychological Methods, 17*(4), 615–622. doi:10.1037/a0030003

Zuckerman, M. (1999). *Vulnerability to psychopathology: A biosocial model*. Washington, DC: American Psychological Association.

Part III

Family/Parenting Level Influences

Parenting and Language in Ethnic Minority and Immigrant Families in North America and the European Union: Toward an Emphasis on Positive Development

Marc H. Bornstein

Bornstein, M.H. Parenting and language in ethnic minority and immigrant families in North America and the European Union: Toward an emphasis on positive development. In N. Cabrera & B. Leyendecker (Eds.), *Handbook of Positive Development of Minority Children* (pp. xx–xx). New York: Springer.

Correspondence to: Marc H. Bornstein, Child and Family Research, *Eunice Kennedy Shriver* National Institute of Child Health and Human Development, National Institutes of Health, Rockledge 1, Suite 8030, 6705 Rockledge Drive, MSC 7971, Bethesda MD 20892-7971, U.S.A. e-mail: Marc_H_Bornstein@nih.gov.

Being an ethnic minority child in an ethnic minority family is challenging on multiple fronts, and being an immigrant child in an immigrant family is a disorganizing experience; thus, both are vulnerable populations that face significant common and unique trials. Among their shared potential vulnerabilities are limited education, constrained finances, small social networks, volatile neighborhoods, and everyday distress. Ethnic minorities and immigrants also face unique developmental circumstances, in legal status and cultural acceptance for the former and for the latter in the ways ethnic socialization efforts distinctively intersect with the broader social contexts where families live. Little wonder that the contemporary public, political, and scientific conversation about ethnic minority and immigrant children and families largely revolves around risks

and struggles for ethnic minorities and migrants themselves and for the majority populations in their homelands and in their countries of destination. Chapters in this part on Family and Parent Level Influences of Cabrera and Lyendecker's *Handbook of Positive Development of Minority Children and Youth* happily turn the focus to positive development in these children and their families, that is, their assets and strengths and factors that promote those assets and strengths. This part offers three chapters on parenting and family and two on language that join together to answer the question: What resources are available to children in and outside the family that foster their positive development and increase their capabilities to participate in the society where they live? Spoiler alert: Across diverse groups, parents teaching children about the history and values of their cultural heritage, and children's adoption of core cultural values, benefit them in terms of academic competence and feelings of cultural belonging and ethnic identity.

In "Parenting and Families in the United States and Canada," Costigan, Taknint, and Miao review the current state of knowledge regarding parenting and family influences on positive development among ethnic minority adolescents in North America. They include research related to the roles of supportive family relationships in fostering children's social connection, parental school involvement in promoting children's academic competence, and positive parenting practices in consolidating children's social and behavioral competencies. They find that families can influence positive development, that family dynamics are associated with children successfully navigating bicultural environments, and that strong relationships with parents and positive approaches to parenting shape positive qualities in children. Moreover, these findings are similar to those in non-minority adolescents, suggesting their universal applicability within families for positive youth development.

"Family Resources for Promoting Positive Development among Minority Children: European Perspectives," is a companion chapter to Costigan and colleagues wherein Walper and Leyendecker continue the discussion of family factors in fostering positive development among minority children in the diverse states of the European Union. These authors distinguish indigenous minority groups from immigrant minority groups. The two have some things in common. For example, diverse minorities share interests in being recognized and respected as distinct cultural groups. However, in many European countries, the former have been successful in obtaining extended legal protections for their culture and language, where by contrast the latter are expected to integrate or assimilate into the majority society and do not enjoy the same privileges for their heritage cultures and languages. These authors acknowledge the extraordinary complexities that attend the contemporary immigrant scene in the EU. Cultural traditions and adaptations are particularly salient in studies comparing immigrants to majority families in their host country and to families in their country of origin.

These first two chapters set minority child development in families. However, much more is known about mothers' than fathers' roles, and more research is needed to fully understand the parts fathers play in these processes. Fathers may exert unique influences on positive child development in minority (and majority as well) children. In "Minority Fathers and Children's Positive Development in the United States," Cabrera, Karberg, and Kuhns begin to fill in the picture by answering three interrelated questions

about the ways ethnic minority fathers interact and provide safe and stimulating experiences to shape their children's positive cognitive and social development. First, how are ethnic minority fathers involved in their children's lives? That is, how much time do these fathers spend with their children and what do they do for them (in terms of economic resources) and with them (in terms of interacting). Second, what factors explain variability in fathers' involvement? Fathers' residence and family structure, their co-parenting relationships, and individual characteristics (education and income), family functioning, cultural beliefs, and the quality of father–child interactions appear to explain variability in ethnic minority father involvement. Third, how is father involvement related to their children's development? How ethnic minority fathers influence their children's development in a strengths-based framework is a relatively new area of inquiry. The authors here review research that identifies the ways in which fathers' assets (e.g., responsiveness) foster positive development among ethnic minority children.

Language is essential in parenting and family life. Without a language to competently use with children, parents cannot satisfactorily execute their parental role. The issue of language becomes particularly clear in minority contexts, where parents might speak a language to children they themselves hardly know, or where children may not speak the language that their parents speak with them. Because of such linguistic variation, minority language background parents may feel insecure in their parenting role, and their children's positive development may be adversely affected. Chapters 4 and 5 of this part are also companion pieces, both focusing on language in the family nexus.

In "Language and Parenting: Minority Languages in North America," McCabe points to the many positives of bilingualism, countering the negative associations of older studies that confounded socioeconomic status with bilingualism. The apprehension that bilingualism is "subtractive" lies behind outmoded notions that once undermined bilingual education. Modern researchers of bilingual language development subscribe to a view that bilingualism can be "additive" so long as there is ample support in families, schools, and larger communities for children speaking and becoming literate in more than one language. The emerging consensus from much research is that dual language exposure not only does not harm children, but the same kinds of input that have been found advantageous for monolingual children might be doubly advantageous for multilingual children.

In "Minority Language Parenting in Europe and Children's Well-being," De Houwer reviews research from various traditions that inform relations between language use by parents with minority language backgrounds and their children's socio-emotional well-being. Children may hear only or mainly a minority language at home in the first years of life, and not until later become bilingual through exposure to a majority language. These children grow up in an Early Second Language Acquisition setting (ESLA). Alternatively, children may hear both a minority and a majority language in the home regularly from birth, a setting known as Bilingual First Language Acquisition (BFLA). Both in Europe and in the United States BFLA likely occurs much more often as ESLA. Parental language use includes language choice in different communicative situations, the frequency with which the minority language is used, and parental discourse strategies in response to children's language choice. In bilingual families where children hear both minority and majority languages, children's minority language acquisition is supported by a high frequency of parental minority language use.

What does the reader of Family and Parent Level Influences learn from this part of the *Handbook of Positive Development of Minority Children and Youth?* Notwithstanding the wide variation in countries, research settings, methods, social levels, minority and majority cultures and languages, many parallel points crop up. Moreover, all chapters acknowledge the centrality of an ecological perspective and the interplay of challenges and support on the personal, relational, institutional, and cultural levels. All chapters in this part address universal as well as culture-specific mechanisms, and all conclude with solid policy implications and novel and constructive suggestions for future research.

The empirical foundations of these chapter integrations derive from a wide variety of methods and sources, self-reports and variable-centered analyses, qualitative interview data and person-centered analyses, representative surveys within and across countries, observational, qualitative, and intervention studies, and admirably each takes a hard look at the advantages and disadvantages of different methods. Although the majority of the research in this still-nascent field relies on cross-sectional correlational designs and samples of convenience, and so the empirical base is limited in assessing relations between family/parenting influences and important aspects of youth development, increasingly research conclusions are based on large and representative community samples, longitudinal designs, and independent reports from parents, youth, and others (e.g., teachers). These currents improve understanding processes and the direction of associations among constructs of interest and enhance validity and generalizability. Standardized tests are also being supplemented by in-depth observations of home interaction in families with young children and use a range of data collection methods, including the diary method, field notes, and/or audio-and/or video recordings, ethnographies of structured and open interviews, questionnaire studies, and surveys. That said, there are still too few studies that experimentally evaluate the impact of parenting and family on children's positive development. In short, close attention to methods is an admirable feature of all these chapters.

Returning to the bottom-line: What have we learned? Research on immigrant families suggests that children do best if they have parents who convey a connection to the culture of origin and maintain a voice of authority, but at the same time encourage children to take advantage of the opportunities offered by the larger society in which they live. The research supports the conclusion that embracing both the heritage and mainstream cultures constitutes an adaptive approach to balancing the two. Reduced conflict and emotional closeness are likely protective factors for minority and immigrant families alike. Where social and economic stresses can undermine positive parenting, warmth and sensitivity are linked to better child outcomes.

These kinds of conclusions have immediate social policy implications. One clear policy recommendations that emerges from these chapters is the value of supporting the transmission of the ethnic culture within minority and immigrant families. As a corollary, policies and programs that provide resources and supports for families and their communities to maintain their heritage culture and feelings of belonging to the majority culture likely contribute to the positive development of minority youth. The minority language is important for family relationships and values, and the majority language is important for public life. Given the weighty role of socioeconomic resources, efforts to improve access to higher levels of education and income should be promoted. Schools, health care, and social services offer institutional opportunity structures, facilitate integration, and promote positive development. Families are the most proximal context of children's development, so parental well-being per se is also vital to positive parenting. Accordingly, more attention should be paid to mental and physical health services, access to

counseling, and support for successfully coping with stress. Families are systems that include mothers, fathers, children, and significant others. Because each member of the family ecology plays a significant proximal part in shaping children's lives, supporting positive involvement of individual members of minority families needs to be a priority for policy makers and practitioners. Notably, fathers' contributions to child welfare are unique over and above the contributions of mothers; excluding fathers from programs or interventions sends the mistaken message that fathers are not worthy.

Together, these five chapters argue for a shift in focus from deficit perspectives on minority and immigrant youth development towards more sophisticated ecological models that consider the effects of culture in conjunction with other salient contexts, such as social class, gender, school, and neighborhoods that focus affirmatively on positive aspects of youth development. Many of the same family factors that promote positive development among minority and immigrant youth also encourage positive adjustment and competence in the face of adversity. Given global demographics, the future of developmental science needs to embrace the study of positive development among minority and immigrant youth.

Parenting and Families in the United States and Canada

Catherine Costigan, Joelle Taknint, and Sheena Miao

Abstract

This chapter reviews the current state of knowledge regarding parenting and family influence on positive development among ethnic minority adolescents in the United States and Canada. First, general family processes that promote positive development are reviewed in relation to the "Five C's" of positive youth development: connection, competence, confidence, character, and caring (Lerner et al. in J Early Adolesc 25 (1):17–71, 2005). The review includes research related to the role of supportive family relationships in promoting connection, parental school involvement in promoting academic competence, and positive parenting practices in promoting social and behavioral competence. Next, culture-related family influences on positive development are identified, including links between family cultural values and academic competence, parents' cultural socialization efforts and adolescents' academic competence and ethnic heritage culture identification, and parents' support for adolescents' competent functioning in the mainstream culture. Third, family dynamics associated with navigating a bicultural environment are addressed. These dynamics include family support of adolescents' biculturalism, the benefits of parent–child similarities in cultural orientations, and the positive developmental correlates of adolescents' language brokering assistance for parents. Finally, research investigating family influences on positive adolescent development in the context of adversity is reviewed. The chapter concludes with a discussion of policy implications and recommendations for future research, including a call to direct research attention to the role of families in promoting a variety of as yet

Joelle Taknint and Sheena Miao contributed equally to this chapter.

C. Costigan (✉) · J. Taknint · S. Miao
Department of Psychology, University of Victoria,
Victoria, BC V8W 3P5, Canada
e-mail: costigan@uvic.ca

© The Editor(s) 2017
N.J. Cabrera and B. Leyendecker (eds.), *Handbook on Positive Development of Minority Children and Youth*, DOI 10.1007/978-3-319-43645-6_10

unstudied domains of positive adolescent development, such as hope, purpose, spirituality, thriving, civic engagement, and media literacy.

Historical Overview and Theoretical Perspectives

This chapter reviews the current state of knowledge regarding parenting and family influence on positive youth development among ethnic minority adolescents in the United States and Canada. Both the United States and Canada have multicultural populations and are large immigrant receiving countries. As a result, the literature on positive youth development spans multiple ethnic backgrounds, with the greatest representation from African, Latino (especially Mexican), and Asian cultural backgrounds. This chapter brings together examples from literature that adopts a strengths-based perspective on ethnic minority adolescent development.

The study of positive development among ethnic minority adolescents in North America is in its infancy. In a review of the literature on ethnic minority families at the start of this century, McLoyd et al. (2000) argued for a shift in focus from deficit models of minority youth development towards more sophisticated ecological models that consider the effects of culture in conjunction with other salient contexts, such as social class, gender hierarchies, and school and neighborhood environments. The cultural ecological model presented by García Coll et al. (1996), which situates a complex, multidimensional view of culture at the core of the development of minority children, embodies this shift. The literature in this chapter builds on these theoretical foundations by shining a spotlight on the adaptive capacities of families. These capacities include the resources and strengths that ethnic minority families possess that are shaped, promoted, or constrained in dynamic interplay with multiple contexts of family life (e.g., Rodriguez et al. 2009). Although much research still focuses on problematic outcomes, such as mental health

problems, substance use, and aggressive behavior, research with ethnic minority youth increasingly incorporates the study of positive developmental outcomes, such as prosocial values and behaviors (e.g., Calderón-Tena et al. 2011; Pina-Watson et al. 2013).

In this chapter, we only include research that addresses affirmatively positive aspects of development, rather than the absence of negative developmental outcomes. In addition, although we consider family influences broadly, the vast majority of literature we review is focused specifically on parental influences. We note whenever possible when the research included mothers, fathers, or both (see also Chap. 20 of this Handbook for a chapter devoted to fathers). Ethnic minority families are included regardless of generation in the United States or Canada, with specific attention to the challenges and strengths of ethnic minority families from immigrant communities as warranted.

Current Research Questions

The research questions that underlie the reviewed literature fall into four broad categories. The first category examines how general family-based assets relate to positive developmental outcomes within ethnic minority families. Research under this umbrella investigates the role of normative family processes, such as supportive family relationships and parental involvement in school, in fostering positive development. Although the importance of cultural context in these processes is recognized, the identified family processes and positive developmental outcomes are not specific to ethnic minority youth. The second category of questions focuses on understanding more specifically the links between cultural processes (e.g., ethnic socialization) and positive youth development. These studies place culture front and center in understanding positive developmental outcomes. A third set of questions addresses how ethnic minority parents help their children navigate a bicultural environment, and how family dynamics related to living in a multicultural environment relate to positive youth development. A final set of questions addresses how ethnic minority families promote positive development in the face of risk (e.g., due to experiences with discrimination). Although resilience research often centers on identifying factors that minimize problematic outcomes associated with adversity, research increasingly addresses the promotion of competence and well-being despite risk (e.g., McMahon et al. 2013).

Research Measurement and Methodology

The majority of the research that we review relies on cross-sectional designs to assess relations between family/parenting influences and important aspects of youth development. Self-report methods of data collection and variable-centered analyses are most common, although qualitative interview data and person-centered analyses occasionally appear. Increasingly, research conclusions are based on large-sized community samples, longitudinal designs, and independent reports from parents, youth, and others (e.g., teachers) which enhance their validity and generalizability.

Positive youth development is predominantly indexed by superior academic performance, school engagement, and psychological well-being (e.g., life satisfaction). Furthermore, unique to the study of positive development among ethnic minority youth, a number of studies evaluates the role of parenting and family relationships in fostering competence and connection for adolescents in their heritage culture and (less commonly) the mainstream society. These developmental outcomes can be mapped onto the "Five C's" of positive youth development (Lerner et al. 2005): connection,

competence, confidence, character, and caring. Multiple aspects of the domain of connection are investigated, including bonding to parents, friends, and schools, as well as the development of feelings of ethnic group affiliation and belonging. Within the domain of competence, academic abilities are by far the most studied outcome in relation to family influences, although some research also addresses social competence. However, with a few exceptions, little research addresses the other three domains of confidence (e.g., self-regard), character (e.g., sense of right and wrong), or caring (e.g., empathy for others).

Empirical Findings

General Family Promotion of Positive Developmental Outcomes

Connection

Across a variety of ethnic groups, a number of studies documents links between closeness with parents and a sense of connection in other aspects of life. For example, Rodríguez et al. (2014), with a sample of Mexican American adolescents, examined the links between perceptions of warmth from mothers and fathers in early adolescence and feelings of friendship intimacy 2 years later. They found that warmth from both mothers and fathers is related to later intimacy in friendships for females, whereas only warmth from fathers was related for males. Similarly, among middle class African American adolescents, more relatedness with mothers and fathers in early adolescence is associated with more supportive romantic relationships in late adolescence (Smetana and Gettman 2006). High relatedness in the context of low autonomy, however, is not as positive. Supportive relationships with parents also predict greater connection to schools. For example, Wang and Ecceles (2012) found that adolescents' reports of greater parent social support in middle school predict greater school compliance, participation in extracurricular activities, school identification, and subjective valuing of learning in high school. These relations were apparent among both African American and European American adolescents, and parent support was generally a stronger predictor than peer support of these indicators of school engagement. Closeness with mothers and fathers is also related to greater religiosity among Asian American adolescents (Zhai and Stokes 2009). Finally, for Filipino adolescents in Canada, family cohesion is associated with more positive attitudes towards school, whereas for Caribbean adolescents, greater family cohesion is related to more positive appraisals of their ethnic group (Rousseau et al. 2009). Collectively, these studies suggest that cohesion and support within minority families is a resource that may promote positive engagement in relationships outside of the home among peers, romantic partners, and school communities.

Competence

Families also play an important role in the development of competence among ethnic minority adolescence across various domains.

Academic Competence

Research into predictors of competence among minority adolescents most commonly focuses on academic competence. One key family predictor of academic competence is parents' involvement in school. Parental involvement includes home activities that support achievement (e.g., talking with children about school work, grades, or other aspects of school, checking on homework, and limiting the adolescent's time going out with friends), as well as parental involvement at school (e.g., attending parent-teacher conferences and volunteering at school; e.g., Corwyn and Bradley 2008; Turney and Kao 2009). These home-based parental involvement activities help structure and support the child's learning, and school-based involvement enhances parents' social capital with children's teachers and provides parents with information about what children are learning and how they are performing (Hill and Tyson 2009; Turney and Kao 2009). By middle school, parental involvement expands further to include "academic socialization," which refers to parents' efforts to communicate

with their children about the value of education, discuss learning strategies, and encourage children's future aspirations (Hill and Tyson 2009). Parents' academic socialization highlights to children the value of achievement and helps children make the connection between their school work and their future goals. Much research (e.g., Areepattamannil and Lee 2014; Corwyn and Bradley 2008; Eng et al. 2008), including meta-analysis (Hill and Tyson 2009; Jeynes 2007), show that parents' involvement, both at home and at school, is related to better educational outcomes (e.g., overall achievement, grades, and standardized test scores). In both meta-analyses, parental involvement related to communicating high academic aspirations showed the strongest relations with achievement, and school-based involvement was more modestly, yet still significantly, related to achievement outcomes. Parental checking on homework, a common home-based form of parental involvement, has the most mixed relations with achievement. Overall, relations between parental involvement and achievement are of similar strength for ethnic minority and European American children, and remain significant after controlling for salient background characteristics such as family income.

Ethnic minority parents, and particularly immigrant parents, are less likely to be involved in their children's education at school, especially when language barriers are present (e.g., Dyson 2001; Leidy et al. 2012; Tang 2015; Turney and Kao 2009). Whereas language barriers limit immigrant parents' direct participation at school, a lack of familiarity with the educational systems can also hinder their ability to guide their children's educational experience (e.g., course selection, extra-curricular activities). In these instances, supportive social networks may effectively compensate. For example, the presence of positive role models in the family is related to the development of academic competence (Roosa et al. 2012). Specifically, in a large sample of Mexican American families, mothers' reports of positive academic and occupational family role models in the immediate or extended family when their children were in elementary school (average 10.4 years old) were associated with higher academic performance among the children after they transitioned into junior high school 2 years later.

Social and Behavioral Competence

Family influences have also been linked to the development of social and behavioral competence among ethnic minority youth. These studies typically focus on the quality of parenting and parent–child relationships. For example, among low-income immigrant Latino families, mothers' (93 %) reports of family cohesion were related to middle school children's higher problem solving skills and social self-efficacy 9 months later (Leidy et al. 2012). In this study, more positive mothering (i.e., limit setting, communication) was also associated with later social self-efficacy. The link between positive mothering (i.e., high warmth and low hostility and conflict) and greater social competence was also found in a separate large sample of Mexican American early adolescents (Corona et al. 2012). The cultural context of parenting within immigrant samples is acknowledged in research that links caregivers' cultural orientations to their parenting. For example, among immigrant Chinese parents (81 % mothers) in the United States, greater English media use is associated with more authoritative parenting (e.g., high in warmth, reasoning, responsiveness, and encouragement of child's democratic participation), which in turn is associated with higher social and behavioral competence among children (Chen et al. 2014). Additionally, families in which parents and children were similar in their high Chinese media use (according to parent reports) were also most likely to report authoritative parenting practices and better child adjustment.

Confidence, Character, and Caring

Little attention has been paid to the development of confidence, character, and caring among minority and immigrant youth. In a notable exception, with respect to character, Calderón-Tena et al. (2011) examined the development of prosocial behavioral tendencies among Mexican American mothers and their early adolescents (mean age 11 years). Adolescents' prosocial behaviors were assessed in terms of behaviors that are intended to benefit others, including comforting others when they are upset, helping others when asked, and assisting others during a crisis. Mothers' use of prosocial parenting behaviors (such as explaining to children why their help around the house is needed and expecting children to take care of younger family members) predicted prosocial behaviors among adolescents. These links were evident for males and females, as well as first and second generation adolescents.

Taken together, the reviewed research suggests that strong relationships with parents and positive approaches to parenting are associated with a variety of positive qualities among ethnic minority adolescents, especially positive emotional connections with others, academic competence, and social self-efficacy. These findings are similar to what is found among non-minority adolescents, suggesting a universal advantage of these qualities within families for positive youth development.

Culture-Related Family Influences on Positive Youth Development

A second set of research questions focuses on how features of the culture itself foster the development of adaptive qualities among ethnic minority adolescents. This body of work links family transmission of core elements of the ethnic heritage culture to positive youth development.

Family Cultural Values and Positive Development

Cultural values are central components of cultural socialization processes. For example, familism is a key Latino cultural value that emphasizes the importance of loyalty, connectedness, and support within the family (Neblett et al. 2012; Pina-Watson et al., 2013). Similarly, family obligation values, which are important across many ethnic groups, also emphasize the importance of providing support to one's family emotionally, practically, and financially (e.g., Fuligni et al. 2002). Parent and youth endorsement of core values such as familism and family obligation is related to more positive development. For instance, in the study by Calderón-Tena et al. (2011) reviewed above, Mexican American mothers' endorsement of familism values predicted their greater use of prosocial parenting practices, which in turn predicted more prosocial behavior among the adolescents (as well as higher familism value endorsement among adolescents). Similarly, Pina-Watson et al. (2013) demonstrated links between Mexican American adolescents' endorsement of familism values and their feelings of greater self-esteem and life satisfaction.

Endorsement of cultural values is also related to academic achievement. For example, in a sample of Asian American adolescents, Kiang et al. (2013) found that a strong sense of family obligation was related to higher academic adjustment (educational aspirations and the importance of academic success) during high school, beyond the influence of socioeconomic status. Similarly, in a large sample of Mexican American youth (average age 12.3 years old), Gonzales et al. (2008) found that stronger endorsement of traditional cultural values was related to higher academic engagement, as reported by both the adolescent and the teacher.

Parental Ethnic Socialization

A related literature explicitly links parents' ethnic socialization efforts to adolescents' positive developmental outcomes. Ethnic socialization (sometimes also referred to as racial socialization) consists of at least two distinct components: cultural socialization and preparation for bias (Peck et al. 2014). *Cultural socialization* efforts refer to various means by which parents transmit to their children the history, values, and practices of their cultural background, as well as a sense of connection to the heritage culture (Hughes et al. 2006). In contrast, *preparation for bias* messages refer to parental efforts to help youth prepare for the experience of discrimination, stereotypes, and other barriers related to their ethnic background (Peck et al. 2014). Parents typically send more

cultural socialization messages than preparation for bias messages (Peck et al. 2014).

In a review, Evans et al. (2012) argued that ethnic minority parents' efforts to teach their children about the values and practices of their ethnic culture should receive greater attention in the positive youth development literature as an central family influence on development. They outline ways in which parents' cultural socialization efforts may contribute to the development of leadership, character, civic engagement, agency, and prosocial attitudes. Although the empirical literature with ethnic minority adolescents has not spanned such diverse positive developmental outcomes, existing research has consistently linked parents' ethnic socialization to adolescents' academic competence and ethnic identity.

Academic Competence

Different aspects of ethnic socialization (e.g., cultural socialization and preparation for bias) may show different relations with academic competence. *Cultural socialization* efforts by parents have generally been linked to higher academic competence among African American youth. For example, children in grades 4–6 (which corresponds to 9–11 years old) who report more cultural socialization messages about African American heritage, history, and pride from their parents also report greater academic engagement and efficacy (Hughes et al. 2009). These authors suggest that parents' cultural socialization efforts (e.g., teaching children the history and values of their heritage culture) might help buffer adolescents from negative stereotypes about their academic potential so that they can apply themselves more fully to their studies. These relations may be more complex later in adolescence, and may depend on gender, according to research by Brown et al. (2009) with a sample of middle-to-late adolescent African American youth from 14 to 19 years old (average age 15.9 years). Specially, these investigators found that cultural socialization messages that emphasize the importance of African American heritage (i.e., to importance of remember one's heritage and encouragement to attend Black cultural events), from both mothers and fathers, were associated with lower grades among females. In contrast, these same cultural heritage messages from fathers were associated with higher grades among male adolescents. In addition, cultural values messages from mothers (i.e., regarding the importance of family and giving back to the Black community) were also associated with higher grades among males. All analyses controlled for family demographics such as parent education and employment. These investigators speculate that messages may be delivered differently or interpreted differently based on gender. For girls, for instance, they suggest that there may be a point where cultural messages are parent-directed rather than adolescent-directed, rendering females hypersensitive to issues of race and ethnicity, which may create anxiety. Brown and colleagues also highlight the different learning environments that African American males and females encounter (e.g., males are more likely to experience a hostile context and be seen as lack aspirations); they suggest that cultural socialization may be useful in countering the negative expectations that males may face at school.

In contrast to cultural socialization efforts related to developing pride and understanding about the heritage background, *preparation for bias* efforts, such as teaching children how to cope with discrimination or identify racism, has mixed relations with achievement. That is, research has found that preparation for bias socialization messages (e.g., that prepare youth for discrimination) are either unrelated to achievement (Brown et al. 2009) or may even have deleterious effects on achievement (e.g., Rodriguez et al. 2009). However, preparation for bias messages may support academic achievement among African Americans when paired with positive parenting. For example, Smalls (2010) found that children from families in which mothers simultaneously prioritized children's needs, fostered a positive emotional climate, and engaged in a high level of ethnic socialization (i.e., encouraging both racial pride and addressing potential barriers) had the highest

levels of academic engagement (e.g., task persistence, class participation). Similarly, Smalls (2009) found that preparation for bias messages were associated with academic persistence and engagement when paired with a maternal democratic parenting style (e.g., youth involvement in decisions, open communication, quality time together).

Another study of the mechanisms by which parents' cultural socialization may influence adolescents' academic competence found that adolescents' higher self-esteem and stronger ethnic identity meditate these links (Hughes et al. 2009). That is, parents' efforts to teach their children about their ethnic culture helps children feel connected to their culture and feel better about themselves, which in turn predict better academic outcomes. A strong sense of ethnic identification is associated with a host of positive developmental qualities, including academic self-efficacy and social competence (e.g., Umaña-Taylor et al. 2014). A strong ethnic identity may also protect youth in the face of adversity (Costigan et al. 2010). Thus, ethnic identity is an important developmental outcome in itself, and can be considered a culture-related aspect of Connection in the 5 C's of positive youth development model. The role of the family in fostering a strong sense of ethnic identity is reviewed next.

Ethnic Identity

Parental cultural socialization is consistently associated with higher levels of ethnic identity, including ethnic identity pride, cultural knowledge, ethnic identity exploration, and ethnic identity resolution among adolescents (e.g., Lo 2010; Umaña-Taylor et al. 2013). For example, among a large sample of Mexican Americans, Knight et al. (2011) found that mothers with stronger Mexican values engaged in more cultural socialization, which was related to their adolescents' higher ethnic identity and stronger endorsement of Mexican values over time. Fathers' cultural socialization efforts did not show similar links, suggesting that the cultural socialization efforts of mothers are more closely linked to the formation of an ethnic identity among adolescents.

A study of parental cultural values among immigrant Chinese Canadians reached similar conclusions (Su and Costigan 2009). Specifically, for mothers only, greater endorsement of family obligation values was associated with higher ethnic identity achievement among early adolescents. This link was mediated through the adolescents' perceptions of their mothers' family obligation values, suggesting that adolescents need to accurately perceive their mothers' values for family values to influence ethnic identity. A study with self-identified Black American adolescents and a parent (93 % mothers) confirmed the important role of children's perceptions of their parents' cultural socialization messages (Peck et al. 2014). In this study, parents' reports of their cultural socialization messages were only indirectly linked to adolescents' ethnic identity via adolescents' reports of parents' cultural socialization messages; youth must accurately perceive parental messages in order for them to be constructed into their identity. In this study, only cultural socialization messages, and not preparation for bias messages, showed significant links with youth ethnic identity.

A longitudinal study suggests that fathers' cultural socialization efforts are related to adolescent ethnic identity formation under certain circumstances (Umaña-Taylor et al. 2014). In this study, the investigators confirmed the important role of mothers' ethnic socialization efforts in fostering the development of a strong sense of ethnic identity among Mexican American adolescents over time. In addition, they found that fathers' ethnic socialization also predicted adolescents' ethnic identity, but only when adolescents attended schools with a low proportion of other Latino students. The authors propose that fathers' influence may be more content-dependent and therefore missed if the broader ethnic composition of adolescents' lives is not considered. Specifically they suggest that fathers may engage in more cultural socialization in contexts where their children are a minority and/or that adolescents may be more likely to draw on multiple socialization messages

(e.g., from mothers and fathers) when they are in the minority compared to when there are large numbers of same-ethnic peers.

Collectively, across diverse ethnic groups, parents' efforts to teach children about the history and values of their cultural heritage, and children's adoption of core cultural values, may confer benefits to adolescents in terms of academic competence and feelings of cultural belonging and ethnic identity. More research is needed to fully understand the role of fathers in these processes, and how ethnic socialization efforts intersect with the broader social context in which families live (e.g., Umaña-Taylor et al. 2014).

Parent Facilitation of Mainstream Cultural Competence

In contrast to the focus on how parents foster a sense of understanding and connection to the ethnic heritage culture, much less attention has been paid to the ways in which minority parents contribute to their children's successful integration into the mainstream US or Canadian cultures. Although relevant to non-immigrant ethnic minority families, most of this research has focused on immigrants. Immigrant parents may play a role in their children's adoption of the mainstream culture via the opportunities they facilitate for their children outside the home, as well as through the adoption of childrearing goals that reflect qualities that are valued in the mainstream society.

Research with immigrant families often assumes that immigrant parents are threatened by their children's increasing involvement in the mainstream society in the years following immigration. Adolescents' involvement in mainstream culture, however, does not inevitably create conflict or distress within immigrant families, even when parents do not share a high orientation to the mainstream culture (e.g., Costigan and Dokis 2006). This is likely because immigrant parents typically desire their children to be successful in the new culture, and their children's ability to speak the new culture's language, form positive relationships within the new culture, and understand nuances in how members of the new culture think and behave, are all indications of successful attainment of this goal. Children's involvement in the mainstream culture may be especially non-problematic if adolescents' adoption of the new culture is not at the expense of maintaining important heritage cultural values and practices.

Parents are introduced to a host of new ideas regarding childrearing after immigration, and they may modify their parenting cognitions to more closely match the larger society in order to socialize their children to be successful in a new multicultural context (Yee et al. 1998). Consistently, value transmission studies within families demonstrate that parents understand what is normatively important in a society and socialize their children towards those values, even when these values do not mirror parents' own (Benish-Weisman et al. 2013; Chen and Chen 2010). Thus, immigrant parents' socialization goals for their children may not perfectly match their own personal values (e.g., Farver et al. 2007), and parents may actively and intentionally foster their children's competencies in the mainstream culture regardless of their own cultural orientation. Parents may also pursue socialization goals that do not match their personal goals by identifying and encouraging other socialization agents (e.g., opportunities at schools, extended family, extra-curricular activities) to assist their children to develop competencies that are salient in the mainstream culture (Tam and Lee 2010). More research is needed to understand how parents' childrearing goals and cultural socialization efforts are related to positive developmental outcomes.

Family Influences on Navigating a Bicultural Environment

A third set of research questions has examined more closely the family processes involved in helping ethnic minority adolescents develop a positive sense of identity and well-being as they find their way in diverse, sometimes conflicting, cultural worlds. Navigating multiple cultural identities can be a challenge for adolescents who experience competing pulls from parents toward the ethnic heritage culture and from peers towards the mainstream society (Giguère et al. 2010). Much research in this area focuses on the stresses and strains (for both youth and their parents) inherent in balancing two cultures, including the risk of heightened family conflict and distress (e.g., Telzer 2011). Less attention has been paid to the ways in which the process of navigating two cultural contexts can contribute to positive youth development.

Family Influences on Bicultural Competence

One domain of positive development associated with the need to navigate two cultural worlds simultaneously is the concept of biculturalism. Biculturalism refers to an individual's comfort interacting in both ethnic and mainstream contexts, ease of switching between the two contexts, and perception of advantages in being able to move between the two contexts (Basilio et al. 2014). Thus, it is relevant to the domain of competence in the Five C's of positive youth development model. Research generally supports the conclusion that embracing both the heritage and mainstream cultures is the most adaptive approach to balancing two cultures (e.g., Nguyen and Benet-Martínez 2013).

As the definition of the concept of biculturalism has advanced, research has begun to investigate how bicultural competence develops, including the role of families. Research with Mexican American adolescents suggests that high parental acceptance, in conjunction with higher friendship intimacy, fosters bicultural competence (i.e., endorsement of both familism values and a high Anglo orientation; Davidson et al. 2011). In a conceptual paper, Mistry and Wu (2010) proposed that one of the ways in which families foster biculturalism is by exposing children to and valuing diverse frames of reference so that children become familiar with and feel comfortable interacting in multiple groups. Schwartz and Unger (2010), operating from a heritage culture focus, argued that parents' ethnic socialization efforts are a key contributor to the development of bicultural competence. Rather than fostering separation from the mainstream culture, they review research suggesting that parents' intentional efforts to teach children about their heritage culture facilitate the development of biculturalism. Parents' role in supporting bicultural competence may be especially strong in community contexts with little cultural diversity, where there is less community support for heritage cultural retention (Schwartz and Unger 2010).

Parent–Child Cultural Dynamics and Positive Youth Development

Navigating two sets of cultural norms and values at the same time has implications for family relationships as well as individual development. In immigrant families, discrepancies often exist in parents' and children's language skills, social contacts, identifications, and values (e.g., Kwak 2003). Previous research has identified these parent–child differences as a significant obstacle to positive adjustment among adolescents and their families (Unger et al. 2009; Wang et al. 2012). For example, acculturation gaps in language abilities can present obstacles to effective communication, making it more difficult to discuss sensitive emotional issues. One significant challenge for work in this area, however, is disentangling parent–child conflict that is related to cultural differences and parent–child conflict that is developmentally normative (e.g., Phinney and Vedder 2006). This is, all families (e.g., immigrant and non-immigrant) experience intergenerational differences to some extent. Furthermore, it is important to remember that not all parent–child conflict is associated with adjustment challenges for adolescents. Considerably less research has been directed at identifying developmental opportunities that may be embedded in the experience of navigating two cultural worlds as a family. There may be benefits to adolescent adjustment related to similarity

in cultural orientations between parents and children (e.g., Lo 2010). For example, when Asian Indian parents (83 % mothers) and their children in the United States reported the same overall cultural orientation, adolescents reported higher self-esteem (Farver et al. 2002). Parent and child similarity in their orientation to the heritage culture appears to be more important than their similarity in orientation to the mainstream culture. For example, a match between adolescents and their mothers in heritage language skills is associated with higher math scores and overall grade point averages among Chinese American families (Liu et al. 2009). Likewise, among Chinese Canadian families, parent–child similarity in orientation to Chinese culture is associated with higher achievement motivation among adolescents (Costigan and Dokis 2006). In this study, adolescents' similarity in Chinese language use with mothers and in Chinese media use with fathers (whether similarly high or low) showed the strongest links with achievement motivation. When adolescents are better able to communicate and share interests with their parents, they may also be more likely to internalize cultural norms related to the importance of achievement, which may translate into greater effort put towards their studies and stronger achievement motivation. In addition, when mothers and adolescents both speak Chinese, mothers can be more involved in their children's education, so that adolescents experience greater support (Costigan and Dokis 2006). Further research is needed into the mechanisms by which similarity in cultural orientations supports adolescents' positive development across multiple domains of functioning.

Within immigrant families, adolescents' bilingual abilities may also indirectly create developmental opportunities by enabling children to serve as "language brokers" for their parents. Language brokering refers to assistance that children provide their parents in translating and interpreting linguistic and cultural material from the mainstream culture (e.g., Chao 2006). This material may be written or spoken, formal or informal. The literature is currently inconsistent with respect to whether language brokering confers risk on children (e.g., placing too much responsibility on them, exposing them to sensitive personal information about a parent) or whether it can benefit children's cognitive and emotional development (e.g., Hua and Costigan 2012). On the positive side, a number of studies document positive correlates of language brokering experiences. For example, among Latino adolescents, more frequent language brokering is associated with greater biculturalism and academic performance (Buriel et al. 1998) and higher ethnic identity and cultural value endorsement (Weisskirch et al. 2011). Among young adults from multiple ethnic backgrounds, more frequent language brokering is associated with enhanced perspective taking and greater empathic concern (Guan et al. 2014). More frequent language brokering is also associated with greater respect for mothers among Mexican and Chinese American youth and for fathers among Mexican and Korean American youth (Chao 2006).

The family context in which language brokering occurs (e.g., as supportive or conflictual) may shape whether or not the experience is related to the development of adaptive qualities (Hua and Costigan 2012; Weisskirch 2007). In addition, adolescents' own cultural orientation may also shape whether language brokering has a positive or negative impact on adolescent development. For example, adolescents who are more oriented to the heritage culture are more likely to feel they matter to their parents and are more likely to experience feelings of efficacy related to language brokering, whereas adolescents who are less oriented to the heritage culture are more likely to feel alienated from their parents and to experience feelings of burden related to language brokering (Wu and Kim 2009).

Overall, there is little research linking parent–child cultural dynamics with positive developmental outcomes; instead, these dynamics are most often conceptualized as risks. When positive correlates are sought, the most typical outcomes continue to be academic competence and ethnic identity. A broader perspective on positive development that considers qualities such as connection, empathy, and leadership may enrich the research agenda in this area.

Family Promotion of Positive Development in the Face of Adversity

The final set of research questions addresses ways in which ethnic minority families promote positive adolescent development in the face of risk. The challenges and risks faced by ethnic minority families are well documented, including discrimination, prejudice, low income, and acculturative stress; much research documents the deleterious effects of these risks on individuals and families (e.g., Garcia Coll and Magnuson 1997; García Coll et al. 1996; Hwang and Ting 2008; Pérez et al. 2008). Increasingly, research is identifying strengths and protective processes that promote positive development despite these challenges (e.g., Neblett et al. 2012; Zhou et al. 2012).

Many of the same family factors that promote positive development among ethnic minority youth overall also encourage positive adjustment and competence in the face of adversity. Neblett et al. (2012) presented a conceptual model highlighting cultural protective factors that promote positive adaptation in the context of discrimination. These protective factors include ethnic socialization, cultural orientations, and ethnic identities. For example, they propose that connections to the family may become more potent when confronting discrimination, such that familial ethnic socialization messages may show particularly strong links with adaptation in these circumstances. Consistently, Kiang et al. (2013) found that strong endorsement of family obligation values among adolescents buffered the effects of low socioeconomic class on adolescents' achievement outcomes; adolescents with high family obligation values maintained high achievement despite economic risks.

Generally supportive family relationships also protect minority and immigrant adolescents in the context of stress. For example, among a sample of African American adolescents who had been exposed to community violence, positive family functioning (i.e., parental communication, parental concern, and parental supervision) was associated with higher scores on a composite measure of the Five C's of positive youth development (McDonald et al. 2011). Similarly, among American Indian early adolescents living on or near reservations, maternal warmth and support protected youth from risks related to poverty and discrimination (LaFromboise et al. 2006). Specifically, these positive maternal characteristics, along with greater community support, were associated with higher levels of pro-social behavior, including a positive school attitude, high academic aspirations, and good grades. Finally, Tiet et al. (2010) identified longitudinal predictors of positive adjustment among a large and diverse sample of ethnic minority adolescents who were considered to be at risk due to living in an inner city environment (e.g., disadvantaged neighborhoods with high crime rates). These researchers found that family bonding (e.g., depending on parents for advice and guidance) predicted later resilience, assessed as higher academic achievement, self-esteem, and psychosocial functioning. In addition, among a subset of youth in this study from two-parent families, higher levels of parental monitoring of youth activities and lower levels of marital discord were also associated with more resilient outcomes over time.

Policy Implications

Perhaps the clearest policy recommendation that emerges from this review is the value of supporting the transmission of the ethnic culture within minority and immigrant families. Across disparate samples and methods, with few exceptions, parents' cultural socialization efforts, children's endorsement of heritage cultural values, and parent–child similarity in ethnic heritage culture orientations were associated with more positive youth development, particularly in the areas of academic achievement, ethnic identification, and bicultural competence. Thus, policies and programs that provide resources and

supports for families and their communities to maintain an understanding of their heritage culture and feeling of belonging should contribute to the positive development of youth in these families (e.g., Hughes et al. 2009; Rodriguez et al. 2009). These efforts require that cultural knowledge and values are seen as assets and resources for families that support bicultural integration and general well-being, rather than treating the heritage culture as unrelated, or even as a threat to integration into the mainstream society.

In addition to fostering ethnic heritage culture assets, general family processes that are adaptive in non-minority families support the positive development of ethnic minority youth as well, both as promotive factors for all youth and as protective factors for youth facing adversity. Thus, policies and programs that build on these strengths within minority and immigrant families can have far-reaching effects on youth development. For example, programs that promote and support positive parenting and build family cohesion would contribute to the positive development of youth (e.g., Corona et al. 2012; Leidy et al. 2012). Programs that assist families in identifying positive roles models of academic and occupational success for youth to emulate are another means of promoting positive development (e.g., Roosa et al. 2012). Finally, school policies and programs that support the involvement of minority and immigrant parents in their children's school work could contribute to academic achievement in these families.

Future Directions

Future research should embrace the study of positive development among minority and immigrant youth. To date, the majority of work on positive youth development has not integrated key aspects of culture (e.g., cultural values, cultural socialization, parent–child cultural similarity) in fostering positive development (Evans et al. 2012). Yet, for ethnic minority youth, heritage cultural factors are integral to their developmental experiences. Research that has included cultural models in the study of positive youth development has been limited in scope with respect to the types of developmental outcomes that are assessed. With few exceptions (e.g., Smetana and Metzger 2005), little or no research addresses the role of parents and families in promoting domains of positive youth development such as vocational competence, hope, empathy, morality, leadership, purpose, spirituality, thriving, civic engagement, or media literacy. In addition, research should address the question of whether positive development is defined differently in diverse ethnic communities. Qualities that are valued in mainstream US and Canadian society may be irrelevant or devalued in certain ethnic groups, and other culture-specific developmental strengths may be overlooked.

Most of the literature reviewed spans the developmental period from early to late adolescence. More attention is needed on the transition into adulthood for ethnic minority youth and how families facilitate the successful navigation of this phase of life. Young adulthood is the stage of life when young people accrue the capacity for growth in economic and social capital that sets the stage for their lifetime contributions as citizens. In young adulthood, youth may experience extra pressures to succeed in order to honor sacrifices their parents made in raising them. In addition, immigrant parents in particular may look to their children's success to validate the risks they took in migrating. A better understanding of the ways in which families continue to support youth development through this transition is critical.

Although short-term longitudinal data are becoming increasingly common, particularly with Latino populations, longer-term longitudinal data that can begin to address the direction of effects among constructs would be valuable. The inclusion of experimental and observational research methods would also expand the scope of the questions that are asked. In addition, although there are notable exceptions, many studies that report of "parental" correlates of youth development are in fact predominantly assessing maternal influences; continued efforts

to include fathers in research will allow researchers to more systematically address shared and unique roles for mothers and fathers in the development of minority and immigrant youth. Finally, more large representative samples are needed across varied community contexts (e.g., based on the ethnic composition of the surrounding community) in order to represent the full diversity of experiences that exist within ethnic groups.

Research methods and questions in this area would also benefit from expanding beyond the study of mono-cultural youth and traditional definitions of the family. The high and growing number of bicultural and multicultural children in the United States and Canada warrants greater attention to the universal and unique family process that promote positive youth development among these children. Similarly, the influence of families on the positive development of minority youth should expand beyond traditional family roles of mothers and fathers to include a broader, more inclusive lens on what constitutes a family by including other types of family structures, such as grandparent-led families, stepfamilies, and extended kinship networks.

Finally, research designs should routinely situate families in their larger ecological contexts. For example, immigrant families enter the United States and Canada through a variety of mechanisms (e.g., refugee, skilled worker, undocumented), and the vulnerabilities and strengths that each context introduces to the task of raising well-adjusted children are different. Non-immigrant ethnic minority families, as well, experience considerable diversity in their day-to-day experiences due to factors such as socioeconomic status. The associated financial resources, social capital, and human capital that families have available to them interact in a dynamic fashion with the capacities of families to nurture children's positive development. The broader social structures in which families are located (e.g., contexts of reception, neighborhood context, power differentials, ethnic composition of communities, support for diversity) similarly shape and constrain minority and immigrant families' socialization efforts. The work of Umaña-Taylor et al. (2014), for instance, exemplifies how the ethnic composition of schools intersects with parental influences on youth development. A full understanding of family influences on positive youth development requires the integration of real-world constraints and opportunities from families' broader ecological context.

Conclusions

The study of parental and family influences on ethnic minority youth development using a strength-based approach is a growing area of inquiry, but many gaps remain. The research reviewed in this chapter identifies general processes (e.g., sense of connection with parents) and culture-specific processes (e.g., cultural socialization efforts) that are essential to fostering positive development among ethnic minority youth. The clear association between parents' efforts to transmit their ethnic culture and adolescents' positive adaptation signals the importance of supporting parents in this vital activity. Cultural processes (e.g., transmission of cultural values, sense of belonging) also buffer the adverse impacts of contextual threats, such as discrimination, on adolescents' positive development. Further, our review suggests that family dynamics related to navigating a bicultural environment are not inherently stressful or detrimental to individual or family functioning. In the future, research that is framed from a positive youth development point of view, rather than a deficit model, may reveal further beneficial aspects of bicultural family dynamics. Areas of positive youth development that have not yet been addressed (e.g., leadership, civic engagement) should also be incorporated into future research. Finally, our understanding of how to best support positive development among ethnic minority youth will be advanced by research that situates family influences on positive development within a broader ecological context that carefully considers social structures, school and neighborhood environments, and immigration pathways.

References

Areepattamannil, S., & Lee, D. L. (2014). Linking immigrant parents' educational expectations and aspirations to their children's school performance. *The Journal of Genetic Psychology: Research and Theory on Human Development, 175*(1), 51–57. doi:10.1080/00221325.2013.799061

Basilio, C. D., Knight, G. P., O'Donnell, M., Roosa, M. W., Gonzales, N. A., Umaña-Taylor, A. J., et al. (2014). The Mexican American biculturalism scale: Bicultural comfort, facility, and advantages for adolescents and adults. *Psychological Assessment, 26*(2), 539–554. doi:10.1037/a0035951

Benish-Weisman, M., Levy, S., & Knafo, A. (2013). Parents differentiate between their personal values and their socialization values: The role of adolescents' values. *Journal of Research on Adolescence, 23*(4), 614–620. doi:10.1111/jora.12058

Brown, T. L., Linver, M. R., Evans, M., & DeGennaro, D. (2009). African-American parents' racial and ethnic socialization and adolescent academic grades: Teasing out the role of gender. *Journal of Youth and Adolescence, 38*(2), 214–227. doi:10.1007/s10964-008-9362-z

Buriel, R., Perez, W., De Ment, T. L., Chavez, D. V., & Moran, V. R. (1998). The relationship of language brokering to academic performance, biculturalism, and self-efficacy among Latino adolescents. *Hispanic Journal of Behavioral Sciences, 20*(3), 283–297.

Calderón-Tena, C. O., Knight, G. P., & Carlo, G. (2011). The socialization of prosocial behavioral tendencies among Mexican American adolescents: The role of familism values. *Cultural Diversity and Ethnic Minority Psychology, 17*(1), 98–106.

Chao, R. K. (2006). The prevalence and consequences of adolescents' language brokering for their immigrant parents. In M. H. Bornstein & L. R. Cote (Eds.), *Acculturation and parent–child relationships: Measurement and development* (pp. 271–296). Mahwah, NJ: Erlbaum.

Chen, X., & Chen, H. (2010). Child's socioemotional functioning and adjustment in the changing Chinese society. In R. K. Silbereisen & X. Chen (Eds.), *Social change and human development: Concepts and results* (pp. 209–227). London: Sage. doi:10.4135/9781446252161.n10

Chen, S. H., Hua, M., Zhou, Q., Tao, A., Lee, E. H., Ly, J., et al. (2014). Parent–child cultural orientations and child adjustment in Chinese American immigrant families. *Developmental Psychology, 50*(1), 189.

Corona, M., McCarty, C., Cauce, A. M., Robins, R. W., Widaman, K. F., & Conger, R. D. (2012). The relation between maternal and child depression in Mexican American families. *Hispanic Journal of Behavioral Sciences, 34*(4), 539–556.

Corwyn, R. F., & Bradley, R. H. (2008). The panethnic Asian label and predictors of eighth-grade student achievement. *School Psychology Quarterly, 23,* 90–106.

Costigan, C. L., & Dokis, D. P. (2006). Relations between parent–child acculturation differences and adjustment within immigrant Chinese families. *Child Development, 77*(5), 1252–1267.

Costigan, C. L., Koryzma, C. M., Hua, J. M., & Chance, L. J. (2010). Ethnic identity, achievement, and psychological adjustment: Examining risk and resilience among youth from immigrant Chinese families in Canada. *Cultural Diversity and Ethnic Minority Psychology, 16*(2), 264–273. doi:10.1037/a0017275

Davidson, A. J., Updegraff, K. A., & McHale, S. M. (2011). Parent-peer relationship patterns among Mexican-origin adolescents. *International Journal of Behavioral Development, 35*(3), 260–270. doi:10.1177/0165025410384926

Dyson, L. L. (2001). Home-school communication and expectations of recent Chinese immigrants. *Canadian Journal of Education, 26*(4), 455–476. doi:10.2307/1602177

Eng, S., Kanitkar, K., Cleveland, H. H., Herbert, R., Fischer, J., & Wiersma, J. D. (2008). School achievement differences among Chinese and Filipino American students: Acculturation and the family. *Educational Psychology, 28*, 535–550.

Evans, A. B., Banerjee, M., Meyer, R., Aldana, A., Foust, M., & Rowley, S. (2012). Racial socialization as a mechanism for positive development among African American youth. *Child Development Perspectives, 6*(3), 251–257. doi:10.1111/j.1750-8606.2011.00226.x

Farver, J. M., Narang, S. K., & Bhadha, B. R. (2002). East meets West: Ethnic identity, acculturation, and conflict in Asian Indian families. *Journal of Family Psychology, 16*(3), 338–350. doi:10.1037/0893-3200.16.3.338

Farver, J. M., Xu, Y., Bhadha, B. R., Narang, S. K., & Lieber, E. (2007). Ethnic identity, acculturation, parenting beliefs, and adolescent adjustment: A comparison of Asian Indian and European American families. *Merrill-Palmer Quarterly, 53*(2), 184–215. doi:10.1353/mpq.2007.0010

Fuligni, A., Yip, T., & Tseng, V. (2002). The impact of family obligation on the daily activities and psychological well-being of Chinese American adolescents. *Child Development, 73*, 302–314.

García Coll, C., Lamberty, G., Jenkins, R., McAdoo, H. P., Crnic, K., Wasik, B. H., et al. (1996). An integrative model for the study of developmental competencies in minority children. *Child Development, 67*(5), 1891–1914. doi:10.2307/1131600

Garcia Coll, C., & Magnuson, K. (1997). The psychological experience of immigration: A developmental perspective. In A. Booth, A. C. Crouter, & N. Landale (Eds.), *Immigration and the family* (pp. 91–132). Mahwah, NJ: Lawrence Erlbaum Associates.

Giguère, B., Lalonde, R. N., & Lou, E. (2010). Living at the crossroads of cultural worlds: The experience of normative conflicts by second generation immigrant youth. *Social and Personality Psychology Compass, 4*, 14–29.

Gonzales, N. A., Germán, M., Kim, S. Y., George, P., Fabrett, F. C., Millsap, R., et al. (2008). Mexican American adolescents' cultural orientation, externalizing behavior and academic engagement: The role of traditional cultural values. *American Journal of Community Psychology, 41*(1–2), 151–164. doi:10.1007/s10464-007-9152-x

Guan, S. S. A., Greenfield, P. M., & Orellana, M. F. (2014). Translating into understanding: Language brokering and prosocial development in emerging adults from immigrant families. *Journal of Adolescent Research, 29*(3), 331–355. doi:10.1177/0743558413520223

Hill, N. E., & Tyson, D. F. (2009). Parental involvement in middle school: A meta-analytic assessment of the strategies that promote achievement. *Developmental Psychology, 45*(3), 740–763. doi:10.1037/a0015362

Hua, J. M., & Costigan, C. L. (2012). The familial context of adolescent language brokering within immigrant Chinese families in Canada. *Journal of Youth and Adolescence, 41*(7), 894–906. doi:10.1007/s10964-011-9682-2

Hughes, D., Rodriguez, J., Smith, E. P., Johnson, D. J., Stevenson, H. C., & Spicer, P. (2006). Parents' ethnic racial socialization practices: A review of research and directions for future study. *Developmental Psychology, 42*, 747–770.

Hughes, D., Witherspoon, D., Rivas-Drake, D., & West-Bey, N. (2009). Received ethnic–racial socialization messages and youths' academic and behavioral outcomes: Examining the mediating role of ethnic identity and self-esteem. *Cultural Diversity and Ethnic Minority Psychology, 15*(2), 112–124. doi:10.1037/a0015509

Hwang, W., & Ting, J. Y. (2008). Disaggregating the effects of acculturation and acculturative stress on the mental health of Asian Americans. *Cultural Diversity and Ethnic Minority Psychology, 14*(2), 147–154.

Jeynes, W. H. (2007). The relationship between parental involvement and urban secondary school student academic achievement: A meta-analysis. *Urban Education, 42*(1), 82–110. doi:10.1177/0042085906293818

Kiang, L., Andrews, K., Stein, G. L., Supple, A. J., & Gonzalez, L. M. (2013). Socioeconomic stress and academic adjustment among Asian American adolescents: The protective role of family obligation. *Journal of Youth and Adolescence, 42*(6), 837–847. doi:10.1007/s10964-013-9916-6

Knight, G. P., Berkel, C., Umaña-Taylor, A. J., Gonzales, N. A., Ettekal, I., Jaconis, M., et al. (2011). The familial socialization of culturally related values in Mexican American families. *Journal of Marriage and Family, 73*, 913–925. doi:10.1111/j.1741-3737.2011.00856.x

Kwak, K. (2003). Adolescents and their parents: A review of intergenerational family relations for immigrant and non-immigrant families. *Human Development, 46*, 115–136.

LaFromboise, T. D., Hoyt, D. R., Oliver, L., & Whitbeck, L. B. (2006). Family, community, and school influences on resilience among American Indian adolescents in the upper Midwest. *Journal of Community Psychology, 34*(2), 193–209. doi:10.1002/jcop.20090

Leidy, M. S., Guerra, N. G., & Toro, R. I. (2012). Positive parenting, family cohesion, and child social competence among immigrant Latino families. *Journal of Latina/o Psychology, 1*(S), 3–13.

Lerner, R. M., Lerner, J. V., Almerigi, J. B., Theokas, C., Phelps, E., Gestsdottir, S., et al. (2005). Positive youth development, participation in community youth development programs, and community contributions of fifth-grade adolescents: Findings from the first wave of the 4-h study of positive youth development. *The Journal of Early Adolescence, 25*(1), 17–71. doi:10.1177/0272431604272461

Liu, L. L., Benner, A. D., Lau, A. S., & Kim, S. Y. (2009). Mother-adolescent language proficiency and adolescent academic and emotional adjustment among Chinese American families. *Journal of Youth and Adolescence, 38*, 572–586. doi:10.1007/s10964-008-9358-8

Lo, Y. (2010). The impact of the acculturation process on Asian American youths' psychological well-being. *Journal of Child and Adolescent Psychiatric Nursing, 23*(2), 84–91.

McDonald, C. C., Deatrick, J. A., Kassam-Adams, N., & Richmond, T. S. (2011). Community violence exposure and positive youth development in urban youth. *Journal of Community Health, 36*, 925–932. doi:10.1007/s10900-011-9391-5

McLoyd, V. C., Cauce, A. M., Takeuchi, D., & Wilson, L. (2000). Marital processes and parental socialization in families of color: A decade review of research. *Journal of Marriage and Family, 62*, 1070–1093.

McMahon, T. R., Baete Kenyon, D., & Carter, J. S. (2013). "My culture, my family, my school, me": Identifying strengths and challenges in the lives and communities of American Indian youth. *Journal of Child and Family Studies, 22*, 694–706. doi:10.1007/s10826-012-9623-z

Mistry, J., & Wu, J. (2010). Navigating cultural worlds and negotiating identities: A conceptual model. *Human Development, 53*(1), 5–25. doi:10.1159/000268136

Neblett, E. J., Rivas-Drake, D., & Umaña-Taylor, A. J. (2012). The promise of racial and ethnic protective factors in promoting ethnic minority youth development. *Child Development Perspectives, 6*(3), 295–303. doi:10.1111/j.1750-8606.2012.00239.x

Nguyen, A. D., & Benet-Martínez, V. (2013). Biculturalism and adjustment: A meta-analysis. *Journal of Cross-Cultural Psychology, 44*(1), 122–159. doi:10.1177/0022022111435097

Peck, S. C., Brodish, A. B., Malanchuk, O., Banerjee, M., & Eccles, J. S. (2014). Racial/ethnic socialization and identity development in black families: The role of parent and youth reports. *Developmental Psychology, 50*(7), 1897–1909.

Pérez, D. J., Fortuna, L., & Alegría, M. (2008). Prevalence and correlates of everyday discrimination among US Latinos. *Journal of Community Psychology, 36*(4), 421–433. doi:10.1002/jcop.20221

Phinney, J. S., & Vedder, P. (2006). Family relationship values of adolescents and parents: Intergenerational discrepancies and adaptation. In J. W. Berry, J. S. Phinney, D. L. Sam, P. Vedder, J. W. Berry, & J. S. Phinney (Eds.), *Immigrant youth in cultural transition: Acculturation, identity, and adaptation across national contexts* (pp. 167–184). Mahwah, NJ: Lawrence Erlbaum Associates Publishers.

Pina-Watson, B., Ojeda, L., Castellon, N. E., & Dornhecker, M. (2013). Familismo, ethnic identity, and bicultural stress as predictors of Mexican American adolescents' positive psychological functioning. *Journal of Latina/o Psychology, 1*(4), 204–217.

Rodríguez, S. A., Perez-Brena, N. J., Updegraff, K. A., & Umaña-Taylor, A. J. (2014). Emotional closeness in Mexican-origin adolescents' relationships with mothers, fathers, and same-sex friends. *Journal of Youth and Adolescence, 43*(12), 1953–1968. doi:10.1007/s10964-013-0004-8

Rodriguez, J., Umaña-Taylor, A., Smith, E., & Johnson, D. (2009). Cultural processes in parenting and youth outcomes: Examining a model of racial-ethnic socialization and identity in diverse populations. *Cultural Diversity and Ethnic Minority Psychology, 15*, 106–111.

Roosa, M. W., O'Donnell, M., Ham, H., Gonzales, N. A., Zeiders, K. H., Tein, J.-Y., et al. (2012). A prospective study of Mexican American adolescents' academic success: Considering family and individual factors. *Journal of Youth and Adolescence, 41*, 307–319.

Rousseau, C., Hassan, G., Measham, T., Moreau, N., Lashley, M., Castro, T., et al. (2009). From the family universe to the outside world: Family relations, school attitude, and perception of racism in Caribbean and Filipino adolescents. *Health Place, 15*, 751–760.

Schwartz, S. J., & Unger, J. B. (2010). Biculturalism and context: What is biculturalism, and when is it adaptive? *Human Development, 53*(1), 26–32. doi:10.1159/000268137

Smalls, C. (2009). African American adolescent engagement in the classroom and beyond: The roles of mother's racial socialization and democratic-involved parenting. *Journal of Youth and Adolescence, 38*, 204–213.

Smalls, C. (2010). Effects of mothers' racial socialization and relationship quality on African American youth's school engagement: A profile approach. *Cultural Diversity and Ethnic Minority Psychology, 16*, 476–484.

Smetana, J. G., & Gettman, D. C. (2006). Autonomy and relatedness with parents and romantic development in African American adolescents. *Developmental Psychology, 42*, 1347–1351.

Smetana, J. G., & Metzger, A. (2005). Family and religious antecedents of civic involvement in middle class African American late adolescents. *Journal of Research on Adolescence, 15*(3), 325–352.

Su, T. F., & Costigan, C. L. (2009). The development of children's ethnic identity in immigrant Chinese families in Canada: The role of parenting practices and children's perceptions of parental family obligation expectations. *Journal of Early Adolescence, 29*, 638–663.

Tam, K., & Lee, S. (2010). What values do parents want to socialize in their children? The role of perceived normative values. *Journal of Cross-Cultural Psychology, 41*(2), 175–181. doi:10.1177/0022022109354379

Tang, S. (2015). Social capital and determinants of immigrant family educational involvement. *The Journal of Educational Research, 108*(1), 22–34. doi:10.1080/00220671.2013.833076

Telzer, E. H. (2011). Expanding the acculturation gap-distress model: An integrative review of research. *Human Development, 53*(6), 313–340. doi:10.1159/000322476

Tiet, Q. Q., Huizinga, D., & Byrnes, H. F. (2010). Predictors of resilience among inner city youths. *Journal of Child and Family Studies, 19*, 360–378. doi:10.1007/s10826-009-9307-5

Turney, K., & Kao, G. (2009). Barriers to school involvement: Are immigrant parents disadvantaged? *The Journal of Educational Research, 102*, 257–271. doi:10.3200/JOER.102.4.257-271

Umaña-Taylor, A. J., O'Donnell, M., Knight, G. P., Roosa, M. W., Berkel, C., & Nair, R. (2014). Mexican-origin early adolescents' ethnic socialization, ethnic identity, and psychosocial functioning. *The Counseling Psychologist, 42*(2), 170–200. doi:10.1177/0011000013477903

Umaña-Taylor, A. J., Zeiders, K. H., & Updegraff, K. A. (2013). Family ethnic socialization and ethnic identity: A family-driven, youth-driven, or reciprocal process? *Journal of Family Psychology, 27*(1), 137–146. doi:10.1037/a0031105

Unger, J. B., Ritt-Olson, A., Soto, D., & Baezconde-Garbanati, L. (2009). Parent–child acculturation discrepancies as a risk factor for substance use among Hispanic adolescents in Southern California. *Journal of Immigrant Minority Health, 11*, 149–157.

Wang, M., & Ecceles, J. S. (2012). Social support matters: Longitudinal effects of social support on three dimensions of school engagement from middle to high school. *Child Development, 83*, 877–895.

Wang, Y., Kim, S. K., Anderson, E. R., Chen, A. C.-C., & Yan, N. (2012). Parent–child acculturation discrepancy, perceived parental knowledge, peer deviance, and adolescent delinquency in Chinese immigrant families. *Journal of Youth and Adolescence, 41*, 907–919.

Weisskirch, R. (2007). Feelings about language brokering and family relations among Mexican American early adolescents. *The Journal of Early Adolescence, 27*(4), 545–561.

Weisskirch, R. S., Kim, S. Y., Zamboanga, B. L., Schwartz, S. J., Bersamin, M., & Umaña-Taylor, A. J. (2011). Cultural influences for college student language brokers. *Cultural Diversity and Ethnic Minority Psychology, 17*(1), 43–51. doi:10.1037/a0021665

Wu, N. H., & Kim, S. Y. (2009). Chinese American adolescents' perceptions of the language brokering experience as a sense of burden and sense of efficacy. *Journal of Youth and Adolescence, 38*(5), 703–718. doi:10.1007/s10964-008-9379-3

Yee, B. W. K., Huang, L. N., & Lew, A. (1998). Family lifespan socialization in a cultural context. In L. C. Lee & N. W. S. Zane (Eds.), *Handbook of Asian American psychology* (pp. 83–135). Thousand Oaks, CA: SAGE.

Zhai, J. E., & Stokes, C. E. (2009). Ethnic, family, and social contextual influences on Asian American adolescents' religiosity. *Sociological Spectrum, 29*, 201–226.

Zhou, Q., Tao, A., Chen, S. H., Main, A., Lee, E., Ly, J., et al. (2012). Asset and protective factors for Asian American children's mental health adjustment. *Child Development Perspectives, 6*, 312–319.

Family Resources for Promoting Positive Development Among Minority Children: European Perspectives

Sabine Walper and Birgit Leyendecker

Abstract

The focus of this chapter is the role of family factors in fostering positive development among minority children in Europe. The historical overview highlights the heterogeneity among minority families in Europe, differences between indigenous minorities and immigrant minorities and related cross-country differences. The focus of the following sections is mainly on immigrant minority families. Current key research questions relate to families' coping with challenges resulting from migration, cultural distance, and socio-economic strain. Empirical studies rely mainly on large representative surveys within one or across several European countries but also include some observational, qualitative, and intervention studies. The findings discussed in this chapter address changing family forms, point to strong family ties among immigrant families, provide evidence for the general benefits of parental involvement and care, and highlight the role of early daycare and parental involvement in children's schooling. The chapter concludes with policy implications and directions for future research.

Introduction

The colonial past of many European countries, including economically driven migration, and the current inflow of refugees from war zones and terror regimes have contributed to considerable ethnic heterogeneity in European countries. From 1980s to 1990s, the inflow of foreigners to (and between) European countries doubled (Hooghe et al. 2008). By 2010, about 6.5 % of the total population among the 27 European countries had foreign nationalities and 9.4 % of the population in Europe were born outside their country of residence, mostly outside of Europe (Vasileva 2011). The recent increase in refugees exceeds these numbers considerably.

Migration may not only increase individuals' opportunities for better prospects in the host country, but it may also benefit their host countries

S. Walper (✉)
Munich, Germany
e-mail: walper@dji.de

B. Leyendecker
Bochum, Germany

by meeting demands of expanding labor markets and/or compensating demographic problems (e.g. arising from low birth rates). Nevertheless, migration poses major challenges to migrants as well as their host countries in coping with migration experiences, ethnic diversity, the risks of segregation and alienation and its implications for the development of minority children. In fact, much of the public and scientific discourse about immigrants and ethnic minorities focuses on risks and problems resulting for ethnic minorities, migrants, and their children (e.g., Hjern et al. 1991; Kouider et al. 2014; Tan et al. 1991) or for the majority population in host countries (e.g., Lancee and Dronkers 2008). Such one-sided views are likely to affect interethnic exchange and institutional responses which may turn out to work as self-fulfilling hypotheses. Accordingly, there has been increasing attention to the so-far neglected reverse side: positive development of minority children and youth, their particular assets and strengths, and factors that promote positive development (Cabrera 2013; Cabrera et al. 2012).

While schools and institutions such as the health care system and social services play an important role in offering opportunities to individuals and promoting positive development, families are the most proximal context of children's development. The focus of this chapter is on the role of family factors in fostering positive development among minority children in Europe. We will take a broad look not only at family resources, a major source of disadvantage among minority youth (Duncan and Magnuson 2005; Karlsen and Nazroo 2002; McNulty and Bellair 2003; Molcho et al. 2010), but also at multiple domains of family socialization (Grusec and Davidov 2010) including attachment with caregivers, parenting, and providing access to stimulating experiences within and outside the family. Because parents influence children directly through interactions and relationships and indirectly through access to other contexts (Lin et al. 2001; Nauck and Lotter 2015), we will also examine the use of day care and informal education.

Unlike recent research efforts in the USA, there has been less attention paid to the positive development and particular strengths of minority youth in Europe. Accordingly, this chapter cannot meet the demands of a comprehensive, theory-driven approach to positive development as presented in relevant conceptualizations (Lerner et al. 2005). However, we will focus on some key issues, such as health and general well-being, including the lack of problem behavior, social competencies and schooling.

In the following section, we start highlighting the heterogeneity among minority families in Europe and related cross-country differences. We differentiate between indigenous minorities and immigrant minorities because these often differ in the support provided by the majority group. Within in the European Union (EU), languages and cultures of indigenous minority groups tend to be more protected than languages and cultures of immigrant groups. The focus of the following sections is mainly on immigrant minority families. We describe the current key research questions in regard to (1) changing family forms and family norms, (2) variations in parenting and the links of parenting to positive child development, and (3) the role of parents, communities and schools in launching and promoting children's pre- and post-natal health as well as their success in the educational system. Our empirical findings rely mainly on large representative studies within one or across several European countries. The chapter concludes with policy implications and directions for future research.

Historical Overview and Theoretical Perspectives

How can we define a minority in Europe? To what extent are different minority groups unique or similar to other minority groups? Across most groups, speaking a language not spoken by the majority of the country they live in is likely to be a common experience. Aside from the language feature, their experiences of belonging to a cultural minority group are likely to vary greatly across the different minority groups. Within the 28 states of the European Union, there appears to be a subtle, yet important divide between indigenous minorities (often referred to as national minorities) and immigrant minorities. This is most evident in terms of the status of the language of a minority group. In many countries, indigenous minority groups were quite successful in obtaining extended legal protection for their culture and language. In contrast, immigrant minority groups are more or less expected to integrate (or even to assimilate) into the majority society (Extra and Gorter 2001; Extra and Yağmur 2011).

The Largest Minority: Roma

The Roma people present the largest European minority group of 10–12 million people (see Dimitrova and Ferrer-Wreder in this volume). Roma (sometimes referred to as Romani people) is an umbrella term which includes numerous groups of people who share, to some degree, the same cultural heritage as well as similar experiences with discrimination (antiziganism), social exclusion and extreme poverty. The Roma people are set apart from other minorities because they have less power and hardly any lobby within Europe. Depending on their country of settlement, they have adopted parts of the language, culture, and to some extent even the religion of each country. Even though they are divided in many different subgroups and scattered all over Europe, most Roma people have continued to speak one of several dialects of the Roma language.

The proposal for effective Roma integration measures (European Commission 2013)[1] intends to eliminate discrimination, to ensure at least primary education for all Roma children, to improve access to healthcare and to minimize the gap between the Roma and the majority population of their country of residence in terms of housing and employment. A related EU report (European Commission 2013)[2] describes that many Roma children live in poverty, do not attend school, and are victims of violence and exploitation both within and outside of their community. Aside from providing support for families and children, encouraging parents' participation, and aiming to raise parents' awareness of the importance of education, EU member states are requested to obtain a better understanding of the history and culture of the Roma, for example, by including their history and culture in school curricula. If these long-term goals are eventually implemented by the member states, and if the intended empowerment of the Roma minority will be taken seriously, these families might have a chance in the long run of an actual integration and to reach a status similar to the ones granted to numerous other European minority groups (see Dimotrova et al., in this Handbook for more information on the Roma population). In 2014, the EU announced after a Roma Summit that the integration yielded results and suggested that the inclusion of the largest minority should be a priority for spending EU funds in the next seven years of the financial period.[3]

Indigenous Minorities in the EU

The top-down support structure that the EU has recently adopted for the Roma has been implanted for other, smaller minorities for many years. Eurominority, an organization devoted to provide information on Stateless Nations and national minorities of Europe, lists an impressive number of minorities in Europe.[4] Some of these are very accomplished and well known and have political institutions and a high degree of autonomy, such as the Basque and Catalan in Spain, the Scottish and Welsh people in the United Kingdom, or the Sardinians in Italy. Others are striving to maintain their cultural identity, such as the French (Wallonia) and Flamish (Flanders)

---

[1]http://europa.eu/rapid/press-release_IP-13-1226_en.htm.

[2]http://ec.europa.eu/justice/discrimination/roma/index_en.htm, accessed Jan. 12, 2015.

[3]http://europa.eu/rapid/press-release_IP-14-371_en.htm, accessed Jan. 12, 2015.

[4]http://www.eurominority.eu/version/eng/, accessed Jan. 12, 2105.

speaking cultural groups in Belgium, the Sorbs or the Danish minority in Germany, or the Frisians in the Netherlands. Some of these groups share that they speak a distinct language not spoken elsewhere, whereas other minorities speak a language common in another country but not in the country in which they live. These diverse indigenous minorities are all united by the common interest to be recognized and respected as a distinct cultural group. They are protected by EU laws, e.g., in terms of the right to speak their own language and to have children taught in the minority language in school. In some regards, the ones who are living in autonomous regions in their respective countries share more features typical for a majority population than for a minority population. In contrast to the Roma minority, there is little indication in the literature that the positive development of children from these indigenous groups is hampered by their minority status.

Immigrant Minorities

The increase of migration within the EU as well as into the EU has resulted in an increase as well as a diversification of immigrant groups. While indigenous minorities are more likely to be protected, immigrant minorities do not enjoy the same privileges for their heritage cultures and languages. Instead, parents and migrant organizations have to pursue a bottom-up approach to ensure that their rights to speak their heritage language and to maintain their heritage culture are recognized and accepted. By EU policies, they are encouraged to learn the culture and language of the host country and, in addition, they may maintain their own culture and language. However, maintaining their own culture and language is mostly delegated to the immigrant families themselves and is not considered a task of the receiving country. This practice in policy suggests that not all languages and cultures are equally valued and protected (Schjerve and Vetter 2012). An example of the differences between indigenous and immigrant minorities is the Moroccans living in Catalonia, a comparably wealthy

autonomous region in Spain at the Mediterranean Sea. The Catalonians take pride in their culture and language, they fiercely protect their rights, and children learn both Catalan as well as Spanish in schools. A linguistic census in 2013 indicated that 51 % of the population prefers to speak Castilian Spanish and 36 % prefer to speak Catalan.[5] Another sizable minority are immigrants from Morocco. They present 20 % of all non-Spanish nationals in Catalonia, making Arabic the third most spoken language in this region. However, in contrast to the indigenous Catalan minority, they are not likely to encounter public policies towards the promotion of Arabic culture and language in the schools or at home. In sum, not all minorities enjoy equal rights and policies protecting their cultural heritage. Instead, there appears to be a hierarchy among the minority groups in Europe. In this chapter, we will focus on immigrant minorities rather than on the more privileged indigenous or national minorities.

The New Status of European Countries as Countries of Immigration

Many European countries have perceived themselves as countries of emigration rather than preferred countries of immigration. This has changed over the last 50 years and by now many European countries have realized that they are target countries for immigration. In 2013, for example, 7 million people living in Germany were foreign nationals and another 8.6 million were immigrants with a German passport. As a result, 20 % of the German population are either foreign-born or have at least one foreign-born parent. Every third child age 5 or younger grows up in an immigrant family (Woellert and Klingholz 2013). OECD data from 2010 (cited in Woellert and Klingholz 2013) indicate that Germany, as well as several other European countries, has higher immigration rates than the

---

[5]http://www.idescat.cat/dequavi/?TC=444&V0=15&V1= 2, retrieved Jan. 15, 2015.

United States. The top three countries in the world are Switzerland with 28 %, Israel with 32 %, and Luxembourg with 42 % foreign born population. In all countries of the EU, part of the population is made up of immigrants from other EU countries. Within the EU, people can choose their country of residence freely and aside from the participation in state elections, they enjoy the same basic rights and access to the labor market as the local majority. In most EU countries, immigrants within the EU do not represent a sizable number from one single country, but are from a wide range of EU countries. They may come for shorter or longer periods of time and manifest a high degree of diversity in terms of education, the timing and the reason for immigration. However, with the exception of the Roma people, they all have in common that they are rarely perceived as a problem; they are accepted by the host society and can move back and forth as much as they please. As a result, these immigrants appear in the national statistics but are largely ignored both by national politics as well as by public research. Until recently, immigration from outside of the EU was severely restricted and basically limited to family unification, to (acknowledged) refugees, or to the coveted highly skilled professionals. Since 2011, the EU has tried to attract the high potentials with a so-called "Blue-Card". However, this group is rather small, very diverse, and very mobile. Starting in summer 2015, large numbers of refugees have entered the European Union and it can be expected that these new immigrants will transform the European societies.

Differences Between Immigrant Minorities in North America and Europe

Much of our knowledge of processes of immigration and adaptation is based on studies from the "old world" to the "new world". Portes and Rumbaut (2001) describe that over the course of two or three generations, immigrants in the US or Canada are likely to become either part of the majority society or part of a minority group but

do not consider themselves to be immigrants anymore. The familiar hyphenated identity of Italian-American or Chinese-Canadian indicates the ethnic background while the main emphasis is on being an American or Canadian citizen. Inter-European migration, however, appears to follow a different pattern. Rather than becoming an integral part of the host society and striving to acquire citizenship, inter-European immigrants often prefer to become an integral part of both: the host country and their country of origin (Leyendecker 2011). Inexpensive flights across Europe, vacation times of 4–6 weeks per year, as well as modern communication facilitate staying connected with the country and the culture of origin, including the former's political and societal institutions.

One indicator of this development is the trend for people from outside of the EU to acquire and to maintain dual citizenship. This new type of hybrid identity appears to be a possible pathway preferred by many new immigrants from outside of the EU (Leyendecker 2011). For children, some European countries have noticed this development and have adopted less restrictive policies in recent years. In Germany, for example, children born to foreign nationals were allowed to have dual citizenship, but they had to decide on one of the passports once they reached the age of 23. A new law established at the end of 2014 allows children to maintain their dual citizenship for as long as they want. In a video announcing this new regulation, Aydan Özguz, the representative of the German government, states that young adults are no longer forced to decide between Germany and their families.[6] As she points out, immigrants and their offspring are likely to have more than one identity and to feel at home in more than one country.

Another aspect that keeps the ties to the country of origin alive is the so-called marriage migration. This is particularly evident in the Turkish community in Europe. Marriage migration between a first and a second generation immigrant is likely to occur when one or all of the following apply: (1) Family reunion is the

---

[6]https://einleben-zweipaesse.de/, retrieved Jan. 15, 2015.

major legal way of entry for new immigrants, (2) immigrant parents prefer their children to marry someone from the country of origin, (3) the home country is easily accessible and families tend to spend vacation time in their country of origin, and (4) those women who have acquired a higher education have a better chance of finding a well-educated husband in their country of origin (Leyendecker et al. 2006). Marriage migration is likely to result in acculturation gaps between mothers and fathers. A study exploring the impact of these acculturation gaps found that they were either unrelated to acculturation stress or even associated with lower levels of stress (Spiegler et al. 2015). In families with at least one first generation parent, culture and language of the country of origin were more likely to be kept alive than in families with two second generation parents. For their offspring, speaking parents' heritage language presents an important task in order to be able to communicate with the first generation parent (Willard et al. 2014).

Overall, there is a tremendous heterogeneity among minority families in Europe. The huge number of indigenous or national minorities is very diverse. Immigrant families differ in many socio-demographic aspects such as their socio-economic status, reason for migration, country of origin, legal status, time of arrival, etc. Additional complexities are created within families. These complexities may be due to the bi- and multi-national context that typically results from intermarriage or due to marriages between first and second generation partners from the same ethnic group.

Current Research Questions and Methodology

Research Themes and Questions

In comparison to the United States and Canada, most European countries have only recently started to invest more in research into minority families. Much of this research is descriptive, looking at differences and similarities between families of minority and majority youth (e.g., in parent-child relationships, parenting, family stress). Focusing on the challenges of migration and/or minority status, most research questions are directed at likely problems and disadvantages of minority youth and their families, but some attention has been paid to family factors that promote integration. Overall, however, the attention to positive development is still scarce.

Immigration has been described as one of the most disorganizing individual experiences (Bornstein et al. 2007). On the one side, immigrant families are more vulnerable and face greater, as well as different, challenges when compared to non-immigrant families. Among the potential risk factors for immigrant families are limited education, constrained financial resources, a smaller social network of available family members and friends, unstable neighborhoods, and increased levels of everyday distress. With these risk factors in mind, many studies have looked at mental health and well-being among minority children in Europe. Available evidence provides some support for increased stress and problem behavior (e.g., Flink et al. 2012), suggesting elevated levels of internalizing and peer problems, but not externalizing problems (Derluyn et al. 2008; Jäkel et al. 2015; Kouider et al. 2014). However, the overall pattern of findings across countries and informants is less clear than might be expected (Stevens and Vollebergh 2008), and most differences disappear once families' economic resources are taken into account (Molcho et al. 2010).

On the other side, immigrants have moved to another country in hopes of improving their living conditions as well as those of their offspring. This has coined the description of "immigrant optimism" and has been used to explain the academic achievement of second generation in the U.S. (Kao and Tienda 1995). Accordingly, considerable attention has been paid to issues of schooling and academic success among minority youth in Europe, be it focusing on the role of early education and school systems in improving integration and providing equal opportunities for immigrant children compared to those for the majority group (Dronkers et al. 2012; Spiess et al. 2003) or focusing on the role of parenting, parents' educational aspirations, and their perceptions of schooling (Nauck and Lotter 2015) and their school involvement (Kohl et al. 2015). In line with the above mentioned notion of "immigrant optimism", a study from Germany confirms that Turkish and Vietnamese minority mothers attribute higher instrumentality to academic success for their children's long-term well-being than German mothers do, but the findings also point to the higher perceived costs of schooling, e.g., by increasing the child's distance to his or her heritage culture (Nauck and Lotter 2015).

Immigrant families are confronted with the task of bridging multiple worlds (Cooper 2011). The majority of immigrant families in Europe have roots in countries characterized by collectivistic cultures, which stress norms of obedience and communion (Kağıtçıbaşı 2007). Parents are faced with the task to raise their children in Western individualized host countries, which emphasize norms and values of independence. From a psychological point of view, a positive attitude of immigrants towards the culture and the language of the host country AND the country of origin are considered to be of vital importance for successful adaptation (Leyendecker 2011). This positive attitude is evident on a much deeper level than superficial preferences for music, food, or specific festivities of either country. Research on immigrant families suggests that children do best if they have parents who convey a connection to the culture of origin and maintain a voice of authority, and at the same time encourage them to take advantage of the opportunities offered by the receiving country (Suárez-Orozco and Suárez-Orozco 2001). For parents and children, this task implies that they have to find a balance between the country of origin and the country of residence (Stuart et al. 2010). Along these lines, some research has addressed issues of intergenerational transmission as well as adaptation to the host culture, e.g. with respect to gender attitudes (Idema and Phalet 2007) and educational success (Nauck and Lotter 2016). Bridging cultures is a task which can not be accomplished by parents alone but rather a task which requires the collaboration of the entire society as bridges can be crossed in both directions. Most European countries have aging societies and as a result, the need to invest into children and youth of immigrant families has been more and more recognized. Given the salience of educational attainment for successful integration into the labor market and social participation in general, even more so for immigrant youth, further research on immigrant families' resources and their match to demands of the educational system, as well as on the support that can be provided by the receiving countries, are particularly worthwhile.

We may hypothesize that a receiving country which respects the families' culture of origin and facilitates their access to these opportunities provides an environment which allows immigrant children to develop their potentials to a higher degree than contexts which confront families with discrimination and ethnic prejudice. Negative effects of racial discrimination, independent of socio-economic resources, have been reported in studies on adult health among ethnic minorities in England and Wales (Karlsen and Nazroo 2002). These negative effects are likely to impact family resources. Furthermore, restricted access to desired resources (such as education and occupation) and perceived discrimination are challenges which call for coping not only at an individual level, but also at a family level, e.g. by preserving a strong family orientation and restricting children's social network to the ingroup. This leads us to our overarching key question: What are the resources available to children within their families that foster their positive development and increase the capabilities to participate in the society they live in?

Family processes play a major role in explaining children's well-being. As evident from numerous studies in family science, this holds for the quality of the interparental relationship (Davies et al. 2002; Grych and Fincham 2001), parents' cooperation or conflict in co-parenting (Margolin et al. 2001; McHale and Lindahl 2011), the quality of sibling relationships (Lamb and Sutton-Smith 2014), and most prominently for the quality of parent-child relationships and parenting (Bornstein 2002; Collins et al. 2000). European research on minority families has primarily focused on similarities and differences in parenting and its links to contextual features and child outcomes. Since parenting is likely to be affected by cultural beliefs and practices inherited from the country of origin (Harkness and Super 2002), comparing minorities from collectivistic cultures to the majority groups in more individualistic European social contexts is of particular interest.

However, differences between more individualistic majority families and minority families from more collectivistic cultures may reflect not only cultural heritage, but also coping processes in managing challenges of migration. Immigration is, as noted by Rumbaut (1997), a "family affair", and the success or positive development of immigrants is likely to be facilitated by social support provided by the nuclear and extended family. Accordingly, family solidarity may be of particular salience and functional value for immigrant families, remaining high even alongside adaptation processes in other domains of family life. As a consequence, adaptation can—like social change—bring about new constellations of values and behaviors. Findings from research on social change in more collectivistic countries are a case in point, suggesting considerable continuity in family orientation despite social trends towards greater personal autonomy and independence. Kağıtçıbaşı (2007), who has studied changes within the Turkish society, found that well-educated parents in urban settings were likely to grant more autonomy to their children. At the same time, however, the importance of the family remained high, pointing to a new pattern of interdependence.

Such findings raise the question how norms and values of immigrant families change, suggesting that minority parents may prefer an integration of both cultural traditions rather than assimilating their values of the majority society. Any family services targeting immigrant families ought to be sensitive to these issues. Along these lines, Kağıtçıbaşı suggests that "interventions may be expected to work better if they take into

consideration the existing human connectedness, as reflected in closely knit family, kinship, and community ties, rather than counteracting them, for example, in building individualistic independence and completion" (Kağıtçıbaşı 2007, p. 4). Last but not least, integration may also affect norms and values of the majority group. Given that, in countries like Germany, more than one third of all children grow up in immigrant families, and immigrants, plus the offspring of immigrants, are an increasingly important part of the work force, this also raises the question to what extend the majority societies will over time accept and adopt norms and values of the minorities.

Research Measurements and Methodology

As mentioned above, most research on minority families is comparative, looking at differences to the majority group. In light of this situation and in light of the enormous heterogeneity of immigrant families in Europe, our report of findings primarily relies on large scale national and international representative studies which allow us to control for relevant background variables and investigate mediating as well as moderating factors to shed light on family processes and their links to positive youth development. In addition, some studies focus on certain ethnic or immigrant subgroups, providing more in-depth insight into their situation, often with particular interest in cultural factors. Only few intensive studies using observational data have been conducted. Finally, we also report few small scale non-representative, partly qualitative studies to illustrate the experiences of children and their parents and to highlight some of our points.

Very few studies allow for a comparison of minority families to families in their country of origin for addressing issues of adaptation (e.g., Daglar et al. 2011; Moscardino et al. 2011). Interestingly, Daglar et al. (2011) chose not only Turkish non-migrants, but also migrants within Turkey as comparison groups to Turkish immigrants in the UK in order to capture effects of mobility. Most available studies compare minority families and children to those of the majority group (see also Kouider et al. 2014; e.g. Molcho et al. 2010; Nauck and Lotter 2015, 2016). Given the prevailing focus on stress and disadvantages, these studies are rather unlikely to shed light on particular strengths of minority families and their children unless they pay attention to moderating factors or special features of migrant families. Rather, they seek to inform about general processes that work for minority families as well as those from the majority group. Studies focusing on processes within minority families are better able to capture particular attributes or experiences of migrant families but are scarce (e.g., Emmen et al. 2013). Intervention studies with minority families targeting families processes, most prominently parenting (e.g. Bjørknes et al. 2012; Yagmur et al. 2014), are of particular interest since they avoid causality problems in interpreting the link between parenting and child well-being.

Several limitations of the available research should be noted. Firstly, minority groups are often not adequately represented in the samples. Despite their advantages, large-scale studies tend to under-represent minority families, particularly when language barriers are involved. This is often the case for first and even second generation immigrants. In written questionnaire assessments using translated versions, issues of literacy may limit participation. Accordingly, personal interviews are better able to reach minority families, particularly if the interviewers are of similar background.

Secondly, the heterogeneity of minority groups is often neglected unless specific subgroups are targeted in the research. Many studies combine immigrants into one group without references to their ethnicity, country of origin, and to their generational status regarding immigration, thus limiting the conclusions that can be derived from the analyses.

Finally, there is still a lack of culturally sensitive measures in European research. Most studies just translate existing indicators and measures into the minority languages using standard translation—back translation procedures. In addition to the lack of suitable measures, group-specific norm values are missing for assessing children's language and overall development. Accordingly, future research efforts should aim at improving access to minority groups, providing a more detailed picture of different subgroups, and developing suitable measures that can be used for a variety of minority groups.

Empirical Findings

In reporting selected findings, we first focus on changes in family forms, particularly due to divorce, and how these apply to minority families. We then turn to the role of family ties which have been pointed out as particularly salient in minority families. With respect to cultural and contextual influences on family processes, we address similarities and differences between minority and majority families in parental sensitivity, a major resource for facilitating children's secure attachment relationships. We then discuss issues of parenting, comparing immigrants not only to the majority group, but also to families in the immigrants' country of origin, and address the cultural framing of parenting by looking at differential effects of parenting on child outcomes. Thereafter, findings on minority families' coping with stress are reviewed. Finally, we look at families' investments in children's education.

Changing Family Forms

Due to increasing divorce rates, declining marriage rates, and increasing child-bearing among non-married parents, families have changed considerably across the past decades. Between 1970 and 2010, the average crude marriage rate for EU-27 dropped from 7.9 marriages per 1000 inhabitants to 4.4, while the crude divorce rate almost doubled from 1.0 to 1.9 (Eurostat 2015). Relative to the number of marriages, the divorce risk amounts to 44 % for EU-27 with particularly high divorce rates in Belgium (71 %) and lower figures for countries in Southeastern Europe (20–30 %) and Ireland (15 %).

As suggested by some findings, divorce risks may differ for immigrants. Longitudinal data from the German Socio-Economic Panel for over 5600 marriages indicate a lower divorce risk for immigrant couples than German-origin majority couples (Milewski and Kulu 2014). However, mixed marriages between a German-born partner and an immigrant had a higher likelihood of divorce than marriages between two German partners or between two immigrants from the same country. This difference can only partly be explained by a large number of background factors including differences in religion or education, although differences in social background and cultural distance contributed to a higher divorce risk.

Divorce rates vary among different immigrant groups. For example, the Dutch Generation R Study, a population-based birth cohort study from Rotterdam, revealed large differences in family structure across the various ethnic minority groups. While only 5 % of the Dutch toddlers and their peers from Moroccan or Turkish-origin families were raised by a single parent, 40 % of the children from Antillean, Cape Verdian, and Surinamese Creole families lived in single-parent families (Flink et al. 2012).

Single parenthood, as well as the formation of a stepfamily through re-partnering, affects family ties, and it seems that this impact is similar across immigrants and non-immigrants. A study based on the German Generations and Gender Survey and the supplementary survey of Turkish citizens in Germany revealed that adult children's contact to parents was lower if both biological parents did not live together, be it that they lived as single or in a new partnership (Steinbach 2013). Although this difference was somewhat reduced when taking numerous background factors into account, it remained significant. Most importantly, while intergenerational contact was more frequent for Turkish families, the same pattern of differences by family type was found.

While the large majority of research suggests that parental divorce has negative effects on children's development, the effects are not uniform (Amato 2010). A number of studies from the US suggests that effects of parental divorce and single parenthood on children are weaker among African American than among European Americans (Amato and Keith 1991; McLanahan and Sandefur 1994). One study from the Netherlands (Kalmijn 2010) tested such differences comparing Caribbean and Dutch adult children from divorced or single parent families to those from nuclear families. The expected differences could be confirmed. Whereas there were no or only minor effects of parental divorce on Caribbeans' own divorce, cohabitation, home leaving, and contact frequency with father, significantly stronger disadvantages emerged for adults from divorced homes in the Dutch majority group. Regarding contact to mother, the effect of parental divorce was even positive among Caribbeans, confirming the strong role of maternal kinship ties, particularly in stressful times such as parental divorce.

A study from Belgium (Derluyn et al. 2008) also suggests that single parents can be a major resource for immigrant youth. The authors compared 1249 recently arrived migrant adolescents from 93 different countries to 602 Belgian peers, finding significantly more traumatic experiences among the immigrant adolescents. Nevertheless, anxiety and externalizing and hyperactivity problems were less prevalent among immigrant youth. However, they reported more peer problems and higher avoidance. As can be expected, immigrants who lived without their parents reported higher rates of depression and emotional problems compared to those living with at least one parent. Immigrants from nuclear families had no additional advantage.

Family Ties

Several studies point to the great importance of family ties in non-Western cultures characterized by more collectivistic cultures which stress solidarity, interdependence, and filial obligations. In line with notions of cultural heritage, immigrants from non-Western countries tend to have stronger feelings of filial obligation than non-migrants and immigrants from Western countries (e.g., Dykstra and Fokkema 2012; Liefbroer and Mulder 2006). At the same time, evidence from the Netherlands suggests that second-generation immigrants tend to differ less from the native population in terms of the strength of filial obligations than first-generation migrants (cf. Dykstra et al. 2013). As pointed out by Dykstra et al., this supports the view that people of non-Dutch descent who grow up in the Netherlands acquire a cultural orientation that is similar to that of people of Dutch descent.

While filial obligations are mostly addressed in research on multigenerational living arrangements, the role of family ties is also evident in studies on minority youth. In a forthcoming report by the Scientific Board on Family Issues of the German Federal Ministry of Family, Seniors, Women, and Youth, two large data sets support the increased importance attributed to family members among youth with migration background compared to their non-migrant peers (Wissenschaftlicher Beirat für Familienfragen 2016). This holds for mothers as well as for fathers and siblings, even when controlling large sets of background factors, and irrespective of how migration background was defined. Parents and siblings are particularly important for adolescents with both parents born abroad, while those who have only one foreign-born parent indicated somewhat lower importance of primary family members but still exceeded their non-immigrant peers. Only in the third generation of immigrants, whose grandparents were born abroad, does this effect of increased family ties disappear. Interestingly, a third data set used in these analyses did not find such differences once importance of parents was combined with issues of independence as suggested by conceptions of individuation. However, questions about emotional closeness resembled the above picture of increased parental importance inasmuch as foreign born adolescents reported higher closeness to their mothers. In addition, two of the analyzed data sets provided support for reduced conflict between adolescents and their parents in immigrant families. Particularly foreign born adolescents reported less conflict with their

mothers. Overall, these findings suggest that family ties remain at elevated levels for first and second generation immigrants but adapt to those of the host country in further generations. Reduced conflict and high emotional closeness are likely to be protective factors for immigrant families.

Parental Sensitivity

The provision of a secure base in parent-child attachment has been pointed out as a particularly relevant resource for children's emotional and social development (Ainsworth et al. 1978; Sroufe et al. 2007). Following Mary Ainsworth's seminal research on maternal sensitivity, numerous studies have addressed how mothers recognize, interpret, and react to their children's signals. This research provides ample evidence that maternal sensitivity is causally related to positive child development, including secure attachment (e.g., Bakermans-Kranenburg et al. 2003), self-regulation (e.g., Eisenberg et al. 2001), social functioning (e.g., Bohlin et al. 2000), and cognitive competence (e.g., Stams et al. 2002). Although some evidence suggests that maternal contingency in mother-infant interaction is rooted in universal aspects of parenting, it has been questioned whether the concept of sensitivity is similarly supported by values characteristic of collectivistic cultures, as these may be less conducive to parents' responsiveness to children's individual needs than norms and values in individualistic cultures (see Mesman et al. 2012). Furthermore, given the evidence for increased stress encountered by minority families, difficult life circumstances could similarly undermine sensitivity among minority parents.

In their review of research addressing parental sensitivity in minority families with young children, Mesman et al. (2012) found six studies from the Netherlands that investigated maternal sensitivity comparing Dutch majority families to minority families of Turkish or Surinamese origin. Overall, the six studies found both Surinamese and Turkish minority mothers show lower levels of sensitivity than native Dutch mothers. Although some of these differences were still evident after controlling for SES, they were substantially diminished, particularly when matching the ethnic groups on SES. As concluded by the authors, it seems unlikely that cultural factors are responsible for these differences. Instead, the evidence rather points towards the central role of social and economic stress in undermining maternal sensitivity in minority groups.

Parenting

Differences in parenting and their consequences for children's development have garnered significant attention. Several studies from Germany, the Netherlands, the UK and Norway suggest that parents from minority families are less likely to show warm, involved, supportive and authoritative parenting (Maynard and Harding 2010; Nauck and Lotter 2015; Yaman et al. 2010). They are more likely to report high control (Maynard and Harding 2010), harsh parenting (Flink et al. 2012), an authoritarian style (Daglar et al. 2011), and physical punishment despite higher permissiveness (Javo et al. 2004).

A study from Germany (Nauck and Lotter 2015) investigated whether ethnic differences in parenting styles reflect different investment strategies in the future welfare of offspring as indicated by parents' expectations about the instrumentality, i.e. perceived costs and benefits, of schooling. Based on a combination of parental warmth/involvement and strictness/control, they distinguished authoritative, authoritarian, indulgent, and neglectful parenting styles. Comparing 544 German mother-child dyads, 508 Vietnamese dyads, and 471 Turkish dyads, the authors found expected differences in parenting styles, reflecting more active control in collectivistic cultures (Vietnam) and a strong emphasis on children's individual needs in individualistic cultures (Germany) with an intermediate position of Turkey. Authoritarian parenting was most prevalent among Vietnamese mothers, while indulgent parenting was the dominant style

among Germans. Turkish mothers showed a more equal distribution of parenting styles with highest frequency of neglectful parenting. As expected, high perceived costs of schooling (e.g., child's increased distance to the culture of origin) predicted authoritarian parenting, whereas perceived benefits of schooling increased the likelihood of authoritative parenting. However, contrary to expectations, the higher likelihood of authoritarian parenting among Vietnamese mothers could not be explained by their higher perceived costs of schooling. Differences in authoritative parenting between Turkish minority and German mothers could fully be accounted for by individual resources such as education, language competence, and social capital. Furthermore, resource-rich mothers were less likely to be neglectful in parenting but instead reported considerably more authoritative or indulgent parenting. This underscores the strong association between mothers' personal resources and their emotional closeness to children.

Contrary to notions of gendered parenting, indicating a role division between fathers and mothers with authoritarian paternal parenting and permissive maternal parenting, the study by Flink et al. (2012) found increased harsh parenting among minority fathers as well as mothers across all ethnic groups (Antillean, Cape Verdian, Maroccon, Surinamese and Turkish origin) when compared to parents from Dutch majority families. However, as suggested by this latter data, differences in parenting account only little for children's increased problem behavior among minority groups compared to children from Dutch majority families, once controlling for background factors such as SES and family structure. Prenatal family stress proved a considerably more powerful factor in explaining ethnic differences in child problem behavior.

Comparing Parenting Among Immigrants and Non-immigrants in the Country of Origin

Issues of cultural traditions and adaptation are particularly salient in studies comparing immigrants not only to majority families in their host country but also to families in their country of origin. A study from Italy focusing on families with infants applied this design comparing Italian families to first generation immigrants from Romania as well as Romanian families in Romania (Moscardino et al. 2011). Investigating mother-infant interaction and childrearing patterns, the authors found immigrant mothers to resemble more closely Italian mothers in the importance attributed to stimulating children's cognitive competence, autonomy, and self-fulfillment, whereas Romanian mothers emphasized values and behaviors related to interdependence/sociocentrism.

Adding a focus on more general (selection or socialization) effects of mobility, a study on Turkish immigrants in the UK with 4- to 6-year-old preschoolers compared these not only to Turkish families with stable residence in Turkey, but also to residentially mobile migrants within Turkey (Daglar et al. 2011). These three groups differed significantly in terms of social background: Immigrants were most likely to come from rural areas, to have less than high school education, and to be unemployed. Based on the Parenting Styles and Dimensions Questionnaire and Baumrind's (1971) classification of parenting styles, parents' dominant parenting style was identified as authoritative, authoritarian, or permissive. Controlling for child gender and parental education, Turkish immigrants to the UK were found to be less permissive and more authoritarian than stable residents in Turkey but were not significantly less likely to report the most favorable authoritative parenting style. Immigrant children had more problems across a variety of domains (externalizing, hyperactivity, internalizing, emotional regulation, social competence) than residentially stable children within Turkey. Controlling for child gender, parental education, and SES, Daglar et al. (2011) found a strong link between parenting and child social adjustment. Permissive and, to a greater degree, authoritarian styles of parenting were significantly linked to children's higher problem scores. However, differences between immigrants and locals remained highly significant, suggesting that additional factors account for immigrant children's elevated problems.

Differential Effects of Parenting on Child Outcomes

It has repeatedly been argued that parenting may have different effects on children from minority groups than majority families due to the cultural framing of parenting practices. Evidence for such differential effects of minority mothers' parenting comes from a Norwegian study (Javo et al. 2004). Among Norwegian majority families, physical punishment was significantly related to children's higher externalizing problem behavior, and teasing/ridiculing was linked to children's higher internalizing problems. However, no such effects were found for the indigenous Sami families. These differences in effects were particularly pronounced among boys.

While this study suggests that some minority children may indeed be less vulnerable to aspects of parenting which are detrimental for Western majority children, other evidence emphasizes similarities in the effects of parenting. Using a large multi-ethnic sample of adolescents from 51 schools in London, subgroup analyses controlling for background factors showed that parental care was similarly linked to lower self-reported psychological difficulties (Strengths and Difficulties Questionnaire) among minority youth from five ethnic groups as found for British majority youth (Maynard and Harding 2010). Similarly, all adolescents profited from low parental control, i.e. higher autonomy granted by parents. Interestingly, contrary to most available data, this study found quite consistent evidence for lower psychological problems among minority youth, even when parental care was low or control was high.

Intervention studies provide additional support for the notion that theoretical models of parenting developed in Western societies can also be applied to minority families. For example, a study from Norway (Bjørknes et al. 2012) used the Parent Management Training—Oregon Model (PMTO) to enhance positive parenting and decrease harsh parenting among a sample of 96 Somali and Pakistani mothers with children ages 3–9 years who were at risk of or had already developed conduct problems. Mothers were randomly assigned to the 18 weekly group sessions or a waiting group. As expected, mothers in the intervention group reported a significantly stronger increase in positive parenting, a stronger reduction in harsh discipline, and a stronger reduction in children's conduct problems (pre-post-comparisons) than mothers in the control group. In line with assumptions of the mediation model, the improvement in children's behavior could be fully explained by mothers' enhanced positive parenting as well as their reduced harsh discipline.

Coping with Family Stress

Given the considerable concern about socio-economic inequalities between minority and majority families, one study from the Netherlands (Emmen et al. 2013) has extended the well-known family stress model (Conger et al. 2000, 2010) to immigrant families (see also Mesman, in this volume). According to the family stress model, low SES triggers economic pressure which, in turn, undermines parental well-being, the quality of the interparental relationships, and—mediated through these latter two factors—the quality of parenting. Emmen et al. (2013) included acculturation stress in addition to daily hassles and parents' psychological distress to account for effects of family SES on observed maternal positive parenting. Findings for 107 Turkish-Dutch families confirmed that low SES contributed to more acculturation stress as well as higher maternal psychological distress which were both linked to less positive parenting. However, high SES had additional, independent advantages for positive parenting. Interestingly, low SES minority families did not report higher levels of daily hassles, suggesting that they were well able to manage everyday tasks and demands even with fewer resources. Furthermore, acculturation distress did not seem to undermine parents' general psychological well-being.

Evidence from the US suggests that experiences of discrimination are more detrimental than acculturation stress (Stein et al. 2012). Such

challenges for minority youth well-being, as pointed out in the study by Stein et al. (2012), have received some attention in research on ethnic-racial socialization. This research addresses specific parenting strategies as means to cope with highly multicultural contexts and related risks of facing discrimination (Hughes et al. 2006). However, available evidence from Europe is rather limited. A small-scale qualitative study from the UK compared non-immigrant White, Indian, and Pakistani families with children between 5–7 years of age (Iqbal 2014). The semi-structured interviews revealed that all parents had experienced some discrimination and frequently engaged in efforts to prepare their children for such bias by making them aware of discrimination and teaching them how to deal with it. Furthermore, qualitative interviews with 53 adolescents of Black African origin in the UK point to the perceived significance of parents and family networks in helping to cope with social discrimination and refraining from problem behavior and unhealthy lifestyles (Ochieng 2014).

Most studies, however, address more general features of family well-being versus family stress. A study from Germany (Jäkel et al. 2015) focused on predictors of Turkish immigrant children's and adolescents' mental health and provides support for the equally negative role of family strain and adversity among migrant children and adolescents as well as among their German peers. This, at the same time, suggests that these effects are limited to the family context. While each feature of family adversity (mothers' daily hassles, maternal depressive symptoms, parents' marital problems) was reported at significantly higher levels by Turkish immigrant mothers compared to German mothers, family adversity was similarly linked to maternal reports of children's problem behavior in both groups, except for emotional problems which were more strongly affected by family adversity in the immigrant group. Interestingly, family adversity proved irrelevant for children's social competencies in both groups. In fact, immigrant mothers reported higher social competencies for their children, providing evidence for positive development among these minority youth, even though there was higher prevalence of emotional symptoms and particularly peer problems. As expected, increased family adversity explained that Turkish-immigrant mothers reported higher problem scores for their children than German mothers. However, teachers' ratings did not reflect any elevated problems among minority youth suggesting that the problems encountered by immigrant mothers could be confined to the family context.

Parental Investments in Education

Several studies have looked at parental investments in promoting children's competence. While immigrant status is mostly only a background factor, these studies are still of some interest. For example, based on a large sample of families with 6- to 8-year-old children from Germany and controlling for many background factors (e.g., parental education, family structure, number of children in the household, maternal employment), migration background as captured by family language was not found to relate to educational activities with the child, involvement in household chores, or parental strictness or warmth (Walper and Grgic 2013). Although mothers from immigrant families reported slightly more child problem behavior, neither prosocial behavior nor language competencies in everyday communication differed from children whose family language was exclusively German.

Given the significance of early preschool education for children's cognitive development (Burger 2010) and their later success in the educational system, minority parents' access to and choice of child care is an important issue. Studies in Germany consistently find that children from immigrant families are less likely to enter public daycare before the age of 3. Even though the fees for daycare depend on parents' income and can be waived for families with no or low income, 25 % of Turkish immigrant families

were found to attend public daycare for 2 years or less (Leyendecker et al. 2014). These differences disappear when taking other factors like family structure and maternal employment into account (Wissenschaftlicher Beirat für Familienfragen 2016). Somewhat stronger differences are evident with respect to the use of non-formal education, e.g. baby swimming, mother-child groups, music or dance instruction, etc. Immigrant parents are less likely to use these options, even when controlling for background factors (Leyendecker et al. 2014).

With regard to parental school involvement, elementary school age children and younger adolescents from immigrant and non-immigrant families alike report equal parental interest in their experiences at school and their achievements (Wissenschaftlicher Beirat für Familienfragen 2016). The large majority of adolescents from immigrant families reported that they receive help with homework assignments and when preparing for exams. No differences or even higher levels of support were observed for mixed families with one immigrant and one non-immigrant parent as well as for families who use German as the family language, suggesting that familiarity with the school system and language plays a role.

Universal Versus Culture-Specific Mechanisms

Although research on minority families in Europe has increased, available data linking parenting to relevant contextual and personal resources as well as to children's development are still largely limited to cross-sectional data. Accordingly, inferences about causal mechanisms can only be drawn with considerable caution. With these limitations in mind, the findings reported in the previous section suggest at least two universal patterns. First, there is consistent evidence with respect to the role of socio-economic and personal resources. Most notably, although the family stress model was developed for Western families, it has proven applicable to minority families, as well. In the study by Emmen et al. (2013), the lack of socio-economic resources was linked to parents' psychological distress which, in turn, predicted less positive parenting. Similarly, findings by Nauck and Lotter (2015) emphasize the role of parental resources—socio-economic as well as personal—in predicting higher warmth and less neglectful parenting. While not all parenting differences between ethnic groups may be explained by socio-economic resources, the latter clearly plays a role in making parenting an easier task for resource-rich parents than deprived parents.

Second, there is considerable evidence that positive parenting and particularly parental warmth and sensitivity are linked to better child outcomes across different ethnic groups (e.g., Maynard and Harding 2010; Mesman et al. 2012). With respect to parental control, however, findings are less conclusive. While the intervention study by Bjørknes et al. (2012) suggested that children from minority families profit from a decrease in harsh parenting, other data suggest cultural differences in children's susceptibility to different types of control (Javo et al. 2004). Given the evidence that authoritarian parenting is considerably framed by cultural factors (Nauck and Lotter 2015), minority children whose families are rooted in a collectivistic country of origin are likely to interpret high parental control as more involved parenting. However, respective research which focuses on children's interpretations of parental child-rearing in cultural context is still missing.

Differences have also been pointed out with respect to the effects of parental separation/divorce on children's well-being. Findings suggest that parental divorce is a substantially less important risk factor for certain ethnic groups compared to white majority families (Kalmijn 2010). This could either imply smaller advantages of nuclear families for these groups due to less paternal involvement or lower economic resources even if both biological parents are present, or parental divorce could be less stressful because certain related risk factors (e.g., interparental conflict) are weaker. So far, European research has shed little light on the specific strains and stressors associated with parental separation and divorce among minority families.

Policy Implications and Future Directions for Research

Implications for policy and practice can be derived from several findings. First, given the important role of socio-economic resources, efforts should be increased to improve access to higher levels of education and better-paid jobs. For first-generation immigrants, this includes better recognition of formal qualifications achieved in the country of origin, because educational resources play an important role in the access to better-paid jobs. Similarly, improved access to higher education for immigrant youth and better integration into job training and the labor market are of vital importance for their life prospects. Such advances may not only help to reduce risks like teenage pregnancy but would most likely also pay off later, in early and middle adulthood, when successful occupational careers provide a better standard of living for young migrants' family of procreation.

Second, parental well-being is vital to positive parenting. Accordingly, more attention should be paid to (mental) health services, access to counseling, and support for successful coping with stress. This ought to be a central focus in seeking to provide for the refugees who currently enter Europe, often with many traumatic experiences prior to or along the way. Accordingly, while a major focus of social services on unaccompanied youth is clearly justified, we also need to monitor and support parents' well-being.

Third, given the higher divorce risk for interethnic marriages, it would seem worthwhile to invest in primary prevention, e.g. by informing more broadly about related challenges or by using pre-marital training courses or counseling. Although some findings suggest that children from some minority groups are well—or even better—able to cope with parental divorce, we still lack information about many other groups and the particular problems involved in interethnic marriages, especially legal conflicts about custody. Accordingly, this problem deserves more attention.

Finally, linked to the previous two points, further development and implementation of parenting programs for minority groups seem particularly promising. Given the often-reported stress-induced or culturally driven differences in child-rearing, parenting programs should aim to convey more supportive, sensitive parenting. Such programs can be expected to successfully promote children's positive development while at the same time facilitate parents' adaptation to the Western context. Furthermore, children may benefit from experiencing more consistent patterns of child-rearing at home and at school.

Future Directions for Research

For future research direction, we want to point to three aspects. The first issue concerns the importance of an ecological perspective. Cooper (2011) suggests that in order to understand how minority children and their families succeed despite adverse conditions, how they forge their sense of identity and find their pathways, one needs to trace the interplay of challenges and support on the personal, relational, institutional and cultural level. Following Cooper's concept, we want to point out the necessity to adopt an ecological perspective for future research in order to understand how multiple levels directly and indirectly interact and influence the conditions of child-rearing and of parenting practices. We need studies which provide examples of how families, peers, schools, and communities can support children's positive development. We need to pay particular attention not only to the unique role of parents, peers, schools, and communities in launching and promoting children's well-being, but also to their joint interplay, e.g. by compensating for the lack of support from either of these contexts and by facilitating family well-being.

The second issue concerns the different status of minority groups in Europe. As we have described in the historical overview of this chapter, the status of national or indigenous minorities is mostly protected under EU laws, whereas immigrant minorities are expected to integrate into the majority society with no or much less support for their heritage culture and heritage language. In addition, some minority groups, most notably the Roma, have hardly any lobby. Studies which differentiate between these different status groups allow one to tease apart the influence of the minority status per se, the support provided by the government, and the various degrees of discrimination children and their families from different minority groups experience.

The third issue relates to the enormous and increasing numbers of refugees entering Europe. Since 2013, Europe has witnessed a sharp increase in the number of asylum seekers. In Germany, more than 35,000 people applied for political asylum in the month of June 2015,[7] and these numbers have increased drastically in the second half of the year. One-third are children, and 5–10 % of the children are unaccompanied minors.[8] There is no indication that war, dictatorial oppression, religious extremism or extreme poverty will decrease in the near future, and many will stay permanently.

Compared with native minority groups and immigrant minority groups, these refugees and especially the unaccompanied minors present a much more vulnerable group. Many were exposed to severe violence and suffer from post-traumatic stress disorders, and all are likely to miss their family and their homes. A stable environment, social support and the perspective of being allowed to stay in the new country are likely to increase the chances for a positive development of these extremely vulnerable children. In a review article on refugee children resettled in high-income countries, Fazel et al. (2012) conclude that in order to understand the positive effects on children's psychological

---

[7]http://www.bamf.de/SharedDocs/Anlagen/DE/Downloads/Infothek/Statistik/Asyl/statistik-anlage-teil-4-aktuelle-zahlen-zu-asyl.pdf?__blob=publicationFile.
[8]http://www.unicef.de/blob/56282/fa13c2eefcd41dfca5d89d44c72e72e3/fluechtlingskinder-in-deutschland-unicef-studie-2014-data.pdf,   accessed August 12, 2015.

functioning, we have to go beyond studies focusing on the associations between adverse exposures and psychological symptoms and focus instead on longitudinal studies with an ecological perspective like the one described by Cooper (2011).

References

Ainsworth, M. D. S., Blehar, M. C., Waters, E., & Wall, S. (1978). *Patterns of attachment: A psychological study of the strange situation*. Hillsdale, NJ: Erlbaum.

Amato, P. R. (2010). Research on divorce: Continuing trends and new developments. *Journal of Marriage and Family, 72*(3), 650–666.

Amato, P. R., & Keith, B. (1991). Parental divorce and adult well-being: A meta-analysis. *Journal of Mariage and the Family, 44*, 73–86.

Bakermans-Kranenburg, M. J., Van Ijzendoorn, M. H., & Juffer, F. (2003). Less is more: Meta-analyses of sensitivity and attachment interventions in early childhood. *Psychological Bulletin, 129*(2), 195.

Bjørknes, R., Kjøbli, J., Manger, T., & Jakobsen, R. (2012). Parent training among ethnic minorities: Parenting practices as mediators of change in child conduct problems. *Family Relations, 61*(1), 101–114.

Bohlin, G., Hagekull, B., & Rydell, A.-M. (2000). Attachment and social functioning: A longitudinal study from infancy to middle childhood. *Social Development, 9*(1), 24–39.

Bornstein, M. H. (Ed.). (2002). *Handbook of parenting. Volume 5: Practical issues in parenting*. Mahwah, NJ: Lawrence Erlbaum.

Bornstein, M. H., Deater-Deckard, K., & Lansford, J. (2007). Introduction. Immigrant families in contemporary society. In M. H. Bornstein, K. Deater-Deckard, & J. Lansford (Eds.), *Immigrant families in contemporary society* (pp. 1–6). New York: Guilford Press.

Burger, K. (2010). How does early childhood care and education affect cognitive development? An international review of the effects of early interventions for children from different social backgrounds. *Early Childhood Research Quarterly, 25*(2), 140–165.

Cabrera, N. J. (2013). *Positive development of minority children*. Society for Research in Child Development.

Cabrera, N. J., Beeghly, M., & Eisenberg, N. (2012). Positive development of minority children: Introduction to the special issue. *Child Development Perspectives, 6*(3), 207–209.

Collins, W. A., Maccoby, E. E., Steinberg, L., Hetherington, E. M., & Bornstein, M. H. (2000). Contemporary research on parenting: The case for nature and nurture. *American Psychologist, 55*(2), 218.

Conger, R. D., Conger, K. J., & Martin, M. J. (2010). Socioeconomic status, family processes, and

individual development. *Journal of Marriage and Family, 72*(3), 685–704.

Conger, K. J., Rueter, M. A., & Conger, R. D. (2000). *The role of economic pressure in the lives of parents and their adolescents: The family stress model*.

Cooper, C. R. (2011). *Bridging multiple worlds: Cultures, Identities, and Pathways to College*.

Daglar, M., Melhuish, E., & Barnes, J. (2011). Parenting and preschool child behaviour among Turkish immigrant, migrant and non-migrant families. *European Journal of Developmental Psychology, 8*(3), 261–279.

Davies, P. T., Harold, G. T., Goeke-Morey, M. C., & Cummings, E. M. (2002). *Child emotional security and interparental conflict*. Boston, MA: Blackwell.

Derluyn, I., Broekaert, E., & Schuyten, G. (2008). Emotional and behavioural problems in migrant adolescents in Belgium. *European Child and Adolescent Psychiatry, 17*(1), 54–62.

Dronkers, J., van der Velden, R., & Dunne, A. (2012). Why are migrant students better off in certain types of educational systems or schools than in others? *European Educational Research Journal, 11*(1), 11–44.

Duncan, G. J., & Magnuson, K. A. (2005). Can family socioeconomic resources account for racial and ethnic test score gaps? *The Future of Children, 15*(1), 35–54.

Dykstra, P. A., & Fokkema, T. (2012). Norms of filial obligation in the Netherlands. *Population-E, 67*, 97–122.

Dykstra, P. A., Broek, T. V. D., Mureşan, C., Hărăguş, M., Hărăguş, P.-T., Abramowska-Kmon, A., et al. (2013). *Intergenerational linkages in families*. Families and Societies Working Paper Series.

Eisenberg, N., Losoya, S., Fabes, R. A., Guthrie, I. K., Reiser, M., Murphy, B., et al. (2001). Parental socialization of children's dysregulated expression of emotion and externalizing problems. *Journal of Family Psychology, 15*(2), 183.

Emmen, R. A., Malda, M., Mesman, J., van IJzendoorn, M. H., Prevoo, M. J., & Yeniad, N. (2013). Socioeconomic status and parenting in ethnic minority families: Testing a minority family stress model. *Journal of Family Psychology, 27*(6), 896.

European Commission. (2013). *Council recommendation on effective Roma integration measures in the Member States*. COM (2013) 460 final. Brussels, 26 June 2013. http://ec.europa.eu/justice/discrimination/files/com_2013_460_en.pdf. Accessed 12 Jan 2015.

Eurostat. (2015). *Statistiken zu Eheschließungen und Scheidungen*. http://ec.europa.eu/eurostat/statistics-explained/index.php/Marriage_and_divorce_statistics/de. Accessed 12 Aug 2015.

Extra, G., & Gorter, D. (2001). Comparative perspectives on regional and immigrant minority languages in multicultural Europe. In G. Extra & D. Gorter (Eds.), *The other languages of Europe. Demographic, sociolinguistic and educational perspectives. (Multilingual matters 118)* (pp. 1–44). Trowbridge, Wiltshire: Cromwell Press Ltd.

Extra, G., & Yağmur, K. (2011). Urban multilingualism in Europe: Mapping linguistic diversity in multicultural cities. *Journal of Pragmatics, 43*(5), 1173–1184.

Fazel, M., Reed, R. V., Panter-Brick, C., & Stein, A. (2012). Mental health of displaced an refugee children resettled in high-income countries: risk and protective factors. *Lancet, 379*, 266–282.

Flink, I. J., Jansen, P. W., Beirens, T. M., Tiemeier, H., van IJzendoorn, M. H., Jaddoe, V. W., et al. (2012). Differences in problem behaviour among ethnic minority and majority preschoolers in the Netherlands and the role of family functioning and parenting factors as mediators: The Generation R Study. *BMC Public Health, 12*(1), 1092.

Grusec, J. E., & Davidov, M. (2010). Integrating different perspectives on socialization theory and research: A domain-specific approach. *Child Development, 81*(3), 687–709.

Grych, J. H., & Fincham, F. D. (2001). *Interparental conflict and child development: Theory, research, and applications.* Cambridge: Cambridge University Press.

Harkness, S., & Super, C. M. (2002). Culture and parenting. *Handbook of Parenting, 2*, 253–280.

Hjern, A., Angel, B., & Höjer, B. (1991). Persecution and behavior: A report of refugee children from Chile. *Child Abuse and Neglect, 15*(3), 239–248.

Hooghe, M., Trappers, A., Meuleman, B., & Reeskens, T. (2008). Migration to European countries: A structural explanation of patterns, 1980–20041. *International Migration Review, 42*(2), 476–504.

Hughes, D., Rodriguez, J., Smith, E. P., Johnson, D. J., Stevenson, H. C., & Spicer, P. (2006). Parents' ethnic-racial socialization practices: A review of research and directions for future study. *Developmental Psychology, 42*(5), 747.

Idema, H., & Phalet, K. (2007). Transmission of gender-role values in Turkish-German migrant families: The role of gender, intergenerational and intercultural relations. *Zeitschrift für Familienforschung. Journal of Family Research 19*(1), 71–105.

Iqbal, H. (2014). Multicultural parenting: Preparation for bias socialisation in British South Asian and White families in the UK. *International Journal of Intercultural Relations, 43*, 215–226.

Jäkel, J., Leyendecker, B., & Agache, A. (2015). Family and individual factors associated with Turkish immigrant and German children's and adolescents' mental health. *Journal of Child and Family Studies, 24*(4), 1097–1105.

Javo, C., Rønning, J. A., Heyerdahl, S., & Rudmin, F. W. (2004). Parenting correlates of child behavior problems in a multiethnic community sample of preschool children in northern Norway. *European Child and Adolescent Psychiatry, 13*(1), 8–18.

Kağıtçıbaşı, Ç. (2007). *Family, self and human development across cultures. Theory and applications.* New Jersey: Lawrence Erlbaum Associates Inc.

Kalmijn, M. (2010). Racial differences in the effects of parental divorce and separation on children: Generalizing the evidence to a European case. *Social Science Research, 39*(5), 845–856.

Kao, G., & Tienda, M. (1995). Optimism and achievement: The Educational Performance of Immigrant Youth. *Social Science Quarterly, 76*(1), 1–19.

Karlsen, S., & Nazroo, J. Y. (2002). Relation between racial discrimination, social class, and health among ethnic minority groups. *American Journal of Public Health, 92*(4), 624–631.

Kohl, K., Jäkel, J., & Leyendecker, B. (2015). Schlüsselfaktor Elterliche Beteiligung: Warum Lehrkräfte türkischstämmige und deutsche Kinder aus belasteten Familien häufig als verhaltensauffällig einstufen (Parental involvement in school is the key to teacher judgments of Turkish immigrant and German children's behavior problems). *Zeitschrift für Familienforschung/Journal of Family Research* (in press), *27*(2), 193–207.

Kouider, E. B., Koglin, U., & Petermann, F. (2014). Emotional and behavioral problems in migrant children and adolescents in Europe: A systematic review. *European Child and Adolescent Psychiatry, 23*(6), 373–391.

Lamb, M. E., & Sutton-Smith, B. (Eds.). (2014). *Sibling relationships: Their nature and significance across the lifespan.* New York: Psychology Press.

Lancee, B., & Dronkers, J. (2008). *Ethnic diversity in neighborhoods and individual trust of immigrants and natives: A replication of Putnam (2007) in a West-European country.* Paper presented at the international conference on theoretical perspectives on social cohesion and social capital, Royal Flemish Academy of Belgium for Science and the Arts, Brussels.

Lerner, R. M., Almerigi, J. B., Theokas, C., & Lerner, J. V. (2005). Positive youth development. *Journal of Early Adolescence, 25*(1), 10–16.

Leyendecker, B. (2011). Children from immigrant families-adaptaion, development, and resilience. Current Trends in the Study of Migration in Europe. *International Journal of Developmental Science, 5*(1), 3–9.

Leyendecker, B., Citlak, B., Schräpler, K., & Schölmerich, A. (2014). Bildungserwartungen beim Übergang in die Grundschule—Ein Vergleich von deutschen und zugewanderten Eltern. *Zeitschrift für Familienforschung/Journal of Family Research, 26*, 70–93.

Leyendecker, B., Schölmerich, A., & Citlak, B. (2006). Similarities and differences between first-and second-generation Turkish migrant mothers in Germany: The acculturation gap. In M. H. Bornstein & L. Cote (Eds.), *Acculturation and parent-child relationships: Measurement and development* (pp. 297–315). Mahwah: Erlbaum.

Liefbroer, A. C., & Mulder, C. H. (2006). Family obligations. In P. A. Dykstra, M. Kalmijn, A. E. Komter, T. C. M. Knijn, A. C. Liefbroer, & C. H. Mulder (Eds.), *Family solidarity in the Netherlands* (pp. 123–146). Amsterdam: Dutch University Press.

Lin, N., Cook, K. S., & Burt, R. S. (2001). *Social capital: Theory and research*. New Brunswick, NJ: Transaction Publishers.

Margolin, G., Gordis, E. B., & John, R. S. (2001). Coparenting: A link between marital conflict and parenting in two-parent families. *Journal of Family Psychology, 15*(1), 3.

Maynard, M., & Harding, S. (2010). Perceived parenting and psychological well-being in UK ethnic minority adolescents. *Child: Care, Health and Development, 36* (5), 630–638.

McHale, J. P., & Lindahl, K. M. (2011). *Coparenting: A conceptual and clinical examination of family systems.* Washington, DC: American Psychological Association.

McLanahan, S., & Sandefur, G. (1994). *Growing up in a single-parent family: What helps, what hurts.* Cambridge, MA: Harvard University Press.

McNulty, T. L., & Bellair, P. E. (2003). Explaining racial and ethnic differences in adolescent violence: Structural disadvantage, family well-being, and social capital. *Justice Quarterly, 20*(1), 1–31.

Mesman, J., van IJzendoorn, M. H., & Bakermans-Kranenburg, M. J. (2012). Unequal in opportunity, equal in process: Parental sensitivity promotes positive child development in ethnic minority families. *Child Development Perspectives, 6*(3), 239–250.

Milewski, N., & Kulu, H. (2014). Mixed marriages in Germany: A high risk of divorce for immigrant-native couples. *European Journal of Population, 30*(1), 89–113.

Molcho, M., Cristini, F., Nic Gabhainn, S., Santinello, M., Moreno, M., Gasper de Matos, M., et al. (2010). Health and well-being among child immigrants in Europe. *Eurohealth, 16*(1), 20.

Moscardino, U., Bertelli, C., & Altoè, G. (2011). Culture, migration, and parenting: A Comparative Study of mother-infant interaction and childrearing patterns in Romanian, Romanian Immigrant, and Italian Families. *International Journal of Developmental Science, 5*(1), 11–25.

Nauck, B., & Lotter, V. (2015). Parenting styles and perceived instrumentality of schooling in native, Turkish, and Vietnamese families in Germany. *Zeitschrift für Erziehungswissenschaft, 18*(14), 845–869. doi:10.1007/s11618-015-0630-x

Nauck, B., & Lotter, V. (2016). Bildungstransmission in Migrantenfamilien (Transmission of education in migrant families). In: C. Diehl, C. Hunkler, & C. Kristen (Eds.), *Ethnische Ungleichheiten im Bildungsverlauf. Mechanismen, Befunde, Debatten* (pp. 117–155). Wiesbaden: Springer.

Ochieng, B. M. N. (2014). Minority Ethnic Adolescents' wellbeing: Child rearing practices and positive family influences. *Health Education Journal, 73*(3), 324–331.

Portes, A., & Rumbaut, R. G. (2001). *Legacies: The story of the immigrant second generation.* Berkeley: University of California Press.

Rumbaut, R. G. (1997). Ties that bind: Immigration and immigrant families. In: A. Booth, A. C. Crouter & N. S. Landale (Eds.), Immigration and the family:

Research and policy on US immigrants (pp. 3–46). Mahwah, New Jersey: Lawrence Erlbaum Associates.

Schjerve, R. R., & Vetter, E. (2012). *European multilingualism: current perspectives and challenges* (Vol. 147). Clevedon: Multilingual matters.

Spiegler, O., Leyendecker, B., & Kohl, K. (2015). Acculturation gaps between Immigrant Turkish Marriage Partners: Resource or source of distress? [Online first]. *Journal of Cross-Cultural Psychology, 46*(5), 667–683. doi:10.117/0022022115578686

Spiess, C. K., Büchel, F., & Wagner, G. G. (2003). Children's school placement in Germany: Does Kindergarten attendance matter? *Early Childhood Research Quarterly, 18*(2), 255–270.

Sroufe, L. A., Egeland, B., Carlson, E. A., & Collins, W. A. (2007). *The development of the person.* New York: Guilford Press.

Stams, G.-J. J., Juffer, F., & van IJzendoorn, M. H. (2002). Maternal sensitivity, infant attachment, and temperament in early childhood predict adjustment in middle childhood: The case of adopted children and their biologically unrelated parents. *Developmental Psychology, 38*(5), 806.

Stein, G. L., Gonzalez, L. M., & Huq, N. (2012). Cultural stressors and the hopelessness model of depressive symptoms in Latino adolescents. *Journal of Youth and Adolescence, 41*(10), 1339–1349.

Steinbach, A. (2013). Family structure and parent–child contact: A comparison of native and migrant families. *Journal of Marriage and Family, 75*(5), 1114–1129.

Stevens, G. W., & Vollebergh, W. A. (2008). Mental health in migrant children. *Journal of Child Psychology and Psychiatry, 49*(3), 276–294.

Stuart, J., Ward, C., & Adam, Z. (2010). Current issues in the development and acculturation of Muslim youth in New Zealand. *ISSBD Bulletin, 58*, 9–13.

Suárez-Orozco, C., & Suárez-Orozco, M. (2001). *Children of immigrants*. Cambridge: Harvard University Press.

Tan, G. G., Ray, M. P., & Cate, R. (1991). Migrant farm child abuse and neglect within an ecosystem framework. *Family Relations, 40*(1), 84–90.

Vasileva, K. (2011). 6.5 % of the EU population are foreigners and 9.4 % are born abroad. *Romania, 21* (462), 462.

Walper, S., & Grgic, M. (2013). Verhaltens-und Kompetenzentwicklung im Kontext der Familie. Zur relativen Bedeutung von sozialer Herkunft, elterlicher Erziehung und Aktivitäten in der Familie. *Zeitschrift für Erziehungswissenschaft, 16*(3), 503–531.

Willard, J., Agache, A., Jäkel, J., Glück, C., & Leyendecker, B. (2014). Family factors predicting vocabulary in Turkish as a heritage language. *Applied Psycholinguistics, 36*(4), 875–898. doi:10.1017/S0142716413000544

Wissenschaftlicher Beirat für Familienfragen. (2016). *Familie und Migration. Kindheit mit Zuwanderungshintergrund*. Wiesbaden: Springer.

Woellert, F., & Klingholz, R. (2013). Neue Potenziale. *Zur Lage der Integration in Deutschland*. http://www.

berlin-institut.org/publikationen/studien/neue-potenziale.html

Yagmur, S., Mesman, J., Malda, M., Bakermans-Kranenburg, M. J., & Ekmekci, H. (2014). Video-feedback intervention increases sensitive parenting in ethnic minority mothers: a randomized control trial. *Attachment & Human Development, 16*(4), 371–386.

Yaman, A., Mesman, J., van IJzendoorn, M. H., Bakermans-Kranenburg, M. J., & Linting, M. (2010). Parenting in an individualistic culture with a collectivistic cultural background: The case of Turkish immigrant families with toddlers in the Netherlands. *Journal of Child and Family Studies, 19*(5), 617–628.

Minority Fathers and Children's Positive Development in the United States

Natasha J. Cabrera, Elizabeth Karberg, and Catherine Kuhns

Abstract

This chapter reviews the literature on fathers and their unique influences on positive child development in minority children in the United States. It begins with an historical overview of the field of fatherhood research that has been conducted primarily with minority (African American and Latino) families in the United States. It then describes the central research questions framing studies on ethnic minority fathers and discusses issues related to measurement and methodology. The majority of the chapter reviews empirical findings on the ways that ethnic minority fathers are engaged with their children, the factors that differentially relate to their involvement, and how father involvement relates to children's adjustment in a number of domains (cognitive, language, social skills, and peer relationships). Finally, the chapter suggests policy implications and directions for future research. The chapter provides an illustrative rather than definite review of theories and empirical research on fathers in minority families aiming to offer a framework in which to conceptualize fathering and children's adjustment.

Historical Overview and Theoretical Perspectives

This chapter reviews the literature on fathers and their influences on positive child development among minority children in the United States. Ethnic minority families are a heterogeneous group and vary significantly in terms of immigration status, country of origin, economic, social, and personal histories. This chapter focuses on research in the United States because of the scarcity of research conducted with minority populations in Western European countries (Mesman et al. 2012). The United States has a diverse and growing ethnic population, and this review focuses particularly on Latino and African American families because they are the largest ethnic minority groups in the United States and therefore the most studied (Humes et al. 2011). Nevertheless, the science based on African American and Latino fathers,

N.J. Cabrera (✉) · E. Karberg · C. Kuhns
University of Maryland, College Park, MD, USA
e-mail: ncabrera@umd.edu

© The Editor(s) 2017

N.J. Cabrera and B. Leyendecker (eds.), *Handbook on Positive Development of Minority Children and Youth*, DOI 10.1007/978-3-319-43645-6_12

especially the ways in which they influence their children in positive ways, is quite limited. Therefore, to draw comparisons or highlight certain aspects of positive development, in some instances, this chapter includes findings from studies with minority mothers or other minority groups.

Positive development refers to the strengths or assets (e.g., being bilingual) that ethnic minority children and their families exhibit in particular contexts (Cabrera 2013). The emphasis on the positive development of minority children is rooted in the positive youth development (PYD) literature that aligns adolescents' contextual strengths (e.g. parental involvement in school) with their individual strengths (e.g., academic motivation) to promote well-being (Lerner et al. 2009). Positive development is distinct from children's resilience. Research on resilience focuses on children who thrive in the face of developmental risk factors and children who do not thrive in optimal conditions (Masten and Wright 2009). The resilience paradigm has been particularly important for understanding the mechanisms that promote children's well-being in the face of adversity, but has been less helpful in understanding the promotive and protective factors that support children who are not experiencing risk. In contrast, research on positive development explores the varied, and sometimes overlooked, assets of ethnic minority populations; offers a more nuanced perspective about the ecology in which minority children grow; and highlights the heterogeneity in this population (Guerra et al. 2011). Although many minority children experience hardship and disadvantage, many children thrive and live in supportive environments that are not characterized by risk (Cabrera 2013).

The research reviewed in this chapter builds broadly on bioecological models of human development that highlight the direct influence of the home microsystem on children's development (Bronfenbrenner and Morris 1998). Ethnic minority fathers have assets (e.g., responsiveness) that foster children's positive development. What fathers do for their children, the way they organize their social environment, and the

multiple ways in which they interact and provide a safe and stimulating set of experiences shape children's cognitive, linguistic, and social development (e.g., Cabrera et al. 2007; Flouri and Buchanan 2004; Sarkadi et al. 2008).

Current Research Questions

Overall, the study of how ethnic minority fathers influence their children's development has been guided by three interrelated questions. First, how are ethnic minority fathers involved in their children's lives? Research addressing this question investigates how much time fathers spend with their children and what they do for them (e.g., provide economic resources) and with them (e.g., quality of father-child interactions). The focus on economic provision is especially important for minority low-income men who are more likely than White fathers to be nonresident and to have a child out of wedlock, conditions that tend to reduce economic and emotional support (Humes et al. 2011). Second, what are the factors that explain variability in father involvement? Understanding why some ethnic minority fathers are more involved than others, even when they do not live with their children, is central to understanding their influence on children's development. Researchers have paid most attention to structural factors, such as education and income, that predict men's ability to fulfill their role of providers. There is less research on how other factors, such as fathers' psychological or personality characteristics, and family functioning processes might predict father involvement in other domains of parenting, such as providing emotional support. Third, how is father involvement related to children's development? To be meaningful, fathering behaviors must predict or relate in significant and positive ways to children's development over time. As with research on mothers' influences on children's development, this question assumes that what fathers do, and the choices they make for their children, are central to the psychological, intellectual, behavioral, and social development of their children (Collins et al. 2000).

Research Measurement and Methodology

The majority of the research reviewed in this chapter relies on cross-sectional designs and samples of convenience (that over represent low-income families). In the United States there are few longitudinal studies of fathers, and there are virtually no studies that collect data on fathers and their children from birth to adulthood. The associations reported in the literature typically range from small to modest and tend to test direct linkages. Moreover, the research on ethnic minority fathers has mostly focused on low-income population; thus, the generalizability of this research to other groups is difficult. There are virtually no studies on middle-class ethnic minority fathers.

A stumbling block in fatherhood research has been the lack of conceptual consensus regarding what is father involvement and how to measure it. In lieu of a grand theory of fathering, researchers have appealed to a potpourri of theoretical approaches (e.g., attachment, family systems) resulting in a body of work that is difficult to integrate into a coherent whole. In efforts to address this gap, Cabrera et al. (2014) developed an heuristic ecological model of fathering (or mothering) that accounts for individual, family, and social influences on parenting, and, consequently, on children's development. In this framework, father involvement varies as a function of changes in other individuals within the family system and reflects both the characteristics and behavior of children as well as events in family history (e.g., paternal job loss). The model stipulates that the father's economic resources may influence not only the father's well-being and capacity to provide for his children, but also that of the mother's, as well as the levels of stress (or well-being) experienced by the whole family. Likewise, child characteristics, including health and disability, may incur costs that decrease the father's economic resources in ways that have spillover effects on the co-parenting system.

Across a variety of conceptual frameworks, research with ethnic minority fathers has used quantitative methodologies, including surveys where mothers (or fathers) report on the frequency of fathers' involvement with their children (Mitchell et al. 2009). Unlike research conducted with mothers, survey research conducted with fathers must first tackle the question: who is the father of the target child? A father can be biological, "social", or other men (e.g., priest) unrelated to the mother, who play a fatherly role in the child's life (Coley 2003; Tach et al. 2010). Moreover, who the father of the target child is will vary as time goes by and as families dissolve and recombine in different ways, posing particular challenges for longitudinal research. Researchers' decisions about which father (biological vs. social) to include in the study will depend on the research question as well as on researchers' resources, with important implications for recruitment, retention, and follow-up.

Although identifying and locating *biological* fathers for research is less arduous than locating non-biological fathers, this process is nevertheless very challenging. For many minority men, in particular men who have a child outside of marriage, residence is fluid, increasing the difficulty (and cost) of engaging them in research. Therefore, in some cases, researchers opt for collecting data on biological fathers from mothers. This approach is also fraught with problems as some mothers may report inaccurately on fathers' behaviors or may not know. Studies have shown that maternal reports of the frequency of father involvement are on average lower than fathers' reports of their own behaviors, but there is more convergence when fathers are resident than nonresident (Coley and Morris 2002; Mikelson 2008). Moreover, regardless of residence status, low-income minority mothers and fathers have more agreement about items of contact (e.g., "how often does father see/visit child?") than about items measuring support of the mother (Coley and Morris 2002). Findings from such studies need to clearly state that they are measuring *mothers' perceptions* of father involvement rather than father involvement per se.

Another salient issue in survey fatherhood research is what to measure about fathers or their behaviors with their children that can capture how it matters for their development. Reflecting the lack of conceptual consensus in the field, father involvement has been measured using an array of questionnaires, many of which do not have psychometric information. A notable effort in this regard is the Developing a Daddy Survey (DADS) that aimed to develop a set of measurement tools for studying fatherhood (Cabrera et al. 2004). DADS consists of coordinated survey modules focusing on various dimensions of father involvement (e.g., accessibility, engagement, responsible, and family functioning) that were developed for and introduced into major national surveys (e.g., the Early Childhood Longitudinal Study—Birth Cohort) that had previously had limited or no content related to fatherhood (Cabrera et al. 2004). The DADS measures are available to the public and can be downloaded from the Department of Health and Human Services website (http://fatherhood.hhs. gov/Research/DADS/newborn/).

Other issues related to the lack of consensus on measurement of father involvement reflect the interdisciplinary nature of the field. Sociologists, demographers, and economists often favor a present versus absent measure, which is rooted in some realities about family life in the United States (Carlson and Magnuson 2011). Families today can be single, cohabiting, married, same-sexed, recombined, and nonresident (Ganong et al. 2015). In these diverse family types, fathers can be resident or nonresident, and this varies by ethnicity: 24 % of African American fathers and 18 % of Latino fathers have a child they do not live with, compared to 8.2 % of White fathers (Jones and Mosher 2013). As a group, nonresident fathers, are far less likely than resident fathers to have contact with their children or to be involved in their rearing (Carlson and Magnuson 2011). By implication, fathers' residential status (resident vs. nonresident) is an important indicator of father involvement.

In contrast, developmental scientists are interested in assessing the quality of father-child relationships. To this end, they use quantitative surveys and, the gold standard, observational methods. In observational research mothers are instructed to play or read with their children while a researcher videotapes (digitalized) the interaction. Observational data provide objective insights into the quality (i.e., sensitive, responsive, intrusive) of the parent-child relationship (Bornstein et al. 2006). The down side of observational research is that it is time-intensive and very expensive. Videotaping interactions of fathers and their children in minority families, especially when fathers do not reside with their children, is a herculean task that often results in very small sample sizes with limited analytical options. Nevertheless, studies using videotaped data of fathers and their children are gaining ground in the field (e.g., Cabrera et al. 2007; Kochanska et al. 2008).

Another methodological approach used in fathering research is qualitative (e.g., focus groups, ethnographies). Qualitative research methods are valuable in providing rich and nuanced descriptions of complex phenomena, clarifying individuals' experiences and interpretations of events, giving voice to those whose views are rarely heard, and conducting initial explorations to develop theories and generate hypotheses. Qualitative and quantitative methods can be complementary, used in sequence or in tandem. A popular and inexpensive method to gather data on fathers is focus groups where fathers' views and perceptions are recorded, transcribed, and analyzed (e.g., Umaña-Taylor and Bámaca 2004). Focus group methodology is useful because it enables investigators to explore themes that arise in new lines of research where theory and past empirical studies cannot inform hypotheses, especially with understudied groups, and enables researchers to contribute to theory and generate hypotheses (Umaña-Taylor and Bámaca 2004). However, focus group samples are small and select, and may provide a skewed perspective of fathers' behaviors or parenting; thus, interpretation needs to be careful and not overreach.

Empirical Findings

How Are Ethnic Minority Fathers Involved in Their Children's Lives?

Before addressing the question of how fathers are involved, it is important to look at the amount of time fathers spend with their children. For a long time fathers have been characterized as being highly involved by economically providing for their children, but less involved in their daily care (Amato and Gilbreth 1999). However, because most children today live in households where both parents work outside the home, it is difficult to imagine contemporary resident fathers not involved in the daily care of their children. Indeed, research finds that in dual earner households, both parents share in the caregiving (e.g., feeding, bathing) of their children as well as in the organization of daily routines, such as taking children to and from school (Coltrane 2000). Nevertheless, there is substantial variation within and across ethnic minority groups in the amount of time that fathers spend (or are able to spend) on activities related to the direct care of their children. National data show that contemporary fathers are more hands-on than they used to be in previous decades and, consequently, more involved in the daily care of their children (Sayer et al. 2004). Although mothers still do more household tasks than fathers (about 17 h per week compared to fathers' 10 h), men and women's time doing chores and other household labor has converged over the last 4 decades (Lachance-Grzela and Bouchard 2010). A similar trend in parents' time is seen with child-specific care. Research based on time diary data conducted in the United States showed that, although mothers spend more time with their children than fathers, on average, fathers' time spent with their children has increased over the last few decades, especially on weekends (Craig 2006; Yeung et al. 2001; Hofferth 2003).

The amount of time fathers spend with their children is also related to the roles they play in families. The multiple family configurations in which ethnic minority fathers live suggest different roles for mothers and fathers (Ganong et al. 2015), especially when fathers are not resident. In these diverse family configurations, with the exception of the provider role, fathers' roles are less defined than mothers' and more dependent on contextual factors. When unions dissolve and fathers become nonresident, a father's role as provider will (hopefully) remain stable, but his role as caregiver or disciplinarian will depend on, among other things, the relationship with his partner and accessibility to his children (Arditti et al. 2005; Fagan and Barnett 2003). If mothers "close the gate" between father and child, fathers' time with his children is reduced making it very difficult for them to be involved in the daily care of their children.

In addressing the question of what fathers do when they are *present* and involved with their children, researchers have compared what fathers do to what mothers do with their children (Belsky et al. 1984; Notaro and Volling 1999). Research focusing on similarities has revealed parallels on a variety of measures (Lewis and Lamb 2003; Lewis 1997). For example, both mothers and fathers seem to engage in more physical play with their sons than with their daughters (Lewis 1997). Overall, both mothers and fathers, across ethnicity and SES, are sensitive to their children's needs, show love and affection, and provide safe and stimulating environments for their children (Cabrera et al. 2014; Fagan et al. 2014).

Researchers focusing on the differences between mothers and fathers have reported that these differences reflect more intensity of engagement rather than type of engagement. For example, fathers are more likely to tease their children, engage in "rough-and-tumble" play, encourage risk-taking, and socialize gender roles than mothers (Fletcher et al. 2013; Grossmann et al. 2008; Paquette and Dumont 2013). There is also evidence that compared to mothers, fathers use higher quality language and are more linguistically challenging partners for their children (Rowe et al. 2004; Pancsofar and Vernon-Feagans 2010; Malin et al. 2012).

Studies that have examined within-group differences generally report differential rates of involvement that vary by ethnicity. A study using the Early Childhood Longitudinal Study—Birth Cohort (ECLS-B), a national sample of babies born in 2001 and their parents, found that ethnic minority fathers reported higher levels of engagement in both caregiving and physical play activities and were reported as being more involved than White fathers (Cabrera et al. 2011; Leavell Smith et al. 2012). When compared to White or other ethnic minority fathers, Latino fathers are rated as being highly engaged (i.e., accessible, engaged, and responsible) with their children, spending, on average, more than 1 h more with them (ages birth to 12 years) during the weekend, and engaging in more responsibility activities (i.e., care-giving, discipline, decision making; Cabrera et al. 2008, 2013).

What Predicts Father Involvement in Minority Populations?

The second research question focuses on the factors that explain variability in father involvement among minority families. Variation in the amount and quality of father involvement is said to reflect multiple factors operating at different levels: individual, family, and societal (Cabrera et al. 2014; Castillo et al. 2011). Fathers' residence and family structure, fathers' individual characteristics, family functioning, cultural beliefs, and the quality of father-child interactions explain variability in father involvement among ethnic minority fathers.

Fathers' Residence and Family Structure
Studies using representative samples of low-income urban minority men show that father residence (i.e., two-parent households) is strongly linked to father's involvement with their children in age-appropriate activities, such as playing peek-a-boo, singing songs, and reading stories (Cabrera et al. 2011; Carlson 2006; Castillo et al. 2011). Fathers who reside with their children, either because they are married or cohabiting, are more likely to be involved and present in their children's lives than fathers who do not. However, the story is not straightforward as there are

mitigating factors that can trump residence. In a study of urban poor families, African American fathers were more likely to be nonresident, but were also more likely to have maintained contact with their child over the first 5 years of life compared with White or Hispanic non-resident fathers because they maintained a supportive coparenting relationship (Carlson et al. 2008).

However, there is also substantial variation among types of two parent households, and so in addition to father's residential status, family structure is an important determinant of child well-being. Compared to minority cohabiting men, married minority men have more resources because of the characteristics of fathers and mothers who select into marriage and because married households tend to be more stable than those in which parents are only cohabiting (Manning and Brown 2006; Osborne et al. 2007). Married fathers are less likely than only cohabiting men to become nonresident and thus less involved in their children's lives.

Fathers' Characteristics
Men's levels of education and income are strong predictors of their involvement. Fathers with higher levels of education and more income are better able to support their children than fathers with less (Carlson and Magnuson 2011; Duncan et al. 2014). Other individual factors that have been implicated in father involvement include fathers' mental and physical health and paternity establishment (Wilson and Brooks-Gunn 2001; Guzzo 2009).

Among nonresident fathers, ability to financially support their children determines in large part how much access they have to their children. Nonresident fathers are involved with their children by providing money through the formal child support system, wherein a child support order is established that requires a father to provide a consistent level of support, and wages are often automatically withheld from fathers' pay to this end (Carlson and Magnuson 2011). Paying child support does not automatically give nonresident fathers access to their children (Koball and Principe 2002). Many states do not have visitation rights contingent on child support payments (e.g., Texas Attorney General 2004).

Some nonresident fathers provide support informally by giving money directly to mothers or providing in-kind (or non-cash) support by paying for necessities, such as diapers, food, or doctor's visits (Grall 2013). Fathers who are able to offer in-kind support are more likely to see and spend more time with their children than those who do not (Kane et al. 2015) and may be actively involved with their children, which is often dictated by formal or informal arrangements with mothers (Choi 2010).

Family Functioning

The ways in which parents get along and relate to one another have important implications for the amount and quality of father involvement (Fagan and Barnett 2003). Fathers who report being happy with their partners also report higher levels of involvement with their young children (Cabrera et al. 2010; Fagan and Palkovitz 2011). Fathers who report conflict with their partners are less likely to have access to their children, which reduces the amount of time with them, especially if fathers become nonresident. In addition, because custodial mothers are often the gatekeepers of children's time, nonresident fathers' relationship with the mother is an important determinant of their involvement. Not surprisingly, nonresident fathers who are on good terms with mothers, and especially those who are still romantically involved with them, are much more likely to be involved across every domain of caregiving (Fagan and Palkovitz 2011).

As important as the quality of the couple relationship seems to be for father involvement, research has shown that the quality of the co-parenting relationship, or parents' ability to work together as parents to rear their children (Feinberg 2003), may be most important. Although direction of causality is unclear, emerging findings suggest that in families where couples who are supportive of each other's parenting, fathers tend to be more involved than in families where fathers are undermined (Cabrera et al. 2010; Fagan and Palkovitz 2011). Fathers who perceive being supported (report more shared

decision making and communication) by their partners in their role of parents were more involved with their children over time than fathers who felt criticized and not supported (Fagan and Palkovitz 2011; Hohmann-Mariott 2011). In a study using the ECLS-B, researchers found that when Mexican American fathers reported conflict with their partner about child rearing (co-parenting conflict) they reported being less involved (e.g., caregiving, physical play) with their toddlers (Cabrera et al. 2010). In other analyses, the quality of the co-parenting relationship appears to be the strongest predictor of involvement especially for nonresident low-income African American (Carlson et al. 2008).

Acculturation and Adaptation

Scholars interested in how minority parents adapt to the cultural norms and values of the host society (acculturation) have focused on the status of adaptation or acculturation (i.e., length of time in the United States, English proficiency). As individuals adapt to the new society, they choose the values, beliefs, and behaviors of the host culture to which they want their children to adapt as well as the norms and values of their country of origin they wish to retain (García Coll et al. 1996). Correlational studies find that levels of acculturation are somewhat associated with father involvement. A study of middle-class, married, Indian immigrant fathers in the United States found that fathers who were more acculturated (e.g., use English more, eat non-Indian food, do not yearn for their homeland) were more engaged with their toddlers than fathers who were less acculturated, controlling for family characteristics (e.g., parents' age, family size; Jain and Belsky 1997). Other studies using national United States data find that Mexican and Chinese American fathers who are more acculturated (i.e., longer residence, United States citizenship, English proficiency) were less warm but engaged in more cognitively stimulating activities than their less acculturated counterparts (i.e., shorter residency, preference for foreign language use; Capps et al. 2010).

Studies that have examined within-group differences find that most differences in type of father engagement between Mexican American and other Latinos (including Puerto Rican, Cuban) disappeared once SES and acculturation (e.g., English proficiency) were controlled (Cabrera et al. 2006). It is difficult to explain why acculturation is negatively related to father involvement because most studies are correlational in nature, vary in how acculturation is measured, and do not often disentangle developmental from acculturation change (Phinney et al. 2000). One possible explanation for the finding that acculturated fathers are more involved is that father involvement in these studies is measured in a way that conforms to American normative parenting practices (e.g., reading to babies). This deficit model approach does not allow for the possibility that ethnic minority fathers from other cultures might be engaged in literacy activities other than reading, for example story telling that also promote literacy. Indeed, research suggests that reading might not be the preferred way to promote literacy in many non-Western countries (Perry 2008). The most we can conclude from these findings is that acculturated fathers (or mothers, as the case may be) have learned American parenting practices but not that less acculturated fathers do not support their children's learning.

Fathers' Cognition: Cultural Beliefs and Values

Scholars interested in fatherhood in minority populations have examined the ways in which specific aspects of culture might relate to positive parenting. Culture is defined as a shared system of commonality, usually operationalized as beliefs, values, norms, and practices (e.g., Harwood 2006; Weisner 2009).

Research on Latino parenting has highlighted the importance of cultural values, such as *familism* (i.e., valuing of family solidarity and family integration) for paternal involvement (Cruz et al. 2011; Morcillo et al. 2011). On average, Latinos have been found to report higher levels of family cohesion (often used interchangeably with *familism*) when compared to individuals of other ethnic groups (Baer and

Schmitz 2007). Studies show that low-income Latino parents who believe that children should grow up in united and strong families have fewer depressive symptoms and are also warm and accepting of their children (Potochnick and Perreira 2010; Smokowski et al. 2008). A study of Mexican American mothers and fathers found that fathers who highly believed in the value of *familism* (i.e., family rituals) and had a stronger Mexican orientation (e.g., I enjoy speaking Spanish; I like to eat Mexican food) also reported being more involved (monitoring and interacting) with their children than fathers who did not (Coltrane et al. 2004).

Cultural beliefs about gender roles and division of labor within the family have also been found to relate to positive parenting behaviors. Fathers who hold less traditional gender roles (i.e., believing that men are more integral to society and the family than women) are more involved in all aspects of parenting (e.g., monitoring, supervising, and interacting with their child) than parents who hold more traditional beliefs (Coltrane et al. 2004). Moreover, fathers whose partners hold less traditional gender roles have more access to their children than fathers whose partners hold more traditional gender roles (Kulik and Tsoref 2010).

Cultural scholars have also turned their attention to the psychosocial function of immigrant parents to understand why some parents who face adversity do not exhibit negative parenting. Optimism, a positive expectation for the future, is considered to be an important psychological resource for those experiencing negative or stressful life circumstances (Carver et al. 2010). Being optimistic may be particularly important for immigrant parents. The "immigrant optimism hypothesis" posits that immigrants have faith in the future despite the many barriers (e.g., language, poverty) to social and economic mobility and therefore have better outcomes (e.g., are happier) than those without faith in the future (Kao and Tienda 1995). Optimistic parents' positive outlook on life may spill over to their parenting views and behaviors showing more sensitivity and patience in their interactions with their children.

How Is Father Involvement Related to Children's Development?

The third set of questions has examined how father involvement is related to children's development. The science on parenting, which is focused mostly on mothers, has unearthed a solid and consistent set of findings about the process by which mothers rear their children and help them thrive in their cultural niches (Bornstein 2015; Bretherton 2010; Grusec and Davidov 2010). Although research on fathers is playing catch-up to the research on mothers and is not as extensive, it has also produced an important set of findings regarding the role that fathers play in their children's development (Cabrera et al. 2000; Flouri and Buchanan 2004; Lamb 2000). As a body of work, however, research on fathers has focused less on the constellation of parenting behaviors, practices, and cognitions that characterize research on parenting (mothering, really) and more on contextual factors that relate to whether fathers are present or absent in their children's lives (Adamson and Johnson 2013; Palkovitz 2007). Nevertheless, below we include some studies that are making headway in these areas. In particular, we highlight correlational data suggesting that key predictors of children's development include family structure, fathers' economic provision, cognitions (e.g., optimism, cultural values) and parenting practices (i.e., family routines).

Social Competence

The benefits of living with fathers for children's social adjustment cannot be overstated (McLanahan et al. 2013; Mead 1991). Social scientists have amassed a large body of evidence showing that children who live with their fathers have better behavioral outcomes, are less likely to be involved in delinquent behaviors, and are more likely to have friends. The adverse effect of father absence on children's social adjustment is well documented in a review of rigorous studies that found evidence for a causal effect (though generally smaller than previously found) of father absence on children's socioemotional adjustment (McLanahan et al. 2013; Sigle-Rushton and McLanahan 2004). In contrast to absent fathers, resident fathers have the opportunity to spend time with their children, which is important for relationship building and hands-on parenting. Although an early meta-analysis found little benefit to nonresident fathers' time spent with children, later studies that have used more refined measures of involvement provide more nuanced results. In a study of African American fathers, Choi (2010) found that mothers who reported high levels of nonresident father contact also reported fewer behavioral problems in their children.

In addition to spending time with their children, resident fathers also influence them through the economic provisions they bring to the household. This association is also true for nonresident fathers. Research shows that nonresident fathers' provision of economic support is associated with fewer externalizing behavior problems (Amato and Gilbreth 1999; Argys et al. 1998; Choi 2010). Although the mechanism is less clear, some findings suggest that child support among nonresident ethnic minority fathers seems to be beneficial for children because it improves mothering behaviors and reduces parenting stress (Choi 2010; Choi and Pyun 2014).

Although less extensively studied, research has shown that ethnic minority fathers' warmth, affection, and responsiveness are positively related to children's social competence (Adamson and Johnson 2013; Cabrera et al. 2014; Flanders et al. 2010). Children whose fathers are responsive to their needs while interacting during play are more likely to have higher cognitive and language skills than children whose fathers are not (Tamis-LeMonda et al. 2004).

Minority fathers can also influence their children's social development through their cognitions, including knowledge and beliefs about how to rear their children. Scholars have argued that having optimism or believing in the future may be a particularly important characteristic of Latino parents that may help to contribute to their children's socioemotional development (Suárez-Orozco and Suárez-Orozco 2001; Taylor et al. 2012). Being optimistic is a a protective factor against adversity and hardship and a promotive factor linked with positive developmental trajectories across ethnic and cultural groups (Carver and Scheier 2014). A study of Mexican American fathers and mothers and their teen children found that both mothers' and fathers' own reports of optimism were directly and concurrently associated with children's peer competence as well as indirectly associated through their partner's reports of positive parenting (Castro-Schilo et al. 2013).

Similarly, Latino mothers and fathers who believe that family cohesion is important (aka *familism*) have children who exhibit good psychosocial functioning (social problem solving skills, social self-efficacy; Gamble and Modry-Mandell 2008; Leidy et al. 2010; Morcillo et al. 2011; Rivera et al. 2008), have fewer depressive symptoms, and are more engaged in school (Stein et al. 2013). *Familism* might also be a protective factor that buffers children from the negative effects of environmental risk on their behaviors (German et al. 2009; Neblett et al. 2012).

There are also hints that Latino children whose parents teach them to be *bien educado* (i.e., proper demeanor and behavior) and to have *respeto* (i.e., obedience and respect to authority figures, deference) are socially competent and regulated in school settings (Calzada et al. 2010; Crosnoe 2007). Children who are polite and respectful of adults and others and show good manners are generally well liked and exhibit good social skills (Calzada et al. 2010). Zucker and Howes (2009) found that found that children whose mothers more frequently mentioned indicators of *bien educado* were reported by their teachers to have higher social skills (i.e., friendly, cooperative, and compliant behavior). Although there are no studies examining whether fathers hold similar beliefs, preliminary data show that fathers, too, endorse beliefs that promote children's skills needed to interact in social situations (Aldoney and Cabrera 2015). These correlational findings are promising and show that many minority children have early experiences that socialize them to be competent and well adjusted. The next step in this line of research is to follow-up with more rigorous designs that includes fathers.

Language Skills

Although low-income minority parents, and fathers in particular, are found to read less often to their children than their middle class counterparts (Duursma and Pan 2011; Malin et al. 2014), studies have pointed to culturally rooted ways that minority fathers and mothers may provide literacy support. Heath (1994) found that Black preschool age children were more likely to develop literacy skills through participation in narrative talk at home with their mothers and fathers than their White counterparts. Black mothers and fathers encouraged their children to begin storytelling at an early age, which increased narrative competence (Sperry and Sperry 1996). A study investigating the use of literate language features (such as noun phrases, adverbs, conjugations, and mental and linguistic verbs) in low-income Black and White preschoolers' oral narratives found no difference between the groups (Curenton and Justice 2004), suggesting that culturally diverse paths to literacy (e.g., through narrative talk or book reading at home) are successful at promoting the same literacy skills.

In addition to using narrative and storytelling, fathers can also influence their children's language skills through the quality of their linguistic interactions with them. Fathers, across minority and SES groups, have an advantage over mothers in the ways they influence the development of language skills in their children (Rowe et al. 2004; Malin et al. 2012; Pancsofar and Vernon-Feagans 2010). A large study of rural African American and White low-income two-parent families with toddlers found that father's use of vocabulary during interactions with his 6-month-old predicted children's expressive language at 3 years old, above the influence of mother's vocabulary and education (Pancsofar and Vernon-Feagans 2010). In another study, fathers use more complex language (e.g., more wh-questions, more requests for clarification) than mothers, which is associated with greater vocabulary development with their 2-year-olds (Rowe et al. 2004). Malin et al. (2012) found that compared to fathers with few depressive symptoms, fathers who reported more depressive symptoms used fewer words and less complex language with their children, which explained their children's poorer linguistic development.

Studies with low-income minority samples suggest that fathers who are responsive and engage in mutually attentive, sensitive interactions have children with stronger language and social skills (Hoff 2006; Tamis-LeMonda et al. 2004; Cabrera et al. 2007). During interactions, black fathers who reported being sensitive and responsive had children rated by their teachers as being more school ready (Black et al. 1999; Downer and Mendez 2010).

Cognitive and Academic Competence

Ethnic minority children who live with their fathers have higher levels of academic achievement and get more schooling than children who do not (McLanahan et al. 2013; Sigle-Rushton and McLanahan 2004). Latino children are more likely than other minority children to live with both parents (Crosnoe 2007).

Indisputably, fathers' income and resources make an important contribution to children's development (Duncan et al. 2014). Fathers' income and education are linked to better cognitive outcomes both directly and indirectly through the influence on the quality of the home experiences mothers provide for their children, including better parent-child interactions (Guo and Harris 2000). According to investment models, ethnic minority fathers who are more educated and have more income are able to provide material goods, such as books, toys, enriching activities, and good schools and colleges for their children that may enrich and encourage their intellectual and academic growth (Duncan et al. 2014; Guo and Harris 2000).

Fathers' economic provision is particularly important for academic outcomes when they do not reside with their children (Amato and Gilbreth 1999; Choi 2010). Informal support (e.g., cash, diapers) given directly to the mother is also related to children's higher cognitive skills (Nepomnyaschy et al. 2012, 2014). Child support among nonresident ethnic minority fathers is beneficial for children because it improves mothering behaviors and reduces parenting stress (Choi 2010; Choi and Pyun 2014).

One important way in which parents shape children's social development is by being emotionally supportive, warm, and affectionate (Feldman and Masalha 2010). Although less extensively studied, research on the quality of minority father involvement has burgeoned over the last decade showing that fathers' warmth and affection are also related to children's cognitive development (Adamson and Johnson 2013; Cabrera et al. 2014; Fagan et al. 2014; Flanders et al. 2010).

Minority fathers also positively impact their children's academic competence through the high expectations they have for their success. A study revealed that East Asian elementary school age children performed better academically than their White counterparts because of high parental (mothers' and fathers') expectations for success (Schneider and Lee 1990). Asian parents (mostly mothers) tend to structure children's extracurricular activities with an academic focus. Whether Asian fathers also structure their children's activities in the same way as mothers is unclear; this is another important area of future research.

Self-Regulatory Behaviors

Fathers' influence seems to be particularly salient in the domain of self-regulation. Reviews of the literature have shown that across a variety of ethnic groups, fathers' involvement is significantly related to children's executive functioning, self-regulation, and social competence (Adamson and Johnson 2013; Amato and Gilbreth 1999; Cabrera et al. 2014; Deater-Deckard et al. 2004; Flanders et al. 2010). A national longitudinal study of American teenagers found that teens' reports of a close, affectively warm relationship with their fathers were associated with more (self-reported) socially competent behaviors; this association was stronger for nonresident fathers (Carlson 2006). A large study of low-income

African American, White, and Latino fathers found that observed father supportiveness during an interaction with his 2-year-old was positively related to children's emotion regulation at 2 and 3 years (Cabrera et al. 2007).

Over the last decade, researchers have turned their attention to play as an important context for fathers and children's social development. Compared to mothers, middle-class fathers spend more time engaged in physical play with their toddlers than in care giving activities (Paquette 2004). One central aspect of this active, physical play (aka rough-and-tumble play; RTP), is the physical dominance that fathers display. When fathers dominate the play they provide key feedback for children to learn to regulate their emotions (Flanders et al. 2010; Fletcher et al. 2013). Observed RTP interactions between 4-year-olds and their fathers were correlated with fewer mother-reported conduct problems (Fletcher et al. 2013). When fathers were observed to be high on RTP and high on dominance during play with their toddlers, fathers rated their children as having fewer aggressive behaviors 5 years later (Flanders et al. 2010).

Policy Implications

The most salient implication emerging from the research summarized in this chapter is that families are systems that include mothers, fathers, children, and, sometimes, other relatives. Because each member of the family ecology plays a significant proximal role in shaping children's lives, supporting positive father involvement in ethnic minority families needs to be a priority for policy makers and practitioners. In numerous studies, varying in scope, methods, and samples, fathers' education, income, residence status, practices, and quality of interaction with their children as well as supportive co-parenting relationship with their partners were associated with children's adjustment, academic achievement, cognitive and language skills, and social behaviors. Many ethnic minority fathers are engaged in parenting that is of enough quality to promote their children's development.

Importantly, findings suggest that fathers' contributions are unique over and above the contributions of mothers, implying that not including them in research might underestimate parenting "effects" on children. Thus, policies and programs that include fathers, provide supports for fathers *and* mothers, and value and encourage resident and nonresident fathers' contribution to their children's well-being, beyond economic provision, should enhance the development of children. Not including fathers into programs or interventions sends a message that fathers are not as important as mothers, potentially discouraging them from continued involvement with their children. Moreover, as Sanders et al. (2007) has shown, single mothers have the highest levels of stress related to parenting, and so including fathers, even when they do not reside with their children, has the potential to indirectly promote child well-being by decreasing maternal parenting stress and thus improving mother-child relationships. These efforts require that fathers be considered assets and an untapped source of support for children and mothers, rather than as insignificant or not worth the investment.

In addition to encouraging and supporting high quality father involvement in various ways and domains, adaptive family functioning processes seen in non-minority families also support the positive development of ethnic minority children, both as promotive factors for all children and as protective factors for children living in disadvantage. Building on these strengths will enhance the efficacy of policies and programs aimed at improving the lives of ethnic minority families and their children. For example, programs that promote positive mothering and fathering and build family cohesion should contribute to children's positive development (e.g., Building Strong Families Project). Programs that assist fathers and mothers in identifying the specific ways in which they promote their children's development are another way of promoting positive development (e.g., Head Start; Fagan and Iglesias 1999). Finally, school policies and programs that acknowledge that many nonresident fathers want to be involved (spend time) in their children's lives could support them and contribute to children's well-being in these families.

Through Responsible Fatherhood Programs (RFPs), a substantial amount of federal money has been allotted to improving father involvement among low-income, minority, and at risk families (Karberg et al. 2016). These programs are specifically targeted to nonresident, low-income, ethnic minority fathers and are aimed at improving fathers' relationships with partners; parenting skills; and, financial responsibility (US HHS 2014). Although the evaluation of these findings is not yet available, the programs' delivery varies from program to program, with many programs not including mothers, for example, or even children (US HHS 2014). Whether or not these programs will be effective is an open question.

The review in this chapter suggests that fathers' levels of education and income, cultural values and beliefs, and the quality of their relationship with their partners are significantly related to increasing positive involvement in their children's lives. Currently funded RFPs already include curricula to improve men's human capital, manage depression stress and improve parenting [e.g., 24/7 Dads; The ABC(3) D approach (2014)], and improve the co-parenting relationship (Avellar et al. 2011; Wood et al. 2014). However, to improve co-parenting both parents must be present (Feinberg et al. 2010), though this is not the case in any current RFPs programs. If the ultimate goal is to improve children's well-being, programmatic efforts that include only one member of the system (either mother or father) may not be as effective as efforts that include both.

Another important implication from this overview is that father' cultural values and beliefs as well as their strong ethnic identity are significantly related to their involvement with their children. Programs that help fathers maintain their cultural identities while adapting to life in America (e.g., learning English) are beneficial for fathers and children. Building ethnic minority fathers' human capital and at the same time helping them to be proud and retain their culture are important ways to improve fathers and

children's well-being. Currently, HHS is investigating the ways in which RFPs address the needs of Latino men and how programs provide services in a cultural context (Avellar et al. 2011; Cabrera et al. 2013).

Future Directions

Research on the specific pathways that link positive fathering to children's positive development is in its infancy, although it is steadily growing. The focus on positive development of minority ethnic children has prompted many scholars to worry that by focusing on positive development, the research community might de-emphasize the adversity that many low-income minority families and their children face. They need not worry. A focus on positive outcome is an effort to provide a balance and comprehensive portrait of the positive and negative outcomes; of the strengths and liabilities. Only by having a clear sense of what is promotive or protective can limited resources be allocated judiciously and effectively to improve children's lives.

To date, research on positive development of ethnic minority children has not examined how specific aspects of culture (e.g., cultural values) foster positive development (Evans et al. 2012). Yet, for ethnic minority children, (bi)cultural factors are integral to their developmental experiences. The high and growing number of bicultural children in the United States demands greater attention to the universal and unique family process that promote positive child development (Costigan and colleagues, this volume). Research that has included cultural models in the study of positive development of young children is just emerging and consequently limited. However, these models often treat culture as static and non-changing and as if culture is only important for minority families. But culture is dynamic and changes all the time, thus models of culture need to account for it by incorporating reflective ways in which parents evaluate the value of cultural norms as being adaptive or maladaptive for rearing children.

With some exceptions (e.g., Cabrera et al. 2007; Deater-Deckard et al. 2004; Flanders et al. 2010; Malin et al. 2012), little research has examined the role of fathers in promoting *domains of positive child development*, such as language skills, social behaviors, self-regulation, and literacy. The myriad ways in which positive development might be defined differently in diverse ethnic groups that are also acculturating to the norms and values of the United States are missing from research. There is cultural variability regarding what cultures value or find relevant at different points in time along the lifespan and under certain conditions. Because American ethnic minority children are developing in a bicultural context, there is a need to understand what parents value of their own country and of their host country to pass on to their children. The immigration context might provide a particular important opportunity for immigrant parents to be reflective about the values they pass on (or not) to their children.

The bulk of the research on positive father involvement focuses on early childhood. More research attention is needed on the transition into middle school and into adulthood for ethnic minority children. Specifically, there is a need to understand how fathers navigate the interface between home and school and how they facilitate successful transitions. As children grow they develop the skills that will help them learn, have positive peer relationships, get along with others and eventually contribute meaningfully to society. Ethnic minority children may experience extra pressures as they become competent in two cultural settings that may necessitate them learning two languages and two sets of social norms. Future research should explore how Latino fathers promote their young children's bilingualism or social skills.

As with the study of parenting, in general, the lack of longitudinal data has been a barrier to understanding processes and the direction of associations among constructs of interest. To date, there are no experimental and observational studies to understand the "impact" of fathering behaviors on children's development. The research base on fathering is mostly correlational

and limited. Studies that report "parental" correlates are mostly based on mothers, which are not parenting research. We need more studies that include both parents to enable researchers to systematically address unique and interaction associations between mothers and fathers and children's development. Additionally, there is a need for more diverse and large representative samples that include varied community contexts and middle class minority families so that we can begin to address the confound that exists today in most research on minority families that is based mostly on low-income samples.

Research methods and questions in this area would also benefit from better conceptualization models of father involvement and what it means to be a father. Until researchers are more able to clearly define father involvement, measurement of the construct will remain vague and overlapping. There is an urgent need to provide the burgeoning field with a set of measures and tools to assess fathering behaviors that capture the developmental needs of children. Measures of father involvement need to be examined side by side with measures of mother involvement to understand what adjustments need to be made and then determine whether these tools help us to understand the unique and shared role of mothers and fathers. Moreover, research methods need to grapple with what constitutes a family by including diverse types of family structures, different roles of different family members, and the interaction among them.

Additionally, more attention needs to be paid to how to conceptualize and assess nonresident father involvement. Although we have made some progress in more clearly delineating the financial and social contributions of nonresident fathers, we would benefit from efforts that include fathers' own reports of the amount and quality of fathers' relationships with their children. These efforts would necessitate federal and policy leadership that purposefully allocates resources to sample fathers and mothers, not just mothers in research designs. Currently, the expense of locating and including fathers into research designs excludes fathers from the onset and makes them optional. The research infrastructure needs to change if we are going to make headway in including both parents in parenting research.

Lastly, research examining how culture, broadly defined, provides a context for fathering should be more theoretically motivated. If there is no theoretical reason to expect differences among cultural groups, then researchers should not compare them. Statistically comparing different groups can lead to deficit thinking in terms of minority families' outcomes.

Conclusions

The study of how ethnic minority fathers influence their children's development using a strengths-based approach is a relatively new area of inquiry, and consequently many questions remain unanswered. The research reviewed in this chapter identifies the ways in which fathers' foster positive development among ethnic minority children. The consistent associations between fathers' education, income, cognitions, parenting practices and relationship with children's positive development underscore the importance of supporting fathers (and mothers) in this process. Cultural values and beliefs (e.g., *familism*) also buffer the adverse impacts of contextual threats, such as depression and anxiety, on children's positive development. Further, the research reviewed in this chapter suggests that minority fathers can and do engage in positive interactions with their children that are promotive, even as they parent in a context of poverty. Future research that is framed from a positive development point of view, rather than a deficit model, may reveal further beneficial aspects to father involvement in a specific cultural context. Areas of positive child development that have not yet been addressed (e.g., social skills) should also be incorporated into future research. Finally, policies and programs to support positive development among ethnic minority children will be advanced by research that acknowledges that fathers are parents, too. Fathers make a unique contribution to children's positive development and in doing so they need to be included in any research on parenting or in any program/intervention aimed at improving children's lives.

References

Adamson, K., & Johnson, S. K. (2013). An updated and expanded meta-analysis of nonresident fathering and child well-being. *Journal of Family Psychology, 27* (4), 589–599.

Aldoney, D., & Cabrera, N. J. (2015). The early cultural socialization context of Latino children in immigrant families.. In B. E. Kurtz-Costes (Chair), *Racial and ethnic socialization and identity development in African American and Latino families.* Paper presented at the Society for Research in Child Development (SRCD), Philadelphia, PA.

Amato, P. R., & Gilbreth, J. G. (1999). Nonresident fathers and children's well-being: A meta-analysis. *Journal of Marriage and Family, 61*(3), 557–573.

Arditti, J. A., Smock, S. A., & Parkman, T. S. (2005). It's been hard to be a father: A qualitative exploration of incarcerated fatherhood. *Fathering, 3*(3), 267–288.

Argys, L. M., Peters, H. E., Brooks-Gunn, J., & Smith, J. R. (1998). The impact of child support on cognitive outcomes of young children. *Demography, 35*(2), 159–173.

Avellar, S., Dio, M. R., Clarkwest, A., Zaveri, H., Asheer, S., Borradaille, K., et al. (2011). *Catalog of research: Programs for low-income fathers (Report 2011–2020).* Washington, DC: Mathematica Policy Research.

Baer, J. C., & Schmitz, M. F. (2007). Ethnic differences in trajectories of family cohesion for Mexican American and non-Hispanic White adolescents. *Journal of Youth and Adolescence, 36*(4), 583–592.

Belsky, J., Rovine, M., & Taylor, D. G. (1984). The pennsylvania infant and family development project, III: The origins of individual differences in infant-mother attachment: Maternal and infant contributions. *Child Development, 55*(3), 718–728.

Black, M. M., Dubowitz, H., & Star, R. H. (1999). African American fathers in low income, urban families: Development, behavior, and home environment of their three-year-old children. *Child Development, 70*(4), 967–978.

Bornstein, M. H. (2015). Children's parents. In M. H. Bornstein & T. Leventhal (Eds.), *Ecological settings and processes in developmental systems.* In R. M. Lerner (Editor-in-chief), *Handbook of child psychology and developmental science* (7th Ed., Vol. 4, pp. 55–132). Hoboken, NJ: Wiley.

Bornstein, M. H., Gini, M., Putnick, D. L., Haynes, O. M., Painter, K. M., & Suwalsky, J. T. D. (2006). Short-term reliability and continuity of emotional availability in mother–child dyads across contexts of observation. *Infancy, 10*(1), 1–16.

Bretherton, I. (2010). Fathers in attachment theory and research: A review. *Early Child Development and Care, 180*(1), 9–23.

Bronfenbrenner, U., & Morris, P. A. (1998). The ecology of developmental processes. In W. Damon & R. M. Lerner (Eds.), *Handbook of child psychology: Theoretical models of human development* (Vol. 1, 5th Ed., pp. 993–1028). Hoboken, NJ: Wiley.

Cabrera, N. (2013). *Positive development of minority children* (Social Policy Review V27, No. 2). Retrieved from Society for Research in Child Development website:http://www.srcd.org/sites/default/files/documents/washington/spr_272_final.pdf

Cabrera, N. J., Aldoney, D., & Tamis-LeMonda, C. S. (2013). Latino fathers. In N. J. Cabrera & C. S. Tamis-LeMonda (Eds.), *Handbook of father involvement: Multidisciplinary perspectives* (2nd ed., pp. 244–260). New York: Taylor & Francis.

Cabrera, N. J., Cook, G. A., McFadden, K. E., & Bradley, R. H. (2011a). Father residence and father-child relationship quality: Peer relationships and externalizing behavioral problems. *Family Science, 2*(2), 109–119.

Cabrera, N. J., Fitzgerald, H. E., Bradley, R. H., & Roggman, L. (2014). The ecology of father-child relationships: An expanded model. *Journal of Family Theory and Review, 6*(4), 336–354.

Cabrera, N. J., Hofferth, S. L., & Chae, S. (2011b). Patterns and predictors of father-infant engagement across race/ethnic groups. *Early Child Research Quarterly, 26*(3), 365–375.

Cabrera, N., Moore, K., Bronte-Tinkew, J., Halle, T., West, J., Brooks-Gunn, J., et al. (2004). The DADS initiative: Measuring father involvement in large-scale surveys. In R. D. Day & M. Lamb (Eds.), *Conceptualizing and measuring father involvement* (pp. 417–452). Mahwah, NJ: Lawrence Erlbaum Associates Inc.

Cabrera, N. J., Ryan, R. M., Mitchell, S. J., Shannon, J. D., & Tamis-LeMonda, C. S. (2008). Low-income, nonresident father involvement with their toddlers: Variation by fathers' race and ethnicity. *Journal of Family Psychology, 22*(4), 643–647.

Cabrera, N. J., Shannon, J. E., & La Taillade, J. J. (2010). Predictors of co-parenting in Mexican American families and direct effects on parenting and child social emotional development. *Infant Mental Health Journal, 30*(5), 523–548.

Cabrera, N. J., Shannon, J. E., & Tamis-LeMonda, C. S. (2007). Fathers' influence on their children's cognitive and emotional development: From toddlers to pre-K. *Applied Developmental Science, 11*(4), 208–213.

Cabrera, N., Shannon, J., West, J., & Brooks-Gunn, J. (2006). Parental interactions with Latino infants: Variation by country of origin and English proficiency. *Child Development, 77*(6), 1190–1207.

Cabrera, N. J., Tamis-LeMonda, C. S., Bradley, R. H., Hofferth, S., & Lamb, M. E. (2000). Fatherhood in the twenty-first century. *Child Development, 71*(1), 127–136.

Calzada, E. J., Fernandez, Y., & Cortes, D. E. (2010). Incorporating the cultural value of respeto into a framework of Latino parenting. *Cultural Diversity & Ethnic Minority Psychology, 16*(1), 77–86.

Capps, R. C., Bronte-Tinkew, J., & Horowitz, A. (2010). Acculturation and father engagement with infants among Chinese and Mexican-origin immigrant fathers. *Fathering, 8*(1), 61–92.

Carlson, M. J. (2006). Family structure, father involvement, and adolescent behavioral outcomes. *Journal of Marriage and Family, 68*(1), 137–154.

Carlson, M. J., & Magnuson, K. A. (2011). Low-income fathers' influence on children. *The ANNALS of the American Academy of Political and Social Science, 635*(1), 95–116.

Carlson, M. J., McLanahan, S. S., & Brooks-Gunn, J. (2008). Coparenting and nonresident fathers' involvement with young children after a nonmarital birth. *Demography, 45*(2), 461–488.

Carver, C. S., & Scheier, M. F. (2014). Dispositional optimism. *Trends in Cognitive Sciences, 18*, 293–299.

Carver, C. S., Scheier, M. F., & Segerstrom, S. C. (2010). Optimism. *Clinical Psychology Review, 30*, 879–889.

Castillo, J., Welch, G., & Sarver, C. (2011). Fathering: The relationship between fathers' residence, fathers' sociodemographic characteristics, and father involvement. *Maternal and Child Health Journal, 15*(8), 1342–1349.

Castro-Schilo, L., Taylor, Z. E., Ferrer, E., Robins, R. W., Conger, R. D., Widaman, K. F. (2013) Parents' optimism, positive parenting, and child peer social competence in Mexican-origin families. *Parenting: Science and Practice 13*(2), 95–112.

Choi, J. (2010). Nonresident fathers' parenting, family processes, and children's development in urban, poor, single-mother families. *Social Service Review, 84*(4), 655–677.

Choi, J., & Pyun, H. (2014). Nonresident fathers' financial support, informal instrumental support, mothers' parenting, and child development in single-mother families with low income. *Journal of Family Issues, 35*(4), 526–546.

Coley, R. L. (2003). Daughter-father relationships and adolescent psychosocial functioning in low-income African American families. *Journal of Marriage and Family, 65*(5), 867–875.

Coley, R. L., & Morris, J. E. (2002). Comparing father and mother reports of father involvement among low-income minority families. *Journal of Marriage and Family, 64*(7), 982–997.

Collins, W. A., Maccoby, E. E., Steinberg, L., Hetherington, E. M., & Bornstein, M. H. (2000). Contemporary research on parenting: The case for nature and nurture. *American Psychologist, 55*(2), 218–232.

Coltrane, S. (2000). Research on household labor: Modeling and measuring the social embeddedness of routine family work. *Journal of Marriage and Family, 62*(4), 1208–1233.

Coltrane, S., Parke, R. D., & Adams, M. (2004). Complexity of father involvement in low-income Mexican American families. *Family Relations, 53*(2), 179–189.

Craig, L. (2006). Does father care mean fathers share? A comparison of how mothers and fathers in intact families spend time with children. *Gender and Society, 20*(2), 259–281.

Crosnoe, R. (2007). Early child care and the school readiness of children from Mexican immigrant families. *International Migration Review, 41*(1), 152–181.

Cruz, R. A., King, K. M., Widaman, K. F., Leu, J., Cauce, A. M., & Conger, R. D. (2011). Cultural influences on positive father involvement in two-parent Mexican-origin families. *Journal of Family Psychology, 25*(5), 731–740.

Curenton, S., & Justice, L. (2004). African American and Caucasian preschoolers' use of decontextualized language: Literate language features in oral narratives. *Language, Speech & Hearing Services in Schools, 35*(3), 240–253.

Deater-Deckard, K., Atzaba-Poria, N., & Pike, A. (2004). Mother- and father-child mutuality in Anglo and Indian British families: A link with lower externalizing problems in middle childhood. *Journal of Abnormal Child Psychology, 32*(6), 609–620.

Downer, J., & Mendez, J. (2010). African American father involvement and preschool children's school readiness. *Early Education and Development, 16*(3), 317–334.

Duncan, G. J., Magnuson, K., & Votruba-Drzal, E. (2014). Boosting family income to promote child development. *The Future of Children, 24*(1), 99–120.

Duursma, E., & Pan, B. A. (2011). Who's reading to children in low-income families? The influence of paternal, maternal and child characteristics. *Early Child Development and Care, 181*(9), 1163–1180.

Evans, A. B., Banerjee, M., Meyer, R., Aldana, A., Foust, M., & Rowley, S. (2012). Racial socialization as a mechanism for positive development among African American Youth. *Child Development Perspectives, 6*(3), 251–257.

Fagan, J., & Barnett, M. (2003). The relationship between maternal gatekeeping, paternal competence, mothers' attitudes about the father role, and father involvement. *Journal of Family Issues, 24*(8), 1020–1043.

Fagan, J., Day, R., Lamb, M., & Cabrera, N. (2014). Should researchers conceptualize fathering and mothering differently? *Journal of Family Theory and Review, 6*(4), 390–405.

Fagan, J., & Iglesias, A. (1999). Father involvement program effects on fathers, father figures, and their Head Start children: A quasi-experimental study. *Early Childhood Research Quarterly, 14*(2), 243–269.

Fagan, J., & Palkovitz, R. (2011). Co-parenting and relationship quality effects on father engagement: Variations by residence, romance. *Journal of Marriage and Family, 73*(3), 637–653.

Feinberg, M. (2003). The internal structure and ecological context of coparenting: A framework for research and intervention. *Parenting: Science and Practice, 3*(1), 95–132.

Feinberg, M., Jones, D. E., Kan, M. L., & Goslin, M. C. (2010). Effects of family foundations on parents and children: 3.5 years after baseline. *Journal of Family Psychology, 24*(5), 532–542.

Feldman, R., & Masalha, S. (2010). Parent-child and triadic antecedents of children's social competence: Cultural specificity, shared process. *Developmental Psychology, 46*(2), 455–467.

Flanders, J. L., Simard, M., Paquette, D., Parent, S., Vitaro, F., Pihl, R. O., et al. (2010). Rough-and-tumble play and the development of physical aggression and emotion regulation: A five year follow-up study. *Journal of Family Violence, 25*(4), 357–367.

Fletcher, R., StGeorge, J., & Freeman, E. (2013). Rough and tumble play quality: Theoretical foundations for a new measure of father-child interaction. *Early Child Development and Care, 183*(6), 746–759.

Flouri, E., & Buchanan, A. (2004). Early father's and mother's involvement and child's later educational outcomes. *British Journal of Educational Psychology, 74*(1), 141–153.

Gamble, W. C., & Modry-Mandell, K. L. (2008). Family relations and the adjustment of young children of Mexican descent: Do cultural values moderate these associations? *Social Development, 17*, 358–379.

Ganong, L., Coleman, M., & Russell, L. T. (2015). Children in diverse families. In M. H. Bornstein & T. Leventhal (Eds.), *Ecological settings and processes in developmental systems*. In R. M. Lerner (Editor-in-chief), *Handbook of child psychology and developmental science* (7th ed., Vol. 4, pp. 133–174). Hoboken, NJ: Wiley.

García Coll, C., Lamberty, G., Jenkins, R., McAdoo, H. P., Crnic, K., Wasik, B. H., et al. (1996). An integrative model for the study of developmental competencies in minority children. *Child Development, 67*(6), 1891–1914.

German, M., Gonzales, N. A., & Dumka, L. (2009). Familism values as a protective factor for Mexican-origin adolescents exposed to deviant peers. *The Journal of Early Adolescence, 29*(1), 16–42.

Grall T. (2013). *Custodial mothers and fathers and their child support: 2011*. http://www.census.gov/prod/2013pubs/p.60-246.pdf

Grossmann, K. E., Grossmann, K., Kindler, H., & Zimmermann, P. (2008). A wider view of attachment and exploration: The influence of mothers and fathers on the development of psychological security from infancy to young adulthood. In J. Cassidy & P. Shaver (Eds.), *Handbook of attachment theory and research*. New York: Guilford.

Grusec, J. E., & Davidov, M. (2010). Integrating different perspectives on socialization theory and research: A domain-specific approach. *Child Development, 81*(5), 687–709.

Guerra, N. G., Graham, S., & Tolan, P. H. (2011). Raising healthy children: Translating research into practice. *Special Issue of Child Development on Raising Healthy Children, 82*(1), 7–16.

Guo, G., & Harris, K. M. (2000). The mechanisms mediating the effects of poverty on children's intellectual development. *Demography, 37*(4), 431–447.

Guzzo, K. B. (2009). Paternity establishment for men's nonmarital births. *Population Research and Policy Review, 28*(6), 853–872.

Harwood, R. L. (2006). Multidimensional culture and the search for universals. *Human Development, 49*(1), 122–128.

Heath, S. B. (1994). What no bedtime story means: Narrative skills at home and school. In B. B. Schieffelin & E. Ochs (Eds.), *Language socialization across cultures* (pp. 97–124). Cambridge, UK: Cambridge University.

Hoff, E. (2006). How social contexts support and shape language development. *Developmental Review, 26*(1), 55–88.

Hofferth, S. L. (2003). Race/ethnic differences in father involvement in two-parent families culture, context, or economy? *Journal of Family Issues, 24*(2), 185–216.

Hohmann-Mariott, B. (2011). Coparenting and father involvement in married and unmarried coresident couples. *Journal of Marriage and Family, 73*(1), 296–309.

Humes, K. R., Jones, N. A., & Ramirez, R. R. (2011). *Overview of race and Hispanic origin: 2010.* http://www.census.gov/prod/cen2010/briefs/c2010br-02.pdf

Jain, A., & Belsky, J. (1997). Fathering and acculturation: A study of immigrant Indian families with young children. *Journal of Marriage and the Family, 59*(4), 873–883.

Jones, J., & Mosher, W. D. (2013). Fathers' involvement with their children: United States, 2006–2010. *National Health Statistics Reports, 71*(1), 1–21.

Kane, J. B., Nelson, T. J., & Edin, K. (2015). How much in-kind support do low-income nonresident fathers provide? A mixed-method analysis. *Journal of Marriage and Family.* Advanced online publication. doi:10.1111/jomf.12188

Kao, G., & Tienda, M. (1995). Optimism and achievement: The educational performance of immigrant youth. *Social Science Quarterly, 76*(1), 1–19.

Karberg, E., Aldoney, D., & Cabrera, N. J. (2016). Fatherhood policies and programs in America. In A. Marin (Ed.), *Families in context.* Westport, CT: Praeger.

Koball, H. L., & Principe, D. (2002). *Do nonresident fathers who pay child support visit their children more* (Report No. B-44)? Retrieved from Urban Institute website: http://www.urban.org/index.cfm

Kochanska, G., Aksan, N., Prisco, T. R., & Adams, E. E. (2008). Mother-child and father-child mutually responsive orientation in the first 2 years and children's outcomes at preschool age: Mechanisms of influence. *Child Development, 79*(1), 30–44.

Kulik, L., & Tsoref, H. (2010). The entrance to the maternal garden: Environmental and personal variables that explain maternal gatekeeping. *Journal of Gender Studies, 19*(3), 263–277.

Lachance-Grzela, M., & Bouchard, G. (2010). Why do women do the lion's share of housework? A decade of research. *Sex Roles, 63*(11/12), 767–780.

Lamb, M. E. (2000). The history of research on father involvement: An overview. *Marriage & Family Review, 29*(2–3), 23–42.

Leavell Smith, A., Tamis-LeMonda, C. S., Ruble, D. R., Zosuls, K., & Cabrera, N. C. (2012). African-American, White, and Latino Fathers' activities with their sons and daughters across early childhood. *Sex Roles, 66*(1), 53–65.

Leidy, M. S., Guerra, N. G., & Toro, R. I. (2010). Positive parenting, family cohesion, and child social competence among immigrant Latino families. *Journal of Family Psychology, 24*(3), 252–260.

Lerner, J. V., Phelps, E., Forman, Y. E., & Bowers, E. P. (2009). *Positive youth development. Handbook of adolescent psychology.* Hoboken, NJ: Wiley.

Lewis, C. (1997). Fathers and preschoolers. In M. E. Lamb (Ed.), *The role of the father in child development* (3rd ed., pp. 121–142). Hoboken, NJ: Wiley.

Lewis, C., & Lamb, M. E. (2003). Fathers' influences on children's development: The evidence from two-parent families. *European Journal of Psychology and Education, 18*(2), 211–228.

Malin, J. L., Cabrera, N. J., & Rowe, M. L. (2014). Low-income minority mothers' and fathers' reading and children's interest: Longitudinal contributions to children's receptive vocabulary skills. *Early Childhood Research Quarterly, 29*(4), 425–432.

Malin, J. L., Karberg, E., Cabrera, N. J., Rowe, M., Cristofaro, T., & Tamis-LeMonda, C. S. (2012). Father-toddler communication in low-income families: The role of paternal education and depressive symptoms. *Family Science, 3*(3–4), 155–163.

Manning, W. D., & Brown, S. (2006). Children's economic well-being in married and cohabiting parent families. *Journal of Marriage and Family, 68*(2), 345–362.

Masten, A. S., & Wright, M. O'. D. (2009). Resilience over the lifespan: Developmental perspectives on resistance, recovery, and transformation. In J. W. Reich, A. J. Zautra, & J. S. Hall (Eds.), *Handbook of adult resilience* (pp. 213–237). New York: Guilford.

McLanahan, S., Tach, L., & Schneider, D. (2013). The causal effects of father absence. *Annual Review of Sociology, 39*(1), 399–427.

Mead, L. (1991). The new politics of poverty. *The Public Interest, 91*(103), 3–20.

Mesman, J., van IJzendoorn, M. H., & Bakermans-Kranenburg, M. J. (2012). Unequal in opportunity, equal in process: Parental sensitivity promotes positive child development in ethnic minority families. *Child Development Perspectives, 6*(3), 239–250.

Mikelson, K. (2008). He said, she said: Comparing mother and father reports of father involvement. *Journal of Marriage and Family, 70*(5), 613–624.

Mitchell, S. J., See, H. M., Tarkow, A. K. H., Cabrera, N., McFadden, K. E., & Shannon, J. D. (2009).

Conducing studies with fathers: Challenges and opportunities. *Applied Developmental Science, 11*(4), 239–244.

Morcillo, C., Duarte, C. S., Shen, S., Blanco, C., Canino, G., & Bird, H. R. (2011). Parental familism and antisocial behaviors: Development, gender and potential mechanisms. *Journal of the American Academy of Child and Adolescent Psychiatry, 50*(5), 471–479.

Neblett, E. W., Rivas-Drake, D., & Umaña-Taylor, A. J. (2012). The promise of racial and ethnic protective factors in promoting ethnic minority youth development. *Child Development Perspective, 6*(3), 295–303.

Nepomnyaschy, L., Magnuson, K. A., & Berger, L. (2012). Child support and young children's development. *Social Service Review, 86*(1), 3–35.

Nepomnyaschy, L., Miller, D. P., Garasky, S., & Nanda, N. (2014). Nonresident fathers and child food insecurity: Evidence from longitudinal data. *Social Service Review, 88*(1), 92–133.

Notaro, P. C., & Volling, B. L. (1999). Parental responsiveness and infant-parent attachment: A replication study with fathers and mothers. *Infant Behavior and Development, 22*(3), 345–352.

Osborne, C., Manning, W., & Smock, P. (2007). Married and cohabiting parents' relationship stability: A focus on race and ethnicity. *Journal of Marriage and Family, 69*(5), 1345–1366.

Palkovitz, R. (2007). Challenges to modeling dynamics in a developmental understanding of father-child relationships. *Journal of Applied Developmental Science, 11*(2), 190–195.

Pancsofar, N., & Vernon-Feagans, L. (2010). Fathers' early contributions to children's language development in families from low-income rural communities. *Early Childhood Research Quarterly, 25*(4), 450–463.

Paquette, D. (2004). Theorizing the father-child relationship: Mechanisms and developmental outcomes. *Human Development, 47*(4), 193–219.

Paquette, D., & Dumont, C. (2013). The father-child activation relationship, sex differences, and attachment disorganization in toddlerhood. *Child Development Research*. http://www.hindawi.com/journals/cdr/2013/102860/

Perry, K. H. (2008). From storytelling to writing: Transforming literacy practices among Sudanese refugees. *Journal of Literacy Research, 40*(2), 317–358.

Phinney, J. S., Ong, A., & Madden, T. (2000). Cultural values and intergenerational value discrepancies in immigrant and non-immigrant families. *Child Development, 71*(2), 528–539.

Potochnick, S. R., & Perreira, K. M. (2010). Depression and anxiety among first-generation immigrant Latino youth: Key correlates and implications for future research. *The Journal of Nervous and Mental Disease, 198*(7), 470–477.

Rivera, F., Guarnaccia, P., Mulvaney-Day, N., Lin, J., Torres, M., & Alegria, M. (2008). Family cohesion and its relationship to psychological distress among Latino Groups. *Hispanic Journal of Behavioral Science, 30*(3), 357–378.

Rowe, M. L., Coker, D., & Pan, B. A. (2004). A comparison of fathers' and mothers' talk to toddlers in low-income families. *Social Development, 13*(2), 278–291.

Sanders, M. R., Bor, W., & Morawska, A. (2007). *J Abnorm Child Psychol, 35,* 983. doi:10.1007/s10802-007-9148-x

Sarkadi, A., Kristiansson, R., Oberklaid, F., & Bremberg, S. (2008). Fathers' involvement and children's developmental outcomes: A systematic review of longitudinal studies. *Acta Paediatrica, 97*(2), 153–158.

Sayer, L. C., Bianchi, S. M., & Robinson, J. P. (2004). Trends in mothers' and fahters' time with children. *American Journal of Sociology, 110*(1), 1–43.

Schneider, B., & Lee, Y. (1990). A model for academic success: The school and home environment of East Asian students. *Anthropology & Education Quarterly, 21*(4), 358–377.

Sigle-Rushton, W., & McLanahan, S. (2004). *Father absence and child well-being: A critical review.* New York: Russell Sage Foundation.

Smokowski, P. R., Rose, R., & Bacallao, M. (2008). Acculturation and Latino family processes: How parent-adolescent acculturation gaps influence family dynamics. *Family Relations, 57*(3), 295–308.

Sperry, L. L., & Sperry, D. E. (1996). Early development of narrative skills. *Cognitive Development, 11*(3), 443–465.

Stein, G. L., Gonzalez, L. M., Cupito, A. M., Kiang, L., & Supple, A. J. (2013). The protective role of familism in the lives of Latino adolescents. *Journal of Family Issues.* http://libres.uncg.edu/ir/uncg/f/A_Supple_Protective_2013.pdf

Suárez-Orozco, C., & Suárez-Orozco, M. (2001). *Children of immigration.* Cambridge, MA: Harvard University Press.

Tach, L., Mincy, R., & Edin, K. (2010). Parenting as a "package deal": Relationships, fertility, and nonresident father involvement among unmarried parents. *Demography, 47*(1), 181–204.

Tamis-LeMonda, C. S., Shannon, J. D., Cabrera, N. J., & Lamb, M. E. (2004). Fathers and mothers at play with their 2-and 3-year-olds: Contributions to language and cognitive development. *Child Development, 75*(6), 1806–1820.

Taylor, Z. E., Widaman, K. F., Robins, R. W., Jochem, R., Early, D. R., & Conger, R. D. (2012). Dispositional optimism: A psychological resource for

Mexican-origin mothers experiencing economic stress. *Journal of Family Psychology, 26*(1), 133–139.

Texas Attorney General. (2004). Retrieved from https://www.texasattorneygeneral.gov/cs/attorneys/crimnonsup/crimnonsuphb_ch11.shtml#ch11_custody

The ABC(3) D approach. (2014). Retreived from, http://www.copes.org/abc3d.php

Umaña-Taylor, A. J., & Bámaca, M. Y. (2004). Conducting focus groups with Latino populations: Lessons from the field. *Family Relations, 53*(3), 261–272.

U.S. Department of Health and Human Services (HHS). (2014). *Promoting responsible fatherhood grants.* http://fatherhood.hhs.gov/2010Initiative/index.shtml

Weisner, T. S. (2009). Culture, development, and diversity: Expectable pluralism and expectable conflict. *Ethos, 37*(2), 181–196.

Wilson, M., & Brooks-Gunn, J. (2001). Health status and behaviors of unwed fathers. *Children and Youth Services Review, 23*(2), 377–401.

Wood, R. G., Moore, Q., Clarkwest, A., & Killewald, A. (2014). The long-term effects of building strong families: A program for unmarried parents. *Journal of Marriage and Family, 76*(2), 446–463.

Yeung, W. J., Sandberg, J. F., Davis-Kean, P. E., & Hofferth, S. L. (2001). Children's time with fathers in intact families. *Journal of Marriage and Family, 63*(1), 136–154.

Zucker, E., & Howes, C. (2009). Respectful relationships: Socialization goals and practices among Mexican Mothers. *Infant Mental Health Journal, 30*(5), 501–522.

Language and Parenting: Minority Languages in North America

Allyssa McCabe

Abstract

Numerous children in North America speak a dialect and/or languages other than those in which they are schooled and can acquire new languages without jeopardizing their heritage languages. Current research questions regarding the impact of bilingualism have documented many positive results, countering the negative findings of older studies that confounded socioeconomic status with bilingualism. Accurate assessment of bilingual children with typical and atypical language development remains challenging despite a great deal of work on this subject and some progress. Early and frequent exposure to high-quality diverse and responsive input from speakers of multiple languages, along with continued support for those languages, results in optimal academic success for bilingual children regardless of whether they are typically or atypically developing. Universal versus culture-specific mechanisms, future directions for research, and policy implications are discussed. Parents should be encouraged to speak frequently and positively with their children using whatever language(s) and/or dialect(s) they are comfortable speaking.

Historical Overview and Theoretical Perspectives

Many North Americans speak a minority language at home at least some of the time. According to the National Center for Education Statistics

(http://nces.ed.gov/fastfacts/display.asp?id=96), the percentage of public school students in the United States who were classified as English Language Learners was "higher in school year 2011–2012 (9.1 %, or an estimated 4.4 million students) than in 2002–2003 (8.7 %, or an estimated 4.1 million students."). Similarly, Canadian Census data reveal numerous individuals—one in five in 2006—whose mother tongue was neither English nor French, but rather an aboriginal or nonaboriginal non-official language (http://www.statcan.gc.ca/daily-quotidien/071204/dq071204a-eng.htm).

A. McCabe (✉)
University of Massachusetts Lowell, Lowell, MA, USA
e-mail: Allyssa_mccabe@uml.edu

© The Editor(s) 2017
N.J. Cabrera and B. Leyendecker (eds.), *Handbook on Positive Development of Minority Children and Youth*, DOI 10.1007/978-3-319-43645-6_13

This chapter will address optimal parenting practices for the millions of North American children who speak minority languages at home.

The Yiddish scholar Max Weinreich reportedly overheard and subsequently made known a wise remark that "A language is a dialect with an army and a navy." Thus, my definition of minority languages in this chapter will include non-standard dialects such as Black English Vernacular (also known as African American English; Labov 1972), Pennsylvania Dutch (Adkins 2011), or Appalachian English. The number of children who speak a non-standard dialect of North American languages is quite large. Add to these, non-oral languages such as American Sign Language for Deaf and Hard of Hearing (DHH) children, and the numbers are even higher.

Whereas Canada is officially a bilingual nation, the United States has had a history of ambivalence or even antagonism towards speaking any language other than English. For example, in 1993, Ron Unz, a wealthy businessman, began his campaign to outlaw bilingual education in the U.S. (Ryan 2002). However, researchers who study multilingualism have documented its many advantages in general and advantages of bilingual education in particular.

Fear of children speaking minority languages stems in part from an unfortunate view that bilingualism is subtractive. That is, that the more children speak a language other than standard English, for example, the less they will become capable of speaking English. There are cases of subtractive bilingualism (Baker and Hornberger 2001). Some children from low socioeconomic backgrounds come to preschool in the United States speaking a language other than English and do in fact fail to acquire enough English to succeed at school, whereas others become adept in English at the expense of their original language. The fear that bilingualism is inevitably subtractive lies behind outmoded notions such as the one that forbade deaf children to use sign language lest it would somehow prevent them from using other forms of communication.

However, modern researchers of bilingual language development, some well-educated and usually affluent parents,—and countries such as Canada—subscribe to a different view, namely that *bilingualism can be additive* so long as there is ample support in families, schools, and larger communities for speaking and becoming literate in more than one language (De Houwer 1990).

In addition to the notion of additive bilingualism, two other theoretical perspectives are important for this chapter: (1) social interactionism is the account of how language is acquired subscribed to by the author, and (2) the Comprehensive Language Account of early literacy (Dickinson et al. 2003) defines the scope of language abilities to be addressed. First, the more children are exposed to any particular language, the more they will become capable of using that language. Children learn a language through social interaction with more competent speakers of a language. Hart and Risley (1995) documented the fact that monolingual children born into lower socioeconomic (SES) groups are exposed to substantially less conversation and substantially less positive conversation than their peers born into higher SES groups and that this difference has an enormous impact on the children's language acquisition. Immigrants to North America are likely to be poor (Hernandez et al. 2008), and numerous older studies (e.g., see Cohen 1970) of bilingual children neglected to take into consideration this common confound between bilingualism and poverty.

Second, people rearing children in multiple languages should be aware that language is a multi-layered construct, with phonology, vocabulary, grammar, narrative, and literacy—i.e., all levels of language—worthy of stimulation and instruction (Dickinson et al. 2003). Thus, parents of children who speak a minority language should, if possible, seek out opportunities for them to acquire literacy in that language(s) in addition to seeking members of extended family and communities for conversation to stimulate acquisition of language-specific phonology, vocabulary, grammar, and narrative structure. True (biliterate) bilingualism is considered an economic asset by most of the world outside the United States and even by many individuals who seek at some considerable expense to themselves to learn a second language within the U.S. (see Hoff 2013).

A great deal of research in language acquisition done over the last 40 years has established the characteristics of optimal linguistic input to monolingual children (see McCabe et al. 2013, for review of this literature). The most important characteristic of optimal child-directed language is that it is *responsive* to children's interests and behavior (Bornstein et al. 2008). Such responsiveness is key probably due to the fact that it occurs at the same time as or shortly after children look at or do or say something and is conceptually related as well (Tamis-LeMonda et al. 2014). Responsive input also labels, describes, and questions about objects or events rather than commanding children to stop doing something. Responsive input is delivered by words and gestures (e.g., pointing; Tamis-LeMonda et al. 2014) and is high-pitched in a manner most likely to capture children's attention (Fernald and Mazzie 1991).

Not only is optimal child-directed language responsive, it is also quite varied. The overall grammatical complexity of input, the informativeness of the context in which it is delivered, and the range of different syntactic constructions in which verbs appear are all positive predictors of vocabulary development (Hoff 2003; Hoff and Naigles 2002), as is mother's co-construction of narratives with their children (Peterson et al. 1999; Rowe 2012). The number of different grammatical forms mothers use predicts children's grammatical development (Huttenlocher et al. 2010). A longitudinal study of children who were typically developing from various SES backgrounds and those with brain injury found numerous very specific effects of parental linguistic input to children in terms of various types of diversity, talk about number and space, and similarity of objects (Goldin-Meadow et al. 2014): Parental (primarily maternal) lexical diversity (i.e., number of different words used with children) predicted children's lexical diversity. Parental constituent diversity predicted child constituent diversity. Parents' cumulative talk about number predicted children's subsequent knowledge of cardinal numbers. Parents' spatial language predicted children's spatial language. Parent talk about similarities (e.g., "the butterfly is like a rainbow" is a global similarity relationship) was related to the acquisition of abstract (e.g., "The crayon is brown like my hair.") similarity relations.

In short, optimal linguistic input labels objects and events that capture a child's attention, uses different types of words, contains complex grammar, and has a positive tone (see review in McCabe et al. 2013). Optimal input to children also includes talking extensively about past events (see Fivush et al. 2006, for review). If parents are comfortably literate in a language, optimal input also involves sharing books interactively with children on a regular basis (e.g., Rodriguez and Tamis-LeMonda 2011); however, the quality of book reading affects children's language and literacy gains (Dickinson and Smith 1994; Whitehurst et al. 1994). What parents say and how they talk about books may well explain the benefits of book reading interactions for early language development (Hoff-Ginsberg 1991). Parents who do not have access to books in their native language (Raikes et al. 2006) or who do not feel comfortable or confident of their literacy skills should take heart from the fact that it is oral conversation in the context of looking at books, rather than reading per se, that is most beneficial to young children.

In summary, numerous children in North America speak a dialect and/or language(s) other than those in which they are schooled. Scholars have moved away from assuming that bilingualism is inevitably subtractive (one language is learned at the expense of another) to recognizing that children can benefit from learning more than one language. Scholars have also pointed to the need to disentangle socioeconomic status from bilingualism.

Current Research Questions

Typically Developing Bilingual Children

As mentioned earlier, key (and related) research questions for some time have been (1) whether dual language exposure harms children, and (2) whether children should be discouraged from speaking their native language at home in favor of the majority language. The emerging consensus from much research is that no, dual language exposure does not harm children (Paradis et al. 2011). Bilingual children develop separate, albeit related, linguistic systems, allowing them to learn a second language without interference from the first (Paradis et al. 2011). However, learning two languages often takes longer than learning one; when the total language of bilingual children is considered, the overall rate of growth is at least equal to the rate of language growth in monolingual children (Hoff et al. 2012). Thus, parents who speak a minority language at home should be encouraged to continue to speak that language with their children. Not only is it not harmful, a study done with a large, representative sample of immigrant families found that immigrant children were at risk of developing poorer cognitive skills *only when English was the only language spoken in the home* (Winsler et al. 2014). That is, use of a heritage language at home served as a protective factor for children of immigrant families; such children had better early cognitive outcomes and preschool math skills. In fact, Winsler et al. (2014) found that children exposed exclusively to the heritage language at home made particularly strong gains in preschool on English literacy relative to children who spoke both a heritage language and English or only English at home. Benefits of speaking the heritage language at home are not limited to literacy acquisition; such children enjoy better relationships with their parents and can communicate with other relatives, who may well only speak the heritage language (Oh and Fuligni 2010; Tabors 1997).

Assessment of Deficit

Assessment of bilingual children is a key current research question and has been so for a number of years. Researchers advise Speech Language Therapists to test bilingual children in both their languages and use a number of different assessments (Peña et al. 2003; Laing and Kamhi 2003). Dynamic Assessment of word learning skills has been recommended especially in identifying language impairment in bilingual children (Kapantzoglou et al. 2012). Assessments mindful of documented cultural differences in narration have also been developed for use with personal narratives told by individuals from diverse cultures and across the lifespan (McCabe and Bliss 2003).

Support for Both Languages

Some current investigations examine the issue of how best to provide therapy and other interventions to children from bilingual families who face special obstacles to language acquisition. Many individuals in the fields of language development and education subscribe to a subtractive model of bilingualism particularly for children with special needs, fearing that the "burden" of an extra language will further delay their progress (see Bunta and Douglas 2013, for review of these claims). Bunta and Douglas (2013) assessed children with Hearing Loss who had received cochlear implants before the age of 5 years, half of whom were from monolingual, half from bilingual, Spanish-English homes. Children were matched on chronological age, length of device use, duration of intervention, type of intervention, and type of device used. Home assignments were given to parents in English in the case of monolingual participants and in Spanish in the case of bilingual participants. Children were tested on the Auditory Comprehension, Expressive Communication, and total language scores of the Preschool Language Scale, fourth Edition (Zimmerman et al. 2002). Despite the fact that the two groups of children could not be matched regarding mother's education level (monolingual English-speaking children's mothers had higher levels) and the findings that poverty is associated with less than optimal linguistic input even for monolingual children (Hart and Risley 1995), the English language skills of the children in the two groups were not significantly different. Spanish and English scores of the bilingual group were also similar. Parents were encouraged to speak whatever language they were comfortable with and fluent in. For these children who faced a double risk for literacy acquisition (e.g., hearing loss and bilingualism; see Snow et al. 1998), parents speaking their native Spanish evidently provided as much of the kind of responsive, varied, optimal input as those speaking their native English—with no deleterious effect on their children's acquisition of English.

Intervention

Studies of successful intervention programs for facilitating multilingual language and literacy acquisition in young learners who are not yet proficient in English are few and far between (August 2013). Nevertheless, the few such studies as do exist support encouraging children to speak their parents' native language as well as English in the United States (August 2013).

Some researchers have noted a vocabulary gap in bilingual children (see McCabe et al. 2013, for review), so a focus on improving their vocabulary is apt. A child's vocabulary in the language of school is best developed at school by methods that (1) take advantage of their first language if that language shares cognates with the school language (*family* in English is a cognate for *familia* in Spanish and vice versa—the two words similar in orthography and meaning), (2) ensure that children learning English know the meaning of basic words (i.e., words like *clock* and *baby* that monolingual English-speaking children would know but which require instruction for children learning English, and (3) include ample time for review and practice (August et al. 2005).

Perozzi and colleagues demonstrated that even when children struggle with language impairment, teaching concepts in two languages resulted in faster acquisition of those concepts in children's second (majority) language compared to teaching such concepts only in their second language (Perozzi 1985; Perozzi and Chavez-Sanchez 1992). Restrepo et al. (2013) tested the impact of bilingual instruction of preschoolers in vocabulary (through shared, interactive book-reading, hands-on activities, and repeated exposure to vocabulary) compared to English-only vocabulary instruction, bilingual mathematics instruction, English-only mathematics instruction, and a no intervention, business-as-usual group of English language learners with typical development. Bilingual instruction in vocabulary of bilingual children with language impairment was equivalent to English-only instruction in promoting English receptive and expressive vocabulary and significantly more effective than all 4 other conditions in promoting Spanish receptive and expressive vocabulary.

In short, both bilingual children with typical and atypical language acquisition benefit from continued support in both their languages.

Research Measurement and Methodology

There are numerous challenges in the study of multilingualism. To begin with, many immigrant children (one in three in the U.S.) are classified as impoverished (Hernandez et al. 2008). Many studies of multilingual children confounded poverty and multilingualism, as noted above. The wide-ranging impact of poverty on measures of well-being has been amply established. The specific impact of poverty on child language acquisition has also been established, as noted (Hart and Risley 1995). Researchers need to tease apart the impact of multilingualism from that of poverty on language acquisition by increased studies of middle-class multilingual families.

In addition, assessment of a child's language and literacy development in multiple languages is far from simple and has important practical and theoretical implications. First, there are many languages for which no appropriately normed, standardized tests of linguistic ability exist. Even when such standardized norm-referenced tests do exist, most speech-language therapists argue that accurate assessment of spoken and written language skills of children who are from culturally and linguistically diverse backgrounds should never depend solely on the use of such tests due to content bias (e.g., some objects are far more common in some cultures than in others), linguistic bias (clinician and child do not speak the same dialect or language), and/or disproportionate representation of some populations in normative samples (see Laing and Kamhi 2003, for review).

Consider the case of the third edition of the much-validated, much-used (in research and clinical practice) Peabody Picture Vocabulary Test (PPVT-III; Dunn and Dunn 1997). Despite the fact that the test's normative sample included minority (34 %) children, and the fact that Washington and Craig (1999) found the PPVT-III to be appropriate for use with African American preschoolers who were deemed at social risk, other researchers (Champion et al. 2003) found that African American Head Start children in the Tampa Bay area showed consistent errors on a few of the PPVT-III items and thus scored significantly below the mean for the normative sample used to establish the test parameters. For example, *trunk* is a word that in African American English means a person's derriere but on the test is exemplified by luggage.

Standardized tests should be supplemented by (1) language sampling, (2) ethnographic interviewing, (3) processing-dependent measures (e.g., repetition of non-words), and (4) dynamic assessment (e.g., testing, teaching a child to name objects and pictures on a standardized test, and then retesting the child). Considerable attention has been paid to the assessment of children who speak African American English (e.g., Taylor and Payne 1983), but children who speak other dialects (e.g., Appalachian English) may also be unfairly scored as answering a question incorrectly with what is an acceptable

form in their dialect (Wolfram 1983). Remarkably, standardized tests have sometimes been found to underestimate the ability even of children who speak Standard English; Prutting et al. (1975) found that such children displayed greater expressive grammatical ability in a free speech sample than on the standardized Northwestern Syntax Screening Test. Moreover, not all free speech sampling situations produce identical results: children produced more utterances and word roots and expressed longer Mean Length of Utterance when interacting with their mothers than when playing alone, particularly during times mothers judged to provide a sample of their children's optimal language (Bornstein et al. 2002). One test has been developed that promises fairer assessment of some dialects—primarily directed at accurate assessment of speakers of African American English—by focusing on whether children deviate from the linguistic patterns in their home language rather than whether they have mastered constructions in Standard English that contrast with their dialect: The Diagnostic Evaluation of Language Variation (Seymour et al. 2005). This test has proven valid for speakers of some other English dialects (such as Cajun English and Appalachian English; see Norbury and Sparks 2013, for review). Similar assessments are underway for children in the United States from Spanish-speaking backgrounds.

Yet another important source of cultural and individual variation is whether or not children's performance in some aspect of language is considered a deficit by their parents and their culture; many children who score low on language tests are not identified as having language difficulties by parents or practitioners, and the benefits versus the costs of identification as deficient must be carefully weighed (Norbury and Sparks 2013).

For researchers attempting to explore such theoretical concerns as the relative rate of language development of bilingual children, comparable assessment in both of their languages is critical. For example, Hoff et al. (2012) found that monolingual children were significantly more advanced than bilingual children on measures of vocabulary and grammar in the majority language (English), but when the bilingual children's vocabulary in both languages was totaled they were comparable to monolingual children.

Many researchers have suggested that linguistic and literacy skills transfer from one language to another. For example, constituents (i.e., number of utterances, orientations, and actions) were correlated in the English and Spanish personal narratives of children with and without typical language development (McCabe and Bliss 2005). Phonological awareness measures in Spanish or English in 4–5-year-old bilingual preschoolers account for a great deal (68 %) of variance in phonological awareness in the other language (Dickinson et al. 2004). Word reading, spelling, vocabulary knowledge, reading comprehension, use of reading strategies, and strategic aspects of writing in one language correlate with the same abilities in the other (see Snow 2006). However, Snow (2006) cautioned that although correlations of similar aspects of language in different languages are consistent with transfer claims, they do not constitute strong, causal proof of those claims. Transfer as a concept has only been defined operationally; evidence supporting or refuting the existence of transfer has not been clearly and unequivocally thought through.

In short, current research questions regarding accurate assessment of the impact of bilingualism remain largely unanswered despite a great deal of work on this subject and some progress.

Empirical Findings Regarding the Impact of Bilingualism on Language and Literacy Acquisition

Bilingual individuals and families—even those who speak a similar heritage language (e.g., Spanish in the U.S.)—are quite diverse. "The Specificity Principle in multiple language learning asserts that the acquisition of multiple languages is moderated" by many specifics (e.g., girls often learn languages faster than boys; Bornstein in McCabe et al. 2013, p. 5). Thus,

research findings below must be understood as generalities with *many* exceptions and caveats.

Disadvantages?

Bilingualism does not in and of itself result in cognitive disadvantages, despite poorly conceived, long-outdated, and unfortunately widely disseminated research to the contrary. In fact, studies in the 1950s and 1960s (and even earlier) that showed negative impacts of bilingualism on mental ability and/or academic accomplishment can be dismissed on methodological grounds (Bialystok 1991; see Hakuta 1986, for review).

Advantages

In fact, the advantages of multilingualism are many. Individuals with fluency and literacy in more than one language are qualified for more jobs and can communicate with more people. Individuals who speak the language of their parents and grandparents can communicate with them more meaningfully than those who do not. In fact, the lack or loss of a heritage family language can have quite poignant effects on family relationships.

Compared to speaking only one language, speaking more than one language confers advantages on tasks that relate to executive function (inhibitory control) and attentional control, metalinguistic awareness, the ability to understand the intentions and knowledge of others, and, sometimes, concepts of print and phonological awareness (see Hoff 2013; McCabe et al. 2013, for review).

Exposure to High-Quality Input

We reviewed what constitutes high-quality linguistic input above, and the same kinds of input that are advantageous for monolingual children are advantageous for multilingual children (also see McCabe et al. 2013, for review). The rate of language development in a bilingual child depends on amount of language exposure to each language (e.g., Place and Hoff 2011). Hearing extensive input in each language from multiple speakers is also important (Place and Hoff 2011). Adults who are proficient in a language provide considerably better input than adults who are less so. Parents who are fluent in a second language induce fluency in that language in their children (Jia et al. 2002; Paradis et al. 2011). Unfortunately, when parents increase their use of second (majority) languages with their children—languages in which they are *not* fluent—they do not necessarily improve their children's skills in that language, but they do decrease their children's skill in the first (native) language (Hammer et al. 2009).

Early Exposure to Appropriate Input

The benefits of early exposure to high-quality input in an accessible language may perhaps best be seen by looking at what happens when such exposure does not occur. Many individuals who are Deaf or Hard of Hearing (DHH) are not exposed to a sign language until they are over 3 years of age; Mayberry and colleagues (see Mayberry 2010, for review) found that such individuals have significant sign language deficits even after 20–40 years of using sign language as their primary means of communication. Throughout the twentieth century, national surveys in the United States found that the average DHH individual graduated from high school reading at the fourth grade level, and this trend extended to DHH individuals in other countries and the present century (see Lederberg et al. 2013, for review). In contrast, DHH children exposed from birth to American Sign Language (ASL) acquire not only that language but also written English grammar and semantics to a near native level and such children (skilled in ASL) also demonstrate English reading achievement between grade 10 and college level (Mayberry 2010). There are few clearer cases than this that bilingualism need not be subtractive; early and fluent signing *facilitated* spoken English despite

the differences in modality, vocabulary, syntax, and discourse between the two languages.

To ensure that bilingual children succeed in becoming fluent and literate at school, it is important to expose them as early as possible to native speakers of the language in which they will be schooled as well as the one their parents use at home. For example, bilingual children exposed to high-quality input in two languages prior to the age of 3 perform better in phonological awareness, reading, and language competence than those first exposed to one of those languages after age 3 (Kovelman et al. 2008).

Continued Support for Both Languages Is Desirable

Support for both languages of a child is highly effective; studies of children in environments that actively support (through both formal, academic and informal, nonacademic, means) both of a child's languages find that bilingual children can perform on par with monolingual children in those languages by the age of 10 years (Gathercole and Thomas 2009). For example, dual-language bilingual schools (such as the Amigos primary school in Cambridge, MA, for children whose native language is English as well as those whose native language is Spanish) offer half their instruction in English and half in Spanish to encourage bilingualism and literacy in both languages in both native English and native Spanish speakers.

Unfortunately, *lack* of support of children's native languages (regardless of whether that native language is European, African, Native American, etc.) is common, regrettable, and has potential negative consequences for literacy acquisition; recall that Winsler et al. (2014) found that controlling for heritage country of origin, family education and income, speaking some heritage language at home (as opposed to English only) was associated with more positive early cognitive outcomes. In the United States, a generational pattern of language usage for immigrants has been noted (see Verdon et al. 2014, for review). The immigrant generation is mostly or exclusively fluent in their first language, their children are also fluent in that language to some degree (depending on which language their parents speak with them), but the third generation—immigrants' grandchildren–speak English exclusively (Fishman 1966). Furthermore, this shift may be taking place more rapidly (Hurtado and Vega 2004). The familial loss of heritage language is unfortunate, especially given the considerable and often less-than-successful emphasis on learning foreign languages at school at older ages. Familial loss of languages involves individual decline in mastering a heritage language orally. Young children in America who are from immigrant, multilingual families often become increasingly English-dominant during their preschool years and decelerate their mastery of their parents' native language due to increases in exposure to English inside and outside their home (Bridges and Hoff 2012). What is crucial for all to realize is that parents who may have low literacy or who may even be illiterate in their native language nonetheless speak that language with far greater skill, complexity, comfort, and frequency than they do a second language acquired later on, and the oral skill, complexity, comfort, and frequency of their conversation in the native language is what is of most social-emotional, cognitive, linguistic, and academic benefit to their children.

A National Literacy Panel surveyed extensive research on language-minority children and youth and concluded that, on the whole, language-minority children are at levels equal, or can be instructed to be equal, to those of their monolingual peers as far as word-level components of literacy (e.g., decoding, spelling) are concerned (August and Shanahan 2006), but that such is not the case for text-level skills, especially reading comprehension (Snow 2006). That same panel also noted that using culturally relevant materials improved comprehension (Goldenberg et al. 2006b), although this practice is not necessarily common nor nearly as extensive as it might be. As Snow (2006) noted, part of this comprehension problem might derive from schools' unfamiliarity with cultural differences in

discourse. In particular, there are notable cultural differences in the way narratives are told (McCabe 1996; McCabe and Bliss 2003), and these differences have a strong impact on narrative comprehension. Having children read stories that originate in the children's home culture and conform to the kind of narrative valued by the children would likely improve those children's reading comprehension as well as their enjoyment of reading.

In short, early and frequent exposure to high-quality input from multiple languages, along with continued support for those languages, results in optimal academic success for bilingual children.

Universal Versus Culture-Specific Mechanisms

In reviewing the work of the National Panel on Language-Minority Children and Youth, Snow (2006) noted the remarkable lack of information available regarding skilled and developing readers of many (probably most) languages other than those who speak the majority languages of North America. Snow (2006, p. 645) argued "the task of learning to read in any language is defined by the orthographic system of that language," an observation that underlies why monolingual and English-as-a-Second-Language students require such similar skills. Skills for reading Chinese or Arabic—with orthographies distinct from European languages—are very different and much under-studied.

Numerous sociocultural variables also affect multilingual acquisition (see Goldenberg et al. 2006a, for review). The readiness of schools to be more compatible with interactions a child has at home affects student engagement in school in that requiring children to do something at school that they have been taught at home is rude (e.g., looking adults directly in the eyes) is unlikely to be successful. As noted above, reading materials congruent with storytelling forms of children's ethnic backgrounds can also improve reading comprehension performance (Goldenberg et al. 2006b; McCabe 1996). Schools might also find more effective ways of engaging immigrant parents in facilitating their children's education. Policies at the district, state/province, and federal levels (e.g., English-only education in the United States) affect students' literacy development. The status or prestige of a minority language versus a majority language also has an impact on children's success at school; academic achievement of children whose minority language is as respected as the majority language is much closer to that of the majority than when the discrepancy in status of the two languages is considerable (Goldenberg et al. 2006a).

Policy Implications of Research Findings on Bilingualism

An interdisciplinary committee of scholars on language acquisition, multilingualism, and pediatrics reviewed current research on best practices and policies for dealing with multilingual children and families (McCabe et al. 2013). They made four specific recommendations for an action plan: (1) collaborations regarding multilingual children across disciplines and involving dialogues between researchers and practitioners (teachers, medical healthcare providers, Speech Language Therapists, policymakers) should be ongoing, both for sharing current research and for addressing concerns of practitioners and parents; the Providence Talks program (http://www.providencetalks.org/) is one such attempt to close the word gap faced by children who grow up in poor households (Hart and Risley 1995). (2) Child professionals and policymakers should routinely engage in making research accessible to practitioners and parents using multiple platforms (e.g., health care settings, home visitation). (3) Federal governments should fund research that advances understanding of basic processes of multilingual children's language and literacy development, with a specific eye to identifying best practices to support such development. (4) Strategies should be developed to address practical obstacles to implementation of recommendations regarding multilingual children's

optimal development in existing professional development requirements of administrators, teachers, and speech-language pathologists.

Future Directions of Research and Policy Regarding Bilingual Families

Most researchers with extensive experience studying multilingualism express dismay that what we do not know about this issue dwarfs what we do know. Hoff (2013) noted several key questions for future research: (1) there is a gap in research documenting trajectories of bilingual development from 2½ years to age 5 or 6 years; that is, many studies find that low-income children who enter school speaking a language other than English in the United States display a "school readiness gap" compared to monolingual and/or middle-class children (Castro et al. 2011). Snow (2006) noted that this age gap in the research is especially egregious in view of the considerable amount of information suggesting that this period is critical for the development of oral language and emergent literacy skills in monolingual children. (2) There is a need to study large samples of children from high-SES bilingual homes in North America and elsewhere in order to tease apart the common confound of SES and multilingualism (Hoff 2013). (3) We need to know whether and when bilingual children catch up to monolingual children in their levels of majority language skill to best support families of bilingual children in preparing their children well for school (Hoff 2013). In an overview of extensive research on the issue of bilingualism, August and Shanahan (2006) pointed to some other critical gaps in the literature: (4) we still do not know exactly what high-quality literacy instruction of multilingual children consists of; even Quebec, which for 50 years has had a exemplary history of endorsing bilingualism in instruction and daily interaction, reports that the actual rate of bilingualism in the province is less than 50 % at present (http://www.statcan.gc.ca/pub/75-006-x/

2013001/article/11795-eng.htm); and (5) we do not know how to build the extensive oral language skills in majority languages that are essential to reading comprehension. August (2013) pointed to a remarkable dearth of studies focusing on intervention to promote multilingual language and literacy development. (6) Snow (2006) pointed also to the need for appropriate assessment of and intervention with older low-income immigrant children who do not have extensive command of a majority language and who may not have had much prior schooling at all in their country of origin.

In addition to such research with families of typically developing children, there is a pressing need for far more extensive research on the developmental trajectories, assessment of, and intervention with children of multilingual families who appear to present with atypical conditions. Thus far, the bulk of such research has been aimed at assessment; specifically, many researchers have been concerned about misdiagnosing differences as deficits or misdiagnosing deficits as differences—both egregious. Research on the optimal treatment of such children, however, is quite scant. A comprehensive survey of research concluded that most reading difficulties can be prevented, that reading disability accounts for about 80 % of all learning disabilities (Snow et al. 1998, p. 13, 89), and that children entering school speaking a minority language—especially when compounded by growing up in an impoverished home—are at risk for successfully acquiring the kinds of literacy required by many jobs in North America. Equipped with knowledge derived from past, present, and future research, families who speak heritage languages at home and practitioners who teach or counsel such families can better guide language-minority children to academic and social success.

Conclusions

Many children in North American and throughout the world enter formal schooling speaking a language and/or dialect other than that in which they will be schooled. Fear that such multilingualism

was detrimental stemmed from outdated studies in which immigrants' poverty was confounded with their multilingualism. Modern studies have to some extent rectified this historic confound and discovered that, like monolingual children, multilingual children benefit from talking extensively with adults. The more language children hear, the more they learn. Optimal linguistic input is conversational, responsive to children, positive in tone, and diverse in vocabulary, syntax, and other aspects of language. Adults who are comfortable with and fluent in a language or dialect best provide such input. In fact, recent well-founded evidence shows that immigrant children learn the language of school best when at least some heritage language is spoken in the home. Not only does such practice benefit children academically, it also improves the quality of their relationships with their families. Assessment of children has been and still is a pressing research concern for many reasons, as has intervention with children who may face additional challenges to language acquisition (e.g., brain injury). Intervention with at-risk children from multilingual backgrounds has also been plagued by the notion that such children may be overburdened with speaking more than one language. However, the scant recent research on bilingual interventions is quite opposed to this notion: parents (and speech language therapists) of children with challenges benefit them best by speaking the language(s) those adults are most comfortable with and, therefore, adept in. Much work remains to devise tests that reveal children's highest abilities, though progress has been made in this regard. Early and frequent opportunities to talk with fluent adults in both heritage and school languages are critical to all children's success, as are continued support for both languages. The most important policy implication is that schools, the medical profession, and others concerned with the well-being of immigrant children not only do not discourage parents from speaking their native language with their offspring but also positively *encourage* them to do so and to do so frequently. Parents who are comfortably literate and who have access to good books written in their native language should be encouraged to read those books with their children. But parents who may have struggled with literacy in their home cultures and/or who do not have access to appropriate books should know that ultimately *speaking with* their children in their native language frequently is much more important than *reading to* those children in any language. We need more information regarding how best to support educational and therapeutic interventions for multilingual and/or multidialectical children given the vast diversity of the children we now find in our school systems.

Acknowledgments The author would like to express her appreciation to Erika Hoff and Marc Bornstein for comments on earlier versions of this chapter.

References

Adkins, T. (2011). "The English Effect" on Amish language literacy practices. *Community Literacy Journal, 5*(2), 25–45.

August, D. (2013). Multilingual children: Developing and disseminations knowledge to support successful language development. A commentary on McCabe, A., Tamis-LeMonda, C. S., Bornstein, M. H., Cates, C. B., Golinkoff, R., Hirsh-Pasek, K., Hoff, E., Kuchirko, Y., Melzi, G., Mendelsohn, A., Paez, M., Song, L., Guerra, A. W. (2013). Multilingual children: Beyond myths and towards best practices. *Society for Research in Child Development Social Policy Report, 27*(4).

August, D., Carlo, M., Dressler, C., & Snow, C. (2005). The critical role of vocabulary development for English Language Learners. The critical role of vocabulary development for English Language Learners. *Learning Disabilities Research & Practice, 20*, 50–57.

August, D., & Shanahan, T. (2006). Introduction and methodology. In D. August & T. Shanahan (Eds.), *Developing literacy in second-language learners: Report of the National Literacy Panel on Language-Minority Children and Youth* (pp. 1–42). Mahwah, NJ: Erlbaum.

Baker, C., & Hornberger, N. H. (Eds.). (2001). *An introductory reader to the writings of Jim Cummins*. Bristol: Multilingual Matters.

Bialystok, E. (1991). *Language processing in bilingual children*. New York: Cambridge University Press.

Bornstein, M. H., Painter, K. M., & Park, J. (2002). Naturalistic language sampling in typically developing children. *Journal of Child Language, 29*, 687–699. doi:10.1017/S030500090200524X

Bornstein, M. H., Tamis-LeMonda, C., Hahn, C., & Haynes, O. M. (2008). Maternal responsiveness to young children at three ages: Longitudinal analysis of a multidimensional, modular, and specific parenting construct. *Developmental Psychology, 44*(3), 867–874. doi:10.1037/0012-1649.44.3.867

Bridges, K., & Hoff, E. (2012). Older sibling influences on the language environment and language development of toddlers in multilingual environments. *Applied Psycholinguistics*. doi:10.1017/S0142716412000379

Bunta, F., & Douglas, M. (2013). The effects of dual-language support on the language skills of bilingual children with hearing loss who use listening devices relative to their monolingual peers. *Language, Speech, and Hearing Services in Schools, 44*, 281–290.

Castro, D. C., Paez, M. N., Dickinson, D. K., & Frede, E. (2011). Promoting language and literacy in young dual language learners: Research practice, and policy. *Child Development Perspectives, 5*, 15–21. doi:10.1111/j.17508606.2010.00142.x

Champion, T. B., Hyter, Y. D., McCabe, A., & Bland-Stewart, L. M. (2003). A matter of vocabulary: Performances of low-income African American Head Start Children on the PPVT-III. *Communication Disorders Quarterly, 24*(3), 121–127.

Cohen, D. K. (1970). Immigrants and the schools. *Review of Educational Research, 40*(1), 13–27.

De Houwer, A. (1990). *The acquisition of two languages from birth: A case study*. Cambridge: Cambridge University Press.

Dickinson, D. K., McCabe, A., Anastasopoulos, L., Peisner-Feinberg, E., & Poe, M. D. (2003). The comprehensive language approach to early literacy: The interrelationships among vocabulary, phonological sensitivity, and print knowledge among preschool-aged children. *Journal of Educational Psychology, 95*, 465–481. doi:10.1037/0022-0663.95.3.465

Dickinson, D. K., McCabe, A., Clark-Chiarelli, N., & Wolf, A. (2004). Cross-language transfer of phonological awareness in low-income Spanish and English bilingual preschool children. *Applied Psycholinguistics, 25*, 323–347. doi:10.1017/S0142716404001158

Dickinson, D. K., & Smith, M. (1994). Long-term effects of preschool teachers' book readings on low-income children's vocabulary and story comprehension. *Reading Research Quarterly, 29*(2), 104–122.

Dunn, L., & Dunn, L. (1997). *The Peabody picture vocabulary test* (3rd ed.). Circle Pines, MN: American Guidance Service.

Fernald, A., & Mazzie, C. (1991). Prosody and focus in speech to infants and adults. *Developmental Psychology, 27*, 209–221.

Fishman, J. A. (1966). *Reversing language shift (RLS): Theoretical and empirical foundations of assistance to threatened languages*. Clevedon: Multilingual Matters.

Fivush, R., Haden, C. A., & Reese, E. (2006). Elaborating on elaborations: Role of maternal reminiscing style in cognitive and socioemotional development. *Child Development, 77*(6), 1568–1588. doi:10.1111/j.1467-8624.2006.00960.x

Gathercole, V. C. M., & Thomas, E. M. (2009). Bilingual first-language development: Dominant language take-over, threatened minority language take-up.

Bilingualism: Language & Cognition, 12(2), 213–237. doi:10.1017/S1366728909004015

Goldenberg, C., Rueda, R. S., & August, D. (2006a). Synthesis: Sociocultural contexts and literacy development. In D. August & T. Shanahan (Eds.), *Developing literacy in second-language learners: Report of the National Literacy Panel on Language-Minority Children and Youth* (pp. 249–267). Mahwah, NJ: Erlbaum.

Goldenberg, C., Rueda, R. S., & August, D. (2006b). Sociocultural influences on the literacy attainment of language-minority children and youth. In D. August & T. Shanahan (Eds.), *Developing literacy in second-language learners: Report of the National Literacy Panel on Language-Minority Children and Youth* (pp. 269–318). Mahwah, NJ: Erlbaum.

Goldin-Meadow, S., Levine, S. C., Hedges, L. V., Huttenlocher, J., Raudenbush, S. W., & Small, S. L. (2014). New evidence about language and cognitive development based on a longitudinal study: Hypotheses for intervention. *American Psychologist, 69*(6), 588–599. doi:10.1037/a0036886

Hakuta, K. (1986). *Mirror of language: The debate on bilingualism*. New York: Basic Books.

Hammer, C. S., Davison, M. D., Lawrence, F. R., & Miccio, A. W. (2009). The effect of maternal language on bilingual children's vocabulary and emergent literacy development during Head Start and kindergarten. *Scientific Studies of Reading, 13*, 99–121. doi:10.1080/10888430902769541

Hart, B., & Risley, T. R. (1995). *Meaningful differences in the everyday experience of young American children*. Baltimore, MD: Brookes.

Hernandez, D. J., Denton, N. A., & Macartney, S. E. (2008). Children in immigrant families: Looking to America's future. *Social Policy Report, 22*(3), 16–17.

Hoff, E. (2003). The specificity of environmental influence: Socioeconomic status affects early vocabulary development via maternal speech. *Child Development, 74*, 1368–1378. doi:10.1111/1467-8624.00612

Hoff, E. (2013). Interpreting the early language trajectories of children from low-SES and language-minority homes: Implications for closing achievement gaps. *Developmental Psychology, 49*(1), 4–14. doi:10.1037/a0027238

Hoff, E., Core, C., Place, S., Rumiche, R., Señor, M., & Parra, M. (2012). Dual language exposure and early bilingual development. *Journal of Child Language, 39*, 1–27. doi:10.1017/S0305000910000759

Hoff, E., & Naigles, L. (2002). How children use input to acquire a lexicon. *Child Development, 73*(2), 418–433. doi:10.1111/1467-8624.00415

Hoff-Ginsberg, E. (1991). Mother-child conversation in different social classes and communicative settings. *Child Development, 62*, 782–796. doi:10.1111/1467-8624.ep9109162253

Hurtado, A., & Vega, L. A. (2004). Shift happens: Spanish and English transmission between parents and their children. *Journal of Social Issues, 60*(1), 137–155. doi:10.1111/j.0022-4537.2004.00103.x

Huttenlocher, J., Waterfall, H., Vasilyeva, M., Vevea, J., & Hedges, L. V. (2010). Sources of variability in children's language growth. *Cognitive Psychology, 61*(4), 343–365. doi:10.1016/j.cogpsych.2010.08.002

Jia, G., Aaronson, D., & Wu, Y. (2002). Long-term language attainment of bilingual immigrants: Predictive variables and language group differences. *Applied Psycholinguistics, 23*(4), 599–621. doi:10.1017/S0142716402004058

Kapantzoglou, M., Restrepo, M. A., & Thompson, M. S. (2012). Dynamic assessment of word learning skills: Identifying language impairment in bilingual children. *Language, Speech, and Hearing Services in Schools, 43*, 81–96.

Kovelman, I., Baker, S. A., & Petitto, L. (2008). Age of first bilingual language exposure as a new window into bilingual reading development. *Bilingualism: Language and Cognition, 11*(2), 203–223. doi:10.1017/S1366728908003386

Labov, W. (1972). *Language in the inner city: Studies in the Black English vernacular*. Philadelphia: University of Pennsylvania Press.

Laing, S. P., & Kamhi, A. (2003). Alternative assessment of language and literacy in culturally and linguistically diverse populations. *Language, Speech, and Hearing Services in Schools, 34*, 44–55.

Lederberg, A. R., Schick, B., & Spencer, P. E. (2013). Language and literacy development of deaf and hard-of-hearing children: Successes and challenges. *Developmental Psychology, 49*(1), 15–30.

Mayberry, R. I. (2010). Early language acquisition and adult language ability: What sign language reveals about the critical period for language. In M. Marshark & P. E. Spencer (Eds.), *The Oxford Handbook of deaf studies, language, and education* (Vol. 2, pp. 281–291). New York, NY: Oxford University Press.

McCabe, A. (1996). *Chameleon readers: Teaching children to appreciate all kinds of good stories*. New York: McGraw-Hill.

McCabe, A., & Bliss, L. S. (2003). *Patterns of narrative discourse: A multicultural, life-span approach*. Boston: Allyn & Bacon.

McCabe, A., & Bliss, L. S. (2005). Narratives from Spanish-speaking children with impaired and typical language development. *Imagination, Cognition and Personality, 24*(4), 331–346.

McCabe, A., Tamis-LeMonda, C. S., Bornstein, M. H., Cates, C. B., Golinkoff, R., Hirsh-Pasek, K., et al. (2013). Multilingual children: Beyond myths and towards best practices. *Society for Research in Child Development Social Policy Report, 27*(4), 1–36.

Norbury, C. F., & Sparks, A. (2013). Difference or disorder? Cultural issues in understanding neurodevelopmental disorders. *Developmental Psychology, 49*(1), 45–58.

Oh, J. S., & Fuligni, A. J. (2010). The role of heritage language development in the ethnic identity and family relationships of adolescents from immigrant backgrounds. *Social Development, 19*, 202–220. doi:10.1111/j.1467-9507.2008.00530.x

Paradis, J., Genesee, F., & Crago, M. B. (2011). *Dual language development and disorders: A handbook on bilingualism and second language learning* (2nd ed.). Baltimore, MD: Brookes.

Peña, E., Bedore, L. M., & Rappazzo, C. (2003). Comparison of Spanish, English, and bilingual children's performance across semantic tasks. *Language, Speech, and Hearing Services in Schools, 34*, 5–16.

Perozzi, J. A. (1985). A pilot study of language facilitation for bilingual language handicapped children: Theoretical and intervention implications. *Journal of Speech and Hearing Disorders, 50*, 403–406.

Perozzi, J. A., & Chavez-Sanchez, M. O. (1992). The effect of instruction in L1 on receptive acquisition of L2 for bilingual children with language delay. *Language, Speech, & Hearing Services in Schools, 23*, 348–352.

Peterson, C., Jesso, B., & McCabe, A. (1999). Encouraging narratives in preschoolers: An intervention study. *Journal of Child Language, 26*, 49–67.

Place, S., & Hoff, E. (2011). Properties of dual language exposure that influence 2-year-olds' bilingual proficiency. *Child Development, 82*(6), 1834–1849. doi:10.1111/j.1467-8624.2011.01660.x

Prutting, C., Gallagher, T., & Mulac, A. (1975). The expressive portion of the NSST compared to a spontaneous language sample. *Journal of Speech and Hearing Disorders, 40*, 40–48.

Raikes, H., Pan, B. A., Luze, G., Tamis-LeMonda, C. S., Brooks-Gunn, J., Tarullo, L. B., et al. (2006). Mother-child bookreading in low-income families: Correlates and outcomes during the first three years of life. *Child Development, 77*(4), 924–953. doi:10.1111/j.1467-8624.2006.00911.x

Restrepo, M. A., Morgan, G., & Thompson, M. S. (2013). The efficacy of a vocabulary intervention for duel-language learners with language impairment. *Journal of Speech, Language, and Hearing Research, 56*, 748–765.

Rodriguez, E. T., & Tamis-LeMonda, C. (2011). Trajectories of the home learning environment across the first 5 years: Associations with children's vocabulary and literacy skills at prekindergarten. *Child Development, 82*(4), 1058–1075. doi:10.1111/j.1467-8624.2011.01614.x

Rowe, M. L. (2012). A longitudinal investigation of the role of quantity and quality of child-directed speech in vocabulary development. *Child Development, 83*, 1762–1774. doi:10.111/j.1467-8624.2012.01805.x

Ryan, W. (2002). The Unz initiatives and the abolition of bilingual education. *Boston College Law Review, 43*(2), 487–519.

Seymour, H. N., Roeper, T., & deVilliers, J. (2005). *Diagnostic evaluation of language variation.* San Antonio, TX: Psychological Corporation.

Snow, C. E. (2006). Cross-cutting themes and future research directions. In D. August & T. Shanahan (Eds.), *Developing literacy in second-language learners: Report of the National Literacy Panel on Language-Minority Children and Youth* (pp. 631–652). Mahwah, NJ: Erlbaum.

Snow, C. E., Burns, M. S., & Griffin, P. (1998). *Preventing difficulties in young children.* Washington, DC: National Academy Press.

Tabors, P. (1997). *One child, two languages: A guide for preschool educators of children learning English as a second language.* Baltimore, MD: Brookes.

Tamis-LeMonda, C. S., Kuchirko, Y., & Song, L. (2014). Why is infant language learning facilitated by parental responsiveness. *Psychological Science, 23*(2), 121–126.

Taylor, O. L., & Payne, K. T. (1983). Culturally valid testing: A proactive approach. *Topics in Language Disorders, 3*(3), 8–20.

Verdon, S., McLeod, S., & Winsler, A. (2014). Language maintenance and loss in a population study of young Australian children. *Early Childhood Research Quarterly, 29*, 168–181.

Washington, J. A., & Craig, H. K. (1999). Performances of at-risk African American preschoolers on the Peabody Picture Vocabulary Test-III. *Language Speech, and Hearing Services in Schools, 30*, 75–82.

Whitehurst, G. J., Arnold, D. S., Epstein, J. N., & Angell, A. L. (1994). A picture book reading intervention in day care and home for children from low-income families. *Developmental Psychology, 30*(5), 679–689.

Winsler, A., et al. (2014). Early development among dual language learners: The roles of language use at home, maternal immigration, country of origin, and socio-demographic variables. *Early Childhood Research Quarterly.* doi:10.1016/j.ecresq.2014.02.008

Wolfram, W. (1983). Test interpretation and sociolinguistic differences. *Topics in Language Disorders, 3*(3), 21–34.

Zimmerman, I., Steiner, V., & Pond, R. (2002). *Preschool language scale* (4th ed.). San Antonio, TX: Harcourt Assessment.

Minority Language Parenting in Europe and Children's Well-Being

Annick De Houwer

Abstract

Language is of central importance in parenting. This becomes particularly clear in a minority context, where parents may be pressured into speaking a language to children that they hardly know, or where children may not speak the language that their parents speak with them. Because of linguistic issues, minority language background parents may feel insecure in their parenting role, and their children's positive development may be adversely affected. This chapter reviews research from various research traditions in the currently (2015) 28 countries of the European Union that can potentially inform relations between language use by parents with a minority language background as an integral part of parenting on the one hand, and young children's socioemotional well-being on the other. Few European research projects so far have specifically addressed the complex relations between the language related aspects of parenting in minority language background families and children's socioemotional well-being. However, the evidence brought together here supports the notion that children's minority language use and proficiency as mediated by their parents' linguistic choices and practices positively affects both parents' and young children's well-being, thus contributing to harmonious bilingual development.

Introduction

Most children in the European Union (EU) speak the language used at school (De Houwer 2003; Extra and Yağmur 2004). The school or majority language is usually also the main and/or official language of local public life. Many children in the EU in addition speak a minority language (Baker and Eversley 2000; CILT 2005; De Houwer 2003; Extra and Yağmur 2004). Typically, these minority languages are infrequently or never used in education and public life.

Children learn minority languages almost exclusively at home. Children may hear just (or mainly) a minority language at home in the very first years of life and only later become bilingual

A. De Houwer (✉)
University of Erfurt, Mitarbeitergebäude 1,
6th Floor, Nordhäuser Str. 63,
99089 Erfurt, Germany
e-mail: annick.dehouwer@uni-erfurt.de

© The Editor(s) 2017
N.J. Cabrera and B. Leyendecker (eds.), *Handbook on Positive Development of Minority Children and Youth*, DOI 10.1007/978-3-319-43645-6_14

through additional access to the majority language. These children are growing up in an Early Second Language Acquisition setting (ESLA; De Houwer 1990). Alternatively, children may regularly hear both a minority and a majority language in the home from birth, a setting known as Bilingual First Language Acquisition (BFLA; Meisel 1990). Both in Europe and in the United States BFLA likely occurs three times as often as ESLA (De Houwer 2017).

Whether potentially bilingual children have any chance of acquiring a minority language in the home depends on the linguistic choices made by the adults who take care of them, that is, by their parents (De Houwer 1999, 2009).[1] Both parents or one of them may have a minority language background, and may address children in that minority language (or in more than one minority language). Both parents or one of them may in addition have some proficiency in the local majority language and may speak it to children as well. Minority language background parents may not speak the minority language to their children, but may still use it amongst each other. Alternatively, they may not use the minority language at home at all. Parental linguistic choices may be made quite consciously, or may just emerge.

Parental linguistic choices in terms of which language(s) are used at home and with whom are to a large degree dependent on parental attitudes towards each of the languages involved (De Houwer 1999, 2009). At the same time, bilingual settings involving a minority and a majority language form a hierarchical relation that often leads to conflicts at the societal level (Darquennes 2013). Such conflicts may also play out at the family level, and will influence parental language attitudes and their language choices (Anderson 2002; De Houwer 1999, 2015a). For instance, parents may feel pressured into speaking a language to children that they hardly know.

Language development is a core aspect of children's development that parents typically play a foundational role in. In bilingual settings, many children experience what De Houwer (2006, 2015a) has termed "harmonious bilingual development", that is, bilingual language development in the absence of interpersonal conflict and feelings of dissonance attributable to the bilingual setting. Because of linguistic issues, however, many minority language background parents may feel insecure in their parenting role. If parents in a bilingual setting cannot fully fulfill their foundational role in children's language development because of linguistic issues, children's socioemotional well-being may be adversely affected.

This chapter reviews research from various research traditions in the currently (2015) 28 countries of the European Union that can potentially inform relations between language use by minority language background parents as an integral part of parenting, and young children's socioemotional well-being. The focus is on families with children under the age of six.

Historical Overview

Because minority languages are used within a majority language environment the question about the link between parental minority language use and young children's socioemotional well-being is also one about early bilingualism. Even before 1930, Vygotskij (2007 [1928–29]: 73) called for researchers to investigate the influence of early child bilingualism on children's global psychological development, including emotional and personality aspects, rather than "just" on cognition and practical intelligence, as was common prior to the 1930s. Until today, Vygotskij's call has hardly been heeded, with European psychologists still mainly examining the effects of early bilingualism on cognitive aspects (e.g., Blom et al. 2014; Lauchlan et al. 2013) but rarely, if at all, on socioemotional well-being. Linguists working on psycholinguistic aspects of bilingual acquisition have likewise paid little attention to socioemotional aspects.

The very first study on early bilingual acquisition within the family had an enormous impact

---

[1]The term "parent(s)" here refers to any adult responsible for children's day-to-day education and socialization.

on parenting in a bilingual setting. Ronjat (1913) advised the use of the "one parent, one language" principle, whereby each parent should address children in only a single, but different language. Up until today, the "one parent, one language" principle has been upheld as an ideal (e.g., see http://bilingualmonkeys.com/the-best-language-strategy-for-raising-bilingual-children/).

Ronjat's detailed study of his young BFLA son was soon followed by Pavlovitch's (1920) less detailed study of his young ESLA son. Both authors emphasized linguistic developments in the first 2 years of life, and both children were growing up in upper middle class environments with French as the majority language and German and Serbian as minority languages, respectively. Both children interacted more often with people speaking the minority than the majority language. They each spoke the minority language better and more often than the majority one, but children were still very young (under age three) when data collection ended. Uneven development of two languages, with bilingual children showing higher proficiency in one of them, is common (De Houwer 2009).

Rūķe-Draviņa (1959) showed that it is possible for young children growing up with just a minority language at home to have hardly any contact with the majority language in the first years of life and as a result not speak it. This is typical of ESLA.

In Europe it took more than 60 years for the next in-depth longitudinal studies of bilingual acquisition within the family context to appear. Porsché's (1983) study of his BFLA son acquiring English and German in Germany and Taeschner's (1983) study of her two BFLA daughters acquiring German and Italian in Italy expanded on the themes covered by Ronjat (1913) and Pavlovitch (1920). Taeschner (1983) also reported on her daughters' refusal to speak German once they were of preschool age, a phenomenon that von Humboldt had experienced with his 4-year-old daughter in Italy more than 200 years before (De Houwer 2009: 46).

This refusal to speak the minority language was also noted by Métraux (1965), who collected maternal questionnaire data in France on 47 children between zero and 20 years of age growing up in 25 upper middle-class American English-French bilingual families. Probably as a first in the EU, Métraux (1965) documented the incidence of non-minority language transmission in this group: In a third of families, children did not speak English. Métraux (1965) is also likely the first European study that mentions emotional and behavioral problems in children as linked to the use of a particular language, that is, to language choice: Amongst others, some children reportedly showed anger and withdrawal symptoms if pressed to speak or even listen to English. Several decades later, Vasquez (1991) reported on language-related socioemotional problems in a young Argentinian boy in France, who ended up refusing to speak Spanish with his exiled single mother at home, resulting in little communication between mother and child. The boy spoke French fluently and was well-adjusted outside the home.

At the same time that European psycholinguists were studying minority and majority language development on the micro-level of the case study, contact linguists and sociologists were examining patterns of intergenerational minority language transmission. Harrison et al.'s (1981) interview study with 311 Welsh-English mothers of young children in Wales was likely the first attempt to help explain children's lesser use of a minority language through analyzing maternal language use patterns and attitudes. Veltman's (1983) census-based study on the transmission of Alsatian, a regional minority language in France, looked at parental language proficiency in trying to explain children's minority language use. Whereas 78 % of parent pairs could speak Alsatian, only 52 % of children were able to, indicating a large intergenerational language loss. The loss was greater for couples where one parent did not know Alsatian than for parents who both knew Alsatian.

As parents, the von Humboldts and Taeschner were not happy with their daughters' refusal to speak the immigrant minority language. With a lot of effort, the children's mothers managed to motivate their children to speak the minority language to them again instead of the majority language (De Houwer 2009; Taeschner 1983). They did so using what Lanza (1992, 1997) in her bilingual interaction model called "monolingual discourse strategies", that is, conversational strategies encouraging and enabling children to use the minority language. These include, for example, feigning to understand children when they speak the majority language, asking children to repeat their majority language sentence in the minority language, or translating children's majority language word into the minority language and then asking children to repeat what they wanted to communicate.

Up until the mid 1980s scholars reported on their own families (see De Houwer 1990; Taeschner 1983 for reviews). De Houwer's (1983, 1990) and Lanza's (1988, 1992) case studies of bilingual development were the first by family-external researchers. There were also new psycholinguistically oriented studies of bilingually reared children's language development which did not collect data within the family: for instance, Meisel and colleagues (e.g., Meisel 1990) focused on BFLA, while Boeschoten and Verhoeven (1987) focused on ESLA. The latter examined lower-SES children's use of Turkish and Dutch. This shift to also studying children from lower-SES backgrounds and to non-European minority languages marked a trend that continues today, bringing us to the next section, which considers studies of minority language background parents and their children in the EU in the 25-year period between 1990 and 2015.

Research Measurement and Methodology: Focus on Families with Young Children

In preparing this chapter I searched for any EU study offering empirical data of any kind on (1) parental minority language practices with young children in the home, (2) young children's (language) behavior in relation to such practices, and (3) young minority language children's

psycho-social adjustment.[2] Most studies address (1) and/or (2), but rarely (3). Many studies do not limit themselves to the age period in focus here, but include data regarding the parenting of both younger and older children. Such studies combining data on the parenting of both younger and older children are included in this section. Relevant studies concerning parents of primary school-aged children are furthermore occasionally cited in the next section, which discusses findings from the studies listed below. Studies offering data on aspects of parenting and/or child (language) development that are not targeted here are included below as long as they also contain data on topics (1), (2) and/or (3) above. Psycho- or neurolinguistic studies focusing just on bilingual children's language development or processing are excluded, even if they contain global information on the overall language input situation.

Within the framework of this chapter it is impossible to list each study with its separate findings. Instead, selected studies are tabulated according to their main methods, with indications of which minority and majority languages were involved, the kind and number of respondents, and children's ages. Studies come from a large variety of research traditions and disciplines, including developmental psycholinguistics, developmental and educational psychology, contact linguistics, social work, family sociology, and ethnicity studies. Hence, they vary greatly in methodological approaches and theoretical assumptions. However, in spite of these methodological and theoretical differences many of the findings converge (see the summary in the next section).

Some studies are listed more than once because they contain different relevant subparts. Studies are listed alphabetically according to minority language, except when there were several minority languages (then studies are listed according to majority language). Only two studies

---

[2]With few exceptions, the literature reviewed here is limited to publications in English, French and German, with an emphasis on those in English. Many points made in these publications were previously raised by authors writing in other languages. Particularly important European studies from outside the EU are included where relevant.

consider a regional minority language (Gathercole 2007; Smith-Christmas 2014). Indeed, whereas European contact linguistics mostly concerns regional minority languages (e.g., Darquennes 2013) and pan-European minority languages such as Yiddish, surprisingly few studies focus on their use in families with young children. All other studies listed cover immigrant minority languages, though De Houwer's (2007) and De Houwer and Bornstein's (2016) studies in officially Dutch-speaking Flanders, Belgium, also contain information about French, which could be considered a regional minority language.

Longitudinal Observational Case Studies of Spontaneous Family Interaction in the Home

In-depth observational studies of home interaction in families with young children use a range of data collection methods, including the diary method, field notes, and/or audio- and/or video-recordings. The studies in Table 1 employed at least one of these, or relied on a combination. They focus on a range of different topics. Afshar's (1998) rich and insightful study is unusual in many ways, especially because occasionally the author (the children's mother) gives attention to the family's emotional well-being by evaluating aspects of family interaction and children's language use.

Observational Studies of Mother-Child Interaction in the Home Involving Structured Tasks

The studies in Table 2 are longitudinal in the sense that they observed the same persons more than once, but they lack the in-depth empirical basis of the longitudinal studies of home

interaction listed in Table 1. The studies here compensate for that by collecting data on many people rather than just on one or two families. In contrast to the studies in Table 1, data collection in the studies in Table 2 was mostly structured around specific tasks. Observations consisted of videorecordings.

Ethnographic Studies

These studies relied on in-depth interviews that used an ethnographic approach and were qualitatively analyzed (see Table 3).

Interview Studies

The studies in Table 4 are based on structured or more open interviews, whether or not combined with separate data on children's language development. They differ from the ethnographic studies in Table 3 in offering quantitative analyses (with or without additional ethnographic-type qualitative analyses).

In-Depth Maternal Questionnaire Studies

Table 5 lists studies based on written questionnaires, whether or not combined with more in-depth interviews. All studies asked about home literacy activities and included demographic information. Most studies also asked about general maternal language use to children. Scheele et al. (2010) had more specific questions about domains of language use. Jäkel et al. (2011) included a maternal self-report measure of language proficiency in the minority and the majority language.

Table 1 In-depth observational studies of home interaction

Study	Minority language	Majority language	Persons observed	C ages
Juan-Garau and Pérez-Vidal (2001)	English	Catalan	1M, 1F, 1C	B 1;3–4;2
De Houwer (1990)	English	Dutch	1M, 1F, 1INV, 1C	G 2;7–3;4
Lanza (1997)	English	Norwegian	2M, 2F, 1INV, 2C	G 1;11–2;7 B 2;0–2;3
Afshar (1998)	Farsi	German	1M, 1F, 2C	B 1;0–4;8 G 0;0–3;0
Deuchar and Quay (2000)	Spanish	English	1M, 1F, 1C, paternal grandmother	G 0;10–2;3
Garlin (2008)	Spanish	German	1M, 1F, 2C	B 0;1–6;11 G 0;0–5;8

M mother, *F* father, *INV* investigator, *C* child(ren); a number in front of these indicates their number; *G* girl, *B* boy

Table 2 Observational studies of parent-child interaction in (semi-)structured tasks

Study	Minority language	Majority language	Persons observed	C ages
De Houwer (2014)	French	Dutch	16M, 16C	1;1 and 1;8
De Houwer and Bornstein (2016)	French	Dutch	31M, 31C[a]	0;5, 1;8 and 4;5
Lundén and Silvén (2011)	Russian	Finnish	24M, 24 F, 24C[b]	0;7
Prevoo et al. (2011)	Turkish	Dutch	87M, 87C[c]	2;2 and 3;2
Demir-Vegter et al. (2014)	Turkish	Dutch	15 M, 15C[d]	3;2 and 4;2

M mother, *C* child; a number in front of these indicates their number
[a]At age 0;5, recorded M-C interaction was unstructured; at child age 4;5 there were only 25 M-C dyads left in the study; there were also maternal questionnaire data
[b]M-C and F-C dyads were recorded separately; at 1;2, parents also filled out questionnaires on children's communicative development
[c]This study additionally relied on maternal questionnaire data
[d]This study additionally used extensive maternal interviews and vocabulary testing of the children in the minority language at ages 3;2 and 4;2 and in the majority language at age 5;10

Table 3 Ethnographic studies

Study	Majority language	Minority language	Interviews with	C age(s)
Smith-Christmas (2014)	English	Gaelic	1 family	[a]
Drury (2007)[b]	English	Pahari	3 families	4
Okita (2002)	English	Japanese	28 families	1–29
Brizić (2006)	(Austrian) German	Several	Parents	[c]
Selimi (2013)	(Swiss) German	Several	27 families	3–6

C child(ren)
[a]This is an in-depth longitudinal participant observation case study of a single extended family with 3 young children; the data are complemented by audio-recordings made when there were only 2 children (1 aged 7 then, 1 aged 3)
[b]This study combines home recordings in the minority language, recordings at preschool in the majority language, and maternal and teacher interviews with data collection both at the beginning and at the end of a school year. Three girls are the focus children
[c]It is not stated how many parents were interviewed, nor what their children's ages were, but parents talked about themselves and their (pre-)primary school aged children

Table 4 Interview studies

Study	Majority language	Minority language	Interviews with	Child age (s)
Raschka et al. (2002)	English	Cantonese	34 children	5–16
Gathercole (2007)	English	Welsh	302 parents[a]	0–7;11
Gathercole (2007)	English	Welsh	57 children	4;6–7;11
E-Rramdani (2003)	Dutch	Tarifit-Berber	31 mothers	4–6[b]
DJI (2000)	German	55 minority languages	1209 children	5–11
Kratzmann (2011)	German	Turkish	25 families	3–4
Leist-Villis (2004)	German	Greek	50 mothers	4–16
Leist-Villis (2004)	Greek	German	50 mothers	4–16
Sirén (1991)	Swedish	Polish or Spanish	20 sets of parents	4

[a]In addition there were ad hoc observations of many interviewees' home language use with family members and Welsh and English language tests for a portion of the interviewees; this sample includes the parents of the 57 children interviewed in the same study
[b]This study also contains extensive information on the children's proficiency in the minority language as obtained through language testing

Table 5 In-depth maternal questionnaire studies

Study	Minority language	Majority language	Questionnaires filled in by	Child age(s)
Scheele et al. (2010)	Tarifit-Berber	Dutch	46 mothers[a]	3
Scheele et al. (2010)	Turkish	Dutch	55 mothers[a]	3
Prevoo et al. (2014)	Turkish	Dutch	111 mothers[a]	Average 6;1
Jäkel et al. (2011)	Turkish	German	79 parents[b]	3–4;9
Willard et al. (2014)	Turkish	German	119 mothers[c]	5;5–7;3

[a]In addition, children were tested in the minority and majority language
[b]In addition, children were tested on majority language speaking proficiency and were given cognitive tests
[c]This study also tested children's receptive vocabulary in the minority language

Table 6 Surveys

Study	Majority language	Minority language	Data collected for	C age(s)
De Houwer (2007)	Dutch	About 73 different minority languages	1899 FAMS with 4556 C	1–20
Gathercole (2007)	English	Welsh	586 FAMS with 724 C	0–7;11
Okita (2002)	English	Japanese	135 FAMS	Under 5
Sirén (1991)	Swedish	About 66 different minority languages	595 FAMS with 595 C	4

FAMS families, *C* child(ren)

Survey Studies

The survey studies in Table 6 collected information on parental and child language use through written questionnaires. They contain less detailed information than the studies in Table 5 but offer data on a larger scale.

Empirical Findings and Theoretical Perspectives

The findings from the studies in the previous section confirm and expand on the major trends found in the earlier research summarized in the Historical Overview.

Studies confirm that young children in the EU typically hear a minority language in the private sphere. In the rare cases that extra classes in the minority language are offered through pre-schools, minority language parents rarely make use of these (DJI 2000; Selimi 2013; Sirén 1991). Children in a majority language preschool may meet peers there who share the same minority language, though (reports of children visiting bilingual preschools are rare).

Many young children learn to speak the minority language that they hear at home (see mostly the survey studies in Table 6). At the same time, many other children do *not* speak the minority language. The results from most parent report studies in Tables 3 and 4 suggest that the lack of minority language transmission is quite common. The survey studies (Table 6) and the studies with children's self-reports (Table 4) nuance this impression somewhat. Although different methods make it difficult to specify with any certainty what the average proportion is of young children who could be speaking a minority language but do not, a conservative estimate for 4-year-olds based on the available data lies around 20 %. Thus, unlike the 100 % majority language transmission rate in both monolingual and bilingual families, *minority* language transmission is not a given.

At issue is whether the early use versus non-use of a minority language by young children in a minority language family has a relation with children's socioemotional well-being. To date, there are only anecdotal data on this aspect, namely when parents (and some children) refer to children's embarrassment, shame, or anger when they are unable to speak the minority language in interactions with extended family members in the country of origin (see most of the parent reports in Tables 3 and 4; see also De Houwer 2015a). I know of no reports of children who speak the minority language well and who show distress in interactions with minority language speakers. Children who speak both the minority and the majority language are proud of their bilingualism (DJI 2000).

There is overwhelming evidence that *parental* socioemotional well-being is negatively affected when young children do not speak the minority language that parents address them in. Parents show a full range of negative emotions in response to their children's non-use of the minority language: They blame themselves for being a bad parent, feel guilty for failing to transmit their language, feel depressed, feel rejected by their children, feel embarrassed and ashamed towards their own parents, feel that they have failed as a person, and are dissatisfied with their bilingual child rearing. In short: Parents' sense of (cultural) identity appears to be under attack when their children do not speak their (minority) language (Anderson 2002).

It is mostly in bilingual families where children hear both a minority and a majority language that minority language transmission is at risk (De Houwer 2007). It is thus not surprising that negative feelings about their children's non-use of the minority language are mostly expressed by parents in families where two languages are spoken at home, that is, in families where children are growing up with two languages from birth (see the studies in Tables 3 and 4). Children in BFLA settings are more likely, then, to *not* speak the minority language than are ESLA children, who start off hearing only the minority language at home and typically come into first regular contact with the majority language through day care or preschool.

As toddlers, BFLA children often start out speaking both the minority and the majority language at home (De Houwer 2009). Most BFLA children are able to adapt their language choice to their interlocutor soon after their second birthdays, and they adjust their language choice to their interlocutor's language proficiency (see the studies in Table 1; De Houwer 2009). They will usually not speak a majority language to someone who only understands the minority language, or the other way round.

However, once BFLA children start regularly attending a preschool, their language choice patterns often quickly change, and they start to limit themselves to speaking just the majority language, even when parents had done their best to adhere to Ronjat's "one parent, one language" principle (cf. the Historical Overview). This principle is not easy to put into practice (De Houwer and Bornstein 2016; Lippert 2010), and parents often feel particularly confused and upset if they did their very best to follow it and yet did not raise an actively bilingual child (Leist-Villis 2004; Hammer 2014). Only in 75 % of bilingual families using the "one parent, one language" approach do children actually speak the minority language (De Houwer 2007).

Even ESLA children may start to gradually use the majority language at home where previously they had only spoken the minority language, sometimes resulting in complete minority language replacement (Kostyuk 2005).

While children's entry into preschool can lead to minority language loss in BFLA children and thereby to lower levels of socioemotional well-being in parents, the effect of starting with majority language preschool leads to initial low levels of socioemotional well-being in ESLA children who speak only the minority language (no such effect has been reported for BFLA children). It is usually a traumatic experience for children to have to start attending (pre)school in a language they do not know. All of a sudden, they can no longer understand anything, and they themselves are not understood, either. Thus communication is severely hampered. Added to this, children find themselves in unfamiliar surroundings with unfamiliar people. Older children in the large DJI (2000) study talk about how embarrassed and ashamed they felt when they could not understand what was going on. They were also often ridiculed for their poor use of the majority language. Research in Switzerland found that children with low majority language skills in preschool were more likely to be bullied and victimized by their majority language-speaking peers (von Grünigen et al. 2012). The three ESLA children in Drury's (2007) study who heard only the minority language at home were extremely

upset and unhappy in the first 2 months they started to go to a majority language preschool, and did not want to go (see also Kostyuk 2005; Nap-Kolhoff 2010). Drury (2007) explains how many minority language children's strategy to deal with the new majority language is to actively disengage. This disengagement may remain a stance taken throughout the school career, which is not conducive to academic achievement.

In a study of German children between 3 and 17, Hölling et al. (2007) found that 3- to 6-year-olds with a migration background showed more behavioral problems than peers without such a background, and that the migration/non-migration difference was larger in this age range than in any other. The authors give no information on children's language backgrounds, but it is striking that this special vulnerability for preschool-aged migrant background children happens to coincide with the difficult transition to the majority language in an institutional setting if it was not learned in the family.

Parents who started out speaking a minority language to their children may start to speak the majority language to them more and more. This shift in language choice often is a response to children's increased use of the majority language once they start attending (pre)school. Pre-school entry may have another effect: Many of the parents interviewed in the studies listed in Tables 3 and 4 refer to preschool teachers, school nurses and school psychologists advising parents to stop speaking the minority language at home. Such advice makes parents insecure (Vasquez 1991). Some follow it, whereas others do not, and feel guilty for not doing so. Parents are torn because they wish to speak their own language to their children and want their children to speak the minority language, while at the same time they realize and support the importance of the majority language; they want their children to do well in both the minority and the majority language. There is a great deal of parental insecurity about how to make sure that children learn both the minority and the majority language (e.g. Kratzmann 2011).

Not all parents with a minority language background who are in a position to speak a minority language to their young children actually do (De Houwer 2009). Parents often believe that their speaking the majority language to children at home will help children develop majority language skills, and do not consider the role of their own majority language skills (see below). Furthermore, as evidenced in the studies in Tables 3 and 4, many parents believe that exposing children to two languages from an early age will confuse them. As a consequence of these beliefs, parents decide to just speak the majority language to children. Other reasons for individual parents deciding not to use their minority language with children may be that their spouse does not know that language or does not have a positive attitude towards it.

In many families parents speak a minority language amongst each other but address the children solely in the majority language, even if their majority language proficiency is very poor. However, without a language to competently use with children, parents cannot satisfactorily assume their parental role. Communication is hampered. This emerges from many parent interviews. Furthermore, interview studies reporting on parents who could have addressed children in their minority language invariably mention parents' regret at not speaking the minority language to children. Often, parents feel a lack of emotional connection to their children if they speak a language to them that parents did not grow up with themselves (Hammer 2014). Psychoanalysts have argued that not speaking one's "own" language to children can negatively affect parent-child bonding (Couëtoux-Jungman et al. 2010). They work with parents to help them (re-)discover the minority language in interactions with their children. However, trying to switch to using the minority language at home where previously it was never or no longer used is a difficult undertaking (Sirén 1991).

When parents do speak a minority language to young children, children's minority language development is supported by a high frequency of parental minority language use (Anstatt 2008; Klassert and Gagarina 2010). The frequency of parental minority language use is higher when both parents speak the minority language to

children. This may help explain the large difference that De Houwer (2007) found between minority language transmission in bilingual families where both parents spoke the minority language and one parent also spoke the majority language (in 93 % of families using this pattern children spoke the minority language), and in families where both parents spoke the majority language at home and only one parent also spoke the minority language (only in 36 % of families using this pattern did children speak the minority language). Input frequency will also be higher if children have the chance to visit a minority language program at preschool or at a child-care center. Attending such programs may lead to children's increased use of the minority language at home (Sirén 1991).

Although it is often claimed by parents and scholars alike that maternal language input to children weighs more in minority language transmission than does paternal language input, the largest study to date that has addressed this issue showed no relation between parent gender and intergenerational language transmission (De Houwer 2007).

Okita (2002) was the first to uncover the emotionally demanding nature of trying to make sure that children learn to speak a minority language. Many studies have since confirmed the fact that trying to ensure that children speak a minority language is highly stressful. Minority language-speaking mothers married to majority language-speaking fathers refer to the arduous but invisible work they do every day in offering children sufficient minority language learning opportunities. The use of monolingual discourse strategies that support minority language use (see the Historical Overview) can be hard to realize, especially with a child who tends not to speak the minority language. Such discourse strategies are paramount: Juan-Garau and Pérez-Vidal (2001) report on a minority language-speaking father's conscious and ultimately successful efforts to turn around his son Andreu's use of the majority language with him through discourse strategies encouraging Andreu to speak the minority language. The father's use of puppets who, Andreu was told, did not understand him when he spoke the majority language and who provided minority language translations of what Andreu was saying in the majority language was particularly helpful in getting Andreu to start using more of the minority language. The use of such minority language supporting discourse strategies will partly depend on parental "impact beliefs" (De Houwer 1999), that is, on their beliefs as to whether they can exercise some sort of control over their children's linguistic functioning. As illustrated by many of the parental interviews in the previous section, not all parents believe they can.

On the whole, the findings here support De Houwer's (1999) three-tier model of bilingual development. In this bidirectional feedback model, (1) parental attitudes and beliefs regarding languages, early bilingualism and parental impact on children's language learning are crucial in (2) shaping parental language use towards children and ultimately, (3) children's bilingual language use and proficiency.

Universal Versus Specific Mechanisms

Notwithstanding the wide variation in countries, research settings, methods, social level, minority languages, majority languages and specific minority language-majority language combinations in the studies reviewed above the same points come up again and again. Most of the findings find confirmation in Kennedy and Romo's (2013) account of an upper middle class family trying to raise children with Spanish and English in the United States, and many are reflected in Iqbal's (2005) study of middle class Canadian mothers with a French minority language background in an English majority language environment.

Healthy children universally learn to speak the majority language, but not necessarily the minority language. This fact is evidenced by the EU studies reviewed here and by studies in the United States (Pearson 2007) and Australia (Verdon et al. 2014). Parents from a wide variety of cultural backgrounds are very distressed if

their children do not speak the parent's minority language. The fact that generally parents wish their language to be transmitted to their children suggests a potential universal. It seems equally universal that minority language parents want their children to do well in the majority language. Even parents who themselves do not speak the majority language underscore this importance (Kratzmann 2011).

Whereas there are few EU studies that have tested Lanza's (1992, 1997) bilingual interaction model (see the Historical Overview), a longitudinal US-based study with 68 parent-child pairs representing the entire SES range (Park et al. 2012) showed the importance of minority language-supporting parental discourse strategies for fostering children's minority language use and proficiency (these are the monolingual discourse strategies referenced above). This finding suggests that such discourse strategies are crucial, regardless of which minority-majority language combination is involved. At the same time, such discourse strategies supporting minority language use may be at odds with minority language-speaking parents' child rearing beliefs (van Tuijl et al. 2001). How parents' emotional investment in the minority language translates into parental practices supporting intergenerational language transmission may thus depend on parents' cultural backgrounds.

The generally supportive role of the frequency of parental minority language input for children's minority language use and proficiency is not only evidenced for the EU but also for the United States (e.g., Tsai et al.'s 2012 study with 79 Chinese immigrant families with children aged four to seven). Additionally, minority language transmission is influenced by factors external to the family, such as whether families live in close proximity to other families using the same minority language and whether the minority language is valued in society at large (Boyd and Latomaa 1996). The latter attitudinal aspect recurs in all studies of minority language transmission. The German immigrant families that Lippert (2010) interviewed in Italy often heard quite denigrating comments from non-Germans about their use of German. Attitudes towards early bilingualism were often negative, and doctors and teachers often went as far as actually telling parents to stop speaking German at home. Many minority language-speaking parents, regardless of country of origin and regardless of the country they live in, share such experiences. However, a particular minority language may be valued more in one region than in another.

Finally, whenever studies in the EU have looked at minority language children who entered preschool not yet knowing the majority language the reports are of distressed, unhappy, depressed, or aggressive children. These findings are in line with results from a large Australian study (Goldfeld et al. 2014). Children who did not yet know the majority language showed greater levels of vulnerability in several domains, including well-being, as rated by their school teachers in the first month after school entry. This finding suggests that we are, sadly, dealing with a widespread phenomenon.

Policy Implications

A 2014 Council of Europe publication states that programs to promote adult migrants' "linguistic integration" should "encourage them to pass [their mother tongue(s)] on to their children (at least using them within the family)" (Beacco et al. 2014: 12). This is a major break with tradition, where in spite of scholars' long-past exhortations to pay attention to children's minority languages (e.g., Verdoodt 1975) the attention went mainly to the majority language.

Although I have been unable to find any policy documents at the EU level specifically promoting children's use of minority languages, a UNICEF report covering several EU countries stresses the importance of proficient bilingualism for young immigrant children's well-being (Hernandez et al. 2009). The minority language is important for family relationships and values, and the majority language is important for public life. Children should have the chance to attend daycare centers and preschools that introduce children to the majority language but that at the same time value and are open to their minority languages (Hernandez et al. 2009).

Educational policies that acknowledge children's minority languages, value them, and perhaps even incorporate them in the (pre)school curriculum, even to a limited extent, will help minority language background children to feel more self-confident and valued (De Houwer 2015b). Such efforts are important because going to preschool often seems to be the "breaking point" for minority languages, partially because both BFLA and ESLA children experience a devaluation of their identity there (De Houwer 2015b). All of a sudden, ESLA children visiting majority language preschools no longer experience themselves as communicatively and socially competent. Projects using "bridge" persons between schools and homes are promising as well (Agirdag and Van Houtte 2011). Indeed, working together with parents is of utmost importance, and will also make parents feel valued. In addition, the creation of structured programs for parents with a minority language background could help in raising parental awareness of how to best support minority language transmission (Leyendecker et al. 2014). The symbolic value of such programs would be very high, because at present there is generally still little attention to minority languages on the part of social workers or other professionals who are in contact with minority language speakers.

Future Directions

Although there is currently much research interest in the well-being of immigrant families and school-aged children in the EU (e.g., Dimitrova et al. 2013), there has been little attention to the well-being of young children with an immigrant or minority language background. Where young immigrant background children's socioemotional well-being has been studied, their minority language use has not received any consideration (e.g., Hölling et al. 2007), or children were too young to be fluent speakers (Yaman et al. 2010).

This chapter has documented how parental socioemotional well-being is negatively affected by children's lack of minority language proficiency. Anecdotal reports mention children's lack of socioemotional well-being when they cannot speak the minority language or cannot speak it well. Systematic studies are needed to further explore children's socioemotional well-being in relation to minority language use. In these studies, children's language learning environments should be closely documented. In particular, it should be made explicit to what extent children have had the chance to learn the majority language alongside the minority language from birth (BFLA) or not (ESLA). As the findings of the studies reviewed here show, socioemotional well-being is likely more at risk for BFLA children who stop speaking a minority language whereas it is more at risk for ESLA children once they start attending a majority language pre-school. Minority language learning opportunities and social contacts outside the home should also be documented, as they may play a vital role in children valuing their minority language more.

Furthermore, dedicated projects are needed that systematically compare different languages in similar situations and the same languages in different settings so as to tease out attitudinal (status) issues. Given the complexity of the issues involved, studies from different theoretical and disciplinary perspectives are needed.

In conclusion, it is currently not clear from research done in the EU to what extent children's minority language use and proficiency relate to child socioemotional well-being. However, children's minority language use and proficiency are to a large degree determined by parental language use towards children. Parental language use includes language choice in different communicative situations, the frequency with which the minority language is used, and parental discourse strategies in response to children's language choice. Parents are not always aware of the importance of these factors. Parental attitudes towards particular languages and towards early

child bilingualism are the basis for parents' basic decision to use a minority language with children in the first place. The distress that parents experience when their children do not speak the minority language that they wish them to learn makes parents feel insecure in their parenting role. This cannot be of benefit to their children. As such, minority language parents' socioemotional well-being will be a major factor to control for in further explorations of European minority language background children's harmonious bilingual development.

Acknowledgments I thank Jeroen Darquennes for his feedback on an earlier version of the Introduction and Wolf Wölck for comments throughout and help in gaining access to relevant literature. I thank the volume editors and the section editor for their valuable feedback.

References

Afshar, K. (1998). *Zweisprachigkeit oder Zwei-sprachigkeit? Zur Entwicklung einer schwachen Sprache in der deutsch-persischen Familienkommu-nikation*. Münster: Waxmann.

Agirdag, O., & Van Houtte, M. (2011). A tale of two cities: Bridging families and schools. *Educational Leadership, 68*(8), 42–46.

Anderson, M. (2002). 'It's a culture thing': Children, language and 'boundary' in the bicultural family. In P. Gubbins & M. Holt (Eds.), *Beyond boundaries: Language and identity in contemporary Europe* (pp. 111–125). Clevedon: Multilingual Matters.

Anstatt, T. (2008). Russisch in Deutschland: Entwick-lungsperspektiven. *Bulletin der deutschen Slavistik, 14*, 67–74.

Baker, P., & Eversley, J. (2000). *Multilingual capital: The languages of London's schoolchildren and their relevance to economic, social and educational poli-cies*. London: Battlebridge.

Beacco, J.-C., Little, D., & Hedges, C. (2014). *Linguistic integration of adult migrants. Guide to policy devel-opment and implementation*. Strasbourg: Council of Europe Publishing.

Blom, W., Küntay, A., Messer, M., Verhagen, J., & Leseman, P. (2014). The benefits of being bilingual: Working memory in bilingual Turkish-Dutch children. *Journal of Experimental Child Psychology, 128*, 105–119.

Boeschoten, H., & Verhoeven, L. (1987). Language mixing in children's speech: Dutch language use in Turkish discourse. *Language Learning, 37*, 191–215.

Boyd, S., & Latomaa, S. (1996). Language maintenance and language shift among four immigrant minorities in the Nordic region: A reevaluation of Fishman's theory of diglossia and bilingualism. *Nordic Journal of Linguistics, 19*(2), 155–182.

Brizić, K. (2006). The secret life of languages. Origin-specific differences in L1/L2 acquisition by immigrant children. *International Journal of Applied Linguistics, 16*(3), 339–362.

CILT. (2005). *Language trends 2005: Community language learning in England, Wales and Scotland.* London: CILT, the National Centre for Languages.

Couëtoux-Jungman, F., Wendland, J., Aidane, E., Rabain, D., Plaza, M., & Lécuyer, R. (2010). Bilinguisme, plurilinguisme et petite enfance. Intérêt de la prise en compte du contexte lin-guistique de l'enfant dans l'évaluation et le soin des difficultés de développement précoce. *Devenir, 22*(4), 293–307.

Darquennes, J. (2013). Language policy and planning in indigenous language minority settings in the EU. *Revue Française de Linguistique Appliquée, 23,* 103–119.

De Houwer, A. (1983). Some aspects of the simultaneous acquisition of Dutch and English by a three-year-old child. *Nottingham Linguistic Circular, 12,* 106–129.

De Houwer, A. (1990). *The acquisition of two languages from birth: A case study.* Cambridge: Cambridge University Press.

De Houwer, A. (1999). Environmental factors in early bilingual development: The role of parental beliefs and attitudes. In G. Extra & L. Verhoeven (Eds.), *Bilingualism and migration* (pp. 75–96). New York: Mouton de Gruyter.

De Houwer, A. (2003). Home languages spoken in officially monolingual Flanders: A survey. *Plurilingua, 24,* 71–87.

De Houwer, A. (2006). Le développement harmonieux ou non harmonieux du bilinguisme de l'enfant au sein de la famille. *Langage et Société, 116,* 29–49.

De Houwer, A. (2007). Parental language input patterns and children's bilingual use. *Applied Psycholinguistics, 283,* 411–424.

De Houwer, A. (2009). *Bilingual first language acquisition.* Bristol: Multilingual Matters.

De Houwer, A. (2014). The absolute frequency of maternal input to bilingual and monolingual children: A first comparison. In T. Grüter & J. Paradis (Eds.), *Input and experience in bilingual development* (pp. 37–58). Amsterdam: John Benjamins.

De Houwer, A. (2015a). Harmonious bilingual development: Young families' well-being in language contact situations. *International Journal of Bilingualism, 19* (2), 169–184 (first published online June 11, 2013. doi:10.1177/1367006913489202)

De Houwer, A. (2015b). Integration und Interkulturalität in Kindertagesstätten und in Kinder-gärten: Die Rolle der Nichtumgebungssprache für das Wohlbefinden von Kleinkindern. In E. Reichert-Garschhammer,

C. Kieferle, M. Wertfein, & F. Becker-Stoll (Eds.), *Inklusion und Partizipation. Vielfalt als Chance und Anspruch* (pp. 113–125). Göttingen: Vandenhoeck & Ruprecht.

De Houwer, A. (2017). Input, context and early child bilingualism: Implications for clinical practice. In A. Bar-On & D. Ravid (Eds.), *Handbook of communication disorders: Theoretical, empirical, and applied linguistic perspectives.* Berlin: Mouton de Gruyter.

De Houwer, A., & Bornstein, M. H. (2016). Bilingual mothers' language choice in child-directed speech: Continuity and change. *Journal of Multilingual and Multicultural Development, 37*(7), 680–693.

Demir-Vegter, S., Aarts, R., & Kurvers, J. (2014). Lexical richness in maternal input and vocabulary development of Turkish preschoolers in the Netherlands. *Journal of Psycholinguistic Research, 43,* 149–165.

Deuchar, M., & Quay, S. (2000). *Bilingual acquisition: Theoretical implications of a case study.* Oxford: Oxford University Press.

Dimitrova, R., Bender, M., & Van de Vijver, F. (Eds.). (2013). *Global perspectives on well-being in immigrant families.* New York: Springer.

DJI [DJI-Projekt "Multikulturelles Kinderleben"]. (2000). *Wie Kinder multikulturellen Alltag erleben. Ergebnisse einer Kinderbefragung.* München: Deutsches Jugendinstitut.

Drury, R. (2007). *Young bilingual learners at home and school: Researching multilingual voices.* Stoke on Trent: Trentham Books.

E-Rramdani, y. (2003). *Acquiring Tarifit-Berber by children in the Netherlands and Morocco.* Amsterdam: Aksant Academic Publishers.

Extra, G., & Yağmur, K. (Eds.). (2004). *Urban multilingualism in Europe: Immigrant minority languages at home and school.* Clevedon: Multilingual Matters.

Garlin, E. (2008). *Bilingualer Erstspracherwerb: Sprachlich handeln, Sprachprobieren, Sprachreflexion. Eine Langzeitstudie eines deutsch-spanisch aufwachsenden Geschwister-paares.* Münster: Waxmann.

Gathercole, V. (Ed.). (2007). *Language transmission in bilingual families in Wales.* Cardiff: Welsh Language Board.

Goldfeld, S., O'Connor, M., Mithen, J., Sayers, M., & Brinkman, S. (2014). Early developmental outcomes of emerging and English-proficient bilingual children at school entry in an Australian population cohort. *International Journal of Behavioral Development, 38* (1), 42–51.

Hammer, F. (2014). 'Vererbte' Mehrsprachigkeit. Sprachpraktiken und Zugehörigkeitsverständnisse multilingualer Eltern. In M. Scheer (Ed.), *Bindestrich-Deutsche?: Mehrfachzugehörigkeit und Beheimatungspraktiken im Alltag* (pp. 31–62). Tübingen: Tübinger Vereinigung für Volkskunde e.V.

Harrison, G., Bellin, W., & Piette, B. (1981). *Bilingual mothers in Wales and the language of their children.* Cardiff: University of Wales Press.

Hernandez, D., Macartney, S., & Blanchard, V. (2009). *Children in immigrant families in eight affluent countries. Their family, national and international context.* Florence: UNICEF Innocenti Research Centre.

Hölling, H., Erhart, M., Ravens-Sieberer, U., & Schlack, R. (2007). Verhaltensauffälligkeiten bei Kindern und Jugendlichen. *Bundesgesundheitsblatt-Gesundheitsforschung-Gesundheitsschutz, 50,* 784–793.

Iqbal, I. (2005). Mother tongue and motherhood: Implications for French language maintenance in Canada. *The Canadian Modern Language Review, 61,* 305–323.

Jäkel, J., Schölmerich, A., Kassis, W., & Leyendecker, B. (2011). Paternal book reading as a resource for pre-schoolers' cognitive skills. A comparison of Turkish migrant and German non-migrant families. *International Journal of Developmental Science, 5,* 27–39.

Juan-Garau, M., & Pérez-Vidal, C. (2001). Mixing and pragmatic parental strategies in early bilingual acquisition. *Journal of Child Language, 28,* 59–86.

Kennedy, K., & Romo, H. (2013). "All colors and hues": An autoethnography of a multiethnic family's strategies for bilingualism and multiculturalism. *Family Relations, 62,* 109–124.

Klassert, A., & Gagarina, N. (2010). Der Einfluss des elterlichen Inputs auf die Sprachentwicklung bilingualer Kinder: Evidenz aus russischsprachigen Migrantenfamilien in Berlin. *Diskurs Kindheits-und Jugendforschung, 4,* 413–425.

Kostyuk, N. (2005). *Der Zweitspracherwerb beim Kind: eine Studie am Beispiel des Erwerbs des Deutschen durch drei russischsprachige Kinder.* Hamburg: Verlag Dr. Kovač.

Kratzmann, J. (2011). *Türkische Familien beim Übergang vom Kindergarten in die Grundschule. Einschulungsentscheidungen in der Migrationssituation.* Münster: Waxmann.

Lanza, E. (1988). Language strategies in the home: Linguistic input and infant bilingualism. In A. Holmen, E. Hansen, J. Gimbel, & N. Jørgensen (Eds.), *Bilingualism and the individual* (pp. 69–84). Clevedon: Multilingual Matters.

Lanza, E. (1992). Can bilingual two-year-olds code-switch? *Journal of Child Language, 19,* 633–658.

Lanza, E. (1997). *Language mixing in infant bilingualism: A sociolinguistic perspective.* Oxford: Clarendon Press.

Lauchlan, F., Parisi, M., & Fadda, R. (2013). Bilingualism in Sardinia and Scotland: Exploring the cognitive benefits of speaking a minority language. *International Journal of Bilingualism, 17*(1), 43–56.

Leist-Villis, A. (2004). *Zweisprachigkeit im Kontext sozialer Netzwerke. Unterstützende Rahmenbedingungen zweisprachiger Entwicklung und Erziehung am Beispiel griechisch-deutsch.* Münster: Waxmann.

Leyendecker, B., Willard, J., Agache, A., Jäkel, J., Spiegler, O., & Kohl, K. (2014). Learning a host country: A plea to strengthen parents' roles and to encourage children's bilingual development. In R. Silbereisen, Y. Shavit, & P. Titzmann (Eds.), *The challenges of diaspora migration: Interdisciplinary perspectives on research in Israel and Germany* (pp. 291–306). London: Ashgate.

Lippert, S. (2010). *Sprachumstellung in bilingualen Familien. Zur Dynamik sprachlicher Assimilation bei italienisch-deutschen Familien in Italien.* Münster: Waxmann.

Lundén, M., & Silvén, M. (2011). Balanced communication in mid-infancy promotes early vocabulary development: Effects of play with mother and father in mono- and bilingual families. *International Journal of Bilingualism, 15,* 535–559.

Meisel, J. (Ed.). (1990). *Two first languages. Early grammatical development in bilingual children.* Dordrecht: Foris Publications.

Métraux, R. (1965). A study of bilingualism among children of U.S.-French parents. *The French Review, 38*(5), 650–665.

Nap-Kolhoff, E. (2010). *Second language acquisition in early childhood: A longitudinal multiple case study of Turkish-Dutch children.* Utrecht: Netherlands Graduate School of Linguistics LOT.

Okita, T. (2002). *Invisible work. Bilingualism, language choice and childrearing in intermarried families.* Amsterdam: John Benjamins.

Park, H., Tsai, K., Liu, L., & Lau, A. (2012). Transactional associations between supportive family climate and young children's heritage language proficiency in immigrant families. *International Journal of Behavioral Development, 36,* 226–236.

Pavlovitch, M. (1920). *Le langage enfantin. Acquisition du serbe et du français.* Paris: Champion.

Pearson, B. Z. (2007). Social factors in childhood bilingualism in the United States. *Applied Psycholinguistics, 28,* 399–410.

Porsché, D. (1983). *Die Zweisprachigkeit während des primären Spracherwerbs.* Tübingen: Gunter Narr.

Prevoo, M., Malda, M., Mesman, J., Emmen, R., Yeniad, N., van IJzendoorn, M., et al. (2014). Predicting ethnic minority children's vocabulary from socioeconomic status, maternal language and home reading input: Different pathways for host and ethnic language. *Journal of Child Language, 41,* 963–984.

Prevoo, M., Mesman, J., van IJzendoorn, M., & Pieper, S. (2011). Bilingual toddlers reap the language they sow: Ethnic minority toddlers' childcare attendance increases maternal host language use. *Journal of Multilingual and Multicultural Development, 32,* 561–576.

Raschka, C., Li, W., & Lee, S. (2002). Bilingual development and social networks of British-born Chinese children. *International Journal of the Sociology of Language, 153,* 9–25.

Ronjat, J. (1913). *Le développement du langage observé chez un enfant bilingue.* Paris: Champion.

Rūķe-Draviņa, V. (1959). Zur Entstehung der Flexion in der Kindersprache: Ein Beitrag auf der Grundlage des lettischen Sprachmaterials. *International Journal of Slavic Linguistics and Poetics, 1*(2), 201–222.

Scheele, A., Leseman, P., & Mayo, A. (2010). The home language environment of monolingual and bilingual children and their language proficiency. *Applied Psycholinguistics, 31*, 117–140.

Selimi, N. (2013). *Familiäre und institutionelle Einflüsse auf die Sprachentwicklung mehrsprachig aufwachsender Kinder.* Baltmannsweiler: Schneider Verlag Hohengehren.

Sirén, U. (1991). *Minority language transmission in early childhood. Parental intention and language use.* Stockholm: Institute of International Education, Stockholm University.

Smith-Christmas, C. (2014). Being socialised in language shift: The impact of extended family members on family language policy. *Journal of Multilingual and Multicultural Development, 5*(35), 511–526.

Taeschner, T. (1983). *The sun is feminine: A study on language acquisition in bilingual children.* Berlin: Springer.

Tsai, K. M., Park, H., Liu, L. L., & Lau, A. S. (2012). Distinct pathways from parental cultural orientation to young children's bilingual development. *Journal of Applied Developmental Psychology, 33*, 219–226.

van Tuijl, C., Leseman, P., & Rispens, J. (2001). Efficacy of an intensive home-based educational intervention program for 4–6 year old ethnic minority children in the Netherlands. *International Journal of Behavioral Development, 25*(2), 148–159.

Vasquez, A. (1991). Le bilinguisme chez les enfants d'exilés, affectivité et stratégies d'identité. *Enfance, 45* (4), 279–290.

Veltman, C. (1983). La transmission de l'alsacien dans le milieu familial. *Revue des Sciences Sociales de la France de l'Est, 12/12bis,* 125–133.

Verdon, S., McLeod, S., & Winsler, A. (2014). Language maintenance and loss in a population study of young Australian children. *Early Childhood Research Quarterly, 29,* 168–181.

Verdoodt, A. (1975). Les problemes linguistiques des travailleurs migrants adultes et les problèmes sociolinguistiques des enfants des travailleurs migrants scolarisés dans le pays d'accueil. *Cahiers de l'Institut de Linguistique de Louvain, 3,* 66–76.

von Grünigen, R., Kochenderfer-Ladd, B., Perren, B., & Alsaker, F. (2012). Links between local language competence and peer relations among Swiss and immigrant children: The mediating role of social behaviour. *Journal of School Psychology, 50*(2), 195–213.

Vygotskij, L. (2007 [1928–29]). Zur Frage nach der Mehrsprachigkeit im kindlichen Alter (translated into German from the original Russian text published in 1928–29). In K. Meng & J. Rehbein (Eds.), *Kindliche Kommunikation—einsprachig und mehrsprachig* (pp. 40–74). Münster: Waxmann.

Willard, J., Agache, A., Jäkel, J., Glück, C., & Leyendecker, B. (2014). Family factors predicting vocabulary in Turkish as a heritage language. *Applied Psycholinguistics, 27,* 2014. doi:10.1017/S0142716413000544

Yaman, A., Mesman, J., van IJzendoorn, M., & Bakermans-Kranenburg, M. (2010). Perceived family stress, parenting efficacy, and child externalizing behaviors in second-generation immigrant mothers. *Social Psychiatry and Psychiatric Epidemiology, 45,* 505–512.

Part IV
Peers and Friendship Level Influences

The Contribution of Friendship and Peers to Immigrant Youth' Positive Development

Christiane Spiel

University of Vienna, Vienna, Austria

Being integrated in a community and having supportive relationships are key for positive development. Successful integration influences psychological and socio-cultural adaptation, such as personal well-being and academic achievement. During adolescence, the amount of time spent with parents and family decreases and peers become increasingly important to individuals' adaptation. Relationships with peers are shown to play a major role in the development of children's and youth's cognitions, emotions, and behaviors. The establishment of friendships begins early in development, is considered to be a major developmental task for pre-schoolers, and it continues to be important for social relationships during the adolescent years. Successful formation of friendship contributes to self-esteem and socio-emotional support and provides children and adolescents with a sense of acceptance and belonging. Positive friendships may be particularly important for immigrant youth, as parents and peers may represent more contrasting value systems, compared with native adolescents. For immigrants, the peer context provides a major arena for the acquisition of the new language, customs and habits of the society. Social scientists and educators have identified intergroup peer relations among immigrants and natives as central to promoting racial harmony.

However, the milieu of cultural norms, expectations, and stereotypes influence peer relationships and friendships and could—in the worse case scenario—lead to peer victimization, rejection or peer exclusion.

So far, there is a lack of knowledge on the influences peers and friendship have on the positive development of minority children and youth. The chapters in this part of the Handbook present cutting-edge scholarship on the peer and friendship factors that support minority children's social integration, psychosocial adaptation, and school functioning. Furthermore, the part provides knowledge about the mechanism that explains why social adaptation occurs.

The part comprises five chapters. Chapter "Interethnic Friendship Formation" by Titzmann focuses on interethnic friendship formation. Titzmann examines the friendships of immigrant adolescents and presents general theoretical considerations as well as immigrant-specific theories regarding friendships during the adolescent years. Specifically, he discusses empirical findings on issues such as homophily and friendship effects for immigrant and native peers.

Chapter "The Friendships of Racial–Ethnic Minority Youth in Context" by Rogers, Niwa, and Way focuses on friendships of ethnic minority youth in context. Rogers and colleagues review research on the friendships of racial-ethnic minority youth by highlighting how the macro-context of ethnic, racial, gender, and sexuality stereotypes shape the micro-context of friendships. This is an innovative approach as the study of friendship among youth rarely attended to the influence of the macro-context.

In Chapter "Minority and Majority Children's Evaluations of Social Exclusion in Intergroup Contexts", Hitti, Lynn Mulvey, and Killen examine minority and majority children's evaluations of social exclusion in intergroup contexts. Hitti and her colleagues highlight recent research that reveals areas of convergence and divergence regarding peer-based social exclusion. While most children and adolescents view social exclusion based on group membership such as race and ethnicity as wrong, differences emerge between majority and minority perspectives. Based on the literature review the authors discuss implications for interventions to fostering positive peer relationships for both majority and minority youth.

Chapter "Children's Healthy Social–Emotional Development in Contexts of Peer Exclusion" focuses on children's healthy socio-emotional development in contexts of peer

exclusion. Malti, Zuffianò, Cui, Colasante, Peplak, and Young Bae review existing literature on the socio-emotional processes of peer inclusion and exclusion from childhood to adolescence with a specific focus on peer exclusion based on minority status in distinct categories. The authors discuss the specific risks of failing to address peer exclusion in multicultural societies. To overcome these risks they offer guidelines and strategies for prevention and intervention and provide avenues for future research.

In Chapter "Positive Youth Development of Roma Ethnic Minority Across Europe" in this part, Dimitrova and Ferrer-Wreder provide a brief overview about historical and current research as well as empirical findings on Roma children and youth, an underrepresented group in research, within the peer and family contexts. Furthermore, Dimitrova and her colleagues address resources with proximal contexts, such as peers and family, that have the potential to foster positive youth development in Roma ethnic minority populations in Europe. They end the chapter with a set of implications for the development of resource-oriented policy and practice for Roma youth.

Interethnic Friendship Formation

Peter F. Titzmann

Abstract

The establishment of mutual and supporting friendships is considered to be a major developmental task during the adolescent years, and both immigrant and native majority adolescents have to deal with it. Immigrant adolescents, however, often face additional challenges, such as discrimination and prejudice, and experience different cultural norms and values across different life domains. The aim of this chapter is to take a closer look at the friendships of immigrant adolescents; it starts with general theoretical considerations regarding friendships during the adolescent years. These general considerations are complemented by immigrant-specific theories on friendships. Next, the chapter discusses empirical findings on the homophily and friendship experiences of immigrant and native majority peers and methodological concerns, including sampling and assessment issues. The chapter ends with a discussion of current and future research questions as well as implications for policies.

Introduction

During the adolescent years, peer relations become increasingly important for individuals' development—at the same time as the dependency on parents decreases (Brown and Klute 2006; Steinberg and Silverberg 1986). Positive peer relationships such as friendships provide adoles-cents with a sense of acceptance and belonging, play a role in the development of social compe-tences, are first steps towards romantic relation-ships, and instigate changes in cognitions and in emotion regulation (Adams and Berzonsky 2003; Hartup 1996). Its importance is further demon-strated by the fact that successful formation of adolescent friendships contributes to self-esteem and socio-emotional support (Hartup 1996) and facilitates long-term adjustment in other domains of development, such as the work or partnership environment (Roisman et al. 2004). Given the important functions of friendships, it is not sur-prising that the establishment of mature mutual

P.F. Titzmann (✉)
Institute of Psychology, Leibniz Universität Hannover, Hanover, Germany
e-mail: titzmann@psychologie.uni-hannover.de

© The Editor(s) 2017
N.J. Cabrera and B. Leyendecker (eds.), *Handbook on Positive Development of Minority Children and Youth*, DOI 10.1007/978-3-319-43645-6_15

friendships is considered to be a major developmental task for the adolescent years, albeit first and formative friendship experiences are made during the pre-school years (Havighurst 1972).

The aim of this chapter is to take a closer look at the friendships of immigrant adolescents. Immigrant adolescents are confronted with the challenges of a transition into a new cultural context but also undergo the normative changes of growing up. This chapter presents, first, some theoretical considerations that focus on universal and immigration-specific aspects of friendship formation. Second, it presents selected empirical results followed by methodological considerations, current research questions, and future directions for research. The chapter concludes with some thoughts about policy implications.

First and foremost, however, the chapter addresses some definitional considerations of who is an immigrant. The growing body of research on immigrants in Europe focuses on people who temporarily or permanently move from one country to another (IOM 2010). Children or youth are identified as immigrant based on their country of birth, the country of birth of their parents, or their cultural group (e.g. mother tongue, ethnicity, cultural background). This chapter uses the term 'ethnic group' to refer to an immigrant youth's background. Ethnicity is defined broadly as 'the social group a person belongs to, and either identifies with or is identified with by others, as a result of a mix of cultural and other factors including language, diet, religion, ancestry, and physical features' (Bhopal 2004, p. 443). Thus, ethnicity cannot be seen as an unchangeable stable characteristic of a person, because some of these features can change through constant exchange with the majority population or other minorities.

Historical Overview and Theoretical Perspectives

General Considerations

When reflecting on friendships of immigrant adolescents, the general (immigration-unspecific) aspects of adolescent friendships have to be considered. Three such general aspects are (a) the peer ecology in which adolescents and their friendships are embedded, (b) the similarity as a general principle in friendship formation, and (c) the developmental changes in friendships that occur over the adolescent years. These general aspects seem to be universal and the incorporation of these aspects in the study of friendships among immigrant adolescents is crucial, because otherwise general phenomena of growing up may be misattributed to acculturation-related factors.

The first general principle is that friendships are embedded in a complex *ecology of peer relationships*. Based on Bronfenbrenner's (1986) work, Brown (1999) developed a model that depicts adolescents' peer ecology by differentiating between dyadic relations (best friends, romantic relationships), cliques of small friendship groups, crowds, and the overarching youth culture. Although these peer structures are interrelated, each of these peer structures serves a specific function in adolescent development (e.g., Brown 1999; Urberg et al. 1997). The dyadic relationships' function is mutual disclosure and the development of interpersonal skills, whereas cliques (small friendship groups) predominantly provide companionship for joint activities. Crowds are rather cognitive abstractions of groups to which individuals feel attached to and often carry a particular reputation (Brown and Klute 2006). Crowds can be, for example, fans of a particular sports club, people from a particular geographical region, or members of a particular ethnic group. Thus, crowds are less concrete and can be based on formal (neighbourhood, ethnic group) or informal (interests, beliefs) criteria that are shared among members of the crowd. Crowds provide role models for behaviour and identity development. Youth culture, the fourth peer structure, is the most abstract part of Brown's (1999) peer ecology and shares some parallels with Bronfenbrenner's (1986) macro context. It resembles youths' exposure to media and the general adolescent lifestyle at a particular historical period. All adolescents' experiences and behaviours (whether immigrant or not) are shaped to some extent by these peer structures, and adolescents, in turn, influence these structures. Nevertheless, adolescents' ability to influence each structure varies. Whereas adolescents may easily affect best friends, they may be limited in affecting the youth culture by adopting a specific music or clothing style and the related consumption behaviour (Brown 1999) or by their political or social engagement.

The second general aspect concerns the *similarity assumption in friendships* (Hartup and Stevens 1997). Adolescent friends have long been found to be similar in many aspects, particularly in demographic characteristics such as grade, age, gender and ethnicity (Kandel 1978). Three processes are relevant for this similarity: the initial selection of similar peers as friends, mutual socialization resulting in higher similarity over time, or deselection, which means that relationships with dissimilar friends are dissolved over time (van Workum et al. 2013).

The third general aspect in adolescents' friendships is *normative development*. During the adolescent years, individuals are confronted with substantial biological, psychological and social changes (Adams and Berzonsky 2003). These changes pose age-specific developmental tasks on individuals. In the friendship area, one of the most prominent developmental task in adolescence, a developmental task is to develop more mature social relationships with friends (Havighurst 1972). Whereas in early childhood friendships refer to companions for play activities, in adolescence, friends increasingly become confidants with mutual disclosure and trust, and bonding (Epstein 1989; Hartup and Stevens 1997). Furthermore, as the dependency on parents decreases, peer relations become increasingly important for adolescents' further normative development (Brown and Klute 2006; Steinberg and Silverberg 1986).

Friendships of Immigrants

Besides these general characteristics of adolescent friendships, immigrant adolescents are confronted with additional challenges: They often face discrimination, language problems and a substantial lack of resources in terms of finances and social network contacts (Stoessel et al. 2011;

Titzmann et al. 2011). In addition, immigrant adolescents are more likely to be involved in two or more cultural scripts depending on the life domain. Whereas the family environment often represents norms, values and cultural practices of their heritage culture, the school environment represent the norms, values and cultural practices of the dominant majority society. Bridging these cultures can pose a serious challenge for adolescent immigrants. Research has shown, for example that immigrant adolescents' wish to form friendships with native majority peers can be associated with higher levels of family conflict if parents do not support this wish (Titzmann and Sonnenberg 2016). These immigration-specific challenges may be reasons why research consistently and across various countries has shown that immigrant adolescents form friendships primarily within their own ethnic community and much less across ethnic groups (Titzmann 2014), a phenomenon that has been termed friendship homophily (McPherson et al. 2001).

Although ethnic homophily can be explained by the friendship similarity assumption and the many similarities adolescents from one cultural group share, ethnic homophily is not desired from a multicultural society's perspective. Ethnic homophily contradicts multicultural ideologies, hinders cooperation between ethnic groups and can threaten societal cohesion. For this reason, research started to investigate how interethnic relationships can be fostered and ethnic homophily reduced. Various theoretical approaches have been developed in this regard, more than can be presented in a single chapter. Hence, the following theoretical approaches present a selection of theories that have stimulated research in the area of adolescent immigrants' friendships, but they are far from being exhaustive.

A very prominent theoretical approach to interethnic friendships is *intergroup contact theory*. Intergroup contact theory argues that intergroup contact reduces prejudice and discrimination between groups as long as the contact situation ensures an equal status of groups, the support from authorities, intergroup cooperation and common goals (Allport 1954;

Pettigrew and Tropp 2006). Interethnic friendships are seen as the model case for meeting all these conditions and are thus assumed to be the ideal form of intergroup contact: 'friendship potential is an essential, not merely facilitating, condition for positive intergroup contact effects that generalize' (Pettigrew 1998, p. 76). In alignment with these theoretical assumptions, interethnic friendships were found to be associated with better intergroup relations as indicated by lower levels of mutual mistrust, less discrimination and prejudice (Aberson et al. 2004; Aboud et al. 2003; Titzmann et al. 2015). Due to the substantial evidence, including findings from a meta-analysis (Pettigrew and Tropp 2006), contact theory can be seen as one of the best tested intergroup theories. Based on this theory, interethnic friendships can be enhanced by bringing groups into contact situations that fulfil the contact conditions mentioned earlier.

Nevertheless, the focus of intergroup contact theory is primarily on the effects of contact on children and adolescents rather than the predictors of intergroup friendships. A theoretical approach on the predictors of interethnic friendships is the intergroup perspective and particularly *social identity theory* (Tajfel and Turner 1986). Social identity theory assumes that self-ascribed membership in social groups guides individuals' intergroup attitudes and behaviours because individuals try to bring their behaviour in alignment with what they believe is expected from group members. Research from this perspective emphasises cultural identification with the host or heritage culture as an opportunity for, or barrier to, emerging intergroup friendships of immigrants (Stoessel et al. 2012). According to this theory, group boundaries have to be reduced and group permeability and identification with the host society have to be increased in order to decrease levels of friendship homophily. To achieve this goal, the discrimination of immigrants has to stop as an important first step, as it can foster the identification with the heritage group (Jetten et al. 2001).

Somewhat related to the intergroup perspective is the concept of *acculturation orientations or acculturation strategies* (Berry 1997, 2005). This theoretical approach assumes that acculturative processes are worked out along two dimensions: (a) heritage cultural maintenance (contact with the co-ethnic in-group) and (b) participation in the receiving society (contact with the majority out-group) (Berry 1997). Based on these two dimensions, four acculturation orientations can be differentiated. These four acculturation orientations are not only held by individual immigrants, but can also be identified in the larger (receiving) society. High expression in both dimensions, that is, immigrants' maintaining of aspects of the heritage culture while also establishing relationships with people from the majority leads to integration at the level of individual immigrants and to multiculturalism at the level of the larger society. Low expression in both dimensions (i.e., abandoning and/or devaluing both the culture of origin and the new culture) leads to marginalisation when held by the immigrant and exclusion when held by the larger society. The other two combinations lead either to assimilation (immigrant) and the melting pot (larger society) or to separation (immigrant) and segregation (larger society). Based on this theoretical model and further developments of it (e.g., Bourhis et al. 1997), interethnic friendships should become more likely when immigrants and natives have consensual acculturation orientations that include the cooperation of immigrants and the native majority group—for example when immigrants favour integration and the majority favours multiculturalism. If, however, immigrants and natives have conflictual acculturation orientations (e.g. immigrants want to integrate, whereas natives prefer the exclusion of immigrants) the emergence of interethnic friendships is likely to be reduced.

Another theoretical perspective from acculturation research is *sociocultural learning theory*. Sociocultural learning theory would argue that friendships are the behavioural outcome of the acquisition of cultural skills (Masgoret and Ward 2006; Ward 2001). This theoretical approach is in line with general considerations of similarity as being the backbone of all friendships (Hartup and Stevens 1997). According to this perspective, sociocultural adjustment of adolescent immigrants, given that it takes place over time in the new country, can reduce cultural dissimilarity between immigrants and natives and result in a higher likelihood of interethnic friendships. This line of thinking, therefore, emphasises the strengthening of cultural competences, particularly in the linguistic domain, as a means to promote interethnic friendships. A disadvantage of this view, however, may be that the responsibility for positive intergroup relations is predominantly assigned to the immigrant adolescents, although it is the joint responsibility of immigrants and the native majority.

Besides these psychological processes, the developmental contexts in which interethnic friendships may occur have received substantial attention. Theoretically, both Hallinan's *opportunity hypothesis* (Hallinan 1982; Hallinan and Teixeira 1987) and Blau's *macrostructural theory* (Blau 1974, 1977) suggest that friendship homophily is more likely in contexts with a higher share of same-ethnic individuals. Blau argues that humans always prefer in-group contact over out-group contact, but if opportunities for in-group contact become smaller (fewer in-group members in a context), individuals prefer out-group contacts over not having any social interaction. According to this line of thinking, contexts are potential instruments to reduce friendship homophily or to increase interethnic friendships, by avoiding high levels of segregation in schools or neighbourhoods.

All of these theoretical approaches have received empirical support, but none of these theories alone seems to be able to explain the complexity of interethnic friendships. For this reason, more comprehensive approaches have been developed in recent years. These approaches combine different mechanisms and various sources of influence (Motti-Stefanidi et al. 2012; Titzmann 2014). In addition, the theories mentioned differ in their assumptions about the causality of effects. Intergroup contact theory, for example, assumes that contact leads to changes in attitudes, whereas social identity theory sees friendships as the outcome of adolescents' attitudes and group identification. Most probably, however, processes are linked through dynamic interactions with mutually enhancing effects.

Empirical Findings

The theoretical frameworks presented in the previous section have received substantial attention in empirical research. However, the research on interethnic and intraethnic friendships often has been descriptive and not yet fully integrated into a broader framework. Ethnic groups belonging to different ethnic, racial, cultural or immigrant groups have been studied and different methods for data collection have been used, ranging from peer nomination to questionnaires to observational data. Due to space limitation, this chapter does not present an exhaustive overview of the existing literature, but it covers selected empirical findings that have been replicated in various studies.

Intraethnic Friendship Preference

In general, there is robust empirical evidence that adolescents have friends who are similar in age, gender and ethnic background (Kandel 1978). The preference for peers with similar ethnic or religious backgrounds can already be found in preadolescence (Jugert et al. 2011; Verkuyten and Kinket 2000) but remains high during the adolescent years. Harris and Cavanagh (2008) reported, for example, that about 75 % of friends of black youth are also black. In the same study, 55 % of friends of Hispanic adolescents were reported to also have a Hispanic background and about 40 % of friends of Asian adolescents shared their Asian background. These numbers are from research conducted with American samples and predominantly refer to minority adolescents, but the findings are similar among immigrants in the European context. Shortly after immigration nearly all friends of adolescent immigrants from the former Soviet Union in Germany were found to have a similar (Russian) background (Titzmann 2014). Over time in the new country, the proportion of intraethnic friends in immigrants' friendship networks decreased, but after about 7 years, it levelled off at about 65 % without any further significant change, although the proportion of this group in the school context was on average only 24 % (Titzmann and Silbereisen 2009). The studies described here are no exceptions. Similar findings have been revealed in the US (e.g., Aboud et al. 2003; Graham et al. 2009) and Europe (e.g., Baerveldt et al. 2004; Reinders and Mangold 2005; Strohmeier et al. 2006). In addition, the results are stable across different assessment methods, including socio-metric nominations, observational techniques and other methods (Graham et al. 2009). It is noteworthy, however, that ethnic homophily is not an immigrant-specific phenomenon. Non-immigrant (majority) adolescents have been found to show an even higher preference for intra-ethnic friendships than immigrant adolescents (Baerveldt et al. 2004; Strohmeier 2012). In the study by Harris and Cavanagh (2008), the share of intraethnic friends was highest among the white majority with about 85 %.

Predictors of Interindividual Differences in Friendship Homophily

Although friendship homophily is, in principle, a general phenomenon describing an overall tendency for intraethnic social relations, researchers conceptualize it as an individual characteristic that can vary across individuals so that predictors for these interindividual differences can be identified (Titzmann et al. 2012). The crucial question is why some adolescents have more intraethnic friendships than others. To answer these questions empirical results can be used that explain interindividual differences in friendship homophily.

First of all, *demographic characteristics* have to be considered in the formation of interethnic friendships or in the study of friendship homophily. While data concerning gender differences have been inconsistent (Graham et al. 2009), findings repeatedly showed that interethnic friendships decline as adolescents grow older, i.e. ethnic homophily increases with age (Aboud et al. 2003; Graham et al. 2009; Strohmeier 2012; Titzmann and Silbereisen 2009). One potential explanation for this effect might be the change in

friendship quality over the adolescent years. As discussed earlier, friendships in late childhood refer predominantly to companionship and joint playing, whereas friendships in adolescence increasingly include mutual disclosure and support (Epstein 1989; Hartup and Stevens 1997). The latter may be more easily achieved with intraethnic friends, because these friends share similar experiences of the transition from one country to another, often have the same social status and may also face discrimination. These shared characteristics may enhance mutual understanding and support. Nevertheless, the findings are not fully consistent. Shrum et al. (1988) observed a curvilinear relationship between ethnic homophily and grade in a cross-sectional study of grades 3–12 and Titzmann (2014) argued that some age effects may in fact be the result of hidden associations with other variables. Length of residence in the host country is another demographic factor associated with lower levels of homophily in cross-sectional and longitudinal studies (Titzmann 2014; Titzmann and Silbereisen 2009). Most likely, this association points to adaptation processes with increased language and sociocultural competence with time spent in the new society.

In addition, research across a number of studies showed that context matters, particularly the class or school *ethnic composition*. These variables received substantial attention in research on ethnic homophily of adolescents with the opportunity hypothesis (Hallinan 1982; Hallinan and Teixeira 1987) and macrostructural theory (Blau 1974, 1977) as theoretical backgrounds. Both these theories predict lower levels of homophily and a higher likelihood of interethnic friendships in contexts with low proportions of intraethnic peers. This hypothesis has been supported for black and white students (Graham et al. 2009; Hallinan and Teixeira 1987) as well as for immigrants from the former Soviet Union in Germany (Titzmann and Silbereisen 2009). Furthermore, if students were assigned roommates of a different ethnic group, they started to develop more friendships with other members of that group (Mark and Harris 2012). The effect of opportunity structures is also demonstrated by findings showing that the association between friendship homophily and length of residence depended on the proportion of intraethnic peers in the school context (Titzmann 2014). This association was strongest in schools with less than 12 % intraethnic peers ($r = -0.40$), somewhat smaller in schools with 12–30 % intraethnic peers ($r = -0.27$) and not significant in schools with more than 30 % intraethnic peers ($r = -0.10$). All these results indicate that the opportunity for contact is a major factor for interethnic friendships to occur, but the conditions of the contact also matter. Settings that encourage close interactions through repeated and extensive contact have been found to result in high friendship potential (Jugert et al. 2011). In addition, Spiel and Strohmeier (2012) showed the importance of the school context for creating contact opportunities. When friendship homophily was compared between inside and outside school relations, friendship homophily was significantly lower inside schools.

The *sociocultural adaptation* perspective assumes that cultural adaptation to a new context increases the similarity with native majority peers and decreases the cultural distance between immigrants and natives. Accordingly, interethnic friendships (low friendship homophily) should occur in greater likelihood when immigrants develop cultural skills that fit with the majority culture. One of the most prominent predictors in this regard is use of the new language. Across various cross-sectional and longitudinal studies, those individuals who spoke the new language better and more frequently reported lower levels of friendship homophily (Titzmann and Silbereisen 2009; Titzmann et al. 2012). A likely explanation for the strong association between language and friendship homophily can be seen in the fact that language is not just a tool for interpersonal communication and for access to host-culture information, but that it is also a vehicle transporting identity (Caldas and Caron-Caldas 2002; Gudykunst and Schmidt 1987) and self-worth (Schnittker 2002). Among adolescents, language is also used to determine group boundaries (Androutsopoulos and

Georgakopoulou 2003; Stenström and Jørgensen 2009). Thus, language seems to be an important tool that can help ease the communication between immigrant and native majority adolescents with a higher likelihood of emerging interethnic friendships (i.e., lower friendship homophily).

Finally, the *acculturation orientations* have been studied as predictors of interethnic friendship. Empirical research has developed two methodological approaches to assess acculturation orientations. One approach combines the two dimensions of (a) heritage cultural maintenance and (b) participation in the receiving society in single items (Berry et al. 2006a, b) so that adolescents rate statements like "I prefer social activities which involve both [nationals] and [my ethnic group]" or "I prefer social activities which involve [nationals] only" (Berry et al. 2006a, p. 309). Another approach assess both these dimensions as independent constructs (Ryder et al. 2000) so that participants have to rate separate statements for their willingness in heritage and host culture involvement. Both these methods have shown that acculturation orientations are associated with adolescent immigrants' interethnic friendships and friendship homophily (Berry et al. 2006a, b; Titzmann 2014). If immigrant adolescents are willing to have contact with native majority peers, interethnic friendships become more likely whereas the opposite result was found for adolescents preferring contact with their own group. This association was found on various friendship levels (best friends and more distant friends) as well as in comparisons across receiving societies (Titzmann et al. 2007) and may be explained by the theory of planned behaviour (Armitage and Conner 2001; Fishbein and Ajzen 2010). The theory of planned behaviour assumes that individuals try to bring attitudes and behaviour into alignment. For interethnic friendships this means that native majority and immigrant adolescents may actively seek out situations or contexts in which they meet peers of one or the other ethnicity depending on their acculturation orientation. Nevertheless, there is a lack of research to identify the order of effects. Whereas Fishbein and Ajzen (2010) assume that intentions precede the behaviour, others assume and find evidence for the opposite (e.g., Turner and Brown 2008), so, perhaps, transactional processes describe the association between acculturation orientation and interethnic friendship patterns better than causal assumptions in one or the other direction.

Interethnic Friendships: Effects and Friendship Quality

Interethnic friendships are one of the most powerful sources for changing intergroup relations. Intergroup friendships have been found to reduce the level of intergroup prejudice, to decrease implicit and explicit bias, to reduce discrimination and to improve interactions between members of the two groups (Aberson et al. 2004; Antonio 2001; Perry 2013; Pettigrew and Tropp 2006; Titzmann et al. 2015). Furthermore, having native majority friends is helpful for immigrants to enhance their access to resources and information in local organisations, which gives them the opportunity to cope with the new environment more effectively (Bochner et al. 1977; Mollica et al. 2003; Titzmann et al. 2010). In addition, a Swedish study revealed that having native majority friends can reduce levels of maladjustment among immigrant youth: The data showed that immigrant boys who had predominantly immigrant friends exhibited higher levels of norm-breaking behaviour compared to immigrant boys who also had Swedish friends (Svensson et al. 2011). In general, however, it has to be noted that native majority adolescents seem to profit more from interethnic friendships than the immigrant adolescents because effects of interethnic friendships on changes in attitudes were found to be stronger for native majority than for immigrant adolescents (Feddes et al. 2009).

The underlying mechanisms for the association of interethnic friendships and intergroup relations have also received attention. Research has identified several mechanisms, including reduction of intergroup anxiety, increase in intergroup empathy and advancement in intergroup perspective taking (Pettigrew and Tropp 2006; Stephan and Stephan 2001). In addition, contact in the form of interethnic friendships seems to increase knowledge about the out-group and the acquisition of culture-specific information (Bochner et al. 1977; Titzmann et al. 2010).

Given this substantial body of research, it is not surprising that interethnic friendships "have become an important benchmark in efforts to reduce racial segregation and prejudice" (Aboud et al. 2003, p. 165). One has to be careful, however, with regard to the direction of effects, because some longitudinal studies found that interethnic contact precedes changes in intergroup attitudes (Dhont et al. 2012; Feddes et al. 2009), whereas other (also longitudinal) studies have found bidirectional models more appropriate in describing the association between contact and prejudice (Binder et al. 2009; Swart et al. 2011). Again, bidirectional models with simultaneous longitudinal effects from intergroup contact on prejudice and from prejudice on intergroup contact seem to be underlying these associations.

Besides these positive qualities of interethnic friendships and low levels of friendship homophily, research has also demonstrated some vulnerabilities in interethnic friendships. One such vulnerability that has been found repeatedly is the lower stability of interethnic as compared to intraethnic friendships (Aboud et al. 2003; Jugert et al. 2013; Schneider et al. 2007). This finding led to research on differences in friendship quality between interethnic and intraethnic friendships. Aspects of friendship quality that have been studied include, among others, loyalty, emotional security, intimacy, closeness, competition, reciprocity and or spare time activities (Aboud et al. 2003; Kao and Joyner 2004; Reinders and Mangold 2005; Schneider et al. 2007; Strohmeier et al. 2006). Results show both similarities and differences between intraethnic and interethnic friendships. No differences were identified for loyalty and emotional security (Aboud et al. 2003), conflict (Reinders and Mangold 2005; Strohmeier et al. 2006) or mutual care (Strohmeier et al. 2006). At the same time, interethnic friendships seem to be somewhat lower in closeness (Schneider et al. 2007), joint activities (Kao and Joyner 2004; Strohmeier et al. 2006) and intimacy (Aboud et al. 2003). Such differences may pose greater challenges for relationships in interethnic compared with intraethnic friendships. Future research may shed more light on these inconclusive findings and would benefit from studying interethnic friendship quality in combination with the gender composition and specific cultural background of the friends, as both these factors seem to moderate the effects of interethnic friendships on friendship quality (Reinders and Mangold 2005; Strohmeier et al. 2006).

Methodology

Research on immigrant adolescents' interethnic friendship formation is quite a complex issue and various methodological challenges have to be considered. This section will address two aspects in greater detail: the selection of groups for the study of interethnic friendships and the question of the assessment of interethnic friendships in the current literature.

Group Selection

A particular challenge in the research of immigrant peer relations is the selection of groups to be studied. In principle, researchers can choose between two strategies. The first strategy was suggested by Berry et al. (1987). The basic idea of this strategy is to select acculturating groups from various backgrounds and to observe these groups in various receiving contexts. The more groups and receiving societies, the more complete the picture is that can be derived from such a design. Together with the advent of new methodologies, such as multi-level modelling, such a design offers many opportunities for studying the interactive nature of acculturation processes in general and friendship formation processes in particular (Motti-Stefanidi et al. 2012). Although such designs are labour

intensive and require a large network of collaborators, they certainly have a large potential to advance research.

A second strategy suggests studying a small number of well-chosen groups. Fuligni (2001) suggests, for example, comparing an immigrant group with a native majority reference group and with a culturally similar group of individuals in the country of origin. Such a design, allows the estimation of similarities and differences between the groups and differentiation of whether a particular outcome is due to the migration experience, due to cultural background, or due to the normative development and the environmental constraints and opportunities in the country of residence. An additional elaboration of the design would be the inclusion of groups that migrate within the country of origin, in order to have a group without a cultural transition but similar experiences of being cut off from their familiar environment. Ideally, such comparisons should be conducted in longitudinal fashion (Fuligni 2001) because only longitudinal research can uncover the processes of change that are immanent in both acculturation and normative development. A disadvantage of this strategy, however, is that only specific groups are studied and that the generalizability to other groups or contexts is limited. One solution to this problem is suggested by Kohn (1987). Kohn recommends a comparative design, in which results found in one group or context are replicated in another group or context that is fundamentally different and which can challenge the assumptions made from the original results. If the results are replicated, the effects can be assumed to be quite robust.

Both these approaches have been applied in research on immigrant adolescents and also on friendship patterns. One example for the comparison of multiple groups in multiple contexts is the ICSEY project which was conducted in 13 countries (Berry et al. 2006a). Nevertheless, the study of specific ethnic groups with a comparative perspective seems a little more prominent in existing research (Jugert et al. 2011; Motti-Stefanidi and Asendorpf 2012; Titzmann et al. 2012).

Assessment of Interethnic Friendships

The second important decision to be made in the study of interethnic friendships is the choice of the specific indicator for interethnic friendships or friendship homophily. The most common approach is to assess the composition of immigrant adolescents' friendship networks by calculating the percentage of intraethnic friends among all friends for assessing friendship homophily (Chan and Birman 2009; Spiel 2009; Titzmann 2014). Some authors (McCormick et al. 2014; Strohmeier and Spiel 2012) criticise such measures for not taking into account the availability of intraethnic peers in the relevant context, for example, in a classroom. In order to incorporate these arguments, other indices have been developed that take into account the opportunity structure of a given context (Joyner and Kao 2000; Strohmeier 2012). Thus far, indices that control or do not control for opportunity seem to reveal rather similar findings when compared (McCormick et al. 2014), but indices that account for contact opportunities may gain in importance with the growing number of ethnicities in multicultural classrooms. A disadvantage of these indices is, however, that the opportunity structure becomes part of friendship homophily index, although it is one of the most important predictors of it. More recent approaches apply network analyses in the study of interethnic friendship formation that allow taking into account characteristics of the social network, such as reciprocity and transitivity (Leszczensky and Pink 2015; Smith et al. 2016).

Current Research Questions and Future Directions

The theoretical, empirical and methodological considerations outlined above show that research in the peer environment of adolescent immigrants has been fruitful to increase the understanding of opportunities and risks of interethnic contact. But there is more to do. This section presents some of the issues that deserve more attention in future research.

The first issue is that current research is rather scattered. Various groups of immigrants are typically investigated in various contexts. Given the specific situation of a particular immigrant or ethnic group in a particular context, the generalizability of these results is an issue of debate. Comparative research would help to identify similarities, as well as group-specific aspects (Berry et al. 2006b; Slonim-Nevo et al. 2009). These groups may not necessarily represent specific nationalities. Berry et al. (1987) differentiated immigrant groups (e.g., refugees), native majority people, ethnic minority groups and sojourners. Nowadays, other types of immigrants move into the focus of attention, for example ethnic diaspora migrants or repatriates. Diaspora migrants return to their country of origin after living in a diaspora for quite some time, sometimes even for generations, and face partly different acculturation experiences and conditions than other immigrant groups (Motti-Stefanidi and Asendorpf 2012; Silbereisen et al. 2014; Sussman 2011; Weingrod and Levy 2006). The comparative study of different types of minority and majority groups is one possibility to find groups of immigrants who function similarly or differently. In addition to differentiating types of immigrants, the identification of higher order dimensions on which host societies and acculturating groups differ seems a way forward to reduce the complexity of acculturation research. Such dimensions could be derived from cultural differences (Hofstede 2003), economic prosperity, or national policies for dealing with immigrants (Huddleston et al. 2011). Identification of such underlying macro-level dimensions for successful or challenging adaptation courses would help to make predictions about groups and contexts that are not yet studied.

A second issue is the domain specificity of many results obtained. Research often focuses on single domains, such as success in school or psychological functioning in the family environment. Friendships with native majority peers may, for example, increase the level of educational attainment of adolescent immigrants, because they have better access to information. Adolescent immigrants, however, have to deal with different challenges and cultural scripts in different domains of development. An adaptation to the host-culture dominated peer or school domain, for example, may come at the cost of maladaptation in the heritage-culture dominated family domain (Fillmore 2000; Telzer 2011; Titzmann 2012; Titzmann and Sonnenberg 2016). How adolescents successfully deal with the different demands and cultural scripts needs research covering multiple life domains simultaneously. Promising avenues in how adolescents can successfully navigate through a multicultural society are biculturalism (Schwartz and Unger 2010), models on the situational variations in ethnic identity (Zhang and Noels 2013) and the development of several cultural scripts or working models (Oppedal 2006).

A third aspect is the strengthening of the developmental perspective in research on the adolescents' adaptation to the peer domain. Keeping in mind that a growing number of immigrants are children and youth, the many social, psychological and biological changes that occur at this period of life need to be addressed. Research has already started to investigate the interplay of adolescent age with the immigration process (Cheung et al. 2011) and it does make a difference whether the family migrated with a baby or toddler, a kindergarten child, a school child or an adolescent. A good example in this regard is language acquisition. Whereas language acquisition in the receiving country is assumed to be the learning of a second language after the age of 3 years, it is still considered as first language acquisition before this age, even though children may learn both heritage and host culture language as first languages in this case (Hamers and Blanc 2000; Klein 1987). Similarly, normative development is related to important biographical transitions in life that are culturally and socially structured in societies (Nurmi 1993). In industrialised societies, children start primary school at the age of about five or six. Such 'normative' transitions are of central interest for developmental psychology (Bronfenbrenner 2005; Silbereisen et al. 2012; Walsemann et al. 2009). Children who have to interrupt their school career in one country and who have to restart

schooling in another country obviously face different challenges compared with children who migrated before such formative transitions.

Fourth, despite the many developmental similarities between immigrant and native majority adolescents, mean level differences between both groups can be found in various other characteristics. These differences should be explored more carefully and not simply documented. Ethnic differences in any given outcome are often the result of different levels of well-known risk or protective factors (Feldman and Rosenthal 1994), such as economic disadvantage or lower levels of support. Achievement differences between immigrants and natives turned out to be in favour of immigrants, for example, after analyses accounted for the socio-economic disadvantage the immigrants were confronted with (Kristen et al. 2014). It is a major responsibility of research to disentangle economic, transition-related, context-based, developmental, or cultural factors, because this differentiation is important for a better and less biased understanding of any ethnic differences.

A fifth aspect concerns the increasing diversity in multicultural societies. London, for example, accommodates individuals from as many as 179 countries (Vertovec 2007), which are also present in growingly multicultural schools. Intergroup approaches that only focus on two groups may be limited in understanding such a multicultural complexity. Some research showed, for example, that lowest levels of segregation are observed in settings with moderate (not low, not high) levels of cultural heterogeneity (Moody 2001) and that high levels of cultural heterogeneity relate to fewer interethnic friendships and lower levels of interethnic support (Chan and Birman 2009). Research has to take into account this increasing ethnic and cultural complexity, particularly when studying interethnic friendships.

Finally, more longitudinal research is needed (Fuligni 2001) for documenting and differentiating acculturative and normative changes in friendship patterns, for explaining interindividual differences in these changes, and for studying the order of effects. Although cross-sectional research is an important asset in comparative analyses, it can be misleading. In a study on immigrants from the former Soviet Union, for example, positive associations between age and friendship homophily were uncovered in cross-sectional analyses (Titzmann et al. 2007), whereas negative associations were found in longitudinal data (Titzmann and Silbereisen 2009; Titzmann et al. 2012). The explanation for this contradiction was found in differences between younger and older adolescents (Titzmann 2014). Younger adolescent immigrants were more similar to their native majority peers. Hence, their level of friendship homophily was rather low with little change over time. Older adolescents, in contrast, were more dissimilar to native majority peers but adapted to the native's values over time (Titzmann and Silbereisen 2012). Thus, older adolescents' friendship homophily was significantly higher than that of their younger counterparts with a pronounced decrease over time. In an age-heterogeneous sample, these characteristics result in a positive association between age and the level of homophily and a negative association between age and rate of change in friendship homophily. Only longitudinal research could uncover these effects in greater detail.

Policy Implications

The empirical findings presented above show that there is still a need for more research to fully understand the complexity of the precursors and effects of interethnic friendships. Nevertheless, the existing findings allow deriving strategies for the promotion of positive peer relationships in multicultural settings, such as schools. The major aims of such programmes are to increase intergroup contact (especially friendships) and to improve intergroup attitudes, but the measures to achieve these aims differ. So what can be done?

At the most basic level, contexts (school, neighbourhood, spare time activities) have to be created to allow interethnic contact to emerge. In this regard, it seems beneficial to avoid highly segregated schools or neighbourhoods (Moody

2001; Titzmann 2014). More specifically, as no significant decrease in friendship homophily was found in schools with more than 30 % of intraethnic peers (Titzmann 2014), it seems advisable that the share of a specific ethnic or cultural group in a school context should be lower than that.

Given current knowledge on the effects of interethnic contact, however, it would be negligent to rely just on the effects of a particular school or neighbourhood composition. Schools in particular can create conditions that bolster the effects of interethnic contact. These conditions include equal status of groups, support from authorities (teachers), intergroup cooperation and common goals. Cooperative learning situations, in which small teams of mixed ethnicity work jointly on academic assignments meet most of these conditions and have been found to increase interethnic friendships as well as interethnic friendship reciprocity (Hansell and Slavin 1981). In the past, different versions of cooperative learning have been developed (see Slavin and Cooper 1999, for an overview). All these methods aim at improving cooperation and joint success of small, heterogeneous work groups.

Cooperative learning is an indirect (i.e. does not directly address the intergroup situation) and interactive (i.e. individuals of different ethnicity interact with each other) method (Stephan and Stephan 2001). Other interventions are more direct in addressing cultural diversity and use more didactic teaching methods. One such method is multicultural education or multicultural learning. Multicultural learning approaches systematically integrate learning about other cultures, races and ethnicities into everyday teaching (Sleeter and Grant 2009). The main goals are the acknowledgement and recognition of existing cultural differences as well as the transfer of intercultural knowledge and tolerance (Verkuyten and Thijs 2013). Such interventions have been shown to improve cultural knowledge and understanding across groups and to establish anti-racism norms in multicultural classrooms, which in turn help to improve interethnic relations (Verkuyten and Thijs 2013).

The two interventions just mentioned are only two examples that have been applied in multicultural school settings. Other methods focus on moral education programmes, intergroup dialogues, conflict resolution training, or intercultural training methods (see Stephan and Stephan 2001, for a systematic overview). What is still missing, however, are systematic evaluations of such prevention and intervention programmes as well as knowledge about the underlying mechanisms. Such knowledge is needed to inform practitioners about the differential effects of these programmes to enable them to choose which programme is best for which intergroup situation.

At first sight, the application of theoretical and empirical findings seems challenged by ambiguous findings with regard to the causality of interethnic friendships and their precursors/effects. This chapter showed that some theories and findings assume that contact precedes cultural knowledge and intergroup attitudes, whereas others assume and find the opposite. The most plausible explanation for this seemingly inconsistent evidence is that these processes are intertwined, dynamic and bidirectional. Language competence may, for example, ease communication with native majority peers who, in turn, may help immigrants in further language acquisition. The implication of this bidirectionality assumption is that interventions need not seek causes and consequences, but have two starting points for improving interethnic relations. They could, for example, simultaneously convey the new language and establish situations for interethnic contact.

Of course, most of these approaches should not only target immigrants. More needs to be known about the effects of multicultural classrooms and interethnic friendships on native majority adolescents and how they profit from these relationships. In order to capitalise on the potential of immigrant youth, comprehensive research is needed which includes all students enrolled in multicultural schools. This perspective is in line with interactive models of acculturation (Berry 2005; Bourhis et al. 1997) and with findings showing that adolescents' adaptation can only be understood in light of intraethnic and interethnic peers' attitudes and behaviours in a given school context (Schachner

et al. 2015; Titzmann and Jugert 2015). The goal of sustainable change in the intergroup school climate and school culture, however, may require intervention programmes that target not only adolescents, but the entire school staff. Teachers, typically from the majority population, were found to report reservations about minority students, resulting in teacher–pupil social distance and disaffection (Alexander et al. 1987). Clearly, teacher attitudes also have to be a target of interventions fostering the positive relations between different ethnicities in schools. Furthermore, intervention programmes targeting immigration-unrelated behaviours, such as aggression or bullying, may profit from cultural components. The Viennese Social Competence (ViSC) training, for example, includes training units that directly focus on the intercultural competencies required in modern multicultural school settings (Strohmeier et al. 2012). The general conclusion of this chapter is, hence, that interethnic friendships and positive intergroup relations are desirable and an aim in multicultural societies. Achieving this aim requires the cooperation of all parties involved—the native majority group, the immigrant community and the individual adolescent.

References

Aberson, C. L., Shoemaker, C., & Tomolillo, C. (2004). Implicit bias and contact: The role of interethnic friendships. *Journal of Social Psychology, 144*(3), 335–347.

Aboud, F. E., Mendelson, M. J., & Purdy, K. T. (2003). Cross-race peer relations and friendship quality. *International Journal of Behavioral Development, 27*(2), 165–173.

Adams, G. R., & Berzonsky, M. D. (Eds.). (2003). *Blackwell handbook of adolescence*. Malden: Blackwell Publishing.

Alexander, K. L., Entwisle, D. R., & Thompson, M. S. (1987). School performance, status relations, and the structure of sentiment: Bringing the teacher back in. *American Sociological Review, 52*(5), 665–682. doi:10.2307/2095602

Allport, G. W. (1954). *The nature of prejudice*. Cambridge, MA: Perseus Books.

Androutsopoulos, J. K., & Georgakopoulou, A. (Eds.). (2003). *Discourse constructions of youth identities*. Amsterdam: John Benjamins.

Antonio, A. L. (2001). Diversity and the influence of friendship groups in college. *Review of Higher Education: Journal of the Association for the Study of Higher Education, 25*(1), 63–89.

Armitage, C. J., & Conner, M. (2001). Efficacy of the theory of planned behaviour: A meta-analytic review. *British Journal of Social Psychology, 40*(4), 471–499. doi:10.1348/014466601164939

Baerveldt, C., Van Duijn, M. A. J., Vermeij, L., & Van Hemert, D. A. (2004). Ethnic boundaries and personal choice. Assessing the influence of individual inclinations to choose intra-ethnic relationships on pupils' networks. *Social Networks, 26*(1), 55–74. doi:10. 1016/j.socnet.2004.01.003

Berry, J. W. (1997). Immigration, acculturation, and adaptation. *Applied Psychology: An International Review, 46*(1), 5–34.

Berry, J. W. (2005). Acculturation: Living successfully in two cultures. *International Journal of Intercultural Relations, 29*(6), 697–712. doi:10.1016/j.ijintrel.2005. 07.013

Berry, J. W., Kim, U., Minde, T., & Mok, D. (1987). Comparative studies of acculturative stress. *International Migration Review, 21*(3), 491–511. doi:10. 2307/2546607

Berry, J. W., Phinney, J. S., Sam, D. L., & Vedder, P. (2006a). Immigrant youth: Acculturation, identity, and adaptation. *Applied Psychology: An International Review, 55*(3), 303–332.

Berry, J. W., Phinney, J. S., Sam, D. L., & Vedder, P. (Eds.). (2006b). *Immigrant youth in cultural transition: Acculturation, identity, and adaptation across national contexts*. Mahwah, NJ: Lawrence Erlbaum Associates Publishers.

Bhopal, R. (2004). Glossary of terms relating to ethnicity and race: For reflection and debate. *Journal of Epidemiology and Community Health, 58*(6), 441–445. doi:10.1136/jech.2003.013466

Binder, J., Zagefka, H., Brown, R., Funke, F., Kessler, T., Mummendey, A., et al. (2009). Does contact reduce prejudice or does prejudice reduce contact? A longitudinal test of the contact hypothesis among majority and minority groups in three European countries. *Journal of Personality and Social Psychology, 96*(4), 843–856. doi:10.1037/a0013470

Blau, P. M. (1974). Presidential address: Parameters of social structure. *American Sociological Review, 39*(5), 615–635.

Blau, P. M. (1977). A macrosociological theory of social structure. *American Journal of Sociology, 83*(1), 26–54.

Bochner, S., McLeod, B. M., & Lin, A. (1977). Friendship patterns of overseas students: A functional model. *International Journal of Psychology, 12*, 277–294.

Bourhis, R. Y., Moïse, L. C., Perreault, S., & Senécal, S. (1997). Towards an interactive acculturation model: A social psychological approach. *International Journal of Psychology, 32*(6), 369–386. doi:10.1080/ 002075997400629

Bronfenbrenner, U. (1986). Ecology of the family as a context for human development: Research perspectives. *Developmental Psychology, 22*(6), 723–742. doi:10.1037/0012-1649.22.6.723

Bronfenbrenner, U. (2005). A future perspective (1979). In U. Bronfenbrenner (Ed.), *Making human beings human: Bioecological perspectives on human development* (pp. 50–59). Thousand Oaks, CA: Sage Publications Ltd.

Brown, B. B. (1999). Measuring the peer environment of American adolescents. In S. L. Friedman & T. D. Wachs (Eds.), *Measuring environment across the life span: Emerging methods and concepts* (pp. 59–90). Washington, DC: American Psychological Association.

Brown, B. B., & Klute, C. (2006). Friendships, cliques, and crowds. In G. R. Adams & M. D. Berzonsky (Eds.), *Blackwell handbook of adolescence*. Malden, MA: Blackwell.

Caldas, S. J., & Caron-Caldas, S. (2002). A sociolinguistic analysis of the language preferences of adolescent bilinguals: Shifting allegiances and developing identities. *Applied Linguistics, 23*(4), 490–514.

Chan, W. Y., & Birman, D. (2009). Cross-and same-race friendships of Vietnamese immigrant adolescents: A focus on acculturation and school diversity. *International Journal of Intercultural Relations, 33*(4), 313–324. doi:10.1016/j.ijintrel.2009.05.003

Cheung, B. Y., Chudek, M., & Heine, S. J. (2011). Evidence for a sensitive period for acculturation: Younger immigrants report acculturating at a faster rate. *Psychological Science, 22*(2), 147–152. doi:10. 1177/0956797610394661

Dhont, K., Van Hiel, A., De Bolle, M., & Roets, A. (2012). Longitudinal intergroup contact effects on prejudice using self- and observer-reports. *British Journal of Social Psychology, 51*(2), 221–238. doi:10. 1111/j.2044-8309.2011.02039.x

Epstein, J. L. (1989). The selection of friends: Changes across the grades and in different school environments. In T. J. Berndt & G. W. Ladd (Eds.), *Peer relationships in child development* (pp. 158–187). Oxford: Wiley.

Feddes, A. R., Noack, P., & Rutland, A. (2009). Direct and extended friendship effects on minority and majority children's interethnic attitudes: A longitudinal study. *Child Development, 80*(2), 377–390. doi:10. 1111/j.1467-8624.2009.01266.x

Feldman, S. S., & Rosenthal, D. A. (1994). Culture makes a difference…or does it? A comparison of adolescents in Hong Kong, Australia, and the USA. In R. K. Silbereisen & E. Todt (Eds.), *Adolescence in context* (pp. 99–124). New York: Springer.

Fillmore, L. W. (2000). Loss of family languages: Should educators be concerned? *Theory into Practice, 39*(4), 203–210.

Fishbein, M., & Ajzen, I. (2010). *Predicting and changing behavior: The reasoned action approach*. New York: Psychology Press.

Fuligni, A. J. (2001). A comparative longitudinal approach to acculturation among children from immigrant families. *Harvard Educational Review, 71*, 566–578.

Graham, S., Taylor, A. Z., & Ho, A. Y. (2009). Race and ethnicity in peer relations research. In K. H. Rubin, W. M. Bukowski, & B. Laursen (Eds.), *Handbook of peer interactions, relationships, and groups* (pp. 394–413). New York, NY: Guilford Press.

Gudykunst, W. B., & Schmidt, K. L. (1987). Language and ethnic identity: An overview and prologue. *Journal of Language and Social Psychology, 6*, 157–170.

Hallinan, M. T. (1982). Classroom racial composition and children's friendships. *Social Forces, 61*(1), 56–72.

Hallinan, M. T., & Teixeira, R. A. (1987). Opportunities and constraints: Black–White differences in the formation of interracial friendships. *Child Development, 58*(5), 1358–1371.

Hamers, J. F., & Blanc, M. H. (2000). *Bilinguality and bilingualism*. Cambridge: University Press.

Hansell, S., & Slavin, R. E. (1981). Cooperative learning and the structure of interracial friendships. *Sociology of Education, 54*(2), 98–106. doi:10.2307/2112354

Harris, K. M., & Cavanagh, S. E. (2008). Indicators of the peer environment in adolescence. In B. V. Brown (Ed.), *Key indicators of child and youth well-being: Completing the picture* (pp. 259–278). Mahwah, NJ: Lawrence Erlbaum Associates Publishers.

Hartup, W. W. (1996). The company they keep: Friendships and their developmental significance. *Child Development, 67*(1), 1–13. doi:10.2307/1131681

Hartup, W. W., & Stevens, N. (1997). Friendships and adaptation in the life course. *Psychological Bulletin, 121*(3), 355–370.

Havighurst, R. J. (1972). *Developmental task and education*. New York: David McKay Company Inc.

Hofstede, G. (2003). *Culture's consequences: Comparing values, behaviors, institutions and organizations across nations*. Thousand Oaks, CA: Sage.

Huddleston, T., Niessen, J., Chaoimh, E. N., & White, E. (2011). *Migrant integration policy index III*. Brussels: British Council and the Migration Policy Group.

IOM. (2010). *World migration report 2010*. Geneva: International Organization for Migration.

Jetten, J., Branscombe, N. R., Schmitt, M. T., & Spears, R. (2001). Rebels with a cause: Group identification as a response to perceived discrimination from the mainstream. *Personality and Social Psychology Bulletin, 27*(9), 1204–1213. doi:10.1177/0146167201279012

Joyner, K., & Kao, G. (2000). School racial composition and adolescent racial homophily. *Social Science Quarterly, 81*(3), 810–825. doi:10.2307/42864005

Jugert, P., Noack, P., & Rutland, A. (2011). Friendship preferences among German and Turkish preadolescents. *Child Development, 82*(3), 812–829. doi:10.1111/j.1467-8624.2010.01528.x

Jugert, P., Noack, P., & Rutland, A. (2013). Children's cross-ethnic friendships: Why are they less stable than same-ethnic friendships? *European Journal of Developmental Psychology, 10*(6), 649–662. doi:10.1080/17405629.2012.734136

Kandel, D. B. (1978). Similarity in real-life adolescent friendship pairs. *Journal of Personality and Social Psychology, 36*(3), 306–312. doi:10.1037/0022-3514.36.3.306

Kao, G., & Joyner, K. (2004). Do race and ethnicity matter among friends? Activities among interracial, interethnic, and intraethnic adolescent friends. *The Sociological Quarterly, 45*(3), 557–573. doi:10.2307/4120863

Klein, W. (1987). *Zweitspracherwerb. Eine Einführung [Second language acquisition. An introduction]*. Frankfurt am Main: Athenäum.

Kohn, M. L. (1987). Cross-national research as an analytic strategy: American Sociological Association, 1987 presidential address. *American Sociological Review, 52*(6), 713–731.

Kristen, C., Shavit, Y., Chachashvili-Bolotin, S., Roth, T., & Adler, I. (2014). Achievement differences between immigrant and native fourth graders in Germany and Israel. In R. K. Silbereisen, P. F. Titzmann, & Y. Shavit (Eds.), *The challenges of diaspora migration: Interdisciplinary perspectives on Israel and Germany* (pp. 191–209). Farnham: Ashgate.

Leszczensky, L., & Pink, S. (2015). Ethnic segregation of friendship networks in school: Testing a rational-choice argument of differences in ethnic homophily between classroom-and grade-level networks. *Social Networks, 42*, 18–26. doi:10.1016/j.socnet.2015.02.00

Mark, N. P., & Harris, D. R. (2012). Roommate's race and the racial composition of White college students' ego networks. *Social Science Research, 41*(2), 331–342. doi:10.1016/j.ssresearch.2011.11.012

Masgoret, A.-M., & Ward, C. (2006). Culture learning approach to acculturation. In D. L. Sam & J. W. Berry (Eds.), *The Cambridge handbook of acculturation psychology* (pp. 58–77). New York: Cambridge University Press.

McCormick, M. P., Cappella, E., Hughes, D. L., & Gallagher, E. K. (2014). Feasible, rigorous, and relevant: Validation of a measure of friendship homophily for diverse classrooms. *The Journal of Early Adolescence,*. doi:10.1177/0272431614547051

McPherson, M., Smith-Lovin, L., & Cook, J. M. (2001). Birds of a feather: Homophily in social networks. *Annual Review of Sociology, 27*(1), 415–444.

Mollica, K. A., Gray, B., & Treviño, L. K. (2003). Racial homophily and its persistence in newcomers' social networks. *Organization Science, 14*(2), 123–136. doi:10.1287/orsc.14.2.123.14994

Moody, J. (2001). Race, school integration, and friendship segregation in America. *American Journal of Sociology, 107*(3), 679–716. doi:10.1086/338954

Motti-Stefanidi, F., & Asendorpf, J. B. (2012). Perceived discrimination of immigrant adolescents in Greece: How does group discrimination translate into personal discrimination? *European Psychologist, 17*(2), 93–104. doi:10.1027/1016-9040/a000116

Motti-Stefanidi, F., Berry, J., Chryssochoou, X., Sam, D. L., & Phinney, J. (2012). Positive immigrant youth adaptation in context: Developmental, acculturation, and social–psychological perspectives. In A. S. Masten, K. Liebkind, & D. J. Hernandez (Eds.), *Realizing the potential of immigrant youth* (pp. 117–158). New York: Cambridge University Press.

Nurmi, J.-E. (1993). Adolescent development in an age-graded context: The role of personal beliefs, goals, and strategies in the tackling of developmental tasks and standards. *International Journal of Behavioral Development, 16,* 169–189. doi:10.1177/016502549301600205

Oppedal, B. (2006). Development and acculturation. In D. L. Sam & J. W. Berry (Eds.), *The Cambridge handbook of acculturation psychology* (pp. 97–112). New York: Cambridge University Press.

Perry, S. L. (2013). Racial composition of social settings, interracial friendship, and whites' attitudes toward interracial marriage. *The Social Science Journal, 50* (1), 13–22. doi:10.1016/j.soscij.2012.09.001

Pettigrew, T. F. (1998). Intergroup contact theory. *Annual Review of Psychology, 49*(1), 65–85.

Pettigrew, T. F., & Tropp, L. R. (2006). A meta-analytic test of intergroup contact theory. *Journal of Personality and Social Psychology, 90*(5), 751–783.

Reinders, H., & Mangold, T. (2005). Die Qualität intra- und interethnischer Freundschaften bei Mädchen und Jungen deutscher, türkischer und italienischer Herkunft [Intra- and interethnic friendship quality of boys and girls of German, Turkish, and Italian origin]. *Zeitschrift für Entwicklungspsychologie und Pädagogische Psychologie, 37*(3), 144–155. doi:10.1026/0049-8637.37.3.144

Roisman, G. I., Masten, A. S., Coatsworth, J. D., & Tellegen, A. (2004). Salient and emerging developmental tasks in the transition to adulthood. *Child Development, 75*(1), 123–133. doi:10.1111/j.1467-8624.2004.00658.x

Ryder, A. G., Alden, L. E., & Paulhus, D. L. (2000). Is acculturation unidimensional or bidimensional? A head-to-head comparison in the prediction of personality, self-identity, and adjustment. *Journal of Personality and Social Psychology, 79*(1), 49–65. doi:10.1037/0022-3514.79.1.49

Schachner, M. K., Brenick, A., Noack, P., van de Vijver, F. J. R., & Heizmann, B. (2015). Structural and normative conditions for interethnic friendships in multiethnic classrooms. *International Journal of Intercultural Relations, 47,* 1–12. doi:10.1016/j.ijintrel.2015.02.003

Schneider, B. H., Dixon, K., & Udvari, S. (2007). Closeness and competition in the inter-ethnic and co-ethnic friendships of early adolescents in Toronto and Montreal. *The Journal of Early Adolescence, 27* (1), 115–138.

Schnittker, J. (2002). Acculturation in context: The self-esteem of Chinese immigrants. *Social Psychology Quarterly, 65*(1), 56–76.

Schwartz, S. J., & Unger, J. B. (2010). Biculturalism and context: What is biculturalism, and when is it adaptive? *Human Development, 53*(1), 26–32.

Shrum, W., Cheek, N. H., & Hunter, S. M. (1988). Friendship in school: Gender and racial homophily. *Sociology of Education, 61*(4), 227–239. doi:10.2307/2112441.

Silbereisen, R. K., Titzmann, P. F., Michel, A., Sagi-Schwartz, A., & Lavee, Y. (2012). The role of developmental transitions in psychosocial competence: A comparison of native and immigrant young people in Germany. In A. S. Masten, K. Liebkind, & D. J. Hernandez (Eds.), *Realizing the potential of immigrant youth* (pp. 324–358). New York, NY: Cambridge University Press.

Silbereisen, R. K., Titzmann, P. F., & Shavit, Y. (Eds.). (2014). *The challenges of diaspora migration: Interdisciplinary perspectives on Israel and Germany.* Farnham: Ashgate.

Slavin, R. E., & Cooper, R. (1999). Improving intergroup relations: Lessons learned from cooperative learning programs. *Journal of Social Issues, 55*(4), 647–663. doi:10.1111/0022-4537.00140

Sleeter, C. E., & Grant, C. A. (2009). *Making choices for multicultural education: Five approaches to race, class and gender.* New York: Wiley.

Slonim-Nevo, V., Mirsky, J., Rubinstein, L., & Nauck, B. (2009). The impact of familial and environmental factors on the adjustment of immigrants: A longitudinal study. *Journal of Family Issues, 30,* 92–123.

Smith, S., McFarland, D. A., Tubergen, F. V., & Maas, I. (2016). Ethnic composition and friendship segregation: Differential effects for adolescent natives and immigrants. *American Journal of Sociology, 121*(4), 1223–1272. doi:10.1086/684032

Spiel, C. (2009). Evidence-based practice: A challenge for European developmental psychology. *European Journal of Developmental Psychology, 6*(1), 11–33. doi:10.1080/17405620802485888

Spiel, C., & Strohmeier, D. (2012). Peer relations in multicultural schools. In A. S. Masten, K. Liebkind, D. J. Hernandez, A. S. Masten, K. Liebkind, & D. J. Hernandez (Eds.), *Realizing the potential of immigrant youth* (pp. 376–396). New York, NY: Cambridge University Press.

Steinberg, L., & Silverberg, S. B. (1986). The vicissitudes of autonomy in early adolescence. *Child Development, 57*(4), 841–851. doi:10.2307/1130361

Stenström, A.-B., & Jørgensen, A. M. (2009). Youngspeak in a multilingual perspective: Introduction. In A.-B. Stenström & A. M. Jørgensen (Eds.), *Youngspeak in multilingual perspective* (pp. 1–9). Amsterdam: John Benjamins Publishing Company.

Stephan, W. G., & Stephan, C. W. (2001). *Improving intergroup relations.* Thousand Oaks, CA: Sage.

Stoessel, K., Titzmann, P. F., & Silbereisen, R. K. (2011). Children's psychosocial development following the transitions to kindergarten and school: A comparison between natives and immigrants in Germany.

International Journal of Developmental Science, 5(1–2), 41–55.

Stoessel, K., Titzmann, P. F., & Silbereisen, R. K. (2012). Young diaspora immigrants' attitude and behavior toward the host culture: The role of cultural identification. *European Psychologist, 17*(2), 143–157. doi:10.1027/1016-9040/a000113

Strohmeier, D. (2012). Friendship homophily among children and youth in multicultural classes. In M. Messer, R. Schroeder, & R. Wodak (Eds.), *Migrations: Interdisciplinary perspectives* (pp. 99–109). Wien: Springer.

Strohmeier, D., Hoffmann, C., Schiller, E.-M., Stefanek, E., & Spiel, C. (2012). ViSC social competence program. In D. Strohmeier, G. G. Noam, D. Strohmeier, & G. G. Noam (Eds.), *Evidence-based bullying prevention programs for children and youth* (pp. 71–84). San Francisco, CA: Jossey-Bass.

Strohmeier, D., Nestler, D., & Spiel, C. (2006). Freundschaftsmuster, Freundschaftsqualität und aggressives Verhalten von Immigrantenkindern in der Grundschule [Friendship patterns, friendship quality, and aggressive behavior of immigrant children in primary school]. *Diskurs Kindheits- und Jugendforschung, 1*(1), 21–37.

Strohmeier, D., & Spiel, C. (2012). Peer relations among immigrant adolescents: Methodological challenges and key findings. In M. Messer, R. Schroeder, & R. Wodak (Eds.), *Migrations: Interdisciplinary perspectives* (pp. 57–65). Wien: Springer.

Sussman, N. M. (2011). *Return migration and identity: A global phenomenon, a Hong Kong case.* Hong Kong: Hong Kong University Press.

Svensson, Y., Stattin, H., & Kerr, M. (2011). In- and out-of-school peer groups of immigrant youths. *European Journal of Developmental Psychology, 8*(4), 490–507. doi:10.1080/17405629.2011.559804

Swart, H., Hewstone, M., Christ, O., & Voci, A. (2011). Affective mediators of intergroup contact: A three-wave longitudinal study in South Africa. *Journal of Personality and Social Psychology, 101*(6), 1221–1238. doi:10.1037/a0024450

Tajfel, H., & Turner, J. C. (1986). The social identity theory of intergroup behavior. In S. Worchel & W. G. Austin (Eds.), *Psychology of intergroup relations* (pp. 7–24). Chicago: Nelson-Hall.

Telzer, E. H. (2011). Expanding the acculturation gap-distress model: An integrative review of research. *Human Development, 53*(6), 313–340. doi:10.1159/000322476

Titzmann, P. F. (2012). Growing up too soon? Parentification among immigrant and native adolescents in Germany. *Journal of Youth and Adolescence, 41*(7), 880–893. doi:10.1007/s10964-011-9711-1

Titzmann, P. F. (2014). Immigrant adolescents' adaptation to a new context: Ethnic friendship homophily and its predictors. *Child Development Perspectives, 8*(2), 107–112. doi:10.1111/cdep.12072

Titzmann, P. F., Brenick, A., & Silbereisen, R. (2015). Friendships fighting prejudice: A longitudinal perspective on adolescents' cross-group friendships with immigrants. *Journal of Youth and Adolescence, 44*(6), 1318–1331. doi:10.1007/s10964-015-0256-6

Titzmann, P. F., & Jugert, P. (2015). Acculturation in context: The moderating effects of immigrant and native peer orientations on the acculturation experiences of immigrants. *Journal of Youth and Adolescence, 44*(11), 2079–2094. doi:10.1007/s10964-015-0314-0

Titzmann, P. F., Michel, A., & Silbereisen, R. K. (2010). Inter-ethnic contact and socio-cultural adaptation of immigrant adolescents in Israel and Germany. *ISSBD Bulletin, 58*(3), 13–17.

Titzmann, P. F., & Silbereisen, R. K. (2009). Friendship homophily among ethnic German immigrants: A longitudinal comparison between recent and more experienced immigrant adolescents. *Journal of Family Psychology, 23*(3), 301–310. doi:10.1037/a0015493

Titzmann, P. F., & Silbereisen, R. K. (2012). Acculturation or development? Autonomy expectations among ethnic German immigrant adolescents and their native German age-mates. *Child Development, 83*(5), 1640–1654. doi:10.1111/j.1467-8624.2012.01799.x

Titzmann, P. F., Silbereisen, R. K., & Mesch, G. S. (2012). Change in friendship homophily: A German Israeli comparison of adolescent immigrants. *Journal of Cross-Cultural Psychology, 43*(3), 410–428. doi:10.1177/0022022111399648

Titzmann, P. F., Silbereisen, R. K., Mesch, G. S., & Schmitt-Rodermund, E. (2011). Migration-specific hassles among adolescent immigrants from the former Soviet Union in Germany and Israel. *Journal of Cross-Cultural Psychology, 42*(5), 777–794. doi:10.1177/0022022110362756

Titzmann, P. F., Silbereisen, R. K., & Schmitt-Rodermund, E. (2007). Friendship homophily among diaspora migrant adolescents in Germany and Israel. *European Psychologist, 12*(3), 181–195. doi:10.1027/1016-9040.12.3.181

Titzmann, P. F., & Sonnenberg, K. (2016). Adolescents in conflict: Intercultural contact attitudes of immigrant mothers and adolescents as predictors of family conflicts. *International Journal of Psychology, 51*(4), 279–287. doi:10.1002/ijop.12172

Turner, R. N., & Brown, R. (2008). Improving children's attitudes toward refugees: An evaluation of a school-based multicultural curriculum and an anti-racist intervention. *Journal of Applied Social Psychology, 38*(5), 1295–1328. doi:10.1111/j.1559-1816.2008.00349.x

Urberg, K. A., Değirmencioğlu, S. M., & Pilgrim, C. (1997). Close friend and group influence on adolescent cigarette smoking and alcohol use. *Developmental Psychology, 33*(5), 834–844.

van Workum, N., Scholte, R. H. J., Cillessen, A. H. N., Lodder, G. M. A., & Giletta, M. (2013). Selection, deselection, and socialization processes of happiness in adolescent friendship networks. *Journal of Research on Adolescence, 23*(3), 563–573. doi:10.1111/jora.12035

Verkuyten, M., & Kinket, B. (2000). Social distances in a multi ethnic society: The ethnic hierarchy among Dutch preadolescents. *Social Psychology Quarterly, 63*(1), 75–85. doi:10.2307/2695882

Verkuyten, M., & Thijs, J. (2013). Multicultural education and inter-ethnic attitudes: An intergroup perspective. *European Psychologist, 18*(3), 179–190. doi:10.1027/1016-9040/a000152

Vertovec, S. (2007). Super-diversity and its implications. *Ethnic and Racial Studies, 30*(6), 1024–1054. doi:10.1080/01419870701599465

Walsemann, K. M., Gee, G. C., & Geronimus, A. T. (2009). Ethnic differences in trajectories of depressive symptoms: Disadvantage in family background, high school experiences, and adult characteristics. *Journal of Health and Social Behavior, 50*, 82–98.

Ward, C. (2001). The ABCs of acculturation. In D. Matsumoto (Ed.), *Handbook of culture and psychology* (pp. 411–445). New York: Oxford University Press.

Weingrod, A., & Levy, A. (2006). Social thought and commentary: Paradoxes of homecoming: The Jews and their diasporas. *Anthropological Quarterly, 79*(4), 691–716.

Zhang, R., & Noels, K. A. (2013). When ethnic identities vary: Cross-situation and within-situation variation, authenticity, and well-being. *Journal of Cross-Cultural Psychology, 44*(4), 552–573. doi:10.1177/0022022112463604

The Friendships of Racial–Ethnic Minority Youth in Context

Leoandra Onnie Rogers, Erika Y. Niwa, and Niobe Way

Abstract

An extensive theoretical and empirical literature suggests that friendships are an important, if not essential, micro-context of adolescent development—shaping youth identity, school and civic engagement, and psychological and physical wellbeing. Friendships are also themselves embedded within, and shaped by, the larger macro-context of culture (Bronfenbrenner in Am Psychol 34:844–850, 1979. doi:10.1037/0003-066X.34.10.844), including racial–ethnic stereotypes (García-Coll et al. in Child Dev 67:1891–1914, 1996; Spencer in Black youth: perspectives on their status in the United States. Praeger, Westport, pp 37–69, 1995). Yet, the study of friendship rarely examines the influence of the macro-context or includes racial–ethnic minority adolescents despite the fact that half of all the youth in American schools are members of a racial-ethnic minority group. In this chapter, we review research on the friendships of racial–ethnic minority adolescents and focus specifically on how the macro-context of socialidentity-based stereotypes shapes the micro-context of friendships.

Human beings are innately designed for relationships. The ability to relate to another person- to feel empathy and intimacy- is a defining feature of being human, and our innate desire for relationship shapes every aspect of who we are and who we become (Bond 2013; Bowlby 1969/ 1982; Chu 2014; de Waal 2006; Gilligan 1982, 2011; Hrdy 2009; Trevarthen 1979; Way 2011). Decades ago, Sullivan (1953) argued that friendship—that intimate emotional bond with one's age peers—was the chief source of a child's sense of security, self-worth, and wellbeing. Yet, our relational nature, though universal, does not exist in a vacuum. Who we befriend and how we experience those relationships are shaped by the norms, expectations, and stereotypes of the context and culture in which we are embedded. In a

L.O. Rogers (✉)
Northwestern University, Evanston, USA
e-mail: lorogers@uw.edu

E.Y. Niwa
Brooklyn College, CUNY, Brooklyn, NY, USA

N. Way
New York University, New York, USA

© The Editor(s) 2017
N.J. Cabrera and B. Leyendecker (eds.), *Handbook on Positive Development of Minority Children and Youth*, DOI 10.1007/978-3-319-43645-6_16

socially stratified society like the U.S., youth are shaped by their "social address"—their race and ethnicity, gender, and nationality—and, more importantly, the beliefs that accompany these social positions (García-Coll et al. 1996; García-Coll and Szalacha 2004; Spencer 1995; Spencer et al. 1997). While a vast empirical literature documents the consequences of friendships for adolescents' social, emotional, and cognitive development and adjustment (see Rubin et al. 2009 for review), it rarely attends to the ways the cultural ecology shapes friendships or the friendship experiences of racial–ethnic minority youth. (For exceptions see: Azmitia and Cooper 2001; Cauce 1986; Graham et al. 2009; Way et al. 2006; Way and Chen 2000; Way and Silverman 2011; Way 2011).

In this chapter, we employ an ecological lens (Bronfenbrenner 1979; García-Coll et al. 1996; Spencer 1995) to understand friendships among racial–ethnic minority youth living in the United States. We utilize data from our research with ethnically diverse American adolescents, collected over the past two decades, to reveal the ways in which the macro-context of ethnic, racial, gender, and sexuality stereotypes shapes the quality and experience of adolescents' friendships (e.g., Niwa et al. 2011; Niwa 2012; Rogers 2012; Rogers and Way 2016; Way 2011; Way et al. 2008, 2014; Way and Rogers 2014). In this chapter, we first discuss the ecological framework as used in our analysis and then review existing research on the friendships of racial–ethnic minority youth. In the remainder of the chapter, we use empirical examples from our research, as well as others, to illustrate the ways that stereotypes shape friendships via two interrelated processes: peer discrimination and identity development.

Historical Overview/Theoretical Perspectives

An Ecological Model of Adolescent Development

An ecological approach to human development assumes that the individual is dependent upon and inextricable from the environment around him or her (Bronfenbrenner 1979; Bronfenbrenner and Morris 1998). Bronfenbrenner's bioecological model contends that development is the result of a dynamic transactional relation between individuals and their environment(s). These reciprocal interactions "are posited as the primary engines of human development" (Bronfenbrenner and Morris 1998, p. 798) in which the unit of analysis is not only the individual but the individual-in-context, attending to the ways that the context shapes the person's development and experiences. The environment is operationalized as nested systems that include the *micro-* and *meso-systems*, as those most proximal to the individual, and the *exo-* and *macro-systems* that are more distally situated (Bronfenbrenner 1979). The micro-system is marked by ongoing exchanges that occur *within* the immediate contexts of home, family, school, and neighborhood, and the meso-system consists of the reciprocal interactions *between* the people in those environments: parents, teachers, and peers. The exo-system refers to those contexts in which the individual is not directly located but impact the child's development nonetheless, such as parents' workplace. Finally, the macro-system includes the larger cultural norms, stereotypes, beliefs, expectations and practices as well as governmental laws—all of which impact both the structure and function of settings (e.g., schools), as well as relational dynamics within those settings. An important assumption of the ecological model is that these systems function jointly. As such, the macro-system impacts the individual via the processes that operate within the micro- and meso-systems. Thus, it is through relationships, such as friendships, that values from the macro-system are manifested, enacted, and experienced.

Two key scholars have extended Bronfenbrenner's ecological systems theory to address the ways in which social status and power influence the dynamics of the ecosystem: Cynthia García Coll and Margaret Beale Spencer.

García-Coll's integrative model of development (1996) places beliefs systems about race, ethnicity, and class at the center of her ecological theory and asserts that developmental processes are deeply affected by a child's social position or "social address" (e.g., race/ethnicity, gender) within a social-stratified society (García-Coll and Szalacha 2004). Social position, according to García-Coll, gains meaning through the macro-context and has a direct and indirect effect on individual development as well as the micro-contexts. Importantly, it is not the social category per se that influences development, but the cultural *meaning* associated with that position which influences developmental processes. In other words, it is the stereotypes, norms, and expectations about race–ethnicity that shape development rather than the social positions themselves (Sanchez-Jankowski 1992; Suárez-Orozco 2004).

While García-Coll's (1996) model emphasizes how the meaning of a social position is shaped by the context, Spencer's (1995) P-VEST (Phenomenological Variant of Ecological Systems Theory) incorporates *inter-subjective experience* to focus on how adolescents process or make sense of their social positions. P-VEST asserts that "… the individual's ability to understand societal expectations, stereotypes and biases—even those that they themselves endorse or fulfill" frames their experiences within and responses to the context (Gordon and Gergen 1968; Spencer et al. 1997, p. 818). In this way, P-VEST asserts the role of identity as a mechanism through which the macro-context is manifested at the level of individual development. Race–ethnicity, then, is a lens through which adolescents experience the world—shaping how they see themselves (i.e., identity) and interact with others (i.e., their friendships).

Taken together, ecological systems theory and its theoretical extensions highlight three relevant points in the examination of adolescent friendships. First, contexts make indelible imprints on the relationships that youth develop and experience. Second, socio-historical and cultural forces alter the very geography of adolescents' relationships. Finally, explorations of adolescent friendships should include the perceptions of the adolescents themselves (i.e., identity), who are active agents in their own development.

Friendships Among Racial–Ethnic Minority Youth

Sullivan (1953) theorized that establishing close and intimate connections with peers or "chums" during adolescence is essential for psychological and emotional development, for "… it is during this period that a child begins to develop a real sensitivity to what matters to another person (p. 245)." In other words, friendships or "chumships" lay the groundwork for social skills and perspective-taking, while also providing opportunities for self-worth and a blueprint for future romantic relationships. Empirical research on American adolescents' friendships has primarily assessed *friendship quality* (e.g., intimacy, affection, companionship, satisfaction) and how friendship quality is linked to adolescent wellbeing (see Bukowski et al. 1996; Furman 1996; Rubin et al. 2009). Decades of theory and research demonstrate the link between friendships and a range of social, academic, and cognitive outcomes. Adolescents who report higher quality friendships report better psychological wellbeing, academic performance, social skills, and health (Berndt 2004; Crockett et al. 1984; Csikszentmihalyi and Larson 1984; Hartup 1996; Osterman 2000; Rubin et al. 2009; Savin-Williams and Berndt 1990; Way 2011).

Although friendships appear to be critical for *all* adolescents (Berndt 2004; Hinde 1987; Petterson et al. 2000), the majority of the research has been conducted with White, middle-class, American adolescents. In fact, a recent content analysis of the friendship literature found that less than 7 % of the studies on friendships referenced racial–ethnic minority adolescents (Graham et al. 2009). Yet, 37 % of the U.S. population is of ethnic minority status (Latinos, Asians, Blacks; Pew Research Center 2014), and in the last decade, from 2000 to 2010, ethnic minorities accounted for 91.7 % of America's total population growth (Pew Research Center 2011). This increase is concentrated among youth as half (50.3 %) of students enrolled in American public schools are ethnic minorities (Pew Research Center 2014). These demographic trends raise concerns about the generalizability of research findings that are based on White, middle-class youth to any youth outside of those demographic categories, including racial–ethnic minority, immigrant, non-American, or poor and working-class adolescents.

The literature that has included racial–ethnic minority adolescents focuses mostly on *ethnic differences* or specific topics within the study of friendships. For example, studies find ethnic differences in the importance of friendships (e.g., Gupta and Sirin 2010), levels of friendship quality (e.g., Azmitia and Cooper 2001; Azmitia et al. 2006; Jia et al. 2009; Way et al. 2006), and friendship support (e.g., Kao and Joyner 2004; Way and Chen 2000; Way and Greene 2006). The study of cross-race friendships, which necessarily includes racial–ethnic minority youth, suggests that adolescents prefer same-race friends (DuBois and Hirsch 1990; Hamm et al. 2005; Mouw and Entwisle 2006) and that cross-race friendships tend to be less stable over time (McGill et al. 2012). Research on peer social status suggests that White students garner popularity for prosocial behaviors (being cooperative and cool) whereas African American students (particularly boys) are esteemed for tough, aggressive and antisocial behaviors (e.g., Luther and McMahon 1996; Rodkin et al. 2000). The topic of antisocial or delinquent peer groups focuses almost exclusively on African American boys who are also disproportionately labeled as aggressive by adults and peers and suspended and expelled for behavioral problems (e.g., Noguera 2008). Prior studies find that youth with more antisocial friends exhibit more antisocial behaviors (e.g., Dodge et al. 2006), due to process called "deviancy training" whereby youth "train" their peers in rule breaking and bad behaviors to solidify a delinquent peer culture (Dishion and Piehler 2009). Interestingly, in a study of adolescents' susceptibility to such negative peer pressure, or deviancy training, Steinberg and Monahan (2007) found that African American adolescents were actually the most likely to

resist the influence of negative peers compared to other racial–ethnic groups.

Other friendship research involving racial–ethnic minority youth examines how different levels of context (e.g., family, school) shape friendship processes. For example, in terms of the family context, research suggests that maternal support or acceptance of one's friends is strongly associated with more positive friendship quality (Updegraff et al. 2001; Way and Silverman 2011; Way 2011). In a longitudinal analysis of friendship quality, Way and Greene (2006) found that adolescents who reported the lowest levels of maternal support reported the sharpest increases in friendship support over time, suggesting that the family context significantly impacts adolescents' friendships. Parents' attitudes are also predictive of the quality of adolescents' friendships, where supportive parental attitudes predict more positive friendship quality over time (Way and Silverman 2011; Way 2011). Yet, the influence of parental attitudes towards friendships varies across cultures and cultural variations in parenting beliefs and practices impact how adolescents experience their friendships (e.g., Gupta and Sirin 2010).

The school context also impacts adolescents' friendships. For example, positive school climate and sense of belonging shapes not only adolescents' own self-perceptions (identity) but also their social interactions and relationships (Crosnoe et al. 2003; Eccles and Roeser 1999). In hostile school environments, adolescents are less likely to develop positive and supportive friendships (Crosnoe et al. 2003), and school-level practices that reify stereotypes (e.g., tracking) disrupt positive peer relationships and incite peer discrimination (e.g., Lei 2003; Rosenbloom and Way 2004). Studies of cross-race friendships also note the relevance of context, finding that the likelihood of cross-race friendships is "opportunity-based"—youth in more diverse schools are more likely to befriend peers from a different ethnic–racial group (e.g., Hallinan and Teixeira 1987; Moody 2001). At the same time, other ecological factors, such as ability tracking, instructional practices, and teacher expectations, can disrupt these opportunities. For example, Hallinan and Williams (1987) found that cross-race friendships between Black and White students were significantly less likely when teachers structured their classroom and instructional practices around levels of academic achievement (e.g., ability grouping).

While prior studies highlight relevance of ecological factors in adolescents' friendships, the study of context has been largely limited to the meso-system (family or schools) with little attention given to the mechanisms through which macro-cultural forces, such as stereotypes and expectations, impact the friendships of racial–ethnic minority adolescents in the United States.

Stereotypes and Adolescent Friendships

Stereotypes are widely held cultural beliefs and expectations, generalized attitudes or evaluations about individuals who share a social address or position, such as ethnicity, race, gender, social class, or nationality (Stangor and Schaller 1996). Stereotypes offer a lens through which one can observe the impact of macro level forces (e.g., culture) on micro level contexts, such as friendships. African-American adolescents, for example, are stereotyped as rhythmic and athletic, but also lazy and dumb. African-American males, specifically, are stereotyped as violent, aggressive, and hypersexual whereas African-American females are stereotyped as overweight, loud and angry (Fordham 1993; Ghavami and Peplau 2013; Stevenson 1997). Latino males are similarly stereotyped as lazy and dumb, as well as gangsters and drug lords whereas Latina females are stereotyped as the hyper-sexualized "mamasita" (López 2003). Asian-American youth, in contrast, are stereotyped as "model minorities"—smart, quiet, and obedient (Lee 1994; Lei 2003), but also weak and feminine (Lei 2003; Ghavami and Peplau 2013). At the same time, Asian immigrant youth are viewed as dirty and poor (Chua and Fujino 2008;

Lei 2003; Shek 2006). Notably, stereotypes are not limited to ethnic minorities. Whites are stereotyped as wealthy, smart and successful, but also weak or "soft" and for White males, gay (Ghavami and Peplau 2013; Pascoe 2007). Such racial-ethnic (as well as gender and sexuality) stereotypes make up the very "fabric of the [American] society" (Stangor and Schaller 1996, p. 10).

Stereotypes are inherently relational, such that beliefs about one group are defined in relationship to another (Lesko 2001; Nasir 2011). For example, "acting Black" refers to speaking in slang, dressing in urban style, and listening to hip hop music (Carter 2006), whereas "acting White" refers to speaking proper English and excelling in school (Fordham and Ogbu 1986; Carter 2006). Nasir and Shah (2011) describe these racial and ethnic contrasts in this way:

> As with 'Asians are good at math', the notion that 'White men can't jump' exemplifies how racialized narratives tend to be inherently relational in character. The inability of White men to jump is only visible because of the (presumed) certainty that non-White men (usually African American men) *can* jump (p. 30).

Stereotypes, then, not only shape how youth see themselves, but also how they see others (Way and Rogers 2016). Adolescents from different racial–ethnic groups encounter unique yet related cultural ecologies in the form of stereotypes that shape all aspects of their development, including their peer interactions and friendships.

Current Research and Method

The data we present in this chapter come primarily from the studies with racially–ethnically diverse American adolescents conducted by Niobe Way and her students over the past 20 years, and the dissertation research conducted independently by Onnie Rogers. We draw from four longitudinal mixed-method studies involving, in total, over one thousand youth attending six middle schools and three high schools located in two cities in the United States. Our samples include: African-American, European-American,

Chinese-American, Dominican-American, and Puerto Rican adolescents, most of whom attended schools where the majority of the students qualified for the free/reduced lunch program.

The first two projects, *Connections* and *Relationships Among Peers (RAP)*, were conducted by Niobe Way and funded by the National Science Foundation and The William T. Grant Foundation. These longitudinal studies took place in a co-educational high school in a city in the Northeast, and focused on adolescents' identity development and friendships. The third project, called Project *RAP,* was another longitudinal project conducted by Niobe Way and Diane Hughes at the Center for Research on Culture, Development, and Education at New York University and was funded by the National Science Foundation.[1] This was a 6-year longitudinal project that included six middle schools with a total of 1034 students involved in the survey component and 250 students and their mothers in the interview component that took place from 6th through 11th grade (for more information about the samples, see Niwa et al. 2014; Rogers and Way 2016; Way 2011; Way et al. 2008). The project focused on the ways in which the contexts of school, families and peers, shape the social, emotional, and academic development of ethnically diverse urban youth. Lastly, The *Identity Project*, funded by The Spencer Foundation, was a 2-year mixed-method study conducted by Onnie Rogers at an all-Black, all-male high school in a city in the Midwest. The *Identity Project* used in-depth interview, survey and observation methods to examine adolescent racial and gender identity development.

Our research repeatedly demonstrates that racial–ethnic, gender, and sexuality stereotypes are salient and integral in adolescents' daily experiences and interactions with friends (Niwa et al. 2011, 2014; Rogers 2012; Rogers and Way 2016; Way 2011; Way and Rogers 2014, 2016; Way et al. 2008, 2013). These processes are evident in adolescents' friendships through peer discrimination and identity development.

[1]National Science Foundation (NSF) grant number: 021859.

Peer Discrimination

Prior research, including our own, suggests that adolescents use stereotypes to exclude and discriminate against peers in accordance with social norms. For example, Pascoe's (2007) ethnography of masculinity in an urban high school shows how boys enforce masculine stereotypes in their friendships by excluding boys who deviate from masculine norms. Such boys were teased, rejected and sometimes permanently banned from the group because their actions posed a threat to maintenance of masculine norms—tough, crass, athletic, funny, troublemakers. In an analysis of gender, race and schooling, Davis (2001) finds that "Black boys who do not meet the standards of an acceptable masculinity are treated as masculine mistakes," they are teased by their peers, called "gays" and "sissies," and relegated to socialize with girls (p. 147). Studies on the "acting white" phenomenon (Carter 2006; Fordham and Ogbu 1986; Horvat and O'Connor 2006) similarly reveal how peers may police the cultural stereotypes about what it means to be (and not to be) a member of a particular racial-ethnic group. "Acting white" is set of norms about how one ought to behave (e.g., carry him/herself, dress, speak) given his or her race-ethnicity, and it functions to discriminate against certain peers thereby structuring the dynamics of adolescents' friendships.

In Rogers' dissertation study with African-American adolescent boys attending an all-Black male high school, she finds that stereotypes about race, gender, and sexuality structured the friendship dynamics of boys within the school (Rogers 2012). Many of the boys indicated that simply attending an all-male school was "gay." Teddy (African-American) explained that he did not want to attend the all-boys' school "[Be]cause I heard a lot of stuff about all boys schools. …People turn gay. That's what I heard." Brandon (African-American) explained that there was a "good side and a bad side" to attending an all-boys' school and the bad side is "that people be thinkin' you gay or something like that. Yeah, a lot of guys I know be thinkin' that's gay." In this context where simply attending an all-boys' school was framed as a threat to one's heterosexuality, boys avoided other boys who "acted feminine." A common strategy among the boys was to use homophobic language to assert their heterosexual identities and maintain boundaries between themselves and the boys who "acted feminine" (Rogers 2012). For example, Kirk (African-American) said:

> I mean, dudes play around in this school, they go around tappin' other dudes on the butt and stuff like that. I just try to stay away from that stuff. It's just disgusting…It's just – I don't think I'm homophobic it's just that kind of stuff bothers me …{laughter} I kinda, I just get up and move. I try to just keep 'em over there.

Illustrating how stereotypes were used to draw friendship boundaries, Brandon (African-American) explained: "It ain't none of my business I just stay out of it, I'll be like, that's your all opinion. They just stay together. They mind their business, the others mind theirs, I mind mine." Lewis (African-American) also explained:

> Like we're all friendly and stuff… But we still keep it low because we just don't talk about other gay people; we don't do that unless they make us mad or keep on coming by us. But basically, they keep their distance and we keep our distance. They mind their business and we mind ours.

In other words, stereotypes about (African-American) males' sexuality and how they "should act" were both a barrier to building friendships and a tool to exclude particular students. In this way, stereotypes structured the boys' friendship opportunities.

Even for boys who were not blatantly homophobic, the context of stereotypes actively shaped *which* peers boys interacted with and the quality of those friendships. For example, Devin (African American) explained how the expectation for boys "to act more masculine…I guess you could say like straight…" was used in the school to exclude peers who did not conform:

> I mean we have some feminine guys here at the school. I've got one in my [class] and he's gay, you know. I'm not going to say any names, but I'm just saying I don't have anything against him. I talk to him and he's a cool guy, like he ain't stereotypically all gay. You know, *oh you can't even talk to them [gay students] without them thinking about boys and that they just want to go*

> *with you;* that's why some dudes don't talk to them. But he's just like a regular dude. You know, he's gay; he just acts cool.

Devin is acutely aware that "feminine behavior" is problematic for boys, and he feels the need to protect the identity of his gay friend ("I'm not going to say any names"). But Devin also protects himself, explaining that he sometimes "ignores" this friend who is gay by keeping his distance:

> I mean, I don't hang around him like all the time, you know, I say *what's up to him* and all that stuff. I don't just like chill with him, you know. But I say *hey what's up,* you know and I'm cool with him…

Even though Devin challenges the idea that he needs to completely avoid feminine boys, the threat of the stereotype still looms and directly shapes his friendship.

In Way's studies of racial–ethnic minority adolescents in co-educational and diverse school contexts, we similarly find that stereotypes are used to exclude peers and structure adolescents' friendships (e.g., Niwa et al. 2011, 2014; Way et al. 2008; Way 2011). For example, Patricia (Dominican-American) described the "ghetto kids" in a clique at her school as "Spanish and Black people that are in gangs and people that do drugs" and "beat you up." Abel (Dominican-American) said: "one time, some kid was calling me *'Spanish boy, Spanish boy!'* …I think he just hates Latino kids." In contrast, the Chinese-American students were described by their peers (as well as by themselves) as "weak" and "nerdy," and, as a result, were often victimized by their peers (e.g., Niwa 2012; Niwa et al. 2011; Way et al. 2008). For example, Henry (Chinese-American) described the "nerdy Chinese students": "They're weird. They know everything…All of them have glasses…Like math questions, they will always know it … They're smart." These stereotyped descriptions facilitated peer discrimination: "They call the Chinese kids nerds and chinks…they call them chinks." Other students similarly shared examples of racial slurs based on stereotypes. Judy (Chinese-American) explained: "Sometimes people would bully us in school, like not bully, but like say really racist things about Chinese people." In these examples of peer discrimination, stereotypes, or "racist things" are used to exclude, isolate, and victimize thereby shaping adolescents' friendship experiences.

Other students described experiences of implicit discrimination. For example, Cira (Dominican-American) said "since I'm a Dominican [other students] think I'm not going to be as smart as they are." She offered an example from math class:

> Um, two weeks ago or something…we had to measure apartments and we had to do the dimensions and stuff. And I was going to measure it. And [my classmate] was like *oh, let me do that*, and I was like oh, okay. …It hurts. Because, you know, they don't really know if you know [the answer] they just assume you won't because of your ethnicity.

Cira is acutely aware of the racialized expectations regarding her intellectual abilities and this awareness filters her peer interactions. These empircal examples illustrate that the cultural stereotypes related to race–ethnicity, gender, and sexuality that emanate from the macro-context are manifested in adolescents' friendships through instances of peer discrimination (Niwa 2012; Niwa et al. 2014; Rogers and Way 2016).

Identity Development

The second way that we observe the impact of stereotypes on adolescents' friendships is via identity processes (e.g., Way 2011; Way and Rogers, in press). Adolescents are preoccupied with who they are in the eyes of others (Erikson 1968), and friends are a captive audience, in part because adolescents spend much of their free time in the company of peers (Blyth et al. 1982; Brown 2004; Csikszentmihalyi and Larson 1984). For racial–ethnic minority youth, the normative task of identity development is intensified as they work to cultivate a positive sense of self in the face of negative cultural expectations and stereotypes (García-Coll et al. 1996; Spencer 1995). Macro-level stereotypes are like "social mirrors" that color how youth view themselves in the social world (Suárez-Orozco 2004). Prior research shows that adolescents may respond to

stereotypes by positioning themselves in alignment with the stereotypes, endorsing or reinforcing society's expectations for them, or they may actively position themselves in *opposition* to them, challenging the stereotypes and defining themselves as distinct from the stereotypes (Anyon 1984; Spencer et al. 1997; Rogers 2012; Way and Rogers 2014; Way et al. 2008).

In our prior studies we find that the desire *not to be* seen as a stereotype—and to *resist* stereotypes—dominates the identity narratives of racial–ethnic minority adolescents (Way et al. 2008, 2013; Way and Rogers 2014). African American youth in our studies, for example, did not want to be seen as "dumb," "lazy," and "bad"; Chinese American youth did not want to be seen as "nerdy" or "weak," and Dominican American youth did not want to be seen as "gangsters" and "unsuccessful" (Way et al. 2013). Moreover, we find that how youth position themselves relative to these stereotypes—their identities—influences their friendship opportunities and the quality of those friendships. For example, Rogers (2012) found that Black boys who positioned themselves in *opposition* to racial and gender stereotypes, challenging cultural norms that frame them as emotionally stoic and independent, emphasized the value and importance of friendships; they had "best friends," and shared stories of disclosure and intimacy with their friends (markers of high friendship quality). For example, asked if friendship is important, Brandon (African-American) said: "Yeah. Because like say for instance, you need something, like a helping hand or something, it's important. If you don't have no friends you be like, 'man it takes two to do this job,' then you just be out of luck." Monte (African-American), similarly responded: "Yeah, friendship is important through your whole life. Because without friends, you would be lonely, you wouldn't have nobody to talk to." In describing his relationship with his best friend, Monte, said: "it's real, real close. You just feel it. That's how I feel around Terrance." In contrast to racial and gender norms that position African American males as unemotional and autonomous, boys who constructed their identities in opposition to racial and gender stereotypes revealed their vulnerability and desire for intimacy and interdependence with friends.

These stories of desire for intimate friendships were contrasted with boys who aligned themselves more with mainstream racial and gender stereotypes that position Black males as unemotional, hyper-aggressive, and hypersexual (Rogers 2012). For boys in this identity pattern, friends were seen as "acquaintances" and having a best friend was neither desirable nor necessary. As Steven (African-American) explained, "there's no reason to [have a best friend]. Basically everybody is the same." That is, boys whose identities aligned with stereotypes viewed friendships as interchangeable and dispensable. For boys who accommodated to stereotypes, friends were not seen as intimate "chumships" but distant associates to "kick it with," or "who got your back when you in trouble", or "just like to have fun." Thus, stereotypes about how boys "should be" shaped boys' identities, which in turn informed the quality and intimacy of their friendships.

Other research on adolescent boys' friendships also suggests that when boys position themselves in opposition to gender stereotypes—specifically, challenging the belief that they should be autonomous and emotionally stoic, they are more likely to express emotional vulnerability in their friendships and describe their friendships as more supportive (Cunningham and Meunier 2004; Chu 2004; Santos 2010; Way 2011; Way et al. 2014). For example, Cunningham and Meunier (2004) found an inverse relation between vulnerability/relational intimacy and masculine bravado attitudes among African American males, such that boys with less bravado reported greater desire for intimacy and self-disclosure in their friendships. Santos (2010) similarly finds that adolescent boys with higher levels of adherence to norms of masculinity report lower levels of friendship quality (in terms of support) over time. In this way, friendship can function as a micro-context where youth are supported to challenge cultural expectations and resist negative stereotypes about who they "should be" (Chu 2004; Gilligan 2011; Nasir 2011; Way 2011).

This process of identity development as a response to stereotypes is evident in the broader context of peer interactions as well. For example,

the Chinese-American high school students from Way's longitudinal studies (Niwa et al. 2011) sometimes responded to instances of peer discrimination by deliberately defining themselves as strong and tough—as resistance to the the stereotype that Chinese people are weak and passive:

> People are under the impression that I'm passive. Beginning of high school there were a few kids who picked on me, just pushed me out of the way. Thought I was a quiet kid and you know, I just had to do something to display to them that I'm not somebody you just fuck with.

Ronald (African-American) also explained that although others may expect him to conform to the stereotype "to act tough to be accepted or be in a gang," he positions himself differently:

> I know that like if you are about to get in a fight and you walk away from it, that's the right thing, but some, other people, they'll say you're lame for leaving, 'you're scared,' 'you're a punk,' all of that. And I think that's why people try to act tough all the time. But it doesn't matter, I just walk away.

Ronald recognizes that the stereotype to "act tough" among friends is not the "right thing" and cultivates an identity that counters the cultural expectation ("I just walk away"). The adolescents across our studies were actively constructing their identities in response to cultural stereotypes about who they are and should be, and where they positioned themselves within this cultural narrative impacted their friendships. Taking up identities that challenge these macro-level stereotypes shifted the landscape of adolescents' friendships.

Universal and Cultural-Specific Findings

Our data allows us to see how the macro-context of stereotypes shapes relationships across a range of contexts. Friendships, and relationships more broadly, appear to act as a conduit for the macro-context, a mechanism through which macro-level processes of racism, sexism, and homophobia, are manifested in the proximal experiences of relationships between individuals. In this chapter, we focused on peer relationships among racially–ethnically diverse American youth, as an *example* of this link between the macro and micro-context. The link between macro- and micro-, however, can be realized on multiple levels of relationships and thus, these processes may occur within the family, with teachers, and in community/neighborhood relationships. Similarly, the relationship with the self, or identity, is shaped by stereotypes. Long ago, Erikson (1968) argued that self-processes laid the foundation for relational processes. Our data support this reasoning and further show that this does not occur in a vacuum. Instead, identities are affected by cultural stereotypes that, in turn, shape relational pathways. Thus, the dynamic bidirectional relationship between self and other are inextricable from the macro-context of culture and this interaction likely reflects universal *processes* about human development rather than isolated culturally-specific findings.

Our research findings are based on studies with adolescents in both racially–ethnically diverse settings and a racially homogeneous setting. In diverse settings, adolescents interface with youth of different backgrounds and are afforded the opportunity to use and experience stereotypes across groups, thus increasing, for example, the opportunity for peer discrimination across racial–ethnic groups. Our research, however, also includes data from a homogenous context—an all-Black, all-male high school. In this context, we also observed how stereotypes function to stratify adolescents' friendships. Thus, it seems that the process through which the macro-context of stereotypes impacts the micro-context of friendships may be evident in both diverse and homogenous contexts, though the dimensions of judgment and value may differ. For example, in racially diverse schools, adolescents discussed race-ethnic stereotypes and discrimination in their friendships. But, in the all-male school context, adolescents used gender and sexuality stereotypes (interwoven with race) to discriminate and exclude their peers. That is, a specific context may activate particular stereotypes, but the process is likely present across settings. For example, in a predominately White private school, adolescents' friendships may be structured more along the lines of social-class

stereotypes than race–ethnicity. In this way, the *process* of the macro-level context of cultural stereotypes influencing adolescents' friendships may indeed be a universal phenomenon.

Implications and Future Directions

The goal of this chapter was to highlight the impact of the macro-context on adolescents' friendships by examining how cultural stereotypes shape the friendships' of racial–ethnic minority adolescents. Our studies suggest that two paths of such influence are peer discrimination and identity processes. The ecological perspective underscores how social position variables (e.g., race/ethnicity, gender, sexuality) and social processes (e.g., discrimination) shape adolescents' perceptions and responses to themselves and those around them. Our data reveal how stereotypes simultaneously inform self-processes (i.e., identity) and relational processes (i.e., friendships). Placing the study of adolescents' friendships in an ecological paradigm underscores the intersecting nature of micro- and macro-level developmental processes.

The racial–ethnic differences we found in our studies were in the content of the stereotype rather than the process of impact. For example, the Chinese-American adolescents in our studies were stereotyped as weak and passive and as a result were victimized by peers. In contrast, the African-American adolescents, who were stereotyped as tough and aggressive, rarely endured such threats from peers. The significance of this "ethnic difference" is not only that one group is harassed more than another but also in revealing the ways in which negative stereotypes structure the friendship experiences and opportunities of adolescents within each ethnic group. At the same time, our studies make evident that stereotypes and ecologies are not only relevant for racial–ethnic minority adolescents but for *all* adolescents as all adolescents are stereotyped regarding some aspect of their social identities. In addition, stereotypes are relational and formed in response to one another (Nasir and Shah 2011; Way et al. 2008, 2013) and thus the stereotypes that structure the friendships of ethnic minority youth simultaneously inform those of the ethnic majority and vice versa. If, for example, being aggressive and a troublemaker is the stereotype that defines the friendships of Black boys then *not* being aggressive and delinquent (i.e., pro-social and compliant) becomes the framework for the friendships of White boys (e.g., Dishion and Piehler 2009). Examining the ecological context of friendships can deepen the study of friendships among racial–ethnic majority adolescents because it recognizes that the macro-context of stereotypes positions youth in ways that differentially shape their friendship opportunities and experiences and influences the quality of and choices made by adolescents.

Although we know from an extensive literature that friendships are a robust and important predictor of adolescent outcomes (e.g., Rubin et al. 2009), this chapter contributes to our understanding the factors that shape friendships themselves. Given the relevance of friendships to healthy youth adjustment, understanding the factors that undermine positive, high quality friendships is critical for understanding how to foster resistance to those factors so that positive adjustment occurs (Way and Rogers 2016). Our findings suggest that cultural stereotypes can (and, in fact, do) pose a critical barrier to positive peer relationships especially across racial–ethnic groups. Thus, helping youth cultivate friendships that counteract negative messages that emanate from the larger cultural environment is essential. If we take seriously that stereotypes form the context of friendships, it becomes evident why youth often gravitate toward same-ethnic peers while cross-ethnic friendships are rare and less stable (e.g., McGill et al. 2012; Tatum 2003). Increasing cross-ethnic friendships is not merely about the "opportunity" for interaction with peers of other racial–ethnic groups (e.g., Moody 2001), but also, perhaps more critically, about challenging longstanding stereotypes that interfere with positive peer interactions across racial–ethnic groups. This process has significant implications for interventions and programs designed to support positive youth development.

Friendships are essential in the lives of adolescents as they create a space for self-exploration and transformation. And these friendships are intricately woven into the fabric of the environments in which they reside. As so eloquently described by Erikson (1968) many decades ago, individual development is a constant interplay between the psychological and the social, the developmental and the historical. Friendships that exist in the micro-contexts of adolescents' lives are indelibly shaped by the larger macro-contexts, specifically the stereotypes that envelope and give meaning to those micro-contexts. Negative stereotypes threaten to undermine adolescents' friendships by fostering divisions and perpetuating inequality. At the same time, however, friendships offer an opportunity and space for social change when youth challenge negative cultural norms, expectations and stereotypes in their everyday relationships.

References

Anyon, J. (1984). Intersections of gender and class: Accommodation and resistance by working-class and affluent females to contradictory sex role ideologies. *Journal of Education, 166*, 25–48.

Azmitia, M., & Cooper, C. R. (2001). Good or bad? Peer influences on Latino and European American adolescents' pathways through school. *Journal of Education for Students Placed at Risk, 6*, 45–71. doi:10.1207/S15327671ESPR0601-2_4

Azmitia, M., Ittel, A., & Brenk, C. (2006). Latino-Heritage adolescents' friendships. In X. Chen, D. C. French, & B. H. Schneider (Eds.), *Peer relationships in cultural context* (pp. 426–451). New York, NY: Cambridge University Press. doi:10.1017/CBO9780511499739.019

Berndt, T. J. (2004). Children's friendships: Shifts over a half-century in perspectives on their development and their effects. *Merrill-Palmer Quarterly, 50*, 206–223. doi:10.1353/mpq.2004.0014

Blyth, D. A., Hill, J. P., & Thiel, K. S. (1982). Early adolescents' significant others: Grade and gender differences in perceived relationships with familial and nonfamilial adults and young people. *Journal of Youth and Adolescence, 11*, 425–450. doi:10.1007/BF01538805

Bond, M. (2013). Why are you like you are? *New Scientist Magazine, the Great Illusion of the Self, 217*, 41–43. doi:10.1016/S0262-4079(13)60504-7

Bowlby, J. (1969). *Attachment and loss vol. 1: Attachment* (2nd ed.). New York: Basic Books.

Bronfenbrenner, U. (1979). Contexts of child rearing: Problems and prospects. *American Psychologist, 34*, 844–850. doi:10.1037/0003-066X.34.10.844

Bronfenbrenner, U., & Morris, P. A. (1998). The ecology of developmental processes. In W. Damon & R. M. Lerner (Eds.), *Handbook of child psychology: Vol 1. Theoretical models of human development* (5th ed., pp. 993–1028). Hoboken, NJ: Wiley.

Brown, B. B. (2004). Adolescents' relationships with peers. In R. M. Lerner & L. Steinberg (Eds.), *Handbook of adolescent psychology* (2nd ed.) (pp. 363–394). Hoboken, NJ: John Wiley & Sons Inc.

Bukowski, W. M., Newcomb, A. F., & Hartup, W. W. (1996). *The company they keep: Friendship in childhood and adolescence.* New York, NY: Cambridge University Press.

Carter, P. L. (2006). Straddling boundaries: Identity, culture, and school. *Sociology of Education, 79*, 304–328. doi:10.1177/003804070607900402

Cauce, A. M. (1986). Social networks and social competence: Exploring the effects of early adolescent friendships. *American Journal of Community Psychology, 14*, 607–628. doi:10.1007/BF00931339

Chu, J. Y. (2004). A relational perspective on adolescent boys' identity development. In N. Way & J. Y. Chu (Eds.), *Adolescent boys: Exploring diverse cultures of boyhood* (pp. 78–104). New York, NY: New York University Press.

Chu, J. Y. (2014). *When boys become boys: Development, relationships, and masculinity.* New York, NY: New York University Press.

Chua, P., & Fujino, D. C. (2008). Negotiating new Asian-American masculinities: Attitudes and gender expectations. *The Journal of Men's Studies, 7*, 391–413.

Crockett, L., Losoff, M., & Petersen, A. C. (1984). Perceptions of the peer group and friendship in early adolescence. *The Journal of Early Adolescence, 4*, 155–181. doi:10.1177/0272431684042004

Crosnoe, R., Cavanagh, S., & Elder, G. J. (2003). Adolescent friendships as academic resources: The intersection of friendship, race, and school disadvantage. *Sociological Perspectives, 46*, 331–352. doi:10.1525/sop.2003.46.3.331

Csikszentmihalyi, M., & Larson, R. (1984). *Being adolescent: Conflict and growth in the teenage years.* New York, NY: Basic Books.

Cunningham, M., & Meunier, L. N. (2004). The influence of peer experiences on bravado attitudes among African American males. In N. Way & J. Y. Chu (Eds.), *Adolescent boys: exploring diverse cultures of boyhood* (pp. 219–234). New York, NY: New York University Press.

Davis, J. E. (2001). Transgressing the masculine: African American boys and the failure of schools. In W. Martino & B. Meyenn (Eds.), *What about the boys? Issues of masculinity in schools* (pp. 140–153). Maidenhead: Open University Press.

de Waal, F. (2006). *Primates and philosophers: How morality evolved.* Princeton, NJ: Princeton University Press.

Dishion, T. J., & Piehler, T. F. (2009). Deviant by design: Peer contagion in development, interventions, and schools. In K. H. Rubin, W. M. Bukowski, & B. Laursen (Eds.), *Handbook of peer interactions, relationships, and groups* (pp. 589–602). New York, NY: Guilford Press.

Dodge, K., Coie, J., & Lynam, D. (2006). Aggression and antisocial behavior in youth. In N. Eisenberg (Ed.), *Handbook for child psychology: Vol. 3. Social emotional, and personality development* (6th ed., pp. 719–788). Hoboken, NJ: Wiley.

DuBois, D. L., & Hirsch, B. J. (1990). School and neighborhood friendship patterns of Blacks and Whites in early adolescence. *Child Development, 61*, 524–536. doi:10.2307/1131112

Eccles, J. S., & Roeser, R. W. (1999). School and community influences on human development. In M. H. Bornstein & M. E. Lamb (Eds.), *Developmental psychology: An advanced textbook* (4th ed., pp. 503–554). Mahwah, NJ: Lawrence Erlbaum Associates Publishers.

Erikson, E. (1968). *Identity: youth and Crisis.* New York: W.W. Norton & Company.

Fordham, S. (1993). 'Those loud Black girls': (Black) women, silence, and gender 'passing' in the academy. *Anthropology and Education Quarterly, 24*, 3–32. doi:10.1525/aeq.1993.24.1.05x1736t

Fordham, S., & Ogbu, J. U. (1986). Black students' school success: Coping with the 'burden of acting White'. *The Urban Review, 18*, 176–206. doi:10.1007/BF01112192

Furman, W. (1996). The measurement of friendship perceptions: Conceptual and methodological issues. In W. M. Bukowski, A. F. Newcomb, & W. W. Hartup (Eds.), *The company they keep: Friendship in childhood and adolescence* (pp. 41–65). New York, NY: Cambridge University Press.

García-Coll, C. G., & Szalacha, L. A. (2004). The multiple contexts of middle childhood. *The Future of Children, 14*, 81–97. doi:10.2307/1602795

García-Coll, C., Lamberty, G., Jenkins, R., McAdo, H., Crnic, K., Wasik, B. H., et al. (1996). An intergrative model for the study of developmental competencies in minority children. *Child Development, 67*, 1891–1914.

Ghavami, N., & Peplau, L. A. (2013). An intersectional analysis of gender and ethnic stereotypes: Testing three hypotheses. *Psychology of Women Quarterly, 37*, 113–127.

Gilligan, C. (1982). *In a different voice: Psychological theory and women's development.* Boston, MA: Harvard University Press.

Gilligan, C. (2011). *Joining the resistance.* Oxford: Polity Press.

Gordon, C., & Gergen, K. J. (1968). *The self in social interaction: I. Classic & contemporary perspectives.* New York, NY: John Wiley & Sons, Inc.

Graham, S., Taylor, A. Z., & Ho, A. Y. (2009). Race and ethnicity in peer relations research. In K. H. Rubin, W. M. Bukowski, & B. Laursen (Eds.), *Handbook of peer interactions, relationships, and groups* (pp. 394–413). New York, NY: Guilford Press.

Gupta, T., & Sirin, S. (2010). The social development of immigrant children and their families. Paper presented at the NYU Developmental Colloquia. New York, NY.

Hallinan, M. T., & Teixeira, R. A. (1987). Opportunities and constraints: Black-White differences in the formation of interracial friendships. *Child Development, 58,* 1358–1371. doi:10.2307/1130627

Hallinan, M. T., & Williams, R. (1987). The stability of students' interracial friendships. *American Sociological Review, 52,* 653–664.

Hamm, J. V., Brown, B. B., & Heck, D. J. (2005). Bridging the ethnic divide: Student and school characteristics in African American, Asian-descent, Latino, and White adolescents' cross-ethnic friend nominations. *Journal of Research on Adolescence, 15,* 21–46. doi:10.1111/j.1532-7795.2005.00085.x

Hartup, W. W. (1996). The company they keep: Friendships and their developmental significance. *Child Development, 67,* 1–13. doi:10.2307/1131681

Hinde, R. A. (1987). *Individuals, relationships and culture: Links between ethology and the social sciences.* Cambridge: Cambridge University Press.

Horvat, E. M., & O'Connor, C. (2006). *Beyond acting White: Reframing the debate on Black student achievement.* New York: Rowman and Littlefield Publishers.

Hrdy, S. B. (2009). *Mothers and others: The evolutionary origins of mutual understanding.* Cambridge, MA: Harvard University Press.

Jia, Y., Way, N., Ling, G., Yoshikawa, H., Chen, X., Hughes, D., et al. (2009). The influence of student perceptions of school climate on socioemotional and academic adjustment: A comparison of Chinese and American adolescents. *Child Development, 80,* 1514–1530. doi:10.1111/j.1467-8624.2009.01348.x

Kao, G., & Joyner, K. (2004). Do race and ethnicity matter among friends? Activities among interracial, interethnic, and intraethnic adolescent friends. *The Sociological Quarterly, 45,* 557–573. doi:10.1111/j.1533-8525.2004.tb02303.x

Lee, S. J. (1994). Behind the model-minority stereotype: Voices of high- and low-achieving Asian American students. *Anthropology and Education Quarterly, 25,* 413–429. doi:10.1525/aeq.1994.25.4.04x0530j

Lei, J. L. (2003). (Un) necessary toughness? Those "Loud Black Girls" and those "Quiet Asian Boys". *Anthropology and Education Quarterly, 34,* 158–181.

Lesko, N. (2001). *Act your age! A cultural construction of adolescence.* New York, NY: Routledge Falmer.

López, N. (2003). *Hopeful girls, troubled boys: Race and gender disparity in urban education.* New York, NY: Routlege.

Luther, S., & McMahon, T. (1996). Peer reputation among inner-city adolescents: Structure and correlates. *Journal of Research on Adolescence, 6,* 581–603.

McGill, R. K., Way, N., & Hughes, D. (2012). Intra- and interracial best friendships during middle school:

Links to social and emotional well-being. *Journal of Research on Adolescence, 22,* 722–738.

Moody, J. (2001). Race, school integration, and friendship segregation in America. *American Journal of Sociology, 107,* 679–716. doi:10.1086/338954

Mouw, T., & Entwisle, B. (2006). Residential segregation and interracial friendship in schools. *American Journal of Sociology, 112,* 394–441. doi:10.1086/506415

Nasir, N. S. (2011). *Racialized identities: Race and achievement among African American youth.* Stanford, CA: Stanford University Press.

Nasir, N. I. S., & Shah, N. (2011). On defense: African American males making sense of racialized narratives in mathematics education. *Journal of African American Males in Education, 2,* 24–45.

Niwa, E. Y. (2012). The impact of ethnic and racial discrimination on the social and psychological adjustment of early adolescents: A mixed-method, longitudinal study (Doctoral Dissertation). Dissertation Abstracts International: Section B. *The Sciences and Engineering, 73*(10-B), 3511454.

Niwa, E. Y., Way, N., & Hughes, D. (2014). Trajectories of ethnic–racial discrimination among ethnically diverse early adolescents: Associations with psychological and social adjustment. *Child Development, 85* (6), 2339–2354.

Niwa, E. Y., Way, N., Qin-Hilliard, D. B., & Okazaki, S. (2011). Hostile hallways: Asian American adolescents' experiences of peer discrimination in school. In F. T. L. Leong, L. Juang, D. B. Qin, & H. E. Fitzgerald (Eds.), *Asian American and Pacific Islander children and mental health: Vol. I.* (pp. 193–219). Santa Barbara, CA: Praeger.

Noguera, P. A. (2008). *The trouble with black boys: ... And other reflections on race, equity, and the future of public education.* San Francisco, CA: Wiley.

Osterman, K. F. (2000). Students' need for belonging in the school community. *Review of Educational Research, 70,* 323–367. doi:10.2307/1170786

Pascoe, C. J. (2007). *Dude, you're a fag: Masculinity and sexuality in high school.* Berkeley, CA: University of California Press.

Pew Research Center. (2011, March 30). Minorities account for nearly all U.S. population growth. Retrieved January 4, 2015, from http://www.pewresearch.org/daily-number/minorities-account-for-nearly-all-u-s-population-growth/

Pew Research Center. (2014, July 8). A view of the future through kindergarten demographics. Retrieved January 4, 2015, from http://www.pewresearch.org/fact-tank/2014/07/08/a-view-of-the-future-through-kindergarten-demographics/

Rodkin, P. C., Farmer, T. W., Pearl, R., & Van Acker, R. (2000). Heterogeneity of popular boys: Antisocial and prosocial configurations. *Developmental Psychology, 36,* 14–24. doi:10.1037/0012-1649.36.1.14

Rogers, L. O. (2012). Young, Black, and male: Exploring the inter-sections of racial and gender identity in an all-Black, all-male high school. Available from ProQuest Dissertation Abstracts (UMI No. 10197).

Rogers, L. O., & Way, N. (2016). "I have goals to prove all those people wrong and not fit into any one of those boxes": paths of resistance to stereotypes among Black adolescent males. *Journal of Adoelscent Research, 31,* 263–298.

Rosenbloom, S. R., & Way, N. (2004). Experiences of discrimination among African American, Asian American, and Latino adolescents in an urban high school. *Journal of Youth and Society, 35,* 420–451.

Rubin, K. H., Bukowski, W. M., & Laursen, B. (Eds.). (2009). *Handbook of peer interactions, relationships, and groups.* New York: Guilford Press.

Santos, C. E. (2010). *The missing story: resistance to norms of masculinity in the friendships of adolescent boys.* Available from ProQuest Dissertations database. (UMI No. 3426967).

Sanchez-Jankowski, M. (1992). Ethnic identity and political consciousness in different social orders. *New Directions for Child and Adolescent Development, 1992*(56), 79–93. doi: 10.1002/cd.23219925608

Savin-Williams, R. C., & Berndt, T. J. (1990). Friendship and peer relations. In S. S. Feldman & G. R. Elliott (Eds.), *At the threshold: The developing adolescent* (pp. 277–307). Cambridge, MA: Harvard University Press.

Shek, Y. L. (2006). Asian American masculinity: A review of the literature. *The Journal of Men's Studies, 14,* 379–391. doi:10.3149/jms.1403.379

Spencer, M. B. (1995). Old and new theorizing about African American youth: A phenomenological variant of ecological systems theory. In R. L. Taylor (Ed.), *Black youth: Perspectives on their status in the United States* (pp. 37–69). Westport, CT: Praeger.

Spencer, M. B., Dupree, D., & Hartmann, T. (1997). A phenomenological variant of ecological systems theory (PVEST): A self-organization perspective in context. *Development and Psychopathology, 9,* 817–833. doi:10.1017/S0954579497001454

Stangor, C., & Schaller, M. (1996). Stereotypes as individual and collective representations. In C. N. Macrae, M. Hewstone, & C. Stangor (Eds.), *Foundations of stereotypes and stereotyping* (pp. 3–37). New York: Guilford Press.

Steinberg, L., & Monahan, K. (2007). Age differences to peer influence. *Developmental Psychology, 43,* 1531–1543.

Stevenson, H. J. (1997). Missed, dissed, and pissed': Making meaning of neighborhood risk, fear and anger management in urban black youth. *Cultural Diversity and Mental Health, 3,* 37–52. doi:10.1037/1099-9809.3.1.37

Suárez-Orozco, C. (2004). Formulating identity in a globalized world. In M. M. Suárez-Orozco & D. B. Qin-Hilliard (Eds.), *Globalization: Culture and education in the new millennium* (pp. 173–202). Berkeley, CA: University of California Press.

Sullivan, H. S. (1953). *The interpersonal theory of psychiatry.* New York, NY: W W Norton and Co.

Tatum, B. D. (2003). *"Why are all the Black kids sitting together in the cafeteria?" And other conversations about race.* New York, NY: Basic Books.

Trevarthen, C. (1979). Communication and cooperation in early infancy: A description of primary intersubjectivity. In M. Bullowa (Ed.), *Before speech: The beginning of interpersonal communication* (pp. 321–347). New York, NY: Cambridge University Press.

Updegraff, K. A., McHale, S. M., Crouter, A. C., & Kupanoff, K. (2001). Parents' involvement in adolescents' peer relationships: A comparison of mothers' and fathers' roles. *Journal of Marriage and Family, 63,* 655–668.

Way, N. (2011). *Deep secrets: Boys' friendships and the crisis of connection.* Cambridge, MA: Harvard University Press.

Way, N., & Chen, L. (2000). Close and general friendships among African American, Latino, and Asian American adolescents from low-income families. *Journal of Adolescent Research, 15,* 274–301. doi:10.1177/0743558400152005

Way, N., & Greene, M. L. (2006). Trajectories of perceived friendship quality during adolescence: The patterns and contextual predictors. *Journal of Research on Adolescence, 16,* 293–320. doi:10.1111/j.1532-7795.2006.00133.x

Way, N., & Rogers, L. O. (2014). "[T]hey say Black men won't make it, but I know I'm gonna make it": Identity development in the context of cultural stereotypes. In M. Syed & K. McLean (Eds.), *Oxford handbook of identity development* (pp. 269–285). New York, NY: Oxford University Press.

Way, N. & Rogers, L. O. (2016) Resistance to dehumanization: A developmental process. In N. Nasir, C. Wainryb, & E. Turiel (Eds.) *Jean piaget society.* Cambridge: Cambridge University Press. (in press)

Way, N., & Silverman, L. R. (2011). The quality of friendships during adolescence. In P. K. Kerig, M. S. Schulz, & S. T. Hauser (Eds.), *Adolescence and beyond: Family processes and development* (pp. 91–112). New York, NY: Oxford University Press.

Way, N., Becker, B. E., & Greene, M. L. (2006). Friendships among black, Latino, and Asian American adolescents in an urban context. In L. Balter & C. S. Tamis-LeMonda (Eds.), *Child psychology: A handbook of contemporary issues* (2nd ed., pp. 415–443). New York: Psychology Press.

Way, N., Hernández, M. G., Rogers, L. O., & Hughes, D. L. (2013). "I'm not going to become no rapper": Stereotypes as a context of ethnic and racial identity development. *Journal of Adolescent Research, 28,* 407–430. doi:10.1177/0743558413480836

Way, N., Santos, C., Niwa, E. Y., & Kim-Gervey, C. (2008). To be or not to be: An exploration of ethnic identity development in context. *New Directions for Child and Adolescent Development, 2008,* 61–79. doi:10.1002/cd.216

Minority and Majority Children's Evaluations of Social Exclusion in Intergroup Contexts

Aline Hitti, Kelly Lynn Mulvey, and Melanie Killen

Abstract

Social exclusion based on race and ethnicity occurs within the context of peer relationships beginning in childhood. Surprisingly little is known about the minority youth perspective regarding experiences and evaluations of social exclusion. While it is important to investigate and identify how majority youth's biases contribute to social exclusion of ethnic minority individuals, a full understanding of the factors that contribute to social exclusion necessitates examining both the minority and majority perspectives. In this chapter we highlight recent research which has revealed areas of convergence and divergence regarding peer-based social exclusion. Overall, most children and adolescents view social exclusion based on group membership such as race and ethnicity as wrong. Differences emerge between majority and minority perspectives, however, regarding the expression of outgroup attitudes, ingroup bias, and the factors that contribute to social inclusion and exclusion. We review existing research and discuss implications for interventions, such as how to promote positive intergroup contact, social identity development to foster positive peer relationships, and healthy development for minority and majority youth.

A. Hitti (✉)
Department of Psychology, Tulane University, 2007 Percival Hall, New Orleans, LA 70118, USA
e-mail: ahitti@tulane.edu

K.L. Mulvey
Department of Educational Studies, University of South Carolina, 129 Wardlaw, Columbia, SC 29208, USA
e-mail: mulveykl@mailbox.sc.edu

M. Killen
Department of Human Development and Quantitative Methodology, University of Maryland, College Park, 3942 Campus Drive, Suite 3304, College Park, MD 20814-1131, USA
e-mail: mkillen@umd.edu

Introduction

Children from different ethnicities, cultures, and nationalities increasingly encounter one another due to a myriad of factors including increasing mobility and migration of those seeking a better quality of life, refuge from conflict, and economic stability. Diverse environments can potentially lead to increased cross-ethnic or racial friendships which are often beneficial for children (Bagci et al. 2014; Graham et al. 2014; Tropp and Prenovost 2008). At the same time, ethnically and racially diverse environments can lead to social exclusion, rejection, and, in some cases, prejudice and discrimination. Thus, peer relationships and friendships in intergroup contexts are complex. They require that children draw on developing knowledge about individuals who are affiliated with groups that are based on ethnicity, race, religion, and nationality. This information is often laden with stereotypic expectations based on what children infer about a group's identity, beliefs, norms, and social status. At the same time, when it comes to decisions about exclusion or inclusion and inter-individual treatment, children often apply concepts about fairness, concerns for the welfare of others, and justice.

Until recently, the literature on majority and minority youth development in intergroup contexts reflected different research traditions. Historically, research examining intergroup peer relationships in childhood focused on majority children's attitudes with the goal to reduce prejudice and discrimination against minority groups (Aboud 1993; Bigler and Liben 1993; Killen 2007; Nesdale 2004). Although, intergroup research with minority children began in the late 1940s with the seminal work by Clark and Clark (1947), in the past two decades, it has regained momentum and expanded to include research from around the world, with both racial minority children as well as ethnic minority immigrant children (Bigler and Liben 2007; Dunham et al. 2014; Graham et al. 2014; Flanagan et al. 2009; Killen and Rutland 2011; Nesdale 2008; Verkuyten 2008). Further, research methodologies to measure racial attitudes and racial bias in the context of social exclusion have expanded tremendously to include a range of explicit and implicit forms of bias as well as reasoning and judgments about interracial encounters (as we discuss below).

Current intergroup peer relationships research on minority children and adolescents focuses on how ethnic identity often serves as a buffer to victimization and harassment (Phinney et al. 2001). This research finds that minority children from homes with parents who prepare their children for discrimination are better prepared to resist its negative influences (Hughes et al. 2009). Further, peer groups that provide supportive environments help to reduce prejudice and bias in the school social environment (Tropp et al. 2014; Verkuyten and Thijs 2013). In general, current research on minority children's peer relationships provides recommendations for optimizing diverse school environments in ways that promote minority children's well-being (Nesdale and Lawson 2011; Tropp and Prenovost 2008; Verkuyten 2008). These recommendations pertain to the goals of (1) fostering positive ingroup identity for members of disadvantaged groups, who are often minority in number as well as excluded from the predominant society, (2) reducing intergroup bias that may exist with the predominant majority (and advantaged) groups and increasing opportunities for positive intergroup contact; and (3) creating integrated, multicultural school contexts in which authority figures, parents, and students from different backgrounds recognize and support the goals of mutual respect, acceptance, fair and equal treatment of others (Killen et al. 2011; Thijs et al. 2014).

In this chapter, intergroup peer relationships regarding minority and majority status will be examined by focusing on children's evaluations of social exclusion (Killen and Rutland 2011). This includes addressing children's moral judgments and social reasoning regarding situations of intergroup social exclusion, as well as considering the stereotypes and biases that inhibit positive peer group environments. These different aspects of how minority and majority children think about social exclusion form the obstacles (e.g., outgroup prejudice and stereotypes) and the catalysts (e.g., empathy, intergroup contact, common social identities) to children's healthy social development. This perspective offers insight into minority youth's social judgments, which often reflect a strong sense of social justice, empathy, and fairness (also see chapter by Malti et al.). The consequences of being a constant victim of exclusion include depression, social anxiety, and social withdrawal (Juvonen 2013).

Healthy inclusive peer relationships can foster the positive development of minority youth, who experience exclusion more often than majority youth because of their ethnic and racial backgrounds and their minority status (Rosenbloom and Way 2004). Therefore, examining children's evaluations of exclusion is important for identifying ways to encourage inclusivity within peer relationships.

Theoretical Framework

Investigating minority and majority youth's perspectives on social exclusion requires ascertaining judgments and beliefs about the contexts when exclusion is necessary to make groups work well (such as excluding a slow runner from the track team) and when exclusion is unfair (such as excluding a new student from a school club due to their race). An integrative theoretical approach, a social reasoning developmental (SRD) perspective (Rutland et al. 2010), has been applied to the topic of social exclusion and inclusion and has revealed how judgments about social exclusion are multifaceted, involving concerns for fairness and equality, as well as for group identity and group functioning, and psychological considerations of autonomy. SRD integrates theoretical models about social and moral cognitive development (Turiel 2006), referred to as social domain theory (Smetana 2006) with developmental theories about group identity and group dynamics (Abrams and Rutland 2008; Nesdale 2004). In brief, social domain theory identifies three domains of social knowledge: moral (fairness, equality), societal (group functioning), and psychological (personal choice) used by individuals to evaluate social issues. Developmental group identity theory recognizes the ways that ingroup preference and outgroup attitudes interact in intergroup contexts, and how this changes with age (Nesdale 2008; Abrams and Rutland 2008).

As the SRD model explicitly addresses children's social reasoning, the SRD model has been particularly helpful in shedding light on ethnic minority children's perspectives when examining group dynamics from multiple perspectives (majority and minority; ingroup and outgroup). A social reasoning developmental perspective asserts that children balance information about group norms, their loyalty to their group, and their moral principles when approaching complex social situations, such as those which involve outgroup members (Rutland et al. 2010). This framework highlights the instances when factors such as intergroup contact, societal norms about equality, as well as parental messages about egalitarianism, serve as catalysts for applying moral judgments in intergroup contexts. It also recognizes certain obstacles to applying moral judgments that can lead to prejudice and discrimination, such as ingroup biases, stereotypes, exclusive norms of majority groups, and expectations about outgroup homogeneity.

To date, research from this perspective shows that, with age, children begin to weigh concerns related to group dynamics in addition to moral concerns when making judgments about ingroup and outgroup members (Hitti et al. 2014; Killen et al. 2013; Mulvey et al. 2014a, b). This research reveals that, as children gain more experience with groups and greater awareness of societal norms, they display complex thoughts about the factors and issues that must be considered in intergroup relationships. In addition, children's experiences with intergroup exclusion bear on their understanding of what makes it wrong. What factors children from minority and majority backgrounds give priority to is a function of their experiences as members of these groups and how these experiences shape their evaluations of social exclusion will be examined in this chapter.

Current Questions, Measurement, and Methodology

The current questions regarding social exclusion pertain to how ethnic and racial minority and majority youth evaluate social exclusion and inclusion, the messages that children and adolescents receive from adults (expectations about parental views), and the social experiences that bear on evaluations of exclusion. A central question for evaluation of social exclusion pertains to the distinction between intragroup exclusion (excluding someone from the ingroup) and intergroup inclusion (including someone from the outgroup). Affiliation with groups often results in group loyalty, and these loyalties have a powerful impact on how individual members treat one another within their own group. Reducing bias means challenging ingroup members who espouse racial biases, or who reject equal treatment of others, and this can be difficult when the outcome may be exclusion from one's own group. Alternatively, group loyalty also makes it difficult to include members of outgroups, as this can also result in exclusion when ingroup members view this act to be a reflection of group disloyalty. These pressures in childhood begin early and are difficult to maneuver for many children. What makes it feasible is the strong endorsement of fair and equal treatment of others, as we describe below. Thus, the dynamics between loyalty to ingroups, attitudes about outgroups, and principles of fair and equal treatment are complex to coordinate. Additionally, as children's social cognitive development progresses, they increasingly understand that groups often have intentions that differ from those held by individual members (Mulvey et al. 2014b). We will examine both individual level characteristics (e.g., intergroup contact, shared interests in hobbies) as well as group level characteristics (e.g., social norms, status) that are reflected in how children and adolescents experience and evaluate social exclusion. In addition, messages from parents may reinforce ingroup loyalty or focus on inclusion of outgroup members, and experiences with others from outgroups can enhance concepts of fair treatment of others.

The measurements and methods for examining how minority and majority youth evaluate social exclusion are diverse. These involve judgments, behavior, and reasoning about inclusion and exclusion, and are reflected in both implicit and explicit methods. Implicit methods are used to examine the biases unbeknownst to the individual, particularly about race and gender. Explicit methods are used to directly assess motivations, intentions, and reasoning about interracial encounters. Increasingly, researchers have recognized the value of using both types of measures, as methods reflect a continuum from direct and explicit to more indirect and implicit. Age-related changes have been documented using both forms of assessments.

A major change in the research approaches for this topic over the past decade has been to include the racial or ethnic composition of the schools that children are sampled from as a central variable in the research design. Rather than solely focusing on children in homogenous school (and neighborhood) environments, research has studied classroom and school diversity as a factor that contributes to perceptions of school safety (Juvonen et al. 2006), opportunities for contact (Tropp and Prenovost 2008; Feddes et al. 2009) and support from peer groups. Thus, children with varying levels of social experiences (e.g., attend ethnically heterogeneous or homogeneous schools) have been sampled to study the extent to which cross-group friendship is related to an increase in the use of moral reasoning to reject racial exclusion, for example (Crystal et al. 2008; McGlothlin and Killen 2010; Ruck et al. 2011; Ruck et al. 2014). Surveys and semi-structured interviews about morally relevant third-party scenarios are often used in this research to capture children's moral reasoning and whether they reference concerns for fairness, justice, and other's welfare when justifying their judgments (Turiel 2008). Children's judgments about hypothetical scenarios tend to map onto to their judgments and behavior in actual situations (Turiel 2008). Thus these methods offer insight into children's developing social cognitions as well as how they may act when faced with similar situations.

The research reviewed in this chapter focuses on judgments about intergroup exclusion that children often make within the context of their peer groups. Judgments about such situations can vary as a function of children's experiences with cross-ethnic and racial peers. Decisions about including or excluding an ethnic outgroup member highlight tensions between moral judgments and other factors, such as culturally exclusive norms and traditions, as well as personal interests and prerogatives.

Social Exclusion: Empirical Findings

Minority Children's Experiences with Social Exclusion

While both ethnic and racial majority and minority children experience exclusion and prejudice in peer relationships, minority children experience it more than their majority counterparts do (Rosenbloom and Way 2004). This has been documented in racial and ethnic minorities in the United States (Flanagan et al. 2009; Rosenbloom and Way 2004) and in immigrant children in Europe (Monks et al. 2008; Verkuyten and Thijs 2002). Extreme forms of social exclusion can result in long-term negative outcomes in terms of mental health and academic achievement (Buhs et al. 2006). However experiences across different groups of minority children are varied. For example, African American and Latino/a American adolescents report prejudices based on race and ethnicity more than do Arab Americans, who experience prejudice based on religion, language, and personal attributes (Flanagan et al. 2009). Furthermore, Verkuyten and Thijs (2002) reported that Turkish children in the Netherlands more often perceived their own ethnic group to be excluded than did Moroccan and Surinamese children. Minority children are aware that exclusion based on their ethnicity and race does occur and do recognize that it occurs at both the societal level, through inequitable distribution of resources, and in intergroup peer contexts. Both levels of exclusion are important to consider because, as explained in the next section, societal levels of exclusion can impact one's perceptions and judgments about peer relationships.

Societal Levels of Exclusion

One area of research has examined children's awareness of socioeconomic status (SES) as a basis for social exclusion. This variable is often related to ethnic or racial minority status (unfortunately, SES is often confounded with race and ethnicity in many cultural contexts). Children begin to perceive societal levels of income inequalities as early as 6 years of age (Leahy 1983). In his study of social judgments about income inequality, Leahy (1983) found that both European American and African American children across the developmental spectrum (6, 11, 14, and 17 year-olds) challenged wealth differences between the rich and the poor by citing concerns for the poor. Further, increasingly with age, children began to justify inequalities by referencing merit. African American minority children, however, were more likely to perceive the need for social change and were less willing to justify economic stratification than children from advantaged backgrounds (e.g., middle-class European Americans). These findings, suggest that minority children are motivated to challenge social exclusion.

Other recent research shows both African American and European American children (5–11-year olds) who witnessed an inequality of school supplies between schools that differed in racial group membership allocated more resources to the disadvantaged groups (Elenbaas et al. 2016). While younger children (5–6 years) allocated more resources to the disadvantaged group when it was their own racial ingroup, older children (10–11 years) allocated more resources to the disadvantaged group regardless of whether it was their own group or the outgroup. Older children also recognized the societal patterns of disadvantaged status more so than did the younger children. Therefore, as children get older their social awareness of status and social exclusion increases. This awareness can play an important role in motivating both minority and majority children to partake in social change (e.g., rectifying resource allocation inequities).

Prolonged experiences of resource deprivation as well as experiences with societal levels of exclusion are clearly maladaptive for ethnic and racial minorities. For example, when assessing racial and ethnic minority adolescents, Arsenio et al. (2013) found that the extent to which

African American and Latino/a American adolescents perceived their social structure to be unfair was associated with them expressing less negative emotions (e.g., guilt and shame) after a transgression involving a peer. While this sample of minority adolescents thought their current social order needed restructuring, they expected it to get worse in the future. Thus adolescent minority youth recognize that social change is needed to end social exclusion of minorities in society, but their future expectations that change will come are bleak. Although this research suggests that awareness of societal levels of exclusion may help children rely on moral concepts in intergroup peer situations at a young age, it also shows that over time such awareness can be maladaptive for racial and ethnic minority youth, particularly for the development of positive peer relationships.

Peer Group Exclusion and Stereotypes

Minority youth often expect that their majority peers will act in prejudiced ways. In a study with immigrant youth, Malti et al. (2012) found that Serbian 12- and 15-year-olds attributed more positive emotions to a Swiss excluder, implying they expected that Swiss national peers would feel good about only being with other Swiss peers. With age, minority children in the United States expect race-based exclusion in peer contexts would occur more often than their majority counterparts (Killen et al. 2007b), and attribute this to negative stereotypes. For example, in one study Ruck et al. (2011) found that ethnic minority females and older participants (10-, 13-, 16-year-olds) expected majority individuals to use stereotypes to exclude others based on race, more so than did minority males and younger participants, respectively. Therefore, gender-based experiences and experiences of minority youth with time led them to anticipate exclusive behavior by majority ethnic outgroup peers. Expecting exclusivity from majority peers can result in less motivation to interact with and engage in friendships with majority peers. This could be maladaptive for minority children, on the one hand, as it discourages cross-ethnic or racial friendships, but on the other hand, it could

be protective as it helps them avoid situations in which they could be harmed by being excluded.

Racial minority children in the United States reject the negative academic stereotypes that are associated with their race (Copping et al. 2013). Minority youth, however, can also hold stereotypes about and expect ethnically exclusive behavior from other minority peer groups (e.g., Arab Americans, Hitti and Killen 2015). In this study, Hitti and Killen (2015) surveyed both majority and minority youth (12 and 16 years old) regarding their expectations about the ethnic exclusivity of an Arab American outgroup. Minority youth as well as majority youth anticipated that an Arab American peer group would give priority to peers of the same ethnic identity, but also reported low levels of contact with Arab American peers. Therefore, it is important to consider these findings in light of research on cross-group friendships. For instance, while research revealed that children with greater levels of intragroup contact report lower levels of anxiety (Douglass et al. 2014), research also showed that children with higher levels of cross-group friendships reported lower levels of perceived vulnerability than those with lower levels of cross-group friendships (Graham et al. 2014). The next sections highlights instances in which many minority children challenge social exclusion in intergroup peer contexts and demonstrate inclusive orientations. Inclusivity can be protective for minority youth as it is beneficial for forming positive peer relationships.

Minority Children's Perspectives About Exclusion

While majority and minority children share many similar viewpoints about social exclusion, including when it is unfair to exclude someone based solely on group membership (such as race, ethnicity, culture, and sexual orientation), minority children often become exposed to prejudicial behaviors from others earlier than majority children, and these experiences help them to recognize the negative consequences of exclusion and deter many from partaking in it. Research has shown that a large portion of ethnic minority U.S. children, for example, reject exclusion based on race or ethnicity, and cited empathic concerns for the victim when they did so (Crystal et al. 2008; Killen et al. 2002, 2010a; Killen et al. 2007a, b; Ruck et al. 2011, 2014). One's ability to empathize with a victim and use the victim's emotions as an evaluative appraisal of the situation helps in the application of moral judgments (Turiel and Killen 2010). Although this process becomes more complex in intergroup contexts when biases and misattributions of others based on their racial or ethnic group are invoked (Hitti et al. 2013), the ability to empathize with a victim of exclusion has been associated with children's evaluations of how wrong exclusion is (Malti et al. 2012).

In another study, ethnic and racial U.S. minority children compared to their U.S. European-American counterparts were more likely to indicate that non-race based exclusion was wrong (Killen et al. 2007b). Thus, in multifaceted contexts, when group concerns and concerns of fairness are considered, minority children, in this study, were more likely to reject exclusion of an outgroup member based on race when group functioning considerations were low in salience. Additionally, in the context of dyadic friendships, research showed that at an early age (6 years), ethnic and racial U.S. minority children relied on shared interests more than race and ethnicity when perceiving similarity between cross-race and same-race dyads as well as when making decisions about cross-race friendship potential (Margie et al. 2005). Similar findings were shown for ethnic majority children (i.e., European Americans) who attended ethnically heterogeneous schools but not for those who attended ethnically homogeneous schools (McGlothlin and Killen 2006). U.S. European-American majority children with little cross-ethnic social experiences assumed outgroup homogeneity in their judgments about same-race dyads and friendship potential between cross-race and same-race dyads. These findings indicated that cross-ethnic friendships impact children's judgments about peer inclusion

and exclusion. Intergroup contact increased inclusive orientations and is examined in the next section.

Intergroup Contact

Intergroup contact experiences, whether direct or indirect (e.g., through media and storytelling), can reduce anxiety toward the outgroup and promote understanding and perspective taking (Pettigrew and Tropp 2008; Tropp and Prenovost 2008). Evidence exists to support the benefits of contact but mainly for children of majority groups (Feddes et al. 2009). Findings for children of minority groups are mixed. Some findings indicated other factors such as superordinate common identification with the outgroup (i.e., school or classroom identity) play an important role in reducing prejudices (Jugert et al. 2011). Other findings showed that contact increases ethnic minority children's rejection of race- or ethnic-based exclusion (Crystal et al. 2008; Ruck et al. 2011, 2014).

For example, Crystal et al. (2008) found that both majority and minority students with high contact were more likely to perceive race-based exclusion as wrong than those with low contact. This is consistent with other studies with European American children that assessed varying levels of diversity in school environments (Killen et al. 2010a, b). Compared to students in low diversity schools, students in high-diversity schools generally reported more cross-race friendships, rated race-based exclusion as more wrong, and were less likely to use stereotypes to explain what it is about race that makes people uncomfortable. Similarly, urban minority children (African American and Latino/a American) who had high levels of intergroup contact rated race-based exclusion as more wrong than those with low intergroup contact (Ruck et al. 2011).

While there is some evidence indicating that contact with majority outgroups for minority children can be beneficial, more research is warranted to fully understand the range of contexts that have a significant impact. For example, Feddes et al. (2009) found that for Turkish minority children living in Germany, intergroup contact did not affect their attitudes toward

German peers. Recent work by Bagci et al. (2014), however, showed that high quality cross-race friendships among South Asian British children moderated the negative effects of perceived discrimination on children's psychological well-being and resilience. Additionally, other research has found that intergroup contact and cross-race friendships in adolescence, for U.S. racial and ethnic majority and minority samples, can serve as a shield against negative parental messages about race (Edmonds and Killen 2009). More research is warranted which explicitly focuses on identifying the characteristics of intergroup contact which make the experience for minority youth positive. For instance, preliminary evidence suggests that majority-minority peer relationships could benefit from intergroup contact that fosters a common identity among youth from different ethnic backgrounds (Jugert et al. 2011).

Ethnic Identity

Ethnic identification is the extent to which one identifies with their ethnic group and has positive feelings about being a member of this group (Phinney 2008). The role of ethnic identification on children's evaluations of exclusion is still unclear. Findings from a study by Pfeifer et al. (2007) show that ethnic minority children, in the United States, who show high identification with their ethnic group (e.g., "My Mexican culture is important to me.") demonstrated negative biases toward an outgroup. However, ethnic minority and immigrant children who demonstrated identification with a larger American national identity (e.g., "Being American is important to me."), reported less biases overall. Thus identifying more with a superordinate national identity that encompasses people of all ethnic backgrounds and identification with a nation, as opposed to a unique ethnic identity within that nation, was more adaptive. The latter finding is supported by intergroup contact research which focused on emphasizing superordinate identity categories (e.g., schools and classrooms) to promote positive intergroup peer relationships for minority children (Jugert et al. 2011; Guerra et al. 2010). Clearly, more research is needed to understand

the role of ethnic identification on minority children's perceptions and attitudes about cross-ethnic or racial relationships.

Affiliation with a larger common identity, however, serves to mediate intergroup tensions in a heterogeneous society (Jugert et al. 2011; Guerra et al. 2010). Evidence also exists showing that ethnic and racial identification is protective for minority youth who perceive high levels of discrimination (Brown and Chu 2012; Rivas-Drake et al. 2014; Seaton et al. 2014). Identification with a group is not implied through mere membership but develops over time and through a process of internalization (Bennett and Sani 2011; Phinney 2008). This often entails taking on the group's cultural practices, traditions, and norms. These are facilitated through parental ethnic and racial socialization practices. Among ethnic and racial minority children, ethnic and racial socialization often promotes ethnic and racial identity development (Phinney et al. 2001; Umaña-Taylor et al. 2006). Socialization that promotes knowledge about cultural heritage and instills ingroup pride has been found to positively affect early adolescents' cultural identification, self-esteem, academic efficacy, and engagement (Banerjee et al. 2011; Huynh and Fuligni 2008). Further research on the role of multiple identities in evaluations about intergroup social exclusion is needed to better understand the implications of common identities (e.g., national, school, classroom) and ethnic identities on children's social relationships.

Policy Implications and Future Directions

Findings from the research reviewed contribute to our understanding of the positive development of minority children. What is clear across all the bodies of research reviewed is that minority youth often have a unique and different perspective on ethnic-based and race-based social exclusion. The findings suggest that many minority youth exhibit a strong sense of social justice, empathy, and fairness. They are attuned to the possibility of discrimination and the importance of treating others' equitably. While minority children often express more inclusive orientations than their majority peers, with age, they become more aware of societal levels of exclusion, anticipate exclusive behavior from others, and expect stereotypes to drive peer exclusion. Research on intergroup contact, cross-race friendships, and ethnic identification, however, suggests that these external and psychological experiences can be protective and promote positive development in minority youth.

Intergroup contact has implications for policies that can help promote positive peer relationships in diverse settings. For instance, increasing diversity in schools, fostering ethnically inclusive norms, and adopting curricula that focus on multicultural education can all serve to promote positive social cognitive development in intergroup contexts (Nesdale and Lawson 2011; Rutland et al. 2010; Verkuyten 2008). A significant lesson learned from the 1970s and 1980s backlash regarding redistricting and busing of racial minority children to racial majority schools in the U.S. was that a number of conditions need to be met for it to work successfully (Frankenberg and Orfield 2007). Specifically, training is essential for school administrators, teachers, parents, and educators regarding the value of diversity for all children (authority support), and the ways to enable children from different backgrounds to work together (common goals, equal status) as well as supplemental support in terms of curricula training and counselors (Killen et al. 2007a). When these conditions are met then school districts can implement policies which ensure opportunities for positive intergroup contact both through considering income and ethnicity when using algorithms to assign students to schools and considering the ways in which income and ethnicity are often conflated when determining policies (Reardon et al. 2006). Further, school districts should consider implementing heterogeneous grouping and eliminating school tracking policies which have historically led to segregated classrooms (Oakes 2005; Corbett Burris et al. 2006).

Additionally, schools can adopt curricula which encourage children and adolescents to value differences among peers, as such curricula have proven successful in European contexts where they have been adopted (Verkuyten and Thijs 2013). Moreover, research indicates that some of the reasons why school-wide bullying interventions are not very effective in the United States may be because of issues related to negative intergroup contact (Evans et al. 2014). Policies related to bullying prevention, social exclusion, and peer rejection should also aim to recognize the role that negative intergroup relations and prejudice may play in the manifestation of these forms of negative peer relations (Killen et al. 2013). Thus, the research on minority youth perspectives related to social exclusion and peer relations suggest the importance of directed policy actions to better structure our educational systems so that all youth have opportunities for positive, healthy peer interaction. While the current body of research answers many questions about social exclusion among minority and majority youth, it also raises many additional questions.

The findings reviewed in this chapter indicate that the very question of group membership as a minority is complex: minority status could refer to ethnicity, numerical presence, gender, and socioeconomic status among other identities. Research on social identities indicates that children simultaneously hold a myriad of group memberships and that in different contexts these different memberships may be more or less salient (Bennett and Sani 2011; Phinney 2008). Therefore, future research should aim to understand the complex, fluid and dynamic interplay between group identities (for instance gender and ethnicity or ethnicity and religion) in examining children's social cognitions in intergroup contexts. Future research should therefore examine intergroup exclusion in which multiple identities intersect, such as those where children vary not just by ethnicity but also by socioeconomic status. In addition, the perspectives of biracial children, or children who identify with multiple ethnicities should be included and contrasted with other minority and majority perspectives. While research on social cognitive development in intergroup context has expanded to include minority children from different racial and ethnic backgrounds in the United States and abroad, more research with different ethnic groups is also still needed.

Further, additional research is needed on intragroup dynamics within ethnic minority peer relationships. This will identify how minority children evaluate exclusion of or by other ethnic minority groups and reveal intragroup tensions that children have to confront as well as intergroup ones. How do ingroup and outgroup practices and norms contribute to such interpretations? Related to this, much more research needs to be conducted on how intergroup contact impacts children who are part of different minority groups and to identify individual factors related to differential outcomes (i.e., psychological well-being). For example, in the face of increasing social inequalities, intergroup contact among historically advantaged and historically disadvantaged children can be adaptive (Reid and Ready 2013). However, more research is needed to understand the mechanisms at play that promote the positive effects of intergroup friendships. We still know very little about what makes a high quality intergroup experience for minority youth and what factors relate to positive outcomes of intergroup contact for minority youth.

Finally, in our increasingly global world, it is important that research examine a wider range of intergroup experiences as children are increasingly encountering others who do not share their group membership at earlier and earlier ages and in a wider range of contexts. For instance, research could more directly examine the role of exclusive and inclusive peer group norms in intergroup encounters across a range of settings (i.e., home, school, community, cyberspace). Additionally, such research could more directly examine the interplay between parental ethnic socialization and messages about cross-group friendships. The research to date indicates just how complex intergroup cognition is for majority and minority youth and highlights the need for nuanced future research across group categories and settings, especially given evidence showing that children do not treat all intergroup contexts

in the same way (Mulvey et al. 2014a). In sum, the research findings indicate the astute awareness many minority youth have of both the complexity of group dynamics and the unfair nature of bias, prejudice or preferential treatment. The current research suggests that there is still much more work to be done to uncover how best to support positive youth development in intergroup contexts and to understand when intergroup contexts provide opportunities for positive development.

References

Aboud, F. E. (1993). The developmental psychology of racial prejudice. *Transcultural Psychiatric Research Review, 30*, 229–242. doi:10.1177/136346159303000303

Abrams, D., & Rutland, A. (2008). The development of subjective group dynamics. In S. R. Levy & M. Killen (Eds.), *Intergroup relations and attitudes in childhood through adulthood* (pp. 47–65). Oxford: Oxford University Press.

Arsenio, W. F., Preziosi, S., Silberstein, E., & Hamburger, B. (2013). Adolescents' perceptions of institutional fairness: Relations with moral reasoning, emotions, and behavior. In T. Malti (Ed.), *Adolescent emotions: Development, morality, and adaptation* (pp. 95–110). San Francisco, CA: Jossey-Bass.

Bagci, S. C., Rutland, A., Kumashiro, M., Smith, P. K., & Blumberg, H. (2014). Are minority status children's cross-ethnic friendships beneficial in a multiethnic context? *British Journal of Developmental Psychology, 32*, 107–115. doi:10.1111/bjdp.12028

Banerjee, M., Harrell, Z. A. T., & Johnson, D. J. (2011). Racial/ethnic socialization and parental involvement in education as predictors of cognitive ability and achievement in African American children. *Journal of Youth and Adolescence, 40*, 595–605. doi:10.1007/s10964-010-9559-9

Bennett, M., & Sani, F. (2011). The internalisation of group identities in childhood. *Psychological Studies, 56*, 117–124. doi:10.1007/s12646-011-0063-4

Bigler, R. S., & Liben, L. S. (1993). A cognitive-developmental approach to racial stereotyping and reconstructive memory in Euro-American children. *Child Development, 64*, 1507–1518. doi:10.2307/1131549

Bigler, R. S., & Liben, L. S. (2007). Developmental intergroup theory: Explaining and reducing children's social stereotyping and prejudice. *Current Directions in Psychological Science, 16*, 162–166. doi:10.1111/j.1467-8721.2007.00496.x

Brown, C. S., & Chu, H. (2012). Discrimination, ethnic identity, and academic outcomes of Mexican immigrant children: The importance of school context. *Child Development, 83*, 1477–1485. doi:10.1111/j.1467-8624.2012.01786.x

Buhs, E. S., Ladd, G. W., & Herald-Brown, S. L. (2006). Victimization and exclusion: Links to peer rejection, classroom engagement, and achievement. In S. R. Jimerson, S. M. Swearer, & D. L. Espelage (Eds.), *Handbook of bullying in schools: An international perspective* (pp. 163–172). New York, NY: Routledge/Taylor & Francis Group.

Clark, K. B., & Clark, M. P. (1947). Racial identification and preference in Negro children. In H. P. B. Seidenberg (Ed.), *Basic studies in social psychology* (Vol. 1955). New York: Holt Rinehart & Winston.

Copping, K. E., Kurtz-Costes, B., Rowley, S. J., & Wood, D. (2013). Age and race differences in racial stereotype awareness and endorsement. *Journal of Applied Social Psychology, 43*, 971–980. doi:10.1111/jasp.12061

Corbett Burris, C., Heubert, J. P., & Levin, H. M. (2006). Accelerating mathematics achievement using heterogeneous grouping. *American Educational Research Journal, 43*, 105–136.

Crystal, D. S., Killen, M., & Ruck, M. (2008). It is who you know that counts: Intergroup contact and judgments about race-based exclusion. *British Journal of Developmental Psychology, 26*, 51–70. doi:10.1348/026151007X198910

Douglass, S., Yip, T., & Shelton, J. N. (2014). Intragroup contact and anxiety among ethnic minority adolescents: Considering ethnic identity and school diversity transitions. *Journal of Youth and Adolescence, 43*, 1628–1641. doi:10.1007/s10964-014-0144-5

Dunham, Y., Newheiser, A.-K., Hoosain, L., Merrill, A., & Olson, K. R. (2014). From a different vantage: Intergroup attitudes among children from low- and intermediate-status racial groups. *Social Cognition, 32*, 1–21. doi:10.1521/soco.2014.32.1.1

Edmonds, C., & Killen, M. (2009). Do adolescents' perceptions of parental racial attitudes relate to their intergroup contact and cross-race relationships? *Group Processes & Intergroup Relations, 12*, 5–21. doi:10.1177/1368430208098773

Elenbaas, L., Rizzo, M.T., Cooley, S., & Killen, M. (2016). Rectifying or perpetuating resource disparities: Children's responses to social inequalities based on race. *Cognition, 155*, 176–187. doi:10.1016/j.cognition.2016.07.002

Evans, C. B. R., Fraser, M. W., & Cotter, K. L. (2014). The effectiveness of school-based bullying prevention programs: A systematic review. *Aggression and Violent Behavior, 19*, 532–544. doi:10.1016/j.avb.2014.07.004

Feddes, A. R., Noack, P., & Rutland, A. (2009). Direct and extended friendship effects on minority and majority children's interethnic attitudes: A longitudinal study. *Child Development, 80*, 377–390. doi:10.1111/j.1467-8624.2009.01266.x

Flanagan, C. A., Syvertsen, A. K., Gill, S., Gallay, L. S., & Cumsille, P. (2009). Ethnic awareness, prejudice,

and civic commitments in four ethnic groups of American adolescents. *Journal of Youth and Adolescence, 38*, 500–518. doi:10.1007/s10964-009-9394-z

Frankenberg, E., & Orfield, G. (Eds.). (2007). *Lessons in integration: Realizing the promise of racial diversity in American schools.* Charlottesville, VA: University of Virginia Press.

Guerra, R., Rebelo, M., Monteiro, M. B., Riek, B. M., Mania, E. W., Gaertner, S. L., et al. (2010). How should intergroup contact be structured to reduce bias among majority and minority group children? *Group Processes & Intergroup Relations, 13*, 445–460. doi:10.1177/1368430209355651

Graham, S., Munniksma, A., & Juvonen, J. (2014). Psychosocial benefits of cross-ethnic friendships in urban middle schools. *Child Development, 85*, 469–483. doi:10.1111/j.1467-8624.2010.01480.x

Hitti, A., & Killen, M. (2015). Expectations about ethnic peer group inclusivity: The role of shared interests, group norms, and stereotypes. *Child Development.* doi:10.1111/cdev.12393

Hitti, A., Mulvey, K. L., Rutland, A., Abrams, D., & Killen, M. (2014). When is it okay to exclude a member of the ingroup? Children's and adolescents' social reasoning. *Social Development, 23*, 451–469. doi:10.1111/sode.12047

Hitti, A., Noh, J., & Killen, M. (2013). *Ingroups who exclude will feel bad, but outgroups who exclude will not.* Paper presented at the 43rd Annual Meeting of the Jean Piaget Society. Chicago, IL.

Hughes, D., Witherspoon, D., Rivas-Drake, D., & West-Bey, N. (2009). Received ethnic–racial socialization messages and youths' academic and behavioral outcomes: Examining the mediating role of ethnic identity and self-esteem. *Cultural Diversity and Ethnic Minority Psychology, 15*, 112–124. doi:10.1037/a0015509

Huynh, V. W., & Fuligni, A. J. (2008). Ethnic socialization and the academic adjustment of adolescents from Mexican, Chinese, and European backgrounds. *Developmental Psychology, 44*, 1202–1208. doi:10.1037/0012-1649.44.4.1202

Jugert, P., Noack, P., & Rutland, A. (2011). Friendship preferences among German and Turkish preadolescents. *Child Development, 82*, 812–829. doi:10.1111/j.1467-8624.2010.01528.x

Juvonen, J. (2013). Peer rejection among children and adolescents: Antecedents, reactions, and maladaptive pathways. In C. N. DeWall (Ed.), *The Oxford handbook of social exclusion* (pp. 101–110). New York, NY: Oxford University Press.

Juvonen, J., Nishina, A., & Graham, S. (2006). Ethnic diversity and perceptions of safety in urban middle schools. *Psychological Science, 17*(5), 393–400. doi:10.1111/j.1467-9280.2006.01718.x

Killen, M. (2007). Children's social and moral reasoning about exclusion. *Current Directions in Psychological Science, 16*, 32–36. doi:10.1111/j.1467-8721.2007.00470.x

Killen, M., & Rutland, A. (2011). *Children and social exclusion: Morality, prejudice, and group identity*. Chichester: Wiley-Blackwell.

Killen, M., Crystal, D., & Ruck, M. (2007a). The social developmental benefits of intergroup contact for children and adolescents. In E. Frankenberg & G. Orfield (Eds.), *Lessons in integration: Realizing the promise of racial diversity in American schools* (pp. 57–73). Charlottesville, VA: University of Virginia Press.

Killen, M., Henning, A., Kelly, M. C., Crystal, D., & Ruck, M. (2007b). Evaluations of interracial peer encounters by majority and minority U.S. children and adolescents. *International Journal of Behavioral Development*, *31*, 491–500. doi:10.1177/0165025407081478

Killen, M., Kelly, M. C., Richardson, C., Crystal, D., & Ruck, M. (2010a). European American children's and adolescents' evaluations of interracial exclusion. *Group Processes & Intergroup Relations*, *13*, 283–300. doi:10.1177/1368430209346700

Killen, M., Kelly, M. C., Richardson, C., & Jampol, N. S. (2010b). Attributions of intentions and fairness judgments regarding interracial peer encounters. *Developmental Psychology*, *46*, 1206–1213. doi:10.1037/a0019660

Killen, M., Lee-Kim, J., McGlothlin, H., & Stangor, C. (2002). How children and adolescents evaluate gender and racial exclusion. *Monographs of the Society for Research in Child Development*, *67*, vi–vii. doi:10.1111/1540-5834.00218

Killen, M., Rutland, A., & Ruck, M. (2011). Promoting equity, tolerance, and justice: Policy implications. *SRCD Policy Report: Sharing Child and Youth Development Knowledge*, *25*, 1–33.

Killen, M., Rutland, A., Abrams, D., Mulvey, K. L., & Hitti, A. (2013). Development of intra- and intergroup judgments in the context of moral and social-conventional norms. *Child Development*, *84*, 1063–1080. doi:10.1111/cdev.12011

Leahy, R. L. (1983). Development of the conception of economic inequality: II. Explanations, justifications, and concepts of social mobility and change. *Developmental Psychology*, *19*, 111–125. doi:10.1037/0012-1649.19.1.111

Malti, T., Killen, M., & Gasser, L. (2012). Social judgments and emotion attributions about exclusion in Switzerland. *Child Development*, *83*, 697–771. doi:10.1111/j.1467-8624.2011.01705.x

Margie, N. G., Killen, M., Sinno, S., & McGlothlin, H. (2005). Minority children's intergroup attitudes about peer relationships. *British Journal of Developmental Psychology, 23*, 251. doi:10.1348/026151005X26075

McGlothlin, H., & Killen, M. (2006). Intergroup attitudes of European American children attending ethnically homogeneous schools. *Child Development*, *77*, 1375. doi:10.1111/j.1467-8624.2006.00941.x

McGlothlin, H., & Killen, M. (2010). How social experience is related to children's intergroup attitudes.

European Journal of Social Psychology, 40, 625. doi:10.1002/ejsp.733

Monks, C. P., Ortega-Ruiz, R., & Rodríguez-Hidalgo, A. J. (2008). Peer victimization in multicultural schools in Spain and England. *European Journal of Developmental Psychology*, *5*, 507–535. doi:10.1080/17405620701307316

Mulvey, K. L., Hitti, A., Rutland, A., Abrams, D., & Killen, M. (2014a). Context differences in children's ingroup preferences. *Developmental Psychology*. doi:10.1037/a0035593

Mulvey, K. L., Hitti, A., Rutland, A., Abrams, D., & Killen, M. (2014b). When do children dislike ingroup members? Resource allocation from individual and group perspectives. *Journal of Social Issues, 70*, 29–46. doi:10.1111/josi.12045

Nesdale, D. (2004). Social identity processes and children's ethnic prejudice. In M. Bennett & F. Sani (Eds.), *The development of the social self* (pp. 219–245). New York, NY: Psychology Press.

Nesdale, D. (2008). Social identity development and children's ethnic attitudes in Australia. In S. M. Quintana & C. McKown (Eds.), *Handbook of race, racism, and the developing child* (pp. 313–338). Hoboken, NJ: John Wiley & Sons Inc.

Nesdale, D., & Lawson, M. J. (2011). Social groups and children's intergroup attitudes: Can school norms moderate the effects of social group norms? *Child Development*, *82*, 1594–1606. doi:10.1111/j.1467-8624.2011.01637.x

Oakes, J. (2005). *Keeping track: How schools structure inequality*. CT: Yale University Press.

Pettigrew, T. F., & Tropp, L. R. (2008). How does intergroup contact reduce prejudice? Meta-analytic tests of three mediators. *European Journal of Social Psychology, 38*, 922–934. doi:10.1002/ejsp.504

Pfeifer, J. H., Rubble, D. N., Bachman, M. A., Alvarez, J. M., Cameron, J. A., & Fuligni, A. J. (2007). Social identities and intergroup bias in immigrant and nonimmigrant children. *Developmental Psychology, 43*, 496–507. doi:10.1037/0012-1649.43.2.496

Phinney, J. S. (2008). Bridging identities and disciplines: Advances and challenges in understanding multiple identities. *New Directions for Child and Adolescent Development, 2008*, 97–109.

Phinney, J. S., Horenczyk, G., Liebkind, K., & Vedder, P. (2001). Ethnic identity, immigration, and well-being: An interactional perspective. *Journal of Social Issues, 57*, 493–510. doi:10.1111/0022-4537.00225

Reardon, S. F., Yun, J. T., & Kurlaender, M. (2006). Implications of income-based school assignment policies for racial school segregation. *Educational Evaluation and Policy Analysis, 28*, 49–75. doi:10.3102/01623737028001049

Reid, J. L., & Ready, D. D. (2013). High-quality preschool: The socioeconomic composition of preschool classrooms and children's learning. *Early Education and Development, 24*, 1082–1111. doi:10.1080/10409289.2012.757519

Rivas-Drake, D., Seaton, E. K., Markstrom, C., Quintana, S., Syed, M., Lee, R. M., et al. (2014). Ethnic and racial identity in adolescence: Implications for psychosocial, academic, and health outcomes. *Child Development, 85*, 40–57. doi:10.1111/cdev.12200

Rosenbloom, S. R., & Way, N. (2004). Experiences of discrimination among African American, Asian American, and Latino adolescents in an urban high school. *Youth & Society, 35*, 420–451. doi:10.1177/0044118X03261479

Ruck, M. D., Park, H., Crystal, D. S., & Killen, M. (2014). Intergroup contact is related to evaluations of interracial peer exclusion in african american students. *Journal of Youth and Adolescence.* doi:10.1007/s10964-014-0227

Ruck, M. D., Park, H., Killen, M., & Crystal, D. S. (2011). Intergroup contact and evaluations of race-based exclusion in urban minority children and adolescents. *Journal of Youth and Adolescence, 40*, 633–643. doi:10.1007/s10964-010-9600-z

Rutland, A., Killen, M., & Abrams, D. (2010). A new social-cognitive developmental perspective on prejudice: The interplay between morality and group identity. *Perspectives on Psychological Science (Sage Publications Inc.), 5*, 279–291. doi:10.1177/1745691610369468

Seaton, E. K., Upton, R., Gilbert, A., & Volpe, V. (2014). A moderated mediation model: Racial discrimination, coping strategies, and racial identity among Black adolescents. *Child Development, 85*, 882–890. doi:10.1111/cdev.12122

Smetana, J. G. (2006). Social-cognitive domain theory: Consistencies and variations in children's moral and social judgments. In *Handbook of moral development* (pp. 119–154). Mahwah, NJ: Lawrence Erlbaum Associates.

Thijs, J., Verkuyten, M., & Grundel, M. (2014). Ethnic classroom composition and peer victimization: The moderating role of classroom attitudes. *Journal of Social Issues, 70*, 134–150. doi:10.1111/josi.12051

Tropp, L. R., & Prenovost, M. A. (2008). The role of intergroup contact in predicting children's interethnic attitudes: Evidence from meta-analytic and field studies. In S. R. Levy & M. Killen (Eds.), *Intergroup attitudes and relations in childhood through adulthood* (pp. 236–248). New York, NY: Oxford University Press.

Tropp, L. R., O'Brien, T. C., & Migacheva, K. (2014). How peer norms of inclusion and exclusion predict children's interest in cross-ethnic friendships. *Journal of Social Issues, 70*, 151–166. doi:10.1111/josi.12052

Turiel, E. (2006). Thought, emotions, and social interactional processes in moral development. In M. Killen & J. G. Smetana (Eds.), *Handbook of moral development* (1st ed., pp. 7–35). Mahwah, NJ: Lawrence Erlbaum Associates Publishers.

Turiel, E. (2008). Thought about actions in social domains: Morality, social conventions, and social interactions. *Cognitive Development, 23*, 136–154. doi:10.1016/j.cogdev.2007.04.001

Turiel, E., & Killen, M. (2010). Taking emotions seriously: The role of emotions in moral development. In W. Arsenio & E. Lemerise (Eds.), *Emotions in aggression and moral development* (pp. 33–52). Washington, DC: APA.

Umaña-Taylor, A. J., Bhanot, R., & Shin, N. (2006). Ethnic identity formation during adolescence: The critical role of families. *Journal of Family Issues, 27*, 390–414. doi:10.1177/0192513x05282960

Verkuyten, M. (2008). Multiculturalism and group evaluations among minority and majority groups. In S. R. Levy & M. Killen (Eds.), *Intergroup attitudes and relations in childhood through adulthood* (pp. 157–172). New York, NY: Oxford University Press.

Verkuyten, M., & Thijs, J. (2002). Multiculturalism among minority and majority adolescents in the Netherlands. *International Journal of Intercultural Relations, 26*, 91–108. doi:10.1016/S0147-1767(01)00039-6

Verkuyten, M., & Thijs, J. (2013). Multicultural education and inter-ethnic attitudes: An intergroup perspective. *European Psychologist, 18*, 179–190. doi:10.1016/j.ijintrel.2012.04.012

Children's Social–Emotional Development in Contexts of Peer Exclusion

Tina Malti, Antonio Zuffianò, Lixian Cui, Tyler Colasante, Joanna Peplak, and Na Young Bae

Abstract

In this chapter, we review literature on the social–emotional processes of peer inclusion and exclusion from childhood to adolescence with a focus on peer exclusion based on minority status in distinct categories (e.g., ethnicity/nationality, gender, socioeconomic status). We begin with a brief historical review of research on social–emotional development in the context of peer relationships, followed by current research questions and methods. In our review of empirical findings under prevailing integrative developmental theories (i.e., moral emotions theory and social–developmental reasoning theory), we highlight children's feelings and reasoning in contexts of peer exclusion, and the emotional and behavioral outcomes thereof. We then discuss the risks of failing to address peer exclusion in multicultural societies and offer guidelines and strategies for prevention and intervention. Finally, we conclude with a proposed research agenda that aims to address gaps in the literature and provide avenues for future research.

Positive peer relationships play a critical role in ensuring healthy social–emotional development from childhood to adolescence, whereas peer exclusion can have detrimental effects in this domain. While peer victimization and rejection have been longstanding topics in the peer relations literature, recent efforts have focused on children's social–emotional development in contexts of peer exclusion. This integrative developmental research has studied peer exclusion based on ethnicity/nationality and gender (e.g., Malti et al. 2012), as well as atypical behavioral characteristics and developmental

T. Malti (✉) · T. Colasante · J. Peplak · N.Y. Bae
Department of Psychology, University of Toronto, Deerfield Hall, 3359 Mississauga Road North, Mississauga, ON L5L 1C6, Canada
e-mail: tina.malti@utoronto.ca

A. Zuffianò
Department of Psychology, Liverpool Hope University, Liverpool, United Kingdom

L. Cui
NYU-ECNU Institute for Social Development at NYU Shanghai, New York University Shanghai, Shangai, China

© The Editor(s) 2017
N.J. Cabrera and B. Leyendecker (eds.), *Handbook on Positive Development of Minority Children and Youth*, DOI 10.1007/978-3-319-43645-6_18

disabilities (Gasser et al. 2013; Nahmias et al. 2014).

In this chapter, we focus on research from an integrative, moral-developmental perspective, which has examined children's and adolescents' emotion attributions to excluders and excluded individuals, as well as their reasons for anticipated emotions and evaluations within majority and minority groups. After a brief historical account of research on social–emotional development in contexts of peer exclusion, we discuss our research questions and prevailing methods in this area. We then review recent empirical literature under integrative theoretical paradigms (i.e., moral emotions theory and social-developmental reasoning theory) on children's emotional and social-cognitive processes in contexts of peer inclusion and exclusion. Finally, we briefly summarize the developmental and health outcomes of peer exclusion, discuss implications for educational and intervention strategies, and offer suggestions for future research.

History of Research on Social–Emotional Development in Contexts of Peer Victimization and Exclusion

Current literature on children's emotions in contexts of peer exclusion can be traced to early research on social–emotional and moral development. Specifically, the first accounts of the "happy victimizer" phenomenon (Barden et al. 1980; Nunner-Winkler and Sodian 1988) established an experimental paradigm for understanding the development of emotional experiences in contexts of peer victimization. This paradigm has consistently shown that early childhood is characterized by the attribution of positive (e.g., happy) emotions to hypothetical victimizers (e.g., a protagonist who steals another child's chocolate). By age 6 or 7, children increasingly associate negative emotions, such as guilt and sadness, with moral transgressions (Arsenio 2014).

In the 1980s and 1990s, children's emotion attributions to themselves and others as hypothetical victimizers were predominantly studied in contexts of physical harm (e.g., Arsenio and Lover 1995). In line with a stronger focus on the role of peers in children's social–emotional development, research on emotion attributions expanded into contexts of peer exclusion by the 2000s (see Killen and Cooley 2014; Malti and Ongley 2014). Understanding the excluder's emotions has been the main concern of such studies, although emotion attributions to excluded children and bystanders have been considered in recent years (Malti et al. 2015). Importantly, this line of work has also introduced vignettes depicting the inclusion and exclusion of protagonists with minority status in distinct categories, such as ethnicity/race (e.g., Killen et al. 2002), nationality (e.g., Jugert et al. 2011; Verkuyten 2001), gender (e.g., Killen et al. 2002), and mental or physical ability (e.g., Gasser et al. 2013).

A related vein of research on peer relations also emerged in the 1980s under the auspices of the developmental psychopathology movement. It highlighted the psychological risks of peer rejection and culminated with a seminal review thereof (see Parker and Asher 1987). By the 1990s, evidence clearly showed that rejected children are more vulnerable to concurrent and later maladjustment, such as antisocial behavior and academic difficulties (e.g., DeRosier et al. 1994). With a particular emphasis on in-group bias and out-group threat, this area has since examined various forms of peer rejection (Asher et al. 2001) and resulting social withdrawal (Rubin et al. 2011).

In sum, research has traditionally emphasized social–emotional development in contexts of peer victimization and the psychological risks of peer rejection, whereas recent studies have aimed to understand children's feelings and judgments in contexts of peer exclusion. When deciding whom to include and exclude, children are required to distinguish, reflect upon, and balance moral norms, self-interests, and group functioning. The recent conceptual approaches reviewed in this chapter have attempted to reconcile these individual- and group-level factors within an integrative developmental framework that considers children's emotional experiences and motivations in multifaceted contexts of peer exclusion (Killen and Malti 2015).

Current Research Questions

Comprehensive approaches to understanding the various emotions that children attribute to excluders and excluded targets have brought developmental scientists new questions that promise further insight into the antecedents, correlates, and consequences of peer exclusion. We focus on three interrelated research questions throughout this chapter: First, what emotions do children experience as excluders and excluded targets across development? Second, how do these emotions differ when the excluded target is a minority (e.g., in terms of ethnicity/nationality, gender, developmental ability, or behavior)? Third, what are the consequences of peer exclusion for children's social–emotional development and health?

Research Methods

Developmental researchers have typically relied on questionnaires to assess children's social–emotional development and health outcomes in contexts of peer inclusion and exclusion. More recent techniques include peer nominations, class play, and teacher ratings (e.g., Buhs et al. 2006).

In line with a longstanding tradition of clinical-developmental interview methods in developmental psychology (Piaget 1932/1965), such procedures are also used to study children's emotions and reasoning in contexts of peer exclusion. Experimenters depict hypothetical scenarios of peer inclusion and exclusion that children most likely experience, and ask a series of related questions. For example, children are asked to: (1) judge whether it is right or wrong to exclude a peer based on their specific qualities (e.g., gender or ethnicity); (2) attribute emotions to the excluder and the excluded characters (e.g.,

"how does the excluder feel after excluding the peer?" or "how does the excluded child feel?"); and (3) justify their judgments and attributed emotions (e.g., "why would the excluded child feel this way?"; Gasser et al. 2013; Killen et al. 2001; Malti et al. 2012; Wainman et al. 2012). This paradigm has recently shifted from depicting straightforward acts of social exclusion or peer rejection to invoking multifaceted decision making with more complex interview procedures and vignettes. For example, Brenick and Killen (2014) employed forced-choice scenarios asking children to include or exclude in-group or out-group members and justify their decisions. Similar vignettes have also been used to invoke children's reasons for excluding deviant in-group members (e.g., Hitti et al. 2014b). Researchers (e.g., Oxman-Martinez et al. 2012) have also assessed children's feelings of psychological isolation in school contexts and organized groups (e.g., music clubs) to gain more information about peer exclusion in children's everyday lives.

A number of laboratory tasks have also been developed to simulate children's experiences of peer exclusion and study their associated physiological and psychological responses. These include a "Survivor" task (based on the popular television show *Survivor*) and a "Chatroom" task (Guyer et al. 2014). In these interactive tasks, participants are voted in/out of a certain game or chosen/not chosen by virtual peers to talk about a topic in a chat room. Similarly, the Yale Interpersonal Stressor-Child Version (YIPS-C) includes two confederates who gradually use a variety of verbal and nonverbal techniques to exclude the participant from a discussion while connecting and getting along with each other (e.g., Stroud et al. 2009). These controlled paradigms effectively tap into the physiological and psychological underpinnings of distinct aspects of peer exclusion. However, interview procedures using hypothetical vignettes that depict children's everyday life experiences offer an ecologically valid assessment of their multifaceted emotional experiences and associated reasoning.

Empirical Findings

From a young age, children make decisions about the inclusion and exclusion of peers (Killen and Rutland 2011). Understanding how children from minority and majority groups feel about the exclusion of children from other groups can elucidate the development of social attitudes (e.g., prejudice; Nesdale et al. 2007) and motivations underlying their inclusive and exclusive behavior (Killen and Malti 2015; Hitti et al. 2014b). As likely targets of peer exclusion, children with minority status may be prone to depression, withdrawal, and sometimes anger, which may exacerbate intergroup tensions and influence future behavior in the roles of the excluder and excluded.

Research on children's emotion attributions has mostly examined majority children's perceptions of and feelings toward the exclusion of minority group members based on various categories, such as their ethnicity/nationality and gender (e.g., a boy in an all-girls ballet class), as well as their atypical behavior and developmental disabilities (e.g., aggressive behavior and ADHD; Barnett et al. 2012). However, little is known about minority children's perceptions and

feelings in such situations. Throughout this section, we will discuss key findings in this research area based on integrative developmental approaches to the study of emotions and cognitions in contexts of morality and peer exclusion (Killen and Malti 2015; Malti et al. 2015). These frameworks posit that emotions and judgments in various contexts of peer exclusion are inter-related across development and, in interaction with group processes, affect children's subsequent decisions to include or exclude in such contexts.

Children's Emotion Attributions to Excluded Peers and Excluders

Research suggests that children understand the negative affective repercussions for excluded individuals. For example, they understand that others experience negative emotions, such as sadness and anger, when excluded from a group. However, when it comes to the attribution of emotions to excluders, children and adolescents report a variety of positively and negatively valenced feelings, such as happiness, pride, guilt, and sadness (see Fig. 1, reprinted from Malti

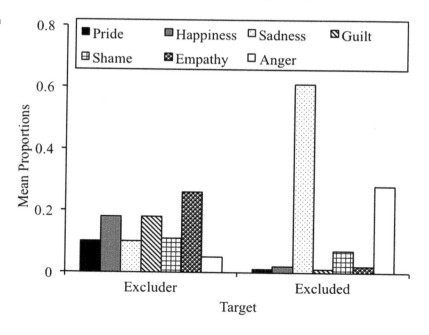

Fig. 1 Emotion attribution by target (excluder versus excluded; reprinted from Malti et al. 2012)

et al. 2012; Nguyen and Malti 2014). In line with integrative developmental models of emotions and reasoning in these contexts (Killen and Malti 2015), this variability reflects the various concerns that typically arise in multifaceted contexts of peer exclusion, since children need to balance moral and social conventional concerns when deciding whether or not to exclude a peer. As a result, these competing considerations may influence whether a child feels positively or negatively—or both—about their own or others' exclusive behavior (Chilver-Stainer et al. 2014; Gasser et al. 2013). Children typically justify negative emotions with moral concerns (i.e., considering the welfare of the other and/or fairness of the situation), suggesting congruence between their affective experiences and cognitive elaborations in contexts of peer exclusion.

There appear to be developmental differences in children's emotion attributions to excluders and excluded minority group members. For instance, Gasser et al. (2013) found that 12-year-olds attributed more negative moral emotions (e.g., guilt, sadness) to the excluder of children with disabilities than 6- and 9-year-olds did. Furthermore, Nguyen and Malti (2014) found that 13-year-olds, compared to 9-year-olds, better understood that a peer excluded based on weight would feel predominantly negative emotions. However, it was also found that 13-year-olds were more likely to differentiate between contexts, as they found it more acceptable to exclude an overweight child when the activity was athletic. This highlights children's increasing ability to balance individual-level concerns of excluding minority others with the group-level costs of including these children (Mulvey et al. 2014), and speaks to the importance of examining context differences in their emotion attributions.

In sum, children recognize the negative consequences of exclusion for others and attribute negatively valenced emotions to excluded children (e.g., sadness and anger). They also tend to assign negative emotions to excluders (e.g., guilt and empathy). However, they attribute positively valenced emotions to excluders as well, such as happiness and pride. Some studies have revealed developmental differences in emotions attributed

to excluders, but further evidence is needed to confirm age differences across different contexts of peer exclusion.

Children's Emotion Attributions in Different Contexts of Exclusion Based on Minority Status

Children and adolescents view the exclusion of others based on ethnicity, nationality, and/or race, as morally wrong (Killen and Rutland 2011) and less legitimate than exclusion based on other characteristics (e.g., gender). Although children frequently attribute negative emotions to the excluder regardless of context, these attributions are often contingent on whether children associate themselves with the majority or minority group. For example, group status matters for the anticipation of emotions in contexts of exclusion based on nationality. This is shown in Malti et al. (2012), where adolescents were shown hypothetical vignettes that depicted a minority group member being excluded from a social activity by a majority group member. One vignette presented a Swiss adolescent choosing to invite a Swiss peer to a Switzerland versus Serbia soccer game, and thereby excluding a Serbian peer. Adolescents who associated themselves more with the minority group member (i.e., the Serbian peer) than the majority group member (i.e., the Swiss peer) attributed more positive emotions (e.g., happiness and pride) to the excluding majority group member.

Research regarding exclusion based on gender has largely focused on children's judgments and reasoning. There is some evidence that children attribute more positive emotions (e.g., happiness and pride) to excluders in contexts of gender (e.g., a girl excluding a boy from ballet class) compared to other contexts (i.e., contexts of race or nationality), for reasons of group functioning and social acceptability (Malti et al. 2012). Interestingly, although the happy victimizer phenomenon is most frequent in early childhood (Arsenio 2014), these findings demonstrate context-dependent happy victimizer effects in adolescence (also see Recchia et al. 2012).

Recently, inclusion/exclusion research has been expanded to encompass contexts of behavioral problems and disability. For example, Gasser et al. (2013) examined children's emotion attributions in contexts of exclusion based on physical and mental disability. Similar to other exclusion contexts, they found that children seldom attributed only happiness to the excluder. The attribution of negative emotions, however, was related to the frequency of children's exposure to the minority group. Specifically, when the excluded minority group member was a child with a disability, children who frequently interacted and had more contact with peers with disabilities (i.e., children who were part of inclusive classrooms) were less likely to attribute positive emotions to the excluder compared to children who did not frequently interact with peers with disabilities (i.e., children who were not part of inclusive classrooms).

Empirical research on children's emotion attributions in contexts of peer exclusion based on behavioral difficulties is largely absent. Yet, the increasing prevalence of behavioral problems, such as aggression and ADHD, speaks to the importance of expanding this line of research. In a related study, Barnett et al. (2012) examined third through fifth grade children's prosocial responding to peers with aggression and symptoms of ADHD. They found that the more children thought a peer's particular characteristics were under personal control, the more they reported they would dislike, tease, or refrain from helping that peer. Specifically, children were less likely to feel positive affect (i.e., like) and respond prosocially towards aggressive children than those with ADHD symptoms, because they believed that aggression was more controllable. Based on these findings, one may speculate that children associate positive emotions with the exclusion of children with behavioral problems, especially if they believe that problematic characteristics are controllable or alterable.

In sum, researchers have predominantly investigated emotion attributions to excluders in contexts of ethnicity/nationality, gender, and, to a lesser extent, disability and behavior problems.

Complementing this line of research, developmental scientists are beginning to shift perspectives to examine group processes of inclusion/exclusion through their exploration of the roles bystanders play in children's exclusion behavior (e.g., Malti et al. 2015). This is important because bystanders are often present in encounters of peer exclusion, particularly in school contexts (Barhight et al. 2013), and may either prevent exclusion or exacerbate its negative effects. Recent research indicates that the presence of bystanders affects children's anticipation of emotions and judgments in these contexts. For example, Malti et al. (2015) found that the presence of on-looking bystanders encouraged adolescents to anticipate more positive emotions (e.g., happiness and pride) to the excluding group. Adolescents may consider on-looking bystanders (i.e., bystanders who observe the situation without engaging) as encouraging the exclusion and consequently attribute more positive emotions to excluders.

As children develop, they increasingly consider a multitude of factors when partaking in inclusive or exclusive behavior. They understand the negative affective consequences of exclusion, particularly in that the excluded predominantly feel negatively valenced emotions (e.g., sadness, anger), but that excluders feel more ambivalent and attribute a variety of positively and negatively valenced emotions. However, there are contextual and developmental differences in the anticipation of emotions to excluders, and further research is warranted to test if and how group status and development are associated with emotional experiences in these contexts.

In addition, much of the research on this topic has focused on how majority children feel about the exclusion of minority group members, but less is known about how children from minority groups feel about the exclusion of majority group members. Accordingly, future research on minority children's evaluations of, and emotions associated with, exclusion is needed to provide a more comprehensive picture of children's social–emotional development in these contexts.

Effects of Peer Exclusion on Children's Social–Emotional Development and Health

Extensive developmental research has demonstrated the long lasting, negative consequences of peer exclusion (both at the inter-personal and inter-group level) on children's and adolescents' social and emotional development and health (see Bynner 2001; Killen and Rutland 2011, for reviews). At the inter-personal level, socially excluded children are more likely to be victimized by their peers (Rubin et al. 2011) and to exhibit externalizing behavior problems, such as aggression, disruptive behavior, and bullying. This, in turn, may lead them to be even more excluded (Killen and Malti 2015). At the inter-group level, the effects of peer exclusion are far more detrimental, leading to widespread prejudice and social discrimination (Killen and Malti 2015). Children belonging to minority groups deserve special attention because they are visible targets of peer exclusion. For instance, studies conducted in the US have reported robust differences in academic performance between children of ethnic minorities (e.g., African American and Hispanic) and children of the majority group (i.e., European American), with the latter group scoring higher on measures of cognitive abilities and academic achievement (Huston and Bentley 2010). Because high percentages of ethnic minority children (under the age of six; 70 % African Americans, 66 % Hispanics; Addy and Wight 2012) in the US live in low-income families, socioeconomic disadvantage has usually been considered as one of the principal reasons for these academic disparities and related negative health outcomes, such as substance abuse (Mays et al. 2007). Similar results have also been found in Europe. Recent data from the Program for International Student Assessment (PISA) showed that European adolescents (i.e., 15-year-olds) from immigrant families scored lower on mathematical skills than their non-migrant counterparts, although this gap was reduced by 30 % when the socio-economic disadvantage of the immigrant adolescents was controlled for (European Commission 2013).

A study conducted in Canada with Asian immigrant children aged 11–13 years showed that 25 % of the minority children reported being discriminated against by their peers (Oxman-Martinez et al. 2012). The results of this study also indicated that the minority children who experienced higher social exclusion had lower social competence, self-esteem, and academic performance.

The negative consequences of peer exclusion on children's social–emotional development and mental health are not limited to group status based on gender or ethnicity/nationality, but extend to children and adolescents with physical and mental disabilities. For example, studies conducted with children (ages 6–13 years; Schenker et al. 2006) and adolescents (ages 12–16 years; Engel-Yeger et al. 2009) with cerebral palsy or developmental coordination disorder (ages 5–7 years; Jarus et al. 2011) indicated lower participation in out-of-school activities (an indicator of well-being) in children with these disabilities compared to typically developing children. Importantly, children with and without disabilities reported similar levels of enjoyment in these out-of-school activities, affirming the negative impact of disability-based exclusion.

Collectively, these studies suggest the presence of a negative link between children's adjustment and peer exclusion across development. Yet, some research questions remain unanswered. For instance, it is unclear if specific types of peer exclusion, such as exclusion based on ethnicity and nationality, are more detrimental to mental health during adolescence than childhood. Some differences depending on timing of experience seem reasonable. That is, as peer groups and social norms become central to the development of one's own identity during adolescence, adolescents may become particularly sensitive to the negative consequences of exclusion. Future research on the long-term effects of exclusion in childhood and adolescence on subsequent health outcomes will help further elucidate how they affect social–emotional development and health across the lifespan.

Universal Versus Culturally-Specific Mechanisms

To date, most studies on children's and adolescents' emotions and reasoning in contexts of peer exclusion have been conducted in North America (e.g., Killen et al. 2007; Oxman-Martinez et al. 2012) or Europe (e.g., Abrams and Rutland 2008; Enesco et al. 2005; Gasser et al. 2013). Only a few studies have included children from Arabic (e.g., Brenick et al. 2010) and Asian countries (e.g., Park and Killen 2010). Overall, there seems to be some evidence for universal negative consequences of peer exclusion on minority children's social–emotional development (Hitti et al. 2014a).

Although a large portion of these studies has investigated the moral judgments underlying peer exclusion, cross-cultural comparisons of the emotions experienced by excluders/excluded children and integrative studies of judgments and emotions in contexts of peer exclusion are still limited (Killen and Malti 2015). Recent studies suggest that children and adolescents from different cultural contexts (e.g., Malti et al. 2012; Nguyen and Malti 2014) may attribute similar, mostly negative, emotions to excluded children (e.g., sadness, anger), whereas excluders are expected to experience a variety of both positively and negatively valenced emotions, depending on the specific context of peer exclusion, group status, and development.

Due to the scarcity of cross-cultural research on emotions in contexts of peer exclusion, we briefly review the related cross-cultural literature on judgments about peer exclusion. Generally, cross-cultural comparisons attest to children's general perception of straightforward peer exclusion as wrong. For example, Rutland et al. (2005) found that children and adolescents regarded peer exclusion based on ethnicity as unfair, although older adolescents were more likely to accept exclusion based on nationality than younger children (see Hitti et al. 2014a). Additionally, children and adolescents tended to perceive exclusion based on ethnicity/nationality and gender as less acceptable than exclusion based on behavioral problems (e.g., aggressive

behavior). Yet, being excluded based on behavioral problems is considered more acceptable in some countries than others. For instance, Park and Killen (2010) found that American children (i.e., 10- to 13-year-olds) were more likely to exclude aggressive peers than Korean children were. The authors argued that the higher salience of overt aggression and its negative consequences in American society (compared to Korean society) might have been driving this cultural difference. However, American children were less likely to exclude peers according to their nationality compared to their Korean counterparts, probably because they are exposed to a stronger multicultural environment.

Some interesting culturally-specific mechanisms have also been found in studies investigating peer exclusion in children living in contexts of conflict and violence. In a study involving Middle Eastern children (4- to 7-year-olds), Brenick et al. (2010) found that Israeli-Jewish, Israeli-Palestinian, Jordanian, and Palestinian children equally evaluated peer exclusion based on nationality as negative, yet Palestinians were more likely to use nationality as a criterion for exclusion. As suggested by the authors, the negative consequences (e.g., poverty, stress) of a long-lasting religious and political conflict on Palestinian children might have enhanced the role of nationality in their judgments about peer exclusion.

Thus far, little attention has been devoted to understanding cross-cultural similarities and differences regarding peer exclusion of minority children based on developmental disability. Although previous research suggests that children are more likely to condone the exclusion of peers with mental or physical disabilities if it benefits group functioning in academic or athletic settings (e.g., Gasser et al. 2013), future studies are needed to better understand if there are cross-cultural differences in children's reasoning and anticipation of emotions in these contexts. These studies should consider the prevalence of disability-based stigma and self-enhancement values, such as competitiveness and need for achievement, as potential influencing factors across cultures.

Implications for Practice and Policy

Research on children's and adolescents' social–emotional development in contexts of peer exclusion provides information on motives that may underlie their actual inclusive/exclusive behavior, which may exacerbate or buffer the negative effects of peer exclusion on developmental and mental health outcomes. Specifically, integrative developmental research that investigates the emotional experiences associated with peer inclusion and exclusion of all participants in these encounters (i.e., excluders, excluded, bystanders) is beneficial to understand: (a) The proximal, developmental processes (e.g., emotions and related judgments and reasoning) associated with the experience of peer exclusion across various social contexts (e.g., classrooms, peer play) that are typical of children's everyday lives; (b) the role of minority group status in these experiences; and (c) the effects of exclusion on social–emotional development and health. As such, these lines of research provide useful knowledge that can inform the design and implementation of educational practices and social policies that aim to reduce the negative consequences of exclusion and promote the benefits of inclusion in peer contexts. Specifically, prevention and intervention practices aimed at enhancing the positive development of minority children should promote their social–emotional skills and moral development while, at the same time, sustaining social environments (e.g., classrooms) in which they can build strong social bonds that will help them create a positive sense of self and identity (see Catalano et al. 2004; Malti and Noam 2008).

For example, it is well documented that excluded children feel negative emotions, sadness in particular. This finding is important because prolonged exclusion and associated sadness may develop into more serious psychopathological problems, such as depression and social anxiety. Children and adolescents also sometimes associate feelings of anger with being excluded, which may contribute to intergroup tension. If the minority group feels oppressed by the majority group and forges their identity on this basis, tensions may culminate in severe forms of intergroup aggression. Thus, a thorough understanding of the emotional experiences of excluded children is necessary to enact better practices aimed to improve the social–emotional development and mental health of minority children.

In addition, considering the full spectrum of emotions associated with excluding others based on a variety of minority statuses may help to tailor intervention strategies to specific contexts of peer exclusion. For example, a positive emotion like pride in the context of peer exclusion based on ethnicity/nationality may be problematic due to high levels of hostility between groups in these categories (Golec de Zavala 2011). The experience of mixed emotions (e.g., feeling both happy and sad), however, may trigger the reflection of contrasting feelings and thereby sharpen the perspective-taking skills of excluders (Malti and Ongley 2014).

In general, past practice against peer exclusion has been developed independently from past practice against bullying and victimization. However, recent research indicates that these boundaries are permeable. Interventions at the individual and group level addressing children's social–emotional functioning and peer group processes associated with minority status may be a promising future avenue (Killen and Malti 2015).

Conclusions and Future Directions

While much research has investigated how children think and reason about peer inclusion and exclusion, more research on the affective processes involved in these experiences is needed. This includes not only research on emotions of the excluder and the excluded, but also on emotions of bystanders. Although some recent research has examined how bystanders in contexts of peer victimization feel (e.g., Malti et al. 2015), little is known about how bystanders feel in *exclusion* contexts. This is particularly important given the powerful role that bystanders play in potentially mitigating or aggravating the effects of victimization.

Importantly, more research on how *minority children* feel about exclusion in multifaceted contexts is needed. Most research has been studying how children from the majority group feel about the exclusion of children from minority groups. However, understanding the perspectives of children from minority groups is critical to foster their resiliency and to offset the risks they face. It is also important to understand the long-term effects of exclusion on minority children's development and health, as one's group status might be an important predictor of atypical development and poor health outcomes.

Applied research is also needed that develops assessment tools to understand children's and adolescents' feelings about peer inclusion and exclusion based on different group categories. Lastly, we urge the design and implementation of intervention programs and educational practices that aim to counteract the exclusion of minority children. Indeed, the ultimate goal is to sustain social environments, at both school and community levels, characterized by inclusion and tolerance in which minority children can build the social–emotional skills that serve as the core of their positive development.

Acknowledgments The first author was funded, in part, by a New Investigator Salary Award from the Canadian Institutes of Health Research (CIHR).

References

Abrams, D., & Rutland, A. (2008). The development of subjective group dynamics. In S. R. Levy & M. Killen (Eds.), *Intergroup relations and attitudes in childhood through adulthood* (pp. 47–65). Oxford, UK: Oxford University Press.

Addy, S., & Wight, V. R. (2012). *Basic facts about low-income children, 2010: Children under age 6.* New York, NY: Columbia University, National Centre for Children in Poverty (NCCP).

Arsenio, W. (2014). Moral emotion attributions and aggression. In M. Killen & J. Smetana (Eds.), *Handbook of moral development* (2nd ed., pp. 235–255). New York, NY: Psychology Press.

Arsenio, W., & Lover, A. (1995). Children's conceptions of sociomoral affect: Happy victimizers, mixed emotions, and other expectancies. In M. Killen & D. Hart (Eds.), *Morality in everyday life: Developmental*

perspectives (pp. 87–128). New York, NY: Cambridge University Press.

Asher, S. R., Rose, A. J., & Gabriel, S. W. (2001). Peer rejection in everyday life. In M. R. Leary (Ed.), *Interpersonal rejection* (pp. 105–142). New York, NY: Oxford University Press.

Barden, R. C., Zelko, F. A., Duncan, S. W., & Masters, J. C. (1980). Children's consensual knowledge about the experiential determinants of emotion. *Journal of Personality and Social Psychology, 39*(5), 968–976. doi:10.1037/0022-3514.39.5.968

Barhight, L. R., Hubbard, J. A., & Hyde, C. T. (2013). Children's physiological and emotional reactions to witnessing bullying predict bystander intervention. *Child Development, 84*(1), 375–390. doi:10.1111/j.1467-8624.2012.01839.x

Barnett, M. A., Sonnentag, T. L., Livengood, J. L., Struble, A. L., & Wadian, T. W. (2012). Role of fault attributions and desire, effort, and outcome expectations in children's anticipated responses to hypothetical peers with various undesirable characteristics. *The Journal of Genetic Psychology: Research and Theory on Human Development, 173*(3), 317–329. doi:10.1080/00221325.2011.610391

Brenick, A., & Killen, M. (2014). Moral judgments about Jewish-Arab intergroup exclusion: The role of cultural identify and contact. *Developmental Psychology, 50*(1), 86–99. doi:10.1037/a0034702

Brenick, A., Killen, M., Lee-Kim, J., Fox, N. A., Leavitt, L. A., Raviv, A., et al. (2010). Social understanding in young Israeli-Jewish, Israeli-Palestinian, Palestinian, and Jordanian children: Moral judgments and stereotypes. *Early Education and Development, 21*, 866–911. doi:10.1080/10409280903236598

Bynner, J. (2001). Childhood risks and protective factors in social exclusion. *Children and Society, 15*(5), 285–381. doi:10.1002/CHI.681

Buhs, E. S., Ladd, G. W., & Herald, S. L. (2006). Peer exclusion and victimization: Processes that mediate the relation between peer group rejection and children's classroom engagement and achievement? *Journal of Educational Psychology, 98*(1), 1–13. doi:10.1037/0022-0663.98.1.1

Catalano, R. F., Berglund, M. L., Ryan, J. A. M., Lonczak, H. S., & Hawkins, J. D. (2004). Positive youth development in the United States: Research findings on evaluations of positive youth development programs. *The Annals of the American Academy of Political and Social Science, 591*, 98–124. doi:10.1177/0002716203260102

Chilver-Stainer, J., Gasser, L., & Perrig-Chiello, P. (2014). Children's and adolescents' moral emotion attributions and judgments about exclusion of peers with hearing impairments. *Journal of Moral Education, 43*(3), 235–249. doi:10.1080/03057240.2014.913515

DeRosier, M., Kupersmidt, J. B., & Patterson, C. J. (1994). Children's academic and behavioral adjustment as a function of the chronicity and proximity of peer rejection. *Child Development, 65*(6), 1799–1813. doi:10.1111/j.1467-8624.1994.tb00850.x

Enesco, I., Navarro, A., Paradela, I., & Guerrero, S. (2005). Stereotypes and beliefs about different ethnic groups in Spain: A study with Spanish and Latin American children living in Madrid. *Journal of Applied Developmental Psychology, 26*(6), 638–659. doi:10.1016/j.appdev.2005.08.009

Engel-Yeger, B., Jarus, T., Anabi, D., & Law, M. (2009). Differences between youth with cerebral palsy and typical youth in community participation. *American Journal of Occupational Therapy, 63*(1), 96–104. doi:10.5014/ajot.63.1.96

European Commission. (2013). *PISA 2012: EU performance and first inferences regarding education and training policies in Europe.* Belgium: Brussels.

Gasser, L., Malti, T., & Buholzer, A. (2013). Children's moral judgments and moral emotions following exclusion of children with disabilities: Relations with inclusive education, age, and contact intensity. *Research in Developmental Disabilities, 34*(3), 948–958. doi:10.1016/j.ridd.2012.11.017

Golec de Zavala, A. (2011). Collective narcissism and intergroup hostility: The dark side of "in-group love". *Social and Personality Psychological Compass, 5*(6), 309–320. doi:10.1111/j1751-9004.2011.00351.x

Guyer, A. E., Caouette, J. D., Lee, C. C., & Ruiz, S. K. (2014). Will they like me? Adolescents' emotional responses to peer evaluation. *International Journal of Behavioral Development, 38*(2), 155–163. doi:10.1177/0165025413515627

Hitti, A., Mulvey, K. L., & Killen, M. (2014a). Social exclusion in adolescence. In R. J. R. Levesque (Ed.), *Encyclopedia of adolescence* (pp. 2783–2792). New York, NY: Springer. doi:10.1007/978-1-4419-1695-2_50

Hitti, A., Mulvey, K. L., Rutland, A., Abrams, D., & Killen, M. (2014b). When is it okay to exclude a member of the ingroup? Children's and adolescents' social reasoning. *Social Development, 23*(3), 451–469. doi:10.1111/sode.12047

Huston, A., & Bentley, A. C. (2010). Human development in societal context. *Annual Review of Psychology, 61*, 411–437. doi:10.1146/annurev.psych.093008.100442

Jarus, T., Lourie-Gelberg, Y., Engel-Yeger, B., & Bart, O. (2011). Participation patterns of school-aged children with and without DCD. *Research in Developmental Disabilities, 32*(4), 1323–1331. doi:10.1016/j.ridd.2011.01.033

Jugert, P., Noack, P., & Rutland, A. (2011). Friendship preferences among German and Turkish preadolescents. *Child Development, 82*(3), 812–829. doi:10.1111/j.1467-8624.2010.01528.x

Killen, M., & Cooley, S. (2014). Morality, exclusion, and prejudice. In M. Killen & J. Smetana (Eds.), *Handbook of moral development* (2nd ed., pp. 340–360). New York, NY: Psychology Press.

Killen, M., & Malti, T. (2015). Moral judgments and emotions in contexts of peer exclusion and victimization. *Advances in Child Development and Behavior, 48*, 249–276. doi:10.1016/bs.acdb.2014.11.007

Killen, M., Henning, A., Kelly, M. C., Crystal, D., & Ruck, M. (2007). Evaluations of interracial peer encounters by majority and minority U.S. children and adolescents. *International Journal of Behavioral Development, 31*(5), 491–500. doi:10.1177/0165025407081478

Killen, M., Lee-Kim, J., McGlothlin, H., & Stangor, C. (2002). How children and adolescents evaluate gender and racial exclusion. *Monographs for the Society for Research in Child Development, 67*(4, Serial No. 271). Oxford: Blackwell Publishers.

Killen, M., Pisacane, K., Lee-Kim, J., & Ardila-Rey, A. (2001). Fairness or stereotypes? Young children's priorities when evaluating group exclusion and inclusion. *Developmental Psychology, 37*(5), 587–596. doi:10.1037/0012-1649.37.5.587

Killen, M., & Rutland, A. (2011). *Children and social exclusion: Morality, prejudice, and group identity.* Oxford, UK: Wiley-Blackwell. doi:10.1002/9781444396317

Malti, T., Killen, M., & Gasser, L. (2012). Social judgments and emotion attributions about exclusion in Switzerland. *Child Development, 83*(2), 697–711. doi:10.1111/j.1467-8624.2011.01705.x

Malti, T., & Noam, G. G. (Eds.). (2008). *Where youth development meets mental health and education: The RALLY approach.* New Directions for Youth Development. No 120.

Malti, T., & Ongley, S. F. (2014). The development of moral emotions and moral reasoning. In M. Killen & J. Smetana (Eds.), *Handbook of moral development* (2nd ed., pp. 163–183). New York, NY: Psychology Press.

Malti, T., Strohmeier, D., & Killen, M. (2015). The impact of on-looking and including bystander behavior on judgments and emotions regarding peer exclusion. *British Journal of Developmental Psychology, 33*, 295–311. doi: 10.1111/bjdp.12090

Mays, V. M., Cochran, S. D., & Barnes, N. W. (2007). Race, race-based discrimination, and health outcomes among African Americans. *Annual Review of Psychology, 58*, 201–205. doi:10.1146/annurev.psych.57.102904.190212

Mulvey, K. L., Hitti, A., Rutland, A., Abrams, D., & Killen, M. (2014). Context differences in ingroup preferences. *Developmental Psychology, 50*(5), 1507–1519. doi:10.1037/a0035593

Nahmias, A. S., Kase, C., & Mandell, D. S. (2014). Comparing cognitive outcomes among children with autism spectrum disorders receiving community-based early intervention in one of three placements. *Autism, 18*(3), 311–320. doi:10.1177/1362361312467865

Nesdale, D., Maass, A., Kiesner, J., Durkin, K., Griffiths, J., & Ekberg, A. (2007). Effects of peer group rejection, group membership, and group norms, on children's outgroup prejudice. *International Journal of Behavioral Development, 31*(5), 526–535. doi:10. 1177/0165025407081479

Nguyen, C., & Malti, T. (2014). Children's judgements and emotions about social exclusion based on weight. *British Journal of Developmental Psychology, 32*(3), 330–344. doi:10.1111/bjdp.12045

Nunner-Winkler, G., & Sodian, B. (1988). Children's understanding of moral emotions. *Child Development, 59*(5), 1323–1328.

Oxman-Martinez, J., Rummens, A. J., Moreau, J., Choi, Y. R., Beiser, M., Ogilvie, L., et al. (2012). Perceived ethnic discrimination and social exclusion: Newcomer immigrant children in Canada. *American Journal of Orthopsychiatry, 82*(3), 376–388. doi:10.1111/j.1939-0025.2012.01161.x

Park, Y., & Killen, M. (2010). When is peer rejection justifiable? Children's understanding across two cultures. *Cognitive Development, 25*(3), 290–301. doi:10. 1016/j.cogdev.2009.10.004

Parker, J. G., & Asher, S. R. (1987). Peer relations and later personal adjustment: Are low-accepted children at risk? *Psychological Bulletin, 102*(3), 357–389. doi:10.1037/0033-2909.102.3.357

Piaget, J. (1965). *The moral judgment of the child*. New York, NY: Free Press. (Original work published in 1932).

Recchia, H., Brehl, B., & Wainryb, C. (2012). Children's and adolescents' reasons for socially excluding others. *Cognitive Development, 27*(2), 195–203. doi:10.1016/j.cogdev.2012.02.005

Rubin, K. H., Bukowski, W., & Laursen, B. (Eds.). (2011). *Handbook of peer interactions, relationships, and groups*. New York, NY: Guilford Press.

Rutland, A., Cameron, L., Milne, A., & McGeorge, P. (2005). Social norms and self-presentation: Children's implicit and explicit intergroup attitudes. *Child Development, 76*(2), 451–466. doi:10.1111/j.1467-8624.2005.00856.x

Schenker, R., Coster, W., & Parush, S. (2006). Personal assistance, adaptations, and participation in students with cerebral palsy mainstreamed in elementary schools. *Disability and Rehabilitation, 28*(17), 1061–1069. doi:10.1080/09638280500526461

Stroud, L. R., Foster, E., Papandonatos, G. D., Handwerger, K., Granger, D. A., Kivlighan, K. T., et al. (2009). Stress response and the adolescent transition: Performance versus peer rejection stressors. *Development and Psychopathology, 21*(1), 47–68. doi:10. 1017/S0954579409000042

Verkuyten, M. (2001). National identification and intergroup evaluations in Dutch children. *British Journal of Developmental Psychology, 19*(4), 559–571. doi:10.1348/026151001166254

Wainman, B., Boulton-Lewis, G., Walker, S., Brownlee, J., Cobb, C., Whiteford, C., et al. (2012). Young children's beliefs about including others in their play: Social and moral reasoning about inclusion and exclusion. *Australasian Journal of Early Childhood, 37*(3), 137–146.

Positive Youth Development of Roma Ethnic Minority Across Europe

Radosveta Dimitrova and Laura Ferrer-Wreder

Abstract

Roma are one of Europe's largest and most vulnerable ethnic minority groups, currently making up nearly 12 million people, and have historically experienced severe marginalization and discrimination. Roma children and youth in particular are globally recognized to be in need of support and their successful adaptation and optimal outcomes are of major interest to practitioners and policy makers. This chapter addresses resources within proximal contexts, such as peers and family contexts that have the potential to foster positive youth development in Roma ethnic minority populations in Europe. Roma are mainly a sedentary indigenous ethnic minority group characterized by strong family, community and peer bonds, thereby creating a unique and underrepresented context to study PYD. In this chapter, we provide a brief historical overview, current research and empirical findings on Roma children and youth within peer and family contexts. We draw on core theoretical models of PYD as well as selected developmental theories of normative development to highlight the applicability of these traditional frameworks to Roma ethnic minority groups. In so doing, we pay careful attention to the cultural, ethnic, and economic characteristics of Roma youth and their family context. In the conclusion, we explored the implications of the reviewed evidence to the development of resource-oriented policy and practice for Roma youth.

Introduction

This chapter addresses the positive youth development (PYD) of Roma ethnic minority populations in Europe by focusing on peer and friendship relations and how they are informed by socialization factors in family, community and school settings. Roma are a large and

R. Dimitrova (✉) · L. Ferrer-Wreder
Department of Psychology, Stockholm University,
Frescati Hagv. 14, SE-106 91 Stockholm, Sweden
e-mail: radosveta.dimitrova@psychology.su.se

© The Editor(s) 2017
N.J. Cabrera and B. Leyendecker (eds.), *Handbook on Positive Development of Minority Children and Youth*, DOI 10.1007/978-3-319-43645-6_19

vulnerable ethnic minority, currently making up nearly 12 million people, and have historically experienced severe marginalization and discrimination (Council of Europe 2010). Roma children and youth in particular are globally recognized to be a group in need of support and their successful adaptation and outcomes are of major interest to practitioners and policy makers due to, in part, the extreme and long-standing marginalization of their community across Europe (European Commission 2013). In fact, well-being, school and social adjustment of Roma youth are particularly salient in post-communist countries which started the process of democratization after 1989. Following the collapse of the communist state system in Europe, many countries hosting Roma who hold the official nationality of their countries of settlement, experienced marked economic and political transitions, rising nationalism, inter-ethnic hostilities, negative attitudes and discrimination toward Roma (Barany 2002). For example, Central-Eastern Europe hosts the largest Roma settlement in the world. The life conditions and chances of Roma youth in this part of the world are partially rooted in historic ethnic tensions and a policy of assimilation of Roma during communist rule, as well as the present-day fluidity of official integration and support efforts for Roma youth.

With this wider context in mind, in this chapter we take a strengths-based, positive youth development (PYD) perspective of adolescence and the social contexts (peers, friendships, family, community) of Roma youth. What cultural resources and key ecologies such as life with peers and family are likely to promote optimal outcomes in Roma youth? Roma populations are indigenous ethnic minority groups characterized by strong family, community and peer bonds, thereby creating a unique and underrepresented context to study positive youth development.

This chapter has three major sections. In the first section, we begin with a brief historical overview and the description of the Roma context. In the second section, we review current research and empirical findings on Roma children and youth within peer and family settings. Although the focus of this chapter is on peers and

friendships, the scarcely available literature on this topic with Roma youth limits our treatment in this area. We therefore present an overview of the most frequently investigated topics of family, community and multiple identity socialization factors that have been indicated as resources for optimal outcomes with relevant consequences on peer relations and friendships among Roma youth. Looking at the contexts of family, community, and neighborhood, and interactions among these settings provides a better understanding of how such settings may be important to peer relationships of Roma children. Roma children and youth spend a majority of their time at home or in the community/neighborhood, making these settings their primary environments (Okely 2008). To best understand and provide a context for Roma peer and friendships, it is important to consider their natural environments in a holistic fashion and to observe how such environments affect Roma as they build relationships with their friends and peers within their community. We draw on core theoretical models of PYD as well as selected developmental theories of normative development to highlight the applicability of these traditional frameworks to Roma ethnic minority groups. In so doing, we briefly discuss measurement and methodology issues, while also paying careful attention to the cultural, ethnic, and economic characteristics of Roma youth and their families. We provide the first review of studies on Roma youth in Europe to discover both universalities and specifics of Roma youth development. In the third section, we derive theoretical implications from the reviewed empirical findings as a step towards informing efforts to promote successful peer and social relations and PYD among Roma youth.

Historical Overview and Theoretical Perspectives

To better understand the specific resources and challenges of many Roma youth, it is important to consider the varying social, political and historical features of Central-Eastern Europe. An important feature of this region is the historical presence of native Roma ethnic minority settlement accompanied with much longer integration (or assimilation) during communist rule, leaving little to no room for acceptance of diversity (Prieto-Flores 2009). Ethnic minority groups such as Roma were not officially recognized and much of their culture was not valued, therefore contributing to extreme marginalization of their communities (Filipescu 2009). The democratic transition following the collapse of the communist state in 1989 has seen reawakened nationalism in many countries, which witnessed the rise of a number of extreme right political parties (Mudde 2000). As a consequence, negative attitudes towards Roma have been heightened by making them a target group to blame for a diversity of socio-economic problems in Europe (Brosig 2010; European Union Agency for Fundamental Rights 2010). Nevertheless, Roma are officially recognized ethnic minority in their respective countries and tolerance, respect and rights of Roma are usually safeguarded (Triandafyllidou 2011).

Accurate data about Roma demographics are difficult to obtain (European Union Agency for Fundamental Rights 2010) primarily because of the absence of census information on ethnic origin in the majority of the European Union (EU) and ethnic mimicry, that is one's refusal to disclose one's ethnicity to avoid stigmatization (Prieto-Flores 2009). Roma are undoubtedly the most significant segment of the ethnic minority population of Europe in terms of the size of their community (9–12 million people) and marginalized social status. The Roma estimates in Europe are presented in Table 1. The highest share of Roma is estimated to live in Bulgaria, the Former Yugoslav Republic of Macedonia, Slovakia, Romania, Serbia and Hungary. The largest Roma settlement is in Romania, and is home to the largest Roma population in the world (Crowe 2008).

Table 1 Roma ethnic minority groups in Europe

Country	Total population	Official census[a]	Average estimate	% of total population (%)
EU Member States				
1. Austria	8.384745	6.273	35.000	0.42
2. Belgium	10.879159	NA	30.000	0.28
3. Bulgaria	7.543325	325.343	750.000	9.94
4. Cyprus	1.103647	502	1.250	0.11
5. Czech Republic	10.525090	11.718	200.000	1.90
6. Denmark	5.544139	NA	2.500	0.05
7. Estonia	1.339646	584	1.050	0.08
8. Finland	5.363624	NA	11.000	0.21
9. France	64.876618	NA	400.000	0.62
10. Germany	81.702329	NA	105.000	0.13
11. Greece	11.319048	NA	175.000	1.55
12. Hungary	10.008703	190.046	750.000	7.49
13. Ireland	4.481430	22.435	37.500	0.84
14. Italy	60.483521	NA	150.000	0.25
15. Latvia	2.242916	8.517	12.500	0.56
16. Lithuania	3.320656	2.571	3.000	0.09
17. Luxembourg	505.831	NA	300	0.06
18. Malta	412.961	NA	0	0.00

(continued)

Table 1 (continued)

Country	Total population	Official census[a]	Average estimate	% of total population (%)
19. Netherlands	16.612213	NA	40.000	0.24
20. Poland	38.187488	12.731	32.500	0.09
21. Portugal	10.642841	NA	52.000	0.49
22. Romania	21.442012	619.007	1.850000	8.63
23. Slovak Republic	5.433456	89.920	490.000	9.02
24. Slovenia	2.052821	3.246	8.500	0.41
25. Spain	46.081574	NA	750.000	1.63
26. Sweden	9.379116	NA	50.000	0.53
27. United Kingdom	62.218761	NA	225.000	0.36
Non-EU Member States				
28. Albania	3.204284	1.261	115.000	3.59
29. Andorra	84.864	NA	0	0.00
30. Armenia	3.92,072	50	2.000	0.06
31. Azerbaijan	9.047932	NA	2.000	0.02
32. Belarus	9.490500	9.927	47.500	0.50
33. Bosnia and Herzegovina	3.760149	8.864	58.000	1.54
34. Croatia	4.424161	9.463	35.000	0.79
35. Georgia	4.452800	1.200	2.000	0.04
36. Iceland	317.398	NA	0	0.00
37. Kosovo	1.815000	45.745	37.500	2.07
38. Liechtenstein	36.032	NA	0	0.00
39. Macedonia	2.060563	53.879	197.000	9.56
40. Moldova	3.562062	12.271	107.100	3.01
41. Monaco	35.407	NA	0	0.00
42. Montenegro	631.490	8.305	20.000	3.17
43. Norway	4.885240	NA	10.100	0.21
44. Russian Federation	141.750000	205.007	825.000	0.58
45. San Marino	31.534	NA	0	0.00
46. Serbia	7.292574	108.193	600.000	8.23
47. Switzerland	7.825243	NA	30.000	0.38
48. Turkey	72.752325	4.656	2.750000	3.78
49. Ukraine	45.870700	47.917	260.000	0.57
Total in Europe	828.510000	1.809631	11.260300	1.36

Authors' own elaboration based on official reports by The Council of Europe (2010), Index Mundi (2012), The World Fact Book (2014) and The World Directory of Minorities and Indigenous People (2014)

NA not available data

[a]Official census data based on self-declared Roma individuals

The World Bank indicated that in Romania, Bulgaria, Slovakia and Macedonia, the Roma proportion of the total population is between 8 and 12 % with an age profile of almost half of Roma being under 18, therefore in these countries, Roma constitute approximately 20 % of the school population (Hawke et al. 2008). Roma children and youth fall behind in education with an average enrolment rate in primary school below 50 % (United Nations Development Project 2011). The lowest preschool coverage for Roma is in South-Eastern Europe, ranging from 0.2 % in Kosovo and 17 % in Romania (UNICEF 2011). Large gaps in Roma school enrolment are also present in Albania, Bosnia and Herzegovina and Montenegro, ranging from 45 to 50 %. Twenty percent of Roma children in Bulgaria and 33 % in Serbia never go to school (Save the Children 2005). In Slovakia, Roma children are 30 times more likely to drop out school than the rest of the school population, and in Bulgaria, most of the 45,000 students who drop out annually are Roma. Roma enrolment beyond primary school is dramatically lower than that of the majority population in several countries. In South-Eastern Europe, for example, only 18 % of Roma attend secondary school, compared with 75 % of the majority, and less than 1 % of Roma attend university. According to recent survey conducted by the United Nations Development Programme (2011), two out of three Roma children do not complete primary school compared with one child out of seven in majority school population in Europe (Ivanov 2006). Only 15 % of young Roma complete upper-secondary education and those who remain beyond primary level have low qualifications and prospects for gainful employment (UNICEF 2011).

Particularly interesting for the purpose of the present chapter are the specific cultural resources and strengths of Roma. Strong family and community cohesion represent essential features of Roma and main vehicle for preservation of their traditions and values, although cultures evolve and adapt to new developments such as technology as also evidenced among young Roma travelers (Daily Mail 2012; Kárpáti 2004). The family remains a central organizing factor of Roma life with socialization norms, including the association of manhood with the role of provider for the family and the virginity of women before marriage. For example, the virginity of single women prior to marriage is relevant in Roma communities to the extent that significant value is often attached to it, and sometimes is a motivation for parents to pull their daughters out of school when they reach puberty (World Bank 2014). Roma are also characterized by increasing birth rates, in particular among teenage girls (Durst 2002). From a young age, children and youth are involved in all family matters (e.g., taking care of younger siblings, helping in domestic work or working to support their family). Roma children are also confronted with death of the family members and allowed to participate in rituals, therefore having firsthand learning experience to support their family and the loss of its members (Okely 2008).

In general, much is known about problematic behavior and development among children and adolescents, including youth from Roma communities. Yet, we are just beginning to gain ground empirically on mapping out positive facets of development and the scarcity of rigorous, large-scale investigations of positive youth development in culturally diverse, minority youth (Spencer and Spencer 2014), is clearly illustrated when considering the evidence base on Roma youth and their families. Research with Roma children and adolescents offers opportunities to deepen our understanding of this under researched community and to provide a better foundation for efforts to ameliorate the life conditions and chances of this group. Future research efforts in this area also promise to yield broader "lessons learned" for developmental science, by providing specific empirical illustrations of how complementary, but different views of human development can be effectively brought to bear to illuminate positive adaptation processes (Masten 2014).

Current Research Questions

The available research on Roma has adopted various approaches with a common goal of improving conditions for Roma youth and families. The European Union promoted the Decade for Roma Inclusion running from 2005 to 2015 to address education, employment, health and housing for Roma. The available findings on Roma children and youth presented in this chapter outline important advancements in the areas of research, theory and practice with these populations, while also raising relevant questions for the future. In the following sections, we highlight key issues that emerged from our literature review in terms of methodological approaches, empirical findings and culture specific mechanisms for PYD among Roma. In so doing, we address the primary goal of this chapter, which is to provide an understanding of the context for Roma youths' relationships with peers and friends and how these relations may be shaped and influenced by major socialization factors within the family, community and neighborhoods. Our goal is to specifically focus on the major topics investigated in the available literature that inform PYD and provide insight into peer/friendship relations among Roma (i.e., family, community and multiple identities as promoting resources for optimal outcomes for Roma youth).

Research Measurement and Methodology

Several methodological challenges characterize research on Roma, which are important to bear in mind when designing and interpreting studies of Roma adolescents and specifically with regards to positive indicators of adjustment and well-being. These challenges are: (a) prevalent conceptual approaches to the study of Roma groups; (b) sample representativeness; (c) the need for more culturally situated theory and research; and (d) multi-method and multidisciplinary perspectives.

Regarding conceptual challenges, the prevalent conceptual approach in studies of Roma youth has been a deficit-oriented one, which emphasizes school-related difficulties, limited levels of education, mental health issues, and a variety of developmental delays. However, increasingly in the overall literature on ethnic minority youth, resource-oriented models have replaced or complemented deficit perspectives with a growing interest in ethnic minority children and youth who succeed as well as factors in their immediate social environment that promote well-being (e.g., García Coll and Marks 2009; Masten 2014). The most salient feature of such a paradigm shift is the focus on positive aspects of development, and resources and strengths, both at individual and context levels. This emerging scholarship is particularly valuable for Roma because it increases the odds of developing strength-based prevention programs and interventions for Roma youth and their families (Dimitrova et al. 2015c).

The second challenge in conducting research on Roma is the difficulty in accessing this group for research (Prieto-Flores 2009). Lack of representation can inflate the potential for selection bias and thereby reduce generalizability. This challenge is multi-faceted and complex. For instance, the meticulous gathering of data on Roma during communist rule poses a barrier to present-day efforts to solicit information from Roma even several generations later because it created mistrust among Roma. Roma's trust in state institutions may also be affected by European Communist regimes' production of official figures about Roma based on governmental sources (official statistics and reports managed by the state), rather than actual survey data from Roma participants (Triandafyllidou 2011). On the other hand, many Roma declare in censuses and surveys a different ethnicity, most often that of the mainstream culture in order to avoid stigmatization (Prieto-Flores 2009). Other issues concerning sample selection include the conditions of Roma youth in important social institutions such as schools. Recruiting Roma youth from schools is a useful research strategy. However, school administrators may be reluctant to endorse research focused on controversial issues such as Roma because of the severe discrimination and negative stereotypes about this group (Doubek and Levinska 2015). By necessity, most research on Roma youth involve young people who attend school and are willing to participate in studies. Yet, the high school dropout rate among Roma makes such studies unrepresentative of all Roma youth (Ringold 2000). Regardless of how the sample is obtained, like other hard to access and severely marginalized groups, Roma adolescents and families who consent to participate in research might differ from adolescents who are unwilling to participate (Font and Méndez 2013).

Another challenge is the need for more culturally situated research among Roma to address the gap in the literature on cultural processes and contexts and how they affect development. Culturally informed research has the power to call attention to the cultural assets and strengths of ethnic minority communities that can help them to rear the next generation in healthy and successful ways (García Coll et al. 1996). Specific cultural values and socialization practices (e.g., family/community cohesion, obligations, connectedness, bicultural identity) can promote positive outcomes among children and youth living in a context of adversity (Dimitrova 2014). More attention is needed on the unique ethnic resources of Roma to promote theory, research, and practice advances that will further the positive adaptation of Roma youth.

Finally, research among Roma is less likely to integrate multidisciplinary perspectives on development and adjustment than research in other ethnic minority groups (Stuart and Rövid 2010). The vast majority of research on Roma is rooted in anthropological, educational, sociological and economical perspectives, leaving little room for multidisciplinary integration or multi-method approaches. Additionally, most data on Roma are likely to come only from official census or self-report questionnaires, with the over reliance on self-reports increasing the potential for common method variance. Studies using different perspectives and methods should be conducted to assess whether similar findings emerge regardless of methodology (Tremlett and McGarry 2013). For example, qualitative and quantitative data, in addition to official reports and focus groups of Roma may broaden insight into their community (Dimitrova et al. 2015b). In this pursuit, mix methods studies employing large community samples of Roma should include both quantitative and ethnographic methods to provide a broader perspective on the complexity of associations among developmental assets for Roma youth.

Empirical Findings

In this section, we review the available relevant literature on Roma children and youth. We focus on key socialization factors investigated in the literature (i.e., family, community and multiple identities) because they have clear implications for peer and friendship relations among Roma. Studying peer relationships cannot be done in isolation of family and community settings, where Roma children spend most of their time and acquire basic social skills that aid them in navigating social networks. How youth form close relations with peers is also informed by multiple identifications they develop and by the way they manage to traverse the complex relations between them and the mainstream culture. In summarizing the relevant literature, our aim is to shed light on peer and friendship relationships among Roma and how these relations are influenced by major socialization factors within family and community as well as in light of the multiple identities that Roma youth may develop.

Family and Community Resources for Roma

Protective factors (e.g., sense of purpose, self-esteem, and family support from multiple levels of influence such as individual, familial, peers, schools, and community; Gaylord-Harden et al. 2012) for Roma youth are clearly identifiable in their family and community relationships. Family and community connectedness have been associated with positive mental, physical, psychological and educational outcomes (Abubakar et al. 2014). In fact, among adolescents from highly marginalized communities such as Roma, family connectedness is particularly salient to their well-being because it moderates the impact of exposure to adverse conditions (Abubakar and Dimitrova 2015). Additional research reports that Roma youth who perceive that their families value their adherence to Roma cultural traditions and customs are more likely to evidence optimal psychological outcomes than their peers who do not have high adherence to such traditions and customs (Dimitrova and Jordanov 2015).

Multiple Identity Resources for Roma

A core developmental task for ethnic minority youth is to develop multiple social identities in a variety of acculturation contexts. Roma youth with multiple or flexible ethnic identities are more likely to be successful in school and in the society at large than those who do not evidence such identity patterns (Dolgozat 2013). Prior research has shown that ethnic, familial, and religious identities are particularly salient for Roma (Dimitrova et al. 2013). Ethnic identity is defined as the process of maintaining positive attitudes and feelings of ethnic group belonging (Erikson 1968; Phinney 1989) and has consistently been found to positively relate to psychological well-being and adjustment in various groups (Rivas-Drake et al. 2014; Schwartz et al. 2009) and Roma, in particular (Dimitrova et al. 2013). Religious identity concerns the sense of group membership to a religion or set of religious convictions, and their importance for individual identity (Nesbitt and Arweck 2010). Particularly among members of ethnic minority (Roma) communities, religious identity can be crucial for enhanced psychological well-being. Familial identity represents the degree of identification with and sense of familial group membership. The family is a core identification domain for Roma youth that provides a sense of relatedness, and commitment. Similarly to ethnic and religious identity, a strong familial identity among Roma groups is often associated with

positive adjustment and health-protective behaviors (Dimitrova et al. 2014a).

A recent study compared multiple identities and well-being in Roma across Bulgaria, the Czech Republic, Kosovo, and Romania. Results suggested overall positive relations between ethnic, familial, and religious identity and well-being among Roma youth, with the strongest and most consistent association between familial identity and well-being (Dimitrova et al. 2017). These findings support the notion that familial identity is a core psychological resource in the context of Roma youth, given the central role of the family within their community. Relatedly, research has shown strong intergenerational continuities of identity among Roma mothers and their offspring and those strong ethnic, mainstream, familial, and religious identities of the Roma are particularly important for their well-being (Dimitrova et al. 2014a). Similar results were confirmed in another study investigating intergenerational transmission of ethnic identity and psychological well-being of Roma adolescents and their mothers and fathers. Results confirmed that ethnic identity was a positive predictor of well-being in both adolescents and parents and that parents' ethnic identity was a predictor of adolescent well-being. The authors concluded that for Roma youth and their parents, ethnic identity represents salient source for well-being and that there was evidence for the intergenerational continuity of identity and well-being (Dimitrova et al. 2015a).

Peers and Friendships Resources for Roma

Adolescence is a developmental period when peer relations are clearly important in that peer groups and close friends are socialization agents and are key contributors to adolescents' overall social interactions (Kroger 2007; Rubin et al. 2011). Peers and friends serve as a significant reference group throughout adolescence and the norms of the peer group play a role in the expression of prejudice and behaviors of adolescents as they adjust to their peer group (Brown 2001). Inevitably, peer relations of Roma youth are affected by intergroup attitudes of majority group adolescents towards the Roma. The literature on this topic suggests that attitudes towards Roma are a relevant factor structuring peer relationships with their majority counterparts. Youth having a coherent attitude concerning the Roma (either clearly prejudiced or clearly tolerant) are more likely to have friends who are similar to them than those whose attitudes are ambivalent. This finding supports the notion that non-Roma adolescents' attitudes towards the Roma are influenced by those of their friends (Váradi 2014).

Several studies have focused on peer relationships of Roma youth across a variety of European contexts. A general characteristic of these studies is that they address peer and family relations in a broader social context of Roma using mostly cross-sectional designs and self-reported measurement methods. Findings from these studies suggest that secure social networks with non-Roma peers, as well as friends from Roma and other minority ethnic backgrounds, were positively linked with retention in secondary school among Roma students (Derrington and Kendall 2004). Findings also suggested that Roma girls in particular, reported feeling more socially secure in the company of other Roma peers at school (Derrington and Kendall 2004) and that some Roma children distanced themselves socially from their majority peers as a coping strategy to avoid social discomfort (Derrington 2007). Related research has shown that peer relationships that provide Roma students with the companionship, help, comfort, and make school more enjoyable, promote their academic success, increase resilience among Roma and their chances of remaining at school (Dimakos and Papakonstantinopoulou 2012). For Roma youth, school can be a significant aspect of their personal experiences and interpersonal relationships with teachers and peers that strongly contributes to their sense of school belonging (Macura-Milovanovic and Pecek 2013). Also, friendship with non-Roma peers can act as a protective factor for Roma in regards to

bullying at school. Roma students who have interethnic friendships are also those who are more integrated into the peer group (Elamé 2013). Strong peer networks can protect Roma youth from risky behaviors. For example, Roma adolescents have been shown to use less alcohol than non-Roma adolescents due to monitoring influences of their parents. A recent study was conducted on 330 Roma and 722 non-Roma youth in Slovakia, analyzing adolescent drunkenness (being drunk at least once in the past four weeks), parental monitoring (parents knowing with whom their children are when they go out) and peer influence (best friend drinking alcohol at least once a week). Results showed that although Roma adolescents reported more parental monitoring and less peer influence when compared with their non-Roma counterparts, stronger parental monitoring and weaker peer influence predicted lower prevalence of drunkenness among Roma adolescents (Babakova et al. 2012).

Universal Versus Culture-Specific Mechanisms

Is PYD conceptualized in the same way or differently for Roma families? A more revealing question is what exactly resonates across diverse youth and what maybe unique in the conceptualization of PYD among Roma youth and their families? This issue also raises the question of how universal theories of development apply to Roma groups and how we interpret group differences in norms of health, success, and competence. In recent years, several studies have been conducted to investigate the specific child and youth socialization practices among Roma based on anthropological and sociological fieldwork.

In Roma communities, children are encouraged to be independent at very early age by participating in economic activities and observing adult verbal and non-verbal communication skills (Kyuchukov 2011; Messing 2008). In fact, Roma socialization practices occur in the extended family network, which provides children with emotional and physical support. Traditional Romani education is community education, where children participate in the communities' every day activities and learn by watching, listening and observing, social, linguistic, and moral codes of their society (Smith 1997). Education within Roma communities differs considerably from educational approaches common in the mainstream population. The highly structured mainstream schools (competitive environments, regulated timetables, learning activities and certain expectations of children and their parents) may not fit favorably with traditional Roma socialization processes. Many Roma parents do not see mainstream education as essential, or necessary for their children, because they may view the educational system as representing a means of controlling their community and children (Lee and Warren 1991). The consequent incompatibility between mainstream and traditional Roma education reflects these opposing structures, values and beliefs. In fact, knowledge in traditional Roma society is passed on orally and is associated with the wisdom of the elderly, who preserve traditional customs and cultural beliefs. Therefore, many Roma parents consider school to be a disruptive influence for their children's lives, because it takes their children away from parental guidance and the cultural, social and economic activities of their traditional education (Lee and Warren 1991). The question is then, are these values and goals still present and salient today in contemporary society, relative to the past or has there been more integration since the 1990s? Recent research has shown that some Roma parents may not value integration or being "bicultural" and this holds true for both mothers and their adolescent offspring (Dimitrova et al. 2014a).

The family and the extended kinship network are the primary influences in a Roma child's life. The socialization and education of Roma children takes place in their community. Roma children are taught to develop self-confidence and acquire culturally appropriate values of their community. They are encouraged to be independent and make a valuable contribution to the community's economic activities. Independent behavior of Roma children is promoted by encouraging children to seek and prepare their own food, dress themselves, go to bed without supervision, and taking care of younger siblings (Berthier 1979). Therefore, Roma children are encouraged to contribute to the real-life economic activities of the community.

A Roma childhood is characterized by being free from many social responsibilities until the onset of puberty, a time when young Roma adults adopt traditional gender-assigned roles. Usually, boys acquire more rights and fewer obligations than girls and often parents will search for a suitable wife for their son as a symbol of his approaching manhood (Berthier 1979; Kyuchukov 2011; Messing 2008). Roma girls in comparison are expected to adopt a series of socially responsible behaviors once they reach puberty (Wood 1973; Sutherland 1975). These traditional gender roles continue today. Traditional Roma families generally pull their daughters from school when they reach 10–12 years of age (World Bank 2014). By the age of 12–13, Roma girls are being prepared for marriage and for their wedding night. Young married women are responsible to their mother-in-law, whom they are obliged to help with cooking, cleaning and child care. In the Roma community, a girl's virginity is of great importance and the lack thereof may expose a girl and her family to social rejection and gossip within the community (Kyuchukov 2011). As a consequence, Roma girls at a very early age face the decision of whether to stay in their communities and accept such restraints or break with tradition, leave their villages, and pursue their lives outside of the Roma community.

Policy Implications

The last decades have seen repeated efforts by the European Union and international organizations to promote evidence-based policy for Roma. Following the end of communist rule in the 1990s, many governments in Eastern Europe officially recognized Roma as a legitimate minority with rights for the preservation and development of their culture. Such recognition was a clear improvement in contrast to previously enacted assimilative policies in these countries. In the early 2000s, the EU elaborated national-level policy documents for the Decade of Roma Inclusion and the subsequent years saw a growth in policy activity in relation to Roma also at regional and local levels. The European Union has increased its engagement on policy toward Roma publishing the *EU Framework for National Roma Integration Strategies* in 2011 as a call to Member States to pursue integration of Roma. On additional positive note, the quality of census data on Roma has begun to improve, presumably due to the increased participation of Roma in the census reports in many European countries.

Nevertheless, attention to successful adaptation and positive outcomes for Roma youth at the level of policy design and implementation are still in need of improvement. Naturally, families and schools are primary social settings for the implementation of research-based policy and practice. School policy should take into consideration bicultural processes as well as the Roma and their values, and to develop socially and culturally responsive educational processes and to make schooling appropriate to meet the needs of Roma pupils. It is crucial that school policies give voice to Roma children who are vulnerable to academic underachievement and to promote the effectiveness of schooling for these children (Marc and Bercus 2007). Related to schooling, issues of discrimination significantly affect Roma minority youth and how they form significant peer and friendship relations. These relations and their implications for well-being of Roma need substantial scholarly and public policy attention to facilitate deeper analysis to the conceptualization and implementation of meaningful social relations and tolerance among marginalized minority youth. These efforts need to be addressed through school programs as well as through stakeholder involvement in the wider local Roma communities. Community participation can be at the core of successful partnerships between schools and Roma communities, where Roma families can play a critical role

(Greenfields and Home 2006; Messing 2008). Ultimately, such local programs should go hand in hand with government policies to ensure adequate institutional and financial means allowing for the implementation of such policies to facilitate good peer (interethnic) relations and ultimately PYD of Roma.

Future Directions

The unique cultural and demographic characteristics of Roma and empirical studies included in this chapter raise a number of issues regarding the conceptualization and theoretical implications for the study of PYD and peer relations of Roma in European countries. The findings provide some support for the conceptual model of PYD and the relevance of cultural assets as sources of psychological well-being and meaningful peer networks of Roma youth across Europe. Even under conditions of adversity, some Roma youth show positive adjustment outcomes (e.g., Dimitrova 2014). Importantly, as for many youth, family, peers, a well-developed identity can provide a source of strength and can be associated with well-being and adjustment for Roma (Dimitrova et al. 2013). Therefore, we should recognize that oppressed minority groups such as Roma have potentially several built-in strengths and researchers need to build on these strengths and not assume that these communities are only characterized by adversity and deficits.

Based on the above considerations, new models need to go beyond prior conceptualizations of Roma minority groups to further theoretical elaborations. These new models should pay close attention to potential factors that resonate across cultures such as the importance of relationships in the family and peers as well as core developmental process such as identity development that can foster positive outcomes and close social relationships. Such conceptualizations should also consider the role of current and past policy towards Roma groups, their sedentary long-term settlement, and history of assimilation and segregation as well as how these factors may influence child and adolescent development, their relations with peers and formation of friendships. These efforts should facilitate exchange and intercultural dialogue among different European youngsters and Roma communities. As the field of positive youth development focuses on resources, including scholarly and public attention to the whole child (e.g., Benson et al. 2012; Bowers et al. 2014; Catalano et al. 2002; Lerner et al. 2005; Moore and Lippman 2005; Silbereisen and Lerner 2007), the fundamental challenge remains to translate intentions into action and to carry out empirical studies that measure aspects of the whole child in context, as well as to better understand what positive youth development is in a diversity of youth living in a wide variety of conditions across the globe (Spencer and Spencer 2014). The overview of research on Roma children and youth in Europe presents a picture reflecting universal and common experiences of their group in how they face and deal with demands and challenges in their local context. The current policy in many European countries sees increasing strategies aimed at the improvement of well-being and conditions for Roma minority groups. This is particularly valuable and relevant because Roma have lived in these countries for centuries and represent sizable and the fastest growing ethnic minority population with an increasingly relevant role in the future of Europe.

Acknowledgments The authors would like to acknowledge the support by a COFAS Forte Marie Curie Grant (Forte-Projekt 2013-2669) to the first author. We also thank members of the European Network for Romani Studies and in particular Margaret Greenfields, Judith Okely, Carol Rogers, Loizos Symeou, Rosamaria Cisneros, Sara Horlai, and Elisabeth Tauber for their help in providing literature on Roma included in the chapter.

References

Abubakar, A., van de Vijver, F. J., Mazrui, L., Murugami, M., & Arasa, J. (2014). Connectedness and psychological well-being among adolescents of immigrant background in Kenya. In R. Dimitrova, M. Bender, & F. van de Vijver (Eds.), *Global perspectives on well-being in immigrant families* (pp. 95–111). New York: Springer.

Abubakar, A., & Dimitrova, R. (2015). Social connectedness, life satisfaction and school engagement: Moderating role of ethnic minority status on resilience processes of Roma youth. *European Journal of Developmental Psychology*, Special Issue on Resilience, *13*, 361–376. doi:10.1080/17405629.2016.1161507

Babakova, D., Kolarcik, P., Geckova, M. A., Klein, D., Reijneveld, S. A., & van Dijk, J. P. (2012). Does the influence of peers and parents on adolescents' drunkenness differ between Roma and non-Roma adolescents in Slovakia? *Ethnicity and Health, 17*, 531–541. doi:10.1080/13557858.2012.678305

Barany, Z. (2002). *The East European gypsies. Regime change, marginality and ethnopolitics*. Cambridge: Cambridge University Press.

Benson, P. L., et al. (2012). Beyond the "village" rhetoric: Creating healthy communities for children and adolescents. *Applied Developmental Science, 16*, 3–23.

Berthier, J.-C. (1979). The socialisation of the Gypsy child. *International Social Science Journal, 4*, 3–12.

Bowers, E. P., Geldhof, G. J., Johnson, S. K., Lerner, J. V., & Lerner, R. M. (2014). Special issue introduction: Thriving across the adolescent years: A view of the issues. *Journal of Youth and Adolescence, 43*, 859–868. doi:10.1007/s10964-014-0117-8

Brosig, M. (2010). The challenge of implementing minority rights in Central Eastern Europe. *Journal of European Integration, 32*, 393–411. doi:10.1080/07036331003797539

Brown, R. (2001). Intergroup relations. In M. Hewstone & W. Stroebe (Eds.), *Introduction to social psychology. A European perspective* (pp. 479–517). Oxford: Blackwell.

Catalano, R. F., et al. (2002). Prevention science and positive youth development: Competitive or cooperative frameworks? *Journal of Adolescent Health, 31*, 230–239.

Council of Europe. (2010). *Statistics*. Retrieved from http://www.coe.int/t/dg3/romatravellers/default_en.asp

Crowe, D. M. (2008). The Roma in post-communist Eastern Europe: Questions of ethnic conflict and ethnic peace. *Nationalities Papers: The Journal of Nationalism and Ethnicity, 36*, 521–552. doi:10.1080/00905990802080752

Daily Mail. (2012). *21st century Gypsies: Stunning pictures show how new-age travellers are now adopting traditional horse-drawn caravans*. Retrieved from http://www.dailymail.co.uk/news/article-2210747/21st-century-Gypsies-New-Age-Travellers-adopt-horse-drawn-caravans-love-Facebook-long-solar-powered.html#ixzz3iVFwjRH2

Derrington, C. (2007). Fight, flight and playing white: An examination of coping strategies adopted by Gypsy Traveller adolescents in English secondary schools. *International Journal of Educational Research, 46*, 357–367. doi:10.1016/j.ijer.2007.06.001

Derrington, C., & Kendall, S. (2004). *Gypsy traveller students in secondary schools: Culture, identity and achievement*. London: Stoke-on-Trent: Trentham Books Ltd.

Dimakos, I., & Papakonstantinopoulou, A. (2012). Providing psychological and counselling services to Roma students: A preliminary report for a three-year longitudinal project. In P. Cunningham & N. Fretwell (Eds.), *Creating Communities: Local, National and Global* (pp. 94–103). London: CiCe.

Dimitrova, R. (2014). *Does your identity make you happy? Collective identifications and acculturation of youth in a post-communist Europe*. Tilburg: Tilburg University. ISBN 978-90-5335-784-2.

Dimitrova, R., Chasiotis, A., Bender, M., & van de Vijver, F. J. R. (2013). Collective identity and well-being of Roma adolescents in Bulgaria. *International Journal of Psychology, 48*, 1–12. doi:10.1080/00207594.2012.682064

Dimitrova, R., Chasiotis, A., Bender, M., & van de Vijver, F. J. R. (2014a). Collective identity and well-being of Bulgarian Roma minority adolescents and their mothers. *Journal for Youth and Adolescence, 43*, 375–386. doi:10.1007/s10964-013-0043-1

Dimitrova, R., van de Vijver, F. J. R., Taušová, J., Chasiotis, A., Bender, M., Buzea, C., Uka, F., & Tair, E. (2017). Ethnic, familial and religious identity and their relations to well-being of Roma in Bulgaria, Czech Republic, Kosovo, and Romania. *Child Development,* Special Issue on Race and Ethnicity, accepted for publication & forthcoming in 2017

Dimitrova, R., & Jordanov, V. (2015). Do family ethnic pressure and national identity enhance psychological well-being among Roma youth in Bulgaria? *Special Issue on Roma youth, The Journal of the International Network for Prevention in Child Maltreatment, 40–41*, 23–35.

Dimitrova, R., Ferrer-Wreder, L., & Trost, K. (2015a). *Intergenerational transmission of ethnic identity and well-being of Roma minority adolescents and their parents* (manuscript under review).

Dimitrova, R., Johnson, D., Adams, B., Thelamour, B., & Sankar, S. (2015b). The influence of ethnic discrimination and identity on emotional and academic Outcomes: A mixed-method study of Roma ethnic minority adolescents (manuscript in preparation).

Dimitrova, R., Sam, D., & Ferrer-Wreder, L. (2015c). (Eds.), *Roma minority youth across cultural contexts: Taking a positive approach to research, policy and practice*. Oxford University Press.

Dolgozat, T. D. (2013). *Minority towards majority—What makes Roma students change their self-reported ethnic identity?*. Hungary: Corvinus University.

Doubek, D., & Levinska, M. (2015). Us and them: What categories reveal about Roma and non-Roma in the Czech Republic. In P. Smeyers, D. Bridges, N. C. Burbules, & M. Griffiths (Eds.), *International handbook of interpretation in educational research*

(pp. 599–622). Dordrecht, Netherlands: Springer Science + Business Media.

Durst, J. (2002). Fertility and childbearing practices among poor gypsy women in Hungary: The intersections of class, race and gender. *Communist and Post-Communist Studies, 35*, 457–474.

Elamé, E. (2013). *Discriminatory bullying. A new intercultural challenge*. Italia: Springer-Verlag.

Erikson, E. (1968). *Identity: Youth and crisis*. New York, NY: Norton.

European Commission (2013). *Roma Integration Concept for 2010-1013*. Retrieved from http://ec.europa.eu/justice/discrimination/files/roma_czech_republic_strategy_en.pdf

European Union Agency for Fundamental Rights (2010). *Addressing the Roma issue in the EU*. Retrieved from http://fra.europa.eu/fraWebsite/roma/roma_en.htm

Filipescu, C. (2009). Revisiting minority integration in Eastern Europe: Examining the case of Roma integration in Romania. *Debate: Journal of Contemporary Central and Eastern Europe, 17*, 297–314. doi:10.1080/09651560903457915

Font, J., & Méndez, M. (2013). *Surveying ethnic minorities and immigrant populations. Methodological challenges and research strategies*. Amsterdam: Amsterdam University Press.

García Coll, C., Crnic, K., Lamberty, G., Wasik, B. H., Jenkins, R., García, H. V., et al. (1996). An integrative model for the study of developmental competencies in minority children. *Child Development, 67*, 1891–1914. doi:10.1111/j.1467-8624.1996.tb01834.x

García Coll, C., & Marks, A. (2009). *The immigrant paradox in children and adolescents: Is becoming American a developmental risk?*. Washington, DC: American Psychological Association.

Gaylord-Harden, N. K., Burrow, A., & Cunningham, J. A. (2012). A cultural-asset framework for investigating successful adaptation to stress in African American youth. *Child Development Perspectives, 6*, 264–271.

Greenfields, M., & Home, R. (2006). Assessing Gypsies and traveler's needs: Partnership working and 'The Cambridge Project'. *Romani Studies, 16*, 105–131.

Hawke, L., Seghedi, A., & Gheorghiu, M. (2008). *Learning from America's mistakes: A proposal for closing the education gap between children and Roma descent and the national averages in the European Union*. Bucharest: Asociata Ovidiu Rom.

Index Mundi (2012). *Country facts*. Retrieved from http://www.indexmundi.com

Ivanov, A. (2006). *At risk: Roma and the displaced in South-East Europe*. UNDP Regional Bureau for Europe.

Kroger, J. (2007). *Identity development: Adolescence through adulthood*. Thousand Oaks, CA: Sage.

Kyuchukov, H. (2011). Roma girls: between traditional values and educational aspirations. *Intercultural*

Education, 22, 97–104. doi:10.1080/14675986.2011.549648

Kárpáti, A. (2004). *Travellers in cyberpace: ICT in Hungarian (Romani) schools*. Retrieved from http://edutech.elte.hu/karpati/en_sajat_irasok/s-5cfaf6458b.pdf#page=140

Lee, K. W., & Warren, W. G. (1991). Alternative education lessons from Gypsy thought and practice. *British Journal of Education Studies, 9*, 311–324.

Lerner, R. M., et al. (2005). Positive youth development, participation in community youth development programs, and community contributions of fifth grade adolescents. *Journal of Early Adolescence, 25*, 17–71.

Macura-Milovanović, S., & Peček, M. (2013). Attitudes of Serbian and Slovenian student teachers towards causes of learning underachievement amongst Roma pupils. *International Journal of Inclusive Education, 17*, 629–645. doi:10.1080/13603116.2012.703247

Marc, A., & Bercus, C. (2007). The Roma Education Fund: A new tool for Roma inclusion. *European Education, 39*, 64–80.

Masten, A. S. (2014). Invited commentary: Resilience and positive youth development frameworks in developmental science. *Journal of Youth and Adolescence, 43*, 1018–1024. doi:10.1007/s10964-014-0118-7.

Messing, V. (2008). Good practices addressing school integration of Roma/Gypsy children in Hungary. *Intercultural Education, 19*, 461–473. doi:10.1080/14675980802531721

Moore, K. A., & Lippman, L. H. (2005). Introduction and framework. In K. A. Moore & L. H. Lippman (Eds.), *What do children need to flourish?* (pp. 1–9). New York: Springer.

Mudde, C. (2000). Extreme-right parties in Eastern Europe. *Patterns of Prejudice, 34*, 5–27. doi:10.1080/00313220008559132

Nesbitt, E., & Arweck, E. (2010). Issues arising from an ethnographic investigation of the religious identity formation of young people in mixed-faith families. *Fieldwork in Religion, 5*, 7–30.

Okely, J. (2008). Knowing without notes. In N. Halstead, E. Hirsch, & J. Okely (Eds.), *Knowing how to know* (pp. 67–70). London: Berghahn.

Phinney, J. S. (1989). Stages of ethnic identity development in minority group adolescents. *Journal of Early Adolescence, 9*, 34–49. doi:10.1177/0272431689091004

Prieto-Flores, Ò. (2009). Does the canonical theory of assimilation explain the Roma case? Some evidence from Central and Eastern Europe. *Ethnic and Racial Studies, 32*, 1387–1405. doi:10.1080/01419870903006988

Ringold, D. (2000). *Roma and the Transition in Central and Eastern Europe*. Washington: World Bank.

Rivas-Drake, D., Syed, M., Umaña-Taylor, A. J., Markstrom, C., French, S., Schwartz, S. J., et al. (2014). Feeling good, happy, and proud: A meta-analysis of positive ethnic-racial affect and adjustment. *Child Development, 85*, 77–102. doi:10.1111/cdev.12175

Rubin, K. H., Bukowski, W. M., & Laursen, B. (Eds.). (2011). *Handbook of peer interactions, relationships, and groups*. NY: Guilford Press.

Save the Children. (2005). *Country Brief 2004/2005*. Retrieved from http://www.savethechildren.org/atf/cf/%7B9def2ebe-10ae-432c-9bd0-df91d2eba74a%7D/ar2005.pdf

Schwartz, S. J., Zamboanga, B. L., Weisskirch, R. S., & Rodriguez, L. (2009). The relationships of personal and ethnic identity exploration to indices of adaptive and maladaptive psychosocial functioning. *International Journal of Behavioral Development, 33*, 131–144. doi:10.1177/0165025408098018

Silbereisen, R. K. & R. M. Lerner (2007). (Eds). *Approaches to positive youth development*. London: Sage.

Smith, T. (1997). Recognising difference: The Romani 'Gypsy' child socialisation and education. *British Journal of Sociology of Education, 18*, 243–256.

Spencer, M. B., & Spencer, T. R. (2014). Invited commentary: Exploring the promises, intricacies and challenges to positive youth development. *Journal of Youth and Adolescence, 43*, 1027–1035.

Stuart, M., & Rövid, M. (2010). *Multi-disciplinary approaches to Romani studies*. Hungary: Central European University Press.

Sutherland, A. (1975). *Gypsies-the hidden Americans*. London: Tavistock.

The World Fact Book. (2014). Retrieved from https://www.cia.gov/library/publications/the-world-factbook/geos/bu.html

Tremlett, A., & McGarry, A. (2013). Challenges facing researchers on Roma minorities in contemporary Europe: Notes towards a research program. European Centre for Minority Issues http://www.ecmi.de/uploads/tx_lfpubdb/Working_Paper_62_Final.pdf

Triandafyllidou, A. (2011). *Addressing cultural, ethnic & religious diversity challenges in Europe. A comparative overview of 15 European countries*. Italy: European University Institute.

UNICEF. (2011). *The Right of Roma children to education: Position paper*. Geneva.

United Nations Development Project. (2011). *Roma data*. Retrieved from http://www.eurasia.undp.org/content/rbec/en/home/ourwork/povertyreduction/roma-in-central-and-southeast-europe/roma-data.html

Váradi, L. (2014). *Youths trapped in prejudice. Hungarian adolescents' attitudes towards the Roma*. Fachmedien Wiesbaden: Springer.

Wood, M. F. (1973). *In the life of a Romany Gypsy*. London: Routledge & Kegan Paul Books.

World Bank. (2014). *Gender dimensions of Roma inclusion: Perspectives from four Roma communities in Bulgaria*. Retrieved from http://www.worldbank.org/content/dam/Worldbank/document/eca/Bulgaria/Roma_Gender-ENG.pdf

World Directory of Minorities and Indigenous People. (2014). *Overview of Europe*. Retrieved from http://www.minorityrights.org/?lid=317

Part V

Early Childhood and School Level Influences

The Positive Development of Minority Children At Home and In School

Allan Wigfield

The authors of the chapters in this section focus on issues of great importance to the positive development of different groups of ethnic minority children: the nature of their self-esteem and influences on it, how ethnic minority parents can be positively involved in their children's education, and the experiences of Canadian immigrant, Aboriginal, and ethnic minority children in Canadian schools. These chapters fit well within the positive psychology framework (e.g., Seligman et al. 2005) in that they focus on "understanding how, why, and under what conditions emotions, positive character, and the institutions that enable them flourish" (p. 410). Likewise, the authors' works are in line with a relational-developmental-systems approach on development (e.g., Lerner et al. 2015) that looks at the positive development of minority children in terms of mutually influential person—context relations; specifically, the family and school contexts.

Thijs and Verkuyten make the crucial point that to understand ethnic minority children's positive development it is critical to understand how their self-esteem develops and the influences on it, because of self-esteem's importance to our overall well-being. In their chapter they focus on ethnic minority children in different European countries, primarily immigrant children. They review research showing that for these (and other) minority children racial/ethnic identity has a strong association with their self-esteem. They also describe three central sources of information for the development of self-esteem in these children: their own self-perceptions, social comparison with other children, and their relational appraisals, or understandings of how others' view their group. These relational assessments may be especially important for European ethnic minority children at the present time, given the migrant crisis affecting many European countries as well as the recent terrorist attacks in Paris and other cities.

Thijs and Verkuyten review research showing that despite histories of experiencing discrimination and prejudice, European ethnic minority children's self-esteem overall is at similar and sometimes higher than that of other non-minority European children. However, they also discuss the importance of examining both explicit (self-reported) self-esteem and implicit self-esteem, reviewing findings showing that stereotyping and discrimination appear to impact these children's implicit but not explicit self-esteem. They also discuss research on how the following variables impact ethnic minority children's self-esteem: schools' ethnic composition, the groups to whom one compares oneself (majority children or one's own group), and the degree of perceived support and discrimination in the school setting. In the final section of their chapter they review work on the direct and indirect effects of multicultural education and teacher–student relationships on minority children's self-esteem. For instance, a positive direct effect of multicultural education is the celebration of different groups' culture. However, a potentially negative indirect effect of multicultural education is the accentuation of differences among groups, which may lead to greater exclusion. Although there is not much research on the direct effects on self-esteem of teachers' relations with ethnic minority children, Thijs and Verkuyten argue that such relations can have a positive impact. Positive relations with teachers also have indirect effects on different positive developmental outcomes by providing ethnic minority children with a sense of trust and support of important adults in their lives.

Ceballo, Jocson, and Alers-Rojas discuss work on the positive development of Latino children in the U.S., focusing in particular on how their parents can be involved in school in ways that support their children's engagement and achievement in school. They review different models of Latino children's development, from "deficit" models to Ogakagi's (2001) triarchic model that emphasizes children and parents' perceptions of education, family cultural norms and beliefs, and children's characteristics as critical factors explaining why some minority children succeed in school and others do not. They also provide an interesting and informative update of Ogbu's (1992) cultural view of why some minority groups do well in American schools and others do not. Latino children primarily fit Ogbu's "voluntary" minority category, yet unlike children from many other voluntary groups many Latino children struggle in school. They discuss how these children's socioeconomic status, attendance at under-resourced schools, maternal education, and discrimination all contribute to the relatively poor achievement outcomes of many Latino children.

In discussing Latino parents' involvement in school Ceballo and her colleagues discuss different barriers these parents face in trying to become involved. They also discuss the importance of *academic socialization* for Latino

children, or the ways in which their parents talk about school and its importance to their children. This socialization goes beyond simply having high expectations for how education will benefit their children. They then take a developmental perspective on parent involvement by discussing how parent involvement changes across elementary, middle, and high school, and the developmental needs of Latino children at each of these levels of schooling. They note important differences in the academic performance of subgroups of Latino children; for instance, Latino girls generally do better than Latino boys. They also note the "immigrant paradox" phenomenon that describes why second generation Latino students often do less well in U.S. schools than children who immigrate to the U.S. on certain outcomes. They close their chapter with a discussion of policy implications and suggestions for how to involve more effectively Latino parents in their children's education.

Perry, Yee, Mazabel-Ortega, Lisaingo and Määttä describe Canadian immigrant, Aboriginal, and language minority children's performance in Canadian schools, focusing on these children in British Columbia. They discuss how many children in these groups continue to do relatively poorly in school, despite the Canadian provincial governments' strong efforts to provide more inclusive education for these children. They note that most teachers in Canada are white, female, middle class and monolingual, and also that teacher training programs still do not deal effectively with the growing minority populations in many schools.

They then turn to a discussion of the particular challenges the different groups face in school. For instance, many Aboriginal children do less well in school than many other children, and are much less likely to graduate from high school. They are more likely to be poor, and often have to travel longer distances to attend schools than do other children. To deal with these and other issues Canadian schools are developing curricula that match better with these students' educational needs.

Perry and her colleagues discuss strategies and practices included in models of self-regulated and co-regulated learning such as those developed by Winne and Hadwin (1998), Zimmerman and Campillo (2003) and McCaslin (2009) that can be used to help minority children do better in school. They describe how these strategies are tools that all learners can utilize, and also that they can be tailored to the educational experiences of different groups. They finish the chapter with a description of how one elementary school teacher embedded these practices in her classroom.

In sum, the authors of the chapters in this section provide important foundational knowledge on factors impacting a wide variety of minority children's self-esteem and their academic achievement. The authors emphasize the challenges many of these children face, but also the conditions under which they can thrive. The authors' suggestions for future research and emphases on different ways of studying the impact of these factors on the positive development of minority children provides many rich ideas for researchers interested in these topics.

References

Lerner, R. M., Lerner, J. V., Bowers, E. P., & Geldhof, G. J. (2015). Positive youth development and relational-developmental systems. In R. M. Lerner (Series Ed.) and W. F. Overton and P. C. M. Molennaar (Vol. ed.), *Handbook of child psychology and developmental science* (7th ed., vol. 1, pp. 607–651). New York: Wiley.

McCaslin, M. M. (2009). Co-regulation of student motivation and emergent identity. *Educational Psychologist, 44*, 137–146.

Ogbu, J. U. (1992). Understanding cultural diversity and learning. *Educational Researcher, 21*, 5–14.

Okagaki, L. (2001). Triarchic model of minority children's school achievement. *Educational Psychologist, 36*, 9–20.

Seligman, M. E., P., Steen, T. A., Park, N., & Peterson, C. (2005). Positive psychology progress: Empirical validation of interventions. *American Psychologist, 60*, 41–421.

Winne, P H., and Hadwin, A. F. (1998). Studying as self-regulated learning. In D. J. Hacker, J. Dunlosky, & A. C. Graesser (eds.), *Metacognition in educational theory and practice* (pp. 277–304). Mahwah, NJ: Erlbaum.

Zimmerman, B. J., & Campillo, M. (2003). Motivating self-regulated problem solvers. In J.E. Davidson & R. J. Sternberg (Eds.), *The Psychology of Problem Solving* (pp. 233–262). Cambridge: Cambridge University Press.

Promoting Positive Self-Esteem in Ethnic Minority Students: The Role of School and Classroom Context

Jochem Thijs and Maykel Verkuyten

Abstract

Self-esteem is considered a core component of psychological well-being, and it has long been assumed that disadvantaged ethnic and racial minority children and adolescents suffer from low self-esteem due to discrimination and the internalization of prejudice. Yet research has contradicted this assumption and shown that they are able to maintain relatively positive self-evaluations and general self-esteem despite the threats of discrimination and prejudice. In this chapter we discuss past and future research on school and classroom characteristics that can promote positive self-esteem among ethnic minority students. We start by giving a broad overview of the nature and antecedents of self-esteem more generally, and then discuss the research on self-esteem in minority children and adolescents. Next, we consider research on three critical aspects of the educational environment that might contribute to the promotion of positive self-esteem among disadvantaged minority students: school ethnic composition, cultural diversity education, and students' relationship with their teachers. We end with a discussion of practical implications and directions for future research.

A handbook on the positive development of ethnic and racial minority[1] children would be incomplete without a discussion of self-esteem.

[1] There is no consensus about how the terms ethnic and racial differ and whether they are applicable to different national contexts. Here we do not have the space to discuss this issue and we follow the ethnic and racial identity (ERI) approach (see Umaña-Taylor et al., 2014) in the use of these terms.

J. Thijs (✉) · M. Verkuyten
Ercomer, Utrecht University, Utrecht,
The Netherlands
e-mail: j.t.thijs@uu.nl

Self-esteem is a core component of psychological well-being and has been extensively studied in developmental and social psychology (see Harter 2006; Mruk 2013). It generally is defined as the person's overall judgment of her worth as a person. Researchers such as Harter (2006) and Marsh, Shavelson, and colleagues (Marsh 1990; Shavelson et al. 1976) distinguish it from self-concept, which concerns individuals' beliefs and evaluations of themselves regarding particular activities (e.g., one's beliefs about one's ability in math). Numerous studies have examined the self-esteem of ethnic and racial minority members, and much of that research was con-

N.J. Cabrera and B. Leyendecker (eds.), *Handbook on Positive Development of Minority Children and Youth*, DOI 10.1007/978-3-319-43645-6_20

ducted among children and adolescents (see Gray-Little and Hafdahl 2000; Harter 2006; Twenge and Crocker 2002). These studies have challenged the assumption of a self-esteem deficit among disadvantaged minority children. Many of them appear to be able to maintain relatively positive self-esteem despite the threats associated with their minority position, such as discrimination and low social status. Particular circumstances and contexts can promote or hamper minority children's positive self-esteem, and in this chapter we consider the role of school and classroom characteristics. For children the educational environment is an important source of information about themselves because it is here that they (further) discover what they are capable of relative to others, and what important others outside the family think of them (see Harter 1999). Moreover, schools are institutions that tend to represent the norms and standards of the culturally dominant majority in society (Motti-Stefanidi and Masten 2013) and therefore education has special relevance to self-esteem development in ethnic minority students.

Before considering the different ways in which schools and educational contexts can affect the self-esteem of minority group children we will first discuss common conceptualizations of self-esteem and theoretical approaches for understanding self-esteem development. Subsequently we will give a short overview of the existing research on self-esteem of ethnic minority children. We focus predominantly on middle to late childhood but will also refer to research on other age groups.

Historical Overview and Theoretical Perspectives on Self-Esteem

Western psychology has taken a strong interest in the study of the self, beginning with the seminal work of James (1890). Especially in the last decennia of the 20th century high self-esteem was considered a panacea for all kinds of individual and social problems, and this idea was, and still is, often endorsed by the general public. Although the research evidence for the claims of the "self-esteem movement" is not as clear or strong as assumed (Baumeister et al. 2003; Emler 2001), self-esteem is still regarded as central to individual happiness and psychological well-being (see Sowislo and Orth 2013).

The Nature of Self-Esteem

Definitions and models

Self-esteem is conceptualized in different ways, such as a motivation or need, as a ratio between one's achievements and one's aspirations, as an evaluative judgment about oneself, and as a self-feeling (Harter 2006). Further, distinctions between (1) trait-like and state-like self-esteem, (2) between global and domain specific self-esteem, and (3) between explicit (conscious) and implicit (unconscious) self-esteem, are made.

State- and trait-like self-esteem

All of us are familiar with temporary increases or decreases in self-esteem due to, for example, a compliment or a criticism. But most of us have also developed a more habitual or stable form of self-esteem. Trait-like self-esteem refers to how one feels about oneself on average or generally, whereas state-like self-esteem is assessed by asking how one feels about oneself right here and now (Heatherton and Polivy 1991). Empirically, Savin-William and Demo (1984, p. 131) found that "Self-feelings are apparently global and context dependent. The largest number of our adolescents had a baseline of self-evaluation from which fluctuations rose or fell mildly, most likely dependent of features of the context". There are several studies that examine situational or state dependent self-esteem. For example, Brown (1998) shows that ethnic stigma is a contextual experience that leads to negative self-feelings in the context of certain relationships. In one of our studies among Turkish-Dutch early adolescents we collected self-reports on experiences with peer victimization, and assessed momentary self-feelings directly after these reports (Verkuyten and Thijs 2001). Results showed that peer victimization had a negative effect on momentary self-feelings, independently of the level of trait-like self-esteem. This suggests that peer discrimination might have a stronger negative impact on situational self-feelings than on trait-like feelings of global self-worth.

Research has shown that global self-esteem starts to develop around age eight and that its trait-like stability increases during adolescence and early adulthood (Harter 2006; Robins and Trzesniewski 2005). Although there is evidence of a drop in self-esteem in early adolescence (particularly if children make a school transition; e.g., Wigfield et al. 1991), longitudinal research has shown a gradual, but small, increase in average self-esteem during adolescence. These trajectories of change generally hold across race and ethnicity (e.g., Greene and Way 2005; Whitesell, et al. 2006) and have also been found for ethnic self-esteem (French et al. 2006). These changes appear to be quite common and cannot explain individual differences in self-esteem. The relative ordering of individuals' self-esteem is quite stable over time, comparable to the stability found for personality traits, and this rank-order stability has been found for different racial and ethnic groups (Trzesniewski et al. 2003).

Global and domain specific self-concept and self-esteem

There are various hierarchical models for the self-concept and most of them assume that it consists of multiple domains or dimensions. For instance, the model of the self-concept by Shavelson, Marsh, and their colleagues (e.g., Byrne et al. 1996; Marsh 1990; Shavelson et al. 1976) posits that (pre)adolescents' global self-worth (or global self-esteem) reflects their self-feelings in the academic, social, physical, emotional realms, which in turn are based on their self-concepts (or self-beliefs or self-perceptions) relating to more specific subareas (e.g., English, history, math, and science, for the academic domain). Other multidimensional models also make the distinction between global and domain-specific self-concepts but are less strictly hierarchical. For instance, Harter's (1982) Self-Perception Profile for Children measures children's perceptions of scholastic competence, athletic competence, peer likability, physical appearance, and behavioral conduct, as well as a their global self-worth. As in the hierarchical models, the former are regarded as sources for the latter. Yet the relative importance of each domain is assumed to vary from child to child, and global self-worth is considered to be more than the sum of the separate perceptions (Harter 1999).

Most of the research on racial and ethnic minority children has treated self-esteem as a general attitude toward the self in which trait-like global feelings of self-worth are examined (e.g., Gray-Little and Hafdahl 2000). In addition, research has focused upon trait-like feelings that children have towards their racial or ethnic group membership: racial or ethnic self-esteem. How a person feels about him- or herself in general is something different to how he or she feels about being a member of a specific ethnic or racial group (Crocker and Luhtanen 1990). Youngsters with high ethnic self-esteem feel good about their ethnic group and are proud of their ethnicity. These feelings are conceptually and empirically different from their global self-esteem. Yet the former may contribute to the latter and research in The Netherlands among preadolescents from different ethnic groups showed that ethnic self-esteem was moderately and positively ($r = 0.33$) related to global self-esteem (Verkuyten and Thijs 2006). Similar findings are reported in studies of African American adolescents in the U.S. (Rowley et al. 1998). The moderate association indicates that ethnic group belonging does not fully determine older children's self-feelings: there are many possible contingencies upon which children can base their global self-esteem (Crocker and Wolfe 2001).

Explicit and implicit self-esteem

In an article on racial identity, Erik Erikson (1966) argued that a sense of identity has conscious as well as unconscious aspects. He pointed out that there are aspects that are accessible only at moments of special awareness or not at all. In line with psychoanalytical ideas he talked about repression and resistance. And he claimed that racial minorities would have more negative self-feelings on an unconscious or implicit level. The implicit-explicit distinction is also made in relation to self-esteem. Explicit self-esteem is the thoughtful response one typically gets on self-report questions that predominate in studies on self-esteem, whereas implicit self-esteem refers to 'the introspectively unidentified...effect of the self-attitude on evaluation of self-associated and self-dissociated objects' (Greenwald and Banaji 1995, p. 11).

An increasing number of researchers have emphasized the importance of the distinction between explicit and implicit self-esteem (e.g. Greenwald and Banaji 1995; Hetts and Pelham 2001). Both may develop differently resulting in a discrepancy in implicit and explicit self-evaluations. The distinction is important because it is possible that stereotypes and discrimination negatively affect the implicit rather than the explicit self-esteem of ethnic minority children. For example, in a study among Turkish-Dutch early adolescents it was found that perceived discrimination was associated with lower implicit ethnic self-esteem but not with explicit self-esteem (Verkuyten 2005).

Origins and antecedents

There are various theoretical propositions about the origins of self-esteem and these are closely connected to the way in which the concept is defined and examined. Roughly at least three broad and complementary processes can be identified (see Mruk 2013; Rosenberg 1979). The first one is the *self-perception process* that holds that children's self-esteem is based on their own perceptions and appraisals of their behaviors or accomplishments. This view has similarities with hierarchical self-concept models (e.g. Shavelson et al. 1976) that propose that global self-esteem is based on domain-specific self-concepts which, in turn, are based on behaviors in specific

situations. The notion that children's self-esteem depends on their behavior does not mean that they always think less of themselves when they do not perform well in a particular domain. James (1890) indicated early on that the importance of a particular outcome for the self depends on one's pretensions for it. Thus even if their academic self-concept is not too positive, children can still have high self-esteem as long as they do not stake it on their academic accomplishments (see Crocker and Wolfe 2001; Harter 1999).

Second, *social comparison processes* are important for developing self-esteem (Festinger 1954). Comparisons with others provide important information about the self. An example is the big-fish-little-pond effect (BFLPE) which is the finding that children's academic self-concept reflects their academic achievement relative to those of their classmates rather than their absolute achievement (Marsh et al. 2008). Similarly, Rosenberg (1979) showed that racial minority children and adolescents (9–17 years) do not tend to have lower self-esteem because they compare themselves selectively with other racial minority children.

The third perspective considers the so-called *reflected appraisal process,* which describes how self-feelings are influenced by the perceived opinions and standards of others. This perspective includes symbolic interactionist theories in sociology (Cooley 1902; Mead 1934) but it is also consistent with sociometer theory (Leary and Baumeister 2000), as well as attachment theory (Bowlby 1982). The core idea is that significant others are a continuous and important source of feedback on one's personal qualities, competences, and worthiness, and that especially children rely on this feedback to develop a sense of self. According to Harter's (1999) developmental model the sensitivity to the judgments of others starts in early childhood and gradually changes over time. From middle childhood on children can assess the opinions and standards of others, internalize them, and use them as a basis for their self-feelings.

Self-Esteem in Minority Group Children

Until the end of the 1960s psychologists and sociologists alike assumed that disadvantaged ethnic and racial minority children and adolescents suffered from relatively low self-esteem. Given the three theoretical processes discussed, this assumption is not an unreasonable one to make. Despite the existence of so-called model minorities, many ethnic minority groups fare relatively poorly in various domains of life, such as education, work or health, and this might negatively affect the self-feelings of children from those groups. Furthermore, children from racial and ethnic minority groups are confronted with unfavorable images of their own group in the media and from others, and they can experience discrimination in school and other settings. Compared to majority group children, they have to deal with these negative messages more often and sometimes on a regular basis. Ethnic devaluation comes from various sources and in early adolescence disadvantaged minority children are clearly aware of the prejudice and discrimination that confronts them as member of their ethnic group (Verkuyten and Thijs 2002). Moreover correlational studies in different countries and among different disadvantaged minority groups have demonstrated that perceived discrimination can threaten the self-esteem of minority children and adolescents (Pascoe and Smart Richman 2009; Schmitt et al. 2014; Verkuyten and Thijs 2006).

The assumption of low self-esteem in children from some minority groups received initial empirical support but the research evidence was indirect, such as in the famous Clark and Clark (1947) doll studies in the 1930s and 1940s done in the U.S., which showed that black children "preferred" to play with white dolls. The interpretation of these findings was that minority group children come to internalize society's negative view about their group and therefore show the 'mark of oppression' (Kardiner and Ovesey 1951). After the 1960s, research in the U.S. started to examine the assumption of low self-esteem among minority groups by using standardized self-esteem scales, such as the well-known Rosenberg's self-esteem scale (Rosenberg 1965). In general, these studies showed that despite the existence of prejudice and discrimination, minority group membership was not systematically related to lower self-esteem. This finding was called the 'puzzle of high self-esteem' (Simmons 1978) and various explanations have been given for it (see Verkuyten 2005). Much of this research involved comparisons between African-American versus European-American youth (children, adolescents, and college students), and a meta-analysis on 257 of those studies concluded that self-esteem was actually higher for the former group (Gray-Little and Hafdahl 2000). A later meta-analysis included more ethnic groups and yielded the same conclusion: the average self-esteem was higher for European-Americans compared to some ethnic groups (Hispanic, Asian, American-Indian) but it was highest for African-Americans. As the latter are arguably the most stigmatized group in American society, these finding cannot be explained in terms of discrimination or low status positions (Twenge and Crocker 2002; Bachman et al. 2011).

There has been far less research on the relation between ethnicity and self-esteem in Europe. Generally speaking, ethnic diversity is less common and less accepted in in European countries in which there is a historically large native majority population, than in traditional immigrant countries like the U.S. and Canada. However, there also considerable differences between the major ethnic minority groups within and between European countries. For example, Pakistani-British, Algerian-French, or Surinamese-Dutch people have a history of colonialism which makes them more culturally similar to natives, than Turkish-German and Turkish- and Moroccan-Dutch people who have a history of labor migration. In addition to this, various ethnic groups differ in terms of socioeconomic status and outward appearances which may make them more or less easy targets of discrimination. Yet despite these differences, there appear to be no systematic self-esteem differences between various ethnic minority and majority groups, but rather a tendency for higher self-esteem among the former (Verkuyten 1994). For example, in a large-scale, nation-wide study in the Netherlands, early adolescents of Turkish, Moroccan and Surinamese background had higher self-esteem than the Dutch (Verkuyten and Thijs 2006). Furthermore, a study that examined global and ethnic self-esteem among almost 40 different ethnic groups in 8 European countries, as well as in Canada, the U.S., Australia and New Zealand, found that all ethnic minority groups scored above the neutral mid-point of the scale suggesting a satisfactory level of self-esteem, and that there were no differences in self-esteem between minority and majority adolescents (Phinney et al. 2006).

These similarly high levels of self-esteem are striking considering the different national contexts with their different histories of slavery, colonialism, immigration and integration policies, as well as the cultural diversity of the immigrant and ethnic minority groups concerned. They indicate that a disadvantaged minority position does not simply lead to lower explicit self-esteem. This is not to say that contextual and cultural differences do not matter for the ways in which minority children and adolescents think and feel about themselves. For example and in relation to cultural differences, research in cross-cultural psychology has shown that the self can have quite diverse cultural connotations related to distinctions such as independence versus interdependence and individualism versus collectivism (Markus and Kitayama 2010; Triandis 2001). One of the research findings is that personal self-esteem is sometimes lower in cultures that prioritize the group over the individual (e.g., Japan) versus cultures that prioritize the individual over the group (e.g., Canada) (Heine et al. 1999; Schmitt and Allik 2005; but for a different outcome, see Verkuyten 2005).[2] Research with implicit measures has shown that this finding cannot be explained by a higher concern with self-modesty in more collectivist cultures (Falk and Heine 2014). Twenge and Crocker (2002) referred to collectivism rather than the experience

of stigmatization in explaining their meta-analytic finding that native, Hispanic and Asian Americans reported lower self-esteem than European-Americans. Yet this interpretation was indirect as it was based on their finding that self-esteem was highest for African Americans, the most stigmatized group in the studies they analyzed. To complicate matters even more, the impact of the original culture may wane in the specific case of immigrants because of their exposure to new cultural norms and values in the host society. For instance, Hetts and colleagues (1999) compared two groups of Asian-Americans: those who were born in the US, and those who recently immigrated. They found that both groups had relatively high *explicit* global self-esteem. Yet they also measured *implicit* self-esteem (to be described below) and found that it was relatively low for the recent immigrants but relatively high for the American-born group. According to the authors, this was an effect of the latter's stronger exposure to the individualistic U.S. culture whereas for the recent immigrants the impact of the original, more collectivist culture was still lingering on a more implicit level.

In considering ethnic group differences in self-esteem it is important to note that most self-esteem measures are self-report scales on which children have to indicate how they feel about themselves. This method can be problematic if children do not yet have the capacity for self-reflection or when they have a tendency to give socially desirable responses (Harter 1999)—a tendency that might be stronger for some cultural groups than for others. In response to this problem, behavioral measures of self-esteem have been proposed (e.g., Savin-William and Demo 1984; Verschueren et al. 1998), as well as implicit measures such as the Implicit Association Test (Buhrmester et al. 2011, p. 366; Falk and Heine 2014). Implicit self-esteem is considered to be unrelated to cultural norms about self-presentation which is relevant when different ethnic groups are compared (Hetts et al. 1999). However, there has been very little research on implicit self-esteem in ethnic minority children. An exception is a study by Pelham and Hetts (1999) that examined the puzzle of high self-esteem among minority

---

[2]There is no systematic evidence that collective self-esteem is higher in collectivistic cultures (Heine et al. 1999).

groups. They suggest that this puzzle may refer to the explicit self-esteem of minority youth and that on an implicit level minority youth might feel less positive about their ethnic group membership. They found that, relative to Anglo Americans, minority youth was lower in implicit ethnic self-esteem. In addition, however, minority group members were not lower on implicit personal self-esteem. A similar result was found in a study among Turkish-Dutch and native Dutch early adolescents (Verkuyten 2005). The Turkish-Dutch early adolescents reported an equally positive (explicit) ethnic identity but suffered from lower implicit ethnic self-esteem which was related to perceived discrimination. Hence, at an explicit or more conscious level, ethnic minority youth can endorse the kind of favorable conceptions of themselves that are common in western societies, whereas at an implicit or unconscious level their ethnic self-feelings can be more consistent with their disadvantaged minority position. Such a discrepancy can result in fragile and defensive high self-esteem (Jordan et al. 2003).

Current Research Questions Regarding the Influence of Education on the Self-Esteem of Disadvantaged Minority Children

The puzzle of high *explicit* self-esteem among disadvantaged minority children is a good example of resilience. The resilience framework resonates well with positive psychology and examines how children are able to receive "good outcomes in spite of serious threats to adaptation or development" (Masten 2001, p. 228). A distinction is made between two kinds of factors that enable children to deal with potential adversities: *promotive factors*, which compensate for the negative impact of the risks children face by having independent positive effects themselves, and *protective factors* which reduces the negative impact of risk factors by interacting with them (Masten 2007; Motti-Stefanidi and Masten 2013). In the case of learning disabilities, for example, academic motivation might be considered a

promotive factor whereas secure attachment can have a protective effect (see Margalit 2004).

Like the risk factors, these so-called resilience factors can involve characteristics of the child but also of the environment. In addition to the home environment, the educational context can play a crucial role. Schools have the important task of helping children to develop intellectually, socially, and emotionally (see Ladd et al. 2010), and from the moment children start formal education they spend many of their waking hours in the presence of their teachers and fellow students.

In the rest of this chapter we discuss current research on the different ways educational contexts can affect self-esteem in ethnic minority children. More specifically, we will consider the questions how schools and classrooms can promote the formation or preservation of positive self-esteem, and how they can protect children's self-esteem against prejudice and discrimination, and individual or group outcomes that are relatively unfavorable and 'disproportionally poor' (see Crocker and Major 1989). But first we will briefly discuss some methodological issues.

Research Methodology: Cluster Sampling and Multilevel Analysis

To examine properly the impact of the educational context on children's self-esteem it is important to use a cluster sampling procedure and to study a whole array of classrooms and schools. Many school and classroom characteristics are interrelated and it is impossible to evaluate their unique contributions based on findings in just a few schools. For instance, in the Netherlands, where schools are relatively free in their implementation of diversity education, multicultural education is more emphasized in schools with an ethnically mixed population than in schools that have a majority of native Dutch pupils (van Geel and Vedder 2010; Verkuyten and Thijs 2002), and classes with a larger proportion of minority students tend to be smaller in size (Verkuyten and Thijs 2002). Studies that sample classrooms (or schools) instead of individual students have hierarchically nested data which should be analysed with multilevel modeling. Multilevel analysis corrects for dependencies between observations (e.g., student data) nested in the same units (e.g., classes), and it can handle variable numbers of observations per unit (Snijders and Bosker 1999). Multilevel research on students typically starts by examining how much of the variance in a particular dependent variable (e.g., self-esteem) depends on the school classes students are nested in, and it seeks to explain this higher-level variance by properties of the classroom context. In addition, this kind of research can examine whether the classroom context makes a difference for the relation between variables at the student level (e.g., perceived discrimination and self-esteem).

The use of cluster sampling also allows researchers to construct more 'objective' classroom (or school) measures based on students' subjective perceptions. For example, in one study (Thijs et al. 2012) we asked children about their teacher's attitudes toward cultural diversity and it appeared that there was considerable agreement among classmates. Taken together the individual judgments in each classroom formed a reliable scale and could be averaged to create a classroom-level variable. Because this aggregate measure reflected classmates' shared perceptions about their teacher it was less biased than individual perceptions. Unfortunately most empirical studies have not used aggregation techniques.

Empirical Finding on the Role of School and Education in Minority Children's Self-Esteem

In this section we discuss research on three critical aspects of the educational environment that might contribute to the promotion of positive self-esteem among disadvantaged minority students: school ethnic composition, cultural diversity education, and students' relationship with their teachers. These three aspects have been found to be important for children's interethnic relations (Verkuyten and Thijs 2013). We will

consider existing research, but also discuss possibilities for future study.

School ethnic composition

In 1954, the U.S. Supreme Court made a historic decision by declaring that it was unjust and illegal to sanction school ethnic segregation by law. Ever since this famous *Brown versus Board of Education* ruling there have been regular and sometimes heated debates about the ethnic or racial composition of schools, not only in the U. S. but also in Europe. In many western countries schools tend to be more segregated than the communities they serve and the segregation tends to be higher in primary than secondary schools.[3] One of the original arguments against law-based segregation was that it sends out a message of inferiority to minority students which would leave a 'mark of oppression' (Kardiner and Ovesey 1951) in the form of self-hatred and low self-esteem (Zirkel 2005). This has led to the more general claim that segregation per se has negative implications for the self-esteem of minority group children. Studies in Europe have shown, however, that there are little to no effects of school ethnic segregation (proportion of minority students) on the global or ethnic self-esteem of ethnic minority children (Agirdag et al. 2012; Kinket and Verkuyten 1997; Verkuyten and Thijs 2004a). And research in the U. S. indicates that African-American students are more, rather than less, likely to have high self-esteem in schools with a higher proportion of African-American students (see the meta-analysis by Gray-Little and Hafdahl 2000). Apparently school ethnic segregation does not undermine the self-esteem of ethnic minority students and there are several reasons for this.

Social comparisons

One self-esteem 'advantage' of segregation is that it decreases the likelihood of making

---

[3]Please note that this is an example of de facto rather than de jure segregation (see Zirkel 2005).

unfavorable comparisons with majority group peers. In general, children from (many) ethnic minority groups would be more likely to have more negative domain-specific self-feelings because on average their individual outcomes are 'disproportionally poor' compared to those of the majority group (see Crocker and Major 1989). However, an important question is whether in their everyday life minority children make such intergroup comparisons. According to Festinger's (1954) social comparison theory, comparisons with others provide relevant information about the self. Yet those others need to be similar to the self because "if the only comparison available is a very divergent one, the person will not be able to make a subjectively precise evaluation of his opinion and ability" (Festinger 1954, p. 121). This means that in more segregated situations minority children may be more likely to compare themselves to their co-ethnic peers rather than to ethnic majority peers (see Crocker and Major 1989; Rosenberg 1979).

The fact that children's self-esteem is typically based on comparisons with others in their direct environments is shown by the earlier mentioned big-fish-little-pond-effect (BFLPE). This implies that an academically weak student can have more positive academic self-esteem than a strong student as long as the former but not the latter outperforms her classmates (Marsh et al. 2008). To our knowledge research on the BFLPE has not explicitly focused on ethnic minority children, but the effect can explain why ethnic school segregation can protect the self-esteem of students that have an ethnic achievement gap. For instance, in our research we examined the academic self-esteem of ethnic minority preadolescents (from either Turkish, Moroccan, or Surinamese backgrounds) compared to that of native Dutch contemporaries (Thijs and Verkuyten 2008). Despite evidence for lower absolute academic achievement among the minority children there were no systematic group differences in academic self-esteem. Importantly, the classrooms involved in this research were relatively segregated—as the average proportion of native Dutch classmates was smaller for the minority than for the majority

children—and in another study we demonstrated that the BFLPE held for both the minority and the majority students (Thijs et al. 2010).[4]

Support and discrimination

There are other reasons why a more segregated context can protect the self-esteem of disadvantaged minority children. In these contexts minority children can experience a stronger sense of ethnic group belonging and stronger peer support, which promotes the development of positive (ethnic) self-esteem. In addition, segregation often implies less direct exposure to prejudice and discrimination (Rosenberg 1979). Both of these possibilities were addressed in our studies among preadolescents and we found most support for the second one. We used a multilevel approach by sampling 182 school classes (grades 5–6) from 82 schools in 30 different cities. We assessed a number of classroom characteristics including the proportion of various ethnic groups in the classroom and we measured students' ethnic and global self-esteem. For minority students, ethnic self-esteem (but not global self-esteem) was higher if they had proportionally fewer native Dutch classmates. Additional analysis showed that there were no effects of the proportion of co-ethnic students which indicated that it was the presence of the majority out-group rather than the ethnic in-group that mattered for children's self-esteem (Verkuyten and Thijs 2004a). Majority group peers are the likeliest perpetrators of discriminatory peer behavior, at least according to children's own perceptions (Verkuyten et al. 1997). Indeed, in an earlier study we found that ethnic minority children with proportionally more native Dutch classmates

---

[4]Even in the absence of tracking there can be strong differences in absolute achievement levels between schools and classrooms, due to factors such as the composition of the student body or the quality of teaching. This means that the absolute achievement differences within classrooms are relatively small, and that the academic achievement gap will not show up in the self-perceptions of minority versus majority children.

reported more experiences with ethnic peer victimization (Verkuyten and Thijs 2002).

However, ethnic composition entails more than the degree of majority-minority segregation. Schools and classrooms also differ in terms of the number of ethnic groups and this can be captured by diversity indexes. For example, higher scores on the Simpson diversity index imply that more different groups are present and also that the sizes of these groups are more equal. Graham and Juvonen and colleagues, in their studies in the U.S., have used this index to evaluate the imbalance of power thesis. This is the idea that school and classroom diversity has positive consequences for students' social relations and psychological well-being because it decreases the likelihood of imbalanced power relations between different ethnic groups. Their findings support the thesis by showing that higher diversity is associated with less peer victimization and higher self-esteem among Latino and African-American students (Graham 2006; Juvonen et al. 2006). This kind of research demonstrates that it is not only the relative presence of the in-group (versus the majority out-group) that matters for the self-esteem of ethnic minority children but that it is also crucial to consider the nature of the relations between different ethnic minority groups at school. Furthermore, questions on the implications of school (de)segregation should not only consider self-esteem and intergroup relations but also the possibilities for intercultural contacts and learning, and academic achievement.

Diversity education

In many western countries there has been the development and implementation of school curricula and educational practices that focus on the acknowledgment, acceptance, and recognition of ethnic and cultural diversity. The variation in this so-called multicultural (or intercultural) education is substantial, but there is quite some agreement that a major goal of these approaches is to foster ethnic tolerance and equality (Kahn 2008; Portera 2008). The vast majority of the theorizing and research on diversity education

has been conducted in the U.S. and is influenced by the country's long history of slavery and continuous immigration. An influential framework is Banks' (2004) conceptualization of five aspects of multicultural education: cultural content integration in the curriculum, learning to question and consider how knowledge is constructed, prejudice reduction, equity pedagogy, and empowering school culture. In the non-settler European countries, the situation is different because there is a historically large native majority group and a relatively recent inflow of labor migrants and ex-colonial minorities. In Europe the notion of multicultural education is less well articulated and there are debates about the need for intercultural and citizenship education rather than forms of multicultural education. Furthermore, although there are some qualitative studies (e.g., Doppen 2007) there is a lack of large-scale quantitative research on cultural diversity education. To our knowledge, one of the exceptions is our research in the Netherlands (see Verkuyten and Thijs 2013). Multicultural education might both directly and indirectly enhance the positive self-esteem of ethnic minority children.

Direct effects of multicultural education

It is likely that multicultural education fosters positive global and ethnic self-esteem in ethnic minority students because it tends to recognize their identity and support their heritage culture. In our study among Turkish-Dutch, Moroccan-Dutch, Surinamese-Dutch, and native Dutch preadolescents (Verkuyten and Thijs 2004a) we measured in different ways the degree of multicultural education in the classroom. We asked teachers how much attention they pay to teaching about cultural differences and discrimination, and we asked students to report on their teacher's educational practices as well as on the (probable) teacher and student reactions to discrimination in the classroom. Results showed that teachers' own reports of multicultural education were unrelated to the global and ethnic self-esteem of the students of different ethnic groups. Yet, there were two effects of children's perceptions that were consistent with our theoretical expectations: Children who perceived more multicultural teaching reported higher global self-esteem, and children who indicated that their teacher and the students would stand up against discrimination reported both higher global and ethnic self-esteem. Interestingly, these results were similar for the ethnic minority and majority children. They therefore suggest that multicultural education and educational practices can have a beneficial impact on the self-feelings of all students regardless of their ethnic background. This was also found in an earlier study among Turkish-Dutch and native Dutch preadolescents (Kinket and Verkuyten 1997).

Indirect effects of multicultural education

A central aim of most forms of multicultural education, both in Europe and North America, is to improve inter-ethnic relations among children by reducing ignorance and misunderstandings about cultural differences and by transmitting norms against prejudice and discrimination (Verkuyten and Thijs 2013). The available evidence in the North American context indicates that multicultural education is moderately successful in reaching these goals (Aboud et al. 2012; Bigler 1999; Stephan et al. 2004). This means, for example, that multicultural education can contribute to less ethnic peer victimization and discrimination at school. By reducing these risks, it may indirectly increase the self-esteem of ethnic minority students.

However, multicultural education can also have unintended effects. By highlighting the differences between ethnic groups, multicultural initiatives may actually increase stereotypical thinking about ethnic others (Bigler and Liben 2007). Thus "curriculum-based interventions may potentially increase children's racial and ethnic bias via the attention they draw to such groups" (Bigler 1999, p. 700). This is especially relevant for younger children who lack multiple classification skills, i.e. the ability to consider

that people belong to different types of nonexclusive categories at the same time (e.g., female, African-American, left-hander) (Aboud 1988). For younger children, ethnic groups may become all-important if multicultural education neglects cross-cutting or overarching categories or the many individual differences that exist within ethnic groups. In addition, multicultural education might backfire if it neglects the cultural distinctiveness and identity of majority students (Tajfel and Turner 1979). Research among white American adults (including university students) has shown that they can be hesitant in embracing multiculturalism when they feel left out and developed a sense of 'what about us' (Plaut et al. 2011). When this happens, multiculturalism can increase rather decrease negative reactions towards ethnic minority groups (Morrison et al. 2010). To our knowledge these processes have not been examined among children and adolescents but it seems an important line of investigation to pursue.

Multicultural education can also have the effect of making children more aware of prejudice and discrimination. In our research, we measured children's own experiences with peer ethnic victimization as well as their perception of the experiences of members of their ethnic group (Verkuyten and Thijs 2002). We related these experiences to teachers' assessments of their multicultural teaching and students' perceptions of this teaching, as well the classroom reactions against discrimination. It appeared that students reported less personal experiences with ethnic victimization in classrooms where discrimination was actively resisted (according to the aggregated student perspective), and perceived less victimization of their ethnic group if their teacher reacted more against discrimination. Yet, the teacher's multicultural teaching as perceived by the children was associated with higher experiences and perceptions of ethnic victimization. This suggests that multicultural education can make children more sensitive and attentive to discrimination and thereby more vulnerable to it.[5]

---

[5]Related to this, there is evidence that minority parents' attempts to prepare their children for discrimination and

Relationships with Teachers

In developmental and educational psychology the student-teacher relationship is seen as a micro-system with important implications for children's adjustment (Pianta et al. 2003). Various studies have shown that the quality of this relationship is uniquely associated with many positive outcomes including higher academic achievement and educational engagement (Roorda et al. 2011), and less social, behavioral, and emotional problems (Baker 2006; Rudasill et al. 2010). Although relatively few studies have examined ethnic group differences in teacher-student relationships, these relationships appear to be more important for the school adjustment of ethnic minority than majority students (e.g., den Brok et al. 2010; Murray et al. 2008). One of the explanations for this finding is that a supportive bond with the teacher can help to bridge the relatively large gap that sometimes exists between the home and school environment (Suárez-Orozco and Pimentel 2009). For example, Suárez-Orozco and Pimentel (2009) interviewed immigrant adolescents about their school experiences. The adolescents reported that teachers who cared for them and helped them with the language barrier made a difference in their cultural transition. Unfortunately, some adolescents also perceived cultural insensitivity and discrimination by teachers.

Direct effects

Very few studies have examined the direct impact of the student-teacher relationship on children's self-esteem, and there is even less research that makes a comparison between minority and majority students. Theoretically, however, self-esteem is one of the more important outcomes of this relationship because it can function as a potential secondary attachment bond (Ainsworth 1989). This means that it can be

an important source of emotional support and comfort that provides children with the necessary security for exploration and initiative (Verschueren and Koomen 2012). Children who are securely attached to their caregivers learn that they are socially accepted and worthy of love and affection, and this promotes the development of high self-esteem (Verschueren and Marcoen 1999).

In line with these propositions, research has shown that children (Verschueren et al. 2012) and early adolescents (Ryan et al. 1994) who have high quality relationships with their teacher also have more positive self-esteem. To our knowledge, only two studies have compared the importance of teachers for the self-esteem of children of different ethnic groups. Both of them found no group differences; however, both were done in the U.S., one study was limited to early adolescent girls from three schools in Texas (Carlson et al. 2000), and the other made the broad distinction between students from western-European versus non-western-European backgrounds (Agirdag et al. 2012). Furthermore, most teachers in both the U.S. and Europe tend to belong to the ethnic majority group (Hamre et al. 2007; Thijs et al. 2012; Zirkel 2008) and research has shown that the quality of the relationship can be compromised when the teacher and the student do not share the same ethnicity (Ewing and Taylor 2009; Saft and Pianta 2001). This is especially likely when there is cultural miscommunication and when teachers have unfavorable attitudes toward ethnic diversity (Thijs et al. 2012). Related to this, research has shown that minority students can feel discriminated by their teachers which leads to lower self-esteem (Wong et al. 2003).

Indirect effects

In addition to promoting positive self-esteem in minority children, the student-teacher relationship might also play an indirect, protective role. Children who can trust their teachers and feel comforted by them are more resilient in dealing with stressful life events (Pianta et al. 2003).

(Footnote 5 continued)
bias can have unintentional negative effects on self-esteem (Hughes et al. 2009).

A longitudinal study among immigrant adolescents from 54 different countries in Sweden shows that this also holds for the risks associated with a minority position. It was found that ethnic victimization predicted lower self-esteem over time, which in turn was related to lower school adjustment. However, these effects were not significant for children who reported positive relationships with their teachers (Bayram Özdemir and Stattin 2014).

Future Directions and Policy Implications

There is a long research tradition on the self-esteem of ethnic and racial minority group children but much less is known about the role that schools and education can play in the development of self-esteem in children of these groups. School is a very important everyday context for children and it is clear that schools matter for how children feel about themselves. It is less clear, however, how schools play a role in self-esteem development and whether this role differs for ethnic minority and majority students, for global and domain-specific self-esteem, for personal and ethnic self-esteem, and for explicit and implicit self-esteem. Research typically focuses on global self-esteem but there are different self-feelings that can be distinguished and therefore provide a more detailed understanding of how ethnic minority children are doing. For example, global self-esteem can be based on different domains for ethnic minority than majority children. It has been suggested for instance that African American adolescents diminish the value of academic achievement on their global self-esteem as a self-worth protection (Osborne 1997) and there is also evidence for this process of disengagement in the Netherlands (Verkuyten and Thijs 2004b). Furthermore, personal self-esteem can be relatively independent of ethnic self-esteem and explicit and implicit self-esteem can differ resulting in a fragile, defensive self-esteem. These distinctions provide various directions for future research that could

greatly advance our understanding of the self-esteem of minority group children.

Future research should also systematically examine the role of various school and educational characteristics for ethnic minority children's self-esteem. The existing research has focused predominantly on ethnic segregation and forms of cultural diversity education, and the findings are not unequivocal. For example, multicultural education with its acceptance and recognition of cultural diversity and group identities can be important for developing positive self-esteem. The evidence, however, is limited and in practice the variation of multicultural ideas, initiatives and programs is substantial (Banks 2004), and not all of these can be expected to have a similar effect on children's self-esteem. Additionally, there might be important contextual and country differences that shape the forms and content of cultural diversity education and thereby have an effect on students' self-esteem. Further, there is the danger that the thinking in terms of groups and group differences, which is inherent in multiculturalism, leads to reified group distinctions that promote group stereotyping and negative inter-ethnic relations which may hamper a positive sense of self. These unintended and subtle processes are not always easy to examine in large-scale quantitative research. In-depth studies that more closely examine what exactly happens on a day-today basis in classrooms and in the educational process might be very useful here. This type of research can give a more detailed understanding of the proximal processes that are involved.

Furthermore, it is important that future research examines different school characteristics in combination with each other. It might be the case, for example, that the effect of the ethnic composition of the classroom (level of segregation or diversity) on children's self-esteem depends on multicultural education. Ethnically mixed classrooms might hamper a positive sense of self when there is not a school climate of acceptance and endorsement of diversity. In such a context ethnic minority students might face more negative stereotypes and discrimination compared to a mixed context in which multiculturalism is endorsed. Similarly, the impact of ethnically mixed classrooms on students' self-esteem might depend on the quality of the teacher-student relationships, and vice versa. For example, a majority group teacher might follow a multicultural curriculum in her classroom but might also have frequent conflictual interactions with her minority group students. This could potentially undermine the perceived consistency and effectiveness of her diversity teachings and could make children insecure about their acceptance and value. To our knowledge, there are no studies on these topics but examining whether teachers 'practice what they preach' is an important task for future research.

There have been many popular ideas and programs about improving children's and adolescents' self-esteem that have been implemented in many schools, especially in the United States. And although the expectations and promises of these programs are substantial, there is little systematic and methodological sound evidence for drawing firm conclusions about what works and why (see Emler 2001). It also is unclear whether interventions work equally well for different ethnic and age groups and in different countries, and whether there are long-term effects. Furthermore, it is important to note that the explicit concern with planned interventions for self-esteem improvement does not exist, or is much less common, in other countries than the United States.

In addition to these initiatives that directly try to address children's self-esteem there are interventions that can improve self-esteem more indirectly. As noted, many studies have demonstrated that negative experiences such as ethnic exclusion, victimization and discrimination tend to have negative effects on minority children's self-esteem. This means that it is important to address these negative behaviors in a systematic and effective way. Unfortunately, the various programs and initiatives for countering ethnic prejudices, peer victimization and harassment are not always very successful (Aboud et al. 2012). One key issue is that it is necessary to have a better understanding about children's own perceptions, interpretations and reasoning about these negative behaviors. Effective interventions are more difficult without such an understanding and an appreciation of the importance of the ways that children among each other negotiate, share and create meanings and interpretations.

Finally, in future research and in developing effective interventions to improve self-esteem it is important to consider the role of parents. Parents have great emotional significance for children and a large influence on the development of self-esteem well into adolescent years (Emler 2001; Harter 1999). The importance of parental acceptance, approval, nurturance and support to self-esteem is found in various (western and eastern) countries (e.g. Faruggia et al. 2004; Scott et al. 1991), and among both ethnic majority and minority groups (e.g. Greenberger and Chen 1996). Furthermore, ethnic minority families are sometimes able to filter out racist and discriminatory messages from the dominant community and to provide positive feedback that will enhance self-esteem (see Hughes et al. 2009). Thus both parents and schools are influential in the development of children's self-feelings. But research on the role of parents tends not take the role of the school into account and vice versa. Yet, it can be expected that for a teacher-student relationship to have a positive effect on the self-esteem of minority children it is of importance that parents also have an emotional supportive relationship with their child. This would mean that there can be important individual differences that are responsible for school and education having a positive effect on the self-esteem of some minority children but not of others.

References

Aboud, F. E. (1988). *Children and prejudice*. New York: Blackwell.

Aboud, F. E., Tredoux, C., Tropp, L. R., Brown, C. S., Niens, U., & Noor, N. M. (2012). Interventions to reduce prejudice and enhance inclusion and respect for ethnic differences in early childhood: A systematic review. *Developmental Review, 32*, 307–336. doi:10.1016/j.dr.2012.05.001

Agirdag, O., Van Houtte, M., & Van Avermaet, P. (2012). Ethnic school segregation and self-esteem: The role of teacher-pupil relationships. *Urban Education, 47*, 1135–1159. doi:10.1177/0042085912452154

Ainsworth, M. D. (1989). Attachments beyond infancy. *American Psychologist, 44*, 709–716.

Bachman, J. G., O'Malley, P. M., Freedman-Doan, P., Trzesniewski, K. H., & Donnellan, M. B. (2011). Adolescent self-esteem: Differences by race/ethnicity, gender, and age. *Self and Identity, 10*, 445–473. doi:10.1080/15298861003794538

Baker, J. A. (2006). Contributions of teacher–child relationships to positive school adjustment during elementary school. *Journal of School Psychology, 44*, 211–229. doi:10.1016/j.jsp.2006.02.002

Banks, J. A. (2004). Multicultural education: Historical development, dimensions, and practice. In J. A. Banks & C. A. M. Banks (Eds.), *Handbook of research on multicultural education* (2nd ed., pp. 3–29). San Francisco: Jossey-Bass.

Baumeister, R. F., Campbell, J. D., Krueger, J. I., & Vohs, K. D. (2003). Does high self-esteem cause better performance, interpersonal success, happiness, or healthier lifestyles? *Psychological Science in the Public Interest, 4*, 1–44. doi:10.1111/1529-1006.01431

Bayram Özdemir, S., & Stattin, H. (2014). Why and when is ethnic harassment a risk for immigrant adolescents' school adjustment? understanding the processes and conditions. *Journal of Youth and Adolescence, 43*(8), 1252–1265. doi:10.1007/s10964-013-0038-y

Bigler, R. S. (1999). The use of multicultural curricula and materials to counter racism in children. *Journal of Social Issues, 55*(4), 687–705. doi:10.1111/0022-4537.00142

Bigler, R. S., & Liben, L. S. (2007). Developmental intergroup theory: Explaining and reducing children's social stereotyping and prejudice. *Current Directions in Psychological Science, 16*, 162–166. doi:10.1111/j.1467-8721.2007.00496.x

Bowlby, J. (1982). *Attachment and loss: Vol. 1 attachment* (2nd ed.). New York: Basic Books.

Brown, L. M. (1998). Ethnic stigma as a contextual experience: A possible selves perspective. *Personality and Social Psychology Bulletin, 24*, 163–172.

Buhrmester, M. D., Blanton, H., & Swann, W. B. (2011). Implicit self-esteem: Nature, measurement, and a new way forward. *Journal of Personality and Social Psychology, 100*, 365–385. doi:10.1037/a0021341

Byrne, B. M., Gavin, M., & Worth, D. A. (1996). The Shavelson model revisited: Testing for the structure of academic self-concept across pre-, early, and late adolescents. *Journal of Educational Psychology, 88*, 215–228. doi:10.1037/0022-0663.88.2.215

Carlson, C., Uppal, S., & Prosser, E. C. (2000). Ethnic differences in processes contributing to the self-esteem of early adolescent girls. *The Journal of Early Adolescence, 20*, 44–67. doi:10.1177/0272431600020001003

Clark, K. B., & Clark, M. P. (1947). Racial identification and preference in Negro children. In T. M. Newcombe & E. L. Hartley (Eds.), *Readings in social psychology* (pp. 169–178). New York: Holt, Rinehart & Winston.

Cooley, C. H. (1902). *Human nature and the social order.* New York: Free Press.

Crocker, J., & Luhtanen, R. (1990). Collective self-esteem and ingroup bias. *Journal of Personality and Social Psychology, 58*, 60–67. doi:10.1037//0022-3514.58.1.60

Crocker, J., & Major, B. (1989). Social stigma and self-esteem: The self-protective properties of stigma. *Psychological Review, 96*, 608–630. doi:10.1037/0033-295X.96.4.608

Crocker, J., & Wolfe, C. T. (2001). Contingencies of self-worth. *Psychological Review, 108*, 593–623. doi:10.1037/0033-295X.108.3.593

den Brok, P., van Tartwijk, J., Wubbels, T., & Veldman, I. (2010). The differential effect of the teacher-student interpersonal relationship on student outcomes for students with different ethnic backgrounds. *British Journal of Educational Psychology, 80*, 199–221. doi:10.1348/000709909X465632

Doppen, F. H. (2007). Now what? Rethinking civic education in The Netherlands. *Education, Citizenship and Social Justice, 2*, 103–118.

Emler, N. (2001). *Self-esteem: The costs and causes of low self-worth.* York, UK: Joseph Rowntree Foundation.

Erikson, E. H. (1966). The concept of identity in race relations: Notes and queries. *Daedalus, 95*, 145–177.

Ewing, A. R., & Taylor, A. R. (2009). The role of child gender and ethnicity in teacher–child relationship quality and children's behavioral adjustment in preschool. *Early Childhood Research Quarterly, 24*, 92–105. doi:10.1016/j.ecresq.2008.09.002

Falk, C. F., & Heine, S. J. (2014). What is implicit self-esteem, and does it vary across cultures? *Personality and Social Psychology Review, 19*, 177–198. doi:10.1177/001872675400700202

Faruggia, S. P., Chen, C., Greenberger, E., Dmitrieva, J., & Macek, P. (2004). Adolescent self-esteem in cross-cultural perspective: Testing measurement equivalence and a mediation model. *Journal of Cross-Cultural Psychology, 35*, 719–733. doi:10.1177/0022022104270114

Festinger, L. (1954). A theory of social comparison processes. *Human Relations, 7*(2), 117–140.

French, S. E., Seidman, E., Allen, L., & Aber, J. L. (2006). The development of ethnic identity during adolescence. *Developmental Psychology, 42*, 1–10. doi:10.1037/0012-1649.42.1.1

Graham, S. (2006). Peer victimization in school: Exploring the ethnic context. *Current Directions in Psychological Science, 15*, 317–321.

Gray-Little, B., & Hafdahl, A. R. (2000). Factors influencing racial comparisons of self-esteem: A quantitative review. *Psychological Bulletin, 126*(1), 26–54. doi:10.1037//0033-2909.126.1.26

Greenberger, E., & Chen, C. (1996). Perceived family relationships and depressed mood in early and late adolescence: A comparison of European and Asian Americans. *Developmental Psychology, 32*, 707–716.

Greene, M. J., & Way, N. (2005). Self-esteem trajectories among ethnic minority adolescents: A growth curve analysis of the patterns and predictors of change. *Journal of Research on Adolescence, 15*, 151–178. doi:10.1111/j.1532-7795.2005.00090.x

Greenwald, A. G., & Banaji, M. R. (1995). Implicit social cognition: Attitudes, self-esteem and stereotypes. *Psychological Review, 102*, 4–27.

Hamre, B. K., Pianta, R. C., Downer, J. T., & Mashburn, A. J. (2007). Teachers' perceptions of conflict with young students: Looking beyond problem behaviors. *Social Development, 17*, 115–136. doi:10.1111/j.1467-9507.2007.00418.x

Harter, S. (1982). The perceived competence scale for children. *Child Development, 53*, 87–97.

Harter, S. (1999). *The construction of the self*. New York: The Guilford Press.

Harter, S. (2006). The self. In W. Damon (Series Ed.) & N. Eisenberg (Vol. Ed.) *Handbook of child psychology: Vol. 3 Social, emotional, and personality development* (6th ed.). Hoboken, NJ: Wiley.

Heatherton, T. F., & Polivy, J. (1991). Development and validation of a scale for measuring state self-esteem. *Journal of Personality and Social Psychology, 60*, 895–910.

Heine, S. J., Lehman, D. R., Markus, H. R., & Kitayama, S. (1999). Is there a universal need for positive self-regard? *Psychological Review, 106*, 794.

Hetts, J. J., & Pelham, B. W. (2001). A case for the nonconscious self-concept. In G. B. Moskowitz (Ed.), *Cognitive social psychology: The Princeton symposium on the legacy and future of social cognition* (pp. 105–123). Mahwah, NJ: Lawrence Erlbaum.

Hetts, J. J., Sakuma, M., & Pelham, B. W. (1999). Two roads to positive regard: Implicit and explicit self-evaluation and culture. *Journal of Experimental Social Psychology, 35*, 512–559. doi:10.1006/jesp.1999.1391

Hughes, D., Witherspoon, D., Rivas-Drake, D., & West-Bey, N. (2009). Received ethnic-racial socialization messages and youths' academic and behavioral outcomes: Examining the mediating role of ethnic identity and self-esteem. *Cultural Diversity & Ethnic Minority Psychology, 15*, 112–124. doi:10.1037/a0015509

James, W. (1890). *Principles of psychology*. Chicago: Encyclopedia Britannica.

Jordan, C. H., Spencer, S. J., Zanna, M. P., Hoshino-Browne, E., & Correll, J. (2003). Secure and defensive high self-esteem. *Journal of Personality and Social Psychology, 85*, 969–978. doi:10.1037/0022-3514.85.5.969

Juvonen, J., Nishina, A., & Graham, S. (2006). Ethnic diversity and perceptions of safety in urban middle schools. *Psychological Science, 17*, 393–400.

Kahn, M. (2008). Multicultural education in the United States: Reflections. *Intercultural Education, 19*, 527–536. doi:10.1080/14675980802568327

Kardiner, A., & Ovesey, L. (1951). *The Mark of oppression*. New York: Norton.

Kinket, B., & Verkuyten, M. (1997). Levels of ethnic self-identification and social context. *Social Psychology Quarterly, 60*, 338–354.

Ladd, G. W., Kochenderfer-Ladd, B., & Rydell, A.-M. (2010). Children's interpersonal skills and school-based relationships. In P. K. Smith & C. H. Hart (Eds.), *The Wiley-Blackwell handbook of childhood social development* (2nd ed., pp. 181–206). Oxford: Wiley-Blackwell.

Leary, M. R., & Baumeister, R. F. (2000). The nature and function of self-esteem: Sociometer theory. In M. Zanna (Ed.), *Advances in experimental social psychology* (Vol. 32, pp. 1–62). San Diego, CA: Academic Press.

Margalit, M. (2004). Second-generation research on resilience: Social-emotional aspects of children with learning disabilities. *Learning Disabilities Research & Practice, 19*, 45–48. doi:10.1111/j.1540-5826.2004.00088.x

Markus, H. R., & Kitayama, S. (2010). Cultures and selves: A cycle of mutual constitution. *Perspectives on Psychological Science, 5*, 420–430. doi:10.1177/1745691610375557

Marsh, H. W. (1990). The structure of academic self-concept. *Journal of Educational Psychology, 82*, 623–636.

Marsh, H. W., Trautwein, U., Lüdtke, O., & Köller, O. (2008). Social comparison and big-fish-little-pond effects on self-concept and other self-belief constructs: Role of generalized and specific others. *Journal of Educational Psychology, 100*, 510–524. doi:10.1037/0022-0663.100.3.510

Masten, A. S. (2001). Ordinary magic: Resilience processes in development. *American Psychologist, 56*, 227–238. doi:10.1037//0003-066X.56.3.227

Masten, A. S. (2007). Resilience in developing systems: Progress and promise as the fourth wave rises. *Development and Psychopathology, 19*, 921–930. doi:10.1017/S0954579407000442

Mead, G. H. (1934). *Mind, self and society*. Chicago: University of Chicago Press.

Morrison, K. R., Plaut, V. C., & Ybarra, O. (2010). Predicting whether multiculturalism positively or negatively influences White Americans' intergroup attitudes: The role of ethnic identification. *Personality and Social Psychology Bulletin, 36*, 1648–1661. doi:10.1177/0146167210386118

Motti-Stefanidi, F., & Masten, A. S. (2013). School Success and school engagement of immigrant children and adolescents. *European Psychologist, 18*, 126–135. doi:10.1027/1016-9040/a000139

Mruk, C. (2013). *Self-esteem and positive psychology: Research, theory, and practice*. New York: Springer.

Murray, C., Waas, G. A., & Murray, K. M. (2008). Child race and gender as moderators of the association between teacher-child relationships and school adjustment. *Psychology in the Schools, 45,* 562–578. doi:10.1002/pits

Osborne, J. W. (1997). Race and academic disidentification. *Journal of Educational Psychology, 89,* 728–735.

Pascoe, E. A., & Smart Richman, L. (2009). Perceived discrimination and health: A meta-analytic review. *Psychological Bulletin, 135,* 531–554. doi:10.1037/a0016059

Pelham, B.W., & Hetts, J. J. (1999). Implicit and explicit personal and social identity: Toward a more complete understanding of the social self. In T. R. Tyler, R. M. Kramer, & O. P. John (Eds.), *The psychology of the social self* (pp. 115–143). Mahwah, NJ: Erlbaum.

Phinney, J. S., Berry, J. W., Vedder, P., & Liebkind, K. (2006). The acculturation experience: Attitudes, identities, and behaviors of immigrant youth. In J. W. Berry, J. S. Phinney, D. L. Sam, & P. Vedder (Eds.), *Immigrant youth in cultural transition: Acculturation, identity, and adaptation across national contexts* (pp. 71–116). Mahwah, NJ: Lawrence Erlbaum.

Pianta, R. C., Hamre, B. K., & Stuhlman, M. (2003). Relationships between teachers and children. In W. M. Reynolds & G. E. Miller (Eds.), *Handbook of psychology* (Vol. 7, pp. 199–234). Hoboken, NJ: Wiley.

Plaut, V. C., Garnett, F. G., Buffardi, L. E., & Sanchez-Burks, J. (2011). "What about me?" Perceptions of exclusion and whites' reactions to multiculturalism. *Journal of Personality and Social Psychology, 101*(2), 337–353. doi:10.1037/a0022832

Portera, A. (2008). Intercultural education in Europe: Epistemological and semantic aspects. *Intercultural Education, 19*(6), 481–491. doi:10.1080/14675980802568277

Robins, R. W., & Trzesniewski, K. H. (2005). Self-esteem development across the lifespan. *Current Directions in Psychological Science, 14,* 158–163. doi:10.1111/j.0963-7214.2005.00353.x

Roorda, D. L., Koomen, H. M. Y., Spilt, J. L., & Oort, F. J. (2011). The Influence of affective teacher-student relationships on students' school engagement and achievement: A meta-analytic approach. *Review of Educational Research, 81,* 493–529. doi:10.3102/0034654311421793

Rosenberg, M. (1965). *Society and the adolescent self-image*. Princeton, NJ: Princeton University Press.

Rosenberg, M. (1979). *Conceiving the self*. New York: Basic Books.

Rowley, S. J., Sellers, R. M., Chavous, T. M., & Smith, M. A. (1998). The relationship between racial identity and self-esteem in African American college and high school students. *Journal of Personality and Social Psychology, 74,* 715–724.

Rudasill, K. M., Reio, T. G., Stipanovic, N., & Taylor, J. E. (2010). A longitudinal study of student-teacher relationship quality, difficult temperament, and risky behavior from childhood to early adolescence. *Journal*

of School Psychology, 48, 389–412. doi:10.1016/j.jsp.2010.05.001

Ryan, R. M., Stiller, J. D., & Lynch, J. H. (1994). Representations of relationships to teachers, parents, and friends as predictors of academic motivation and self-esteem. *Journal of Early Adolescence, 14,* 226–249. doi:10.1177/027243169401400207

Saft, E. W., & Pianta, R. C. (2001). Teachers' perceptions of their relationships with students: Effects of child age, gender, and ethnicity of teachers and children. *School Psychology Quarterly, 16,* 125–141. doi:10.1521/scpq.16.2.125.18698

Savin-William, R. C., & Demo, D. H. (1984). Developmental change and stability in adolescent self-concept. *Developmental Psychology,* 1100–1110. doi:10.1037/0012-1649.20.6.1100

Schmitt, D. P., & Allik, J. (2005). Simultaneous administration of the Rosenberg Self-Esteem Scale in 53 nations: Exploring the universal and culture-specific features of global self-esteem. *Journal of Personality and Social Psychology, 89,* 623–642. doi:10.1037/0022-3514.89.4.623

Schmitt, M. T., Branscombe, N. R., Postmes, T., & Garcia, A. (2014). The consequences of perceived discrimination for psychological well-being: A meta-analytic review. *Psychological Bulletin, 140,* 921–948. doi:10.1037/a0035754

Scott, W. A., Scott, R., & McCabe, M. (1991). Family relationships and children's personality: A cross-cultural, cross-source comparison. *British Journal of Social Psychology, 30,* 1–20. doi:10.1111/j.2044-8309.1991.tb00919.x

Shavelson, R. J., Hubner, J. J., & Stanton, G. C. (1976). Self-concept: Validation of construct interpretations. *Review of Educational Research, 46,* 407–441.

Simmons, R. G. (1978). Blacks and high self-esteem: A puzzle. *Social Psychology, 41,* 54–57.

Snijders, T. A. B., & Bosker, R. J. (1999). *Multilevel analysis: An introduction to basic and advanced multilevel modeling*. London: Sage.

Sowislo, J. F., & Orth, U. (2013). Does low self-esteem predict depression and anxiety? A meta-analysis of longitudinal studies. *Psychological Bulletin, 139,* 213–240. doi:10.1037/a0028931

Stephan, C. W., Renfro, L., & Stephan, W. G. (2004). The evaluation of multicultural education programs: Techniques and meta-analysis. In W. G. Stephan & P. G. Vogt (Eds.), *Education programs for improving intergroup relations: Theory, research, and practice* (pp. 227–242). New York: Teacher College Press.

Suárez-Orozco, C., & Pimentel, A. (2009). The significance of relationships: Academic engagement and achievement among newcomer immigrant youth. *Teachers College Record, 111,* 712–749.

Tajfel, H., & Turner, J. C. (1979). An integrative theory of intergroup conflict. In W. G. Austin & S. Worchel (Eds.), *The social psychology of intergroup relations* (pp. 33–47). Monterey, CA: Brooks/Cole.

Thijs, J., & Verkuyten, M. (2008). Peer victimization and academic achievement in a multiethnic sample: The role of perceived academic self-efficacy. *Journal of Educational Psychology, 100,* 754–764. doi:10.1037/a0013155

Thijs, J., Verkuyten, M., & Helmond, P. (2010). A further examination of the Big-Fish-Little-Pond Effect: Perceived position in class, class size, and gender comparisons. *Sociology of Education, 83,* 333–345. doi:10.1177/0038040710383521

Thijs, J., Westhof, S., & Koomen, H. (2012). Ethnic incongruence and the student-teacher relationship: The perspective of ethnic majority teachers. *Journal of School Psychology, 50*(2), 257–273. doi:10.1016/j.jsp.2011.09.004

Triandis, H. C. (2001). Individualism-collectivism and personality. *Journal of Personality, 69*(6), 907–24. Retrieved from http://www.ncbi.nlm.nih.gov/pubmed/11767823

Trzesniewski, K. H., Donnellan, M. B., & Robins, R. W. (2003). Stability of self-esteem across the life span. *Journal of Personality and Social Psychology, 84,* 205–220. doi:10.1037/0022-3514.84.1.205

Twenge, J. M., & Crocker, J. (2002). Race and self-esteem: Meta-analyses comparing Whites, Blacks, Hispanics, Asians, and American Indians and comment on Gray-Little and Hafdahl (2000). *Psychological Bulletin, 128,* 371–408. doi:10.1037//0033-2909.128.3.371

Umaña-Taylor, A. J., Quintana, S. M., Lee, R. M., Cross, W. E., Rivas-Drake, D., Schwartz, S. J., et al. (2014). Ethnic and racial identity during adolescence and into young adulthood: An integrated conceptualization. *Child Development, 85,* 21–39. doi:10.1111/cdev.12196

van Geel, M., & Vedder, P. (2010). Multicultural attitudes among adolescents: The role of ethnic diversity in the classroom. *Group Processes & Intergroup Relations, 14,* 549–558. doi:10.1177/1368430210379007

Verkuyten, M. (1994). Self-esteem among ethnic minority youth in western countries. *Social Indicators Research, 32,* 21–47.

Verkuyten, M. (2005). The puzzle of high self-esteem among ethnic minorities: Comparing explicit and implicit self-esteem. *Self and Identity, 4,* 171–192. doi:10.1080/13576500444000290

Verkuyten, M., Kinket, B., & van der Wielen, C. (1997). Preadolescents' understanding of ethnic discrimination. *The Journal of Genetic Psychology, 158,* 97–112. doi:10.1080/00221329709596655

Verkuyten, M., & Thijs, J. (2001). Peer victimization and self-esteem of ethnic minority group children. *Journal of Community and Applied Social Psychology, 11,* 227–234. doi:10.1002/casp.628

Verkuyten, M., & Thijs, J. (2002). Racist victimization among children in The Netherlands: The effect of ethnic group and school. *Ethnic and Racial Studies, 25,* 310–331. doi:10.1080/0141987012010950

Verkuyten, M., & Thijs, J. (2004a). Global and ethnic self-esteem in school context: Minority and majority

groups in The Netherlands. *Social Indicators Research, 67,* 253–281.

Verkuyten, M., & Thijs, J. (2004b). Psychological disengagement from the academic domain among ethnic minority adolescents in The Netherlands. *British Journal of Educational Psychology, 74,* 109–125.

Verkuyten, M., & Thijs, J. (2006). Ethnic discrimination and global self-worth in early adolescents: The mediating role of ethnic self-esteem. *International Journal of Behavioral Development, 30,* 107–116. doi:10.1177/0165025406063573

Verkuyten, M., & Thijs, J. (2013). Multicultural education and inter-ethnic attitudes. *European Psychologist, 18,* 179–190. doi:10.1027/1016-9040/a000152

Verschueren, K., Doumen, S., & Buyse, E. (2012). Relationships with mother, teacher, and peers: Unique and joint effects on young children' s self-concept. *Attachment & Human Development, 14,* 233–248. doi:10.1080/14616734.2012.672263

Verschueren, K., & Koomen, H. M. Y. (2012). Teacher-child relationships from an attachment perspective. *Attachment & Human Development, 14,* 205–211. doi:10.1080/14616734.2012.672260

Verschueren, K., & Marcoen, A. (1999). Representation of self and socioemotional competence in kindergartners: Differential and combined effects of attachment to mother and to father. *Child Development, 70,* 183–201.

Verschueren, K., Marcoen, A., & Buyck, P. (1998). Five-year-olds' behaviorally presented self-esteem: Relations to self-perceptions and stability across a three-year period. *The Journal of Genetic Psychology, 159,* 273–279. doi:10.1080/00221329809596151

Whitesell, N. R., Mitchell, C. M., Kaufman, C. E., & Spicer, P. (2006). Developmental trajectories of personal and collective self-concept among American Indian adolescents. *Child Development, 77,* 1487–1503. doi:10.1111/j.1467-8624.2006.00949.x

Wigfield, A., Eccles, J. S., Iver, D. M., Reuman, D. A., & Midgley, C. (1991). Transitions during early adolescence: Changes in children's domain-specific self-perceptions and general self-esteem across the transition to junior high school. *Developmental Psychology, 27,* 552–565.

Wong, C. Eccles, J. S., & Sameroff, A. (2003). The influence of ethnic discrimination and ethnic identification on African American adolescents' school and socioemotional adjustment. *Journal of Personality, 71,* 1197–232. Retrieved from http://www.ncbi.nlm.nih.gov/pubmed/14633063

Zirkel, S. (2005). Ongoing Issues of racial and ethnic stigma in education 50 years after Brown v. Board. *The Urban Review, 37,* 107–126. doi:10.1007/s11256-005-0004-4

Zirkel, S. (2008). The Influence of multicultural educational practices on student outcomes and intergroup relations. *Teachers College Record, 110,* 1147–1181.

Parental Educational Involvement and Latino Children's Academic Attainment

Rosario Ceballo, Rosanne M. Jocson, and Francheska Alers-Rojas

Abstract

A preponderance of research documents the benefits of parental educational involvement on children's academic performance. However, the majority of this work has primarily focused on European American children in middle to upper income homes as well as examining mostly school-based forms of parental involvement. By contrast, this chapter relies on developmental theories and a resilience framework to address parental educational involvement as a protective factor, bolstering the academic performance of low-income, Latino children specifically. We examine parental educational involvement across Latino children's elementary through high school years. Further, we conceptualize parental involvement as a multidimensional construct, incorporating parental behaviors and strategies beyond the traditionally measured aspects of parental participation in school-based activities (e.g., PTO meetings, parent-teacher conferences). Finally, we discuss implications, provide suggestions for future research directions, and highlight the importance of incorporating Latino cultural values in future work.

Historical Overview

Researchers typically define parental educational involvement as encompassing all of the resources, via interactions with their children and schools, that parents devote to their children's academic success (Grolnick and Slowiaczek 1994; Hill and Tyson 2009). A large body of research firmly establishes the benefits of parental educational involvement on children's scholastic achievement, academic motivation, and school engagement (Crosnoe 2001; Fan et al. 2012; Fan and Chen 2001; Hill et al. 2004; Hill and Tyson 2009; Rasinski and Stevenson 2005; Seginer 2006; Sheldon and Epstein 2005). These findings are consistently reported even while controlling for prior academic achievement, in some cases, and with samples across a variety of grade levels. Thus, for decades, social science researchers, educators, and policy experts have lauded the benefits of parental involvement on

R. Ceballo (✉) · R.M. Jocson · F. Alers-Rojas
University of Michigan, Ann Arbor, MI, USA
e-mail: rosarioc@umich.edu

© The Editor(s) 2017   343
N.J. Cabrera and B. Leyendecker (eds.), *Handbook on Positive
Development of Minority Children and Youth*, DOI 10.1007/978-3-319-43645-6_21

children's education. However, the bulk of this research has been conducted with European American children in middle to upper income homes, and few researchers have addressed the role of parental involvement in the educational performance of racial/ethnic minority youth (Fan et al. 2012). To expand upon the work addressing the importance of parent involvement, the present chapter examines parental educational involvement as a protective factor supporting the academic achievement of low-income, Latino children. Before continuing, we should note that when referring to "Latinos," we are specifically referring to Spanish-speaking people who trace their ethnic heritage to Mexico, Central and South America, and the Caribbean. It is, thus, important to highlight the tremendous heterogeneity that exists among Latino families. In addition to differences in national origins, Latino families represent a diversity of immigration histories, socioeconomic statuses, racial phenotypes, and educational backgrounds—within group distinctions that researchers are only now beginning to address with Latino samples.

National data indicates that the educational attainment of Latino youth remains disturbingly low, as evidenced by numerous different indicators of achievement (Hill and Torres 2010). According to data from the National Center for Educational Statistics [NCES] (2007) and the U. S. Census Bureau (2007), Latino youth have lower achievement test scores, higher drop out rates, and lower college attendance compared to European American and African American youth. Within Latino groups, stark gender differences in rates of educational attainment are also present, highlighting a particularly disadvantaged position for Latino males. Compared to Latinas, Latino males have lower reading scores in 12th grade, higher high school drop out rates, lower college enrollments, and lower rates of completing college degrees (Kena et al. 2015). Notably, poverty rates among Latino families are disproportionately high, even for those families with an employed adult living in the home. Whereas 8 % of non-Latino White children live in poverty, over three times more Latino children, 29 %, live below the poverty line (U.S.

Census Bureau 2007). Thus, the conglomeration of social and economic stressors associated with poverty and new immigrant status likely play a potent role in the educational underperformance of Latino youth. The negative impact of growing up in poverty on Latino youth's educational achievement is further compounded by the disproportionate enrollment of Latino students in lower quality, poorly equipped schools, English language barriers, and discriminatory educational practices (Ceballo et al. 2010; Eamon 2005; Hill and Torres 2010; Zambrana 2011). Despite the numerous structural obstacles faced by many Latino children, our chapter will highlight sources of strength in Latino families in support of educational achievement.

Theoretical Perspectives Explaining Latino Youth's Academic Underachievement

Historically, Latino children's academic achievement was explained using deficit-oriented models in which European American, middle class families were exalted as the normative group (Garcia Coll et al. 1996, 2002). Academic "deficiencies" could therefore be explained by the ways in which low-income Latino homes and parents differed from the normative, mostly middle class, European American standard. From this vantage point, the scholastic underachievement of poor Latino youth was attributed to less stimulating home environments, poorer academic motivation, linguistic deficits, lower self-esteem, poorer cognitive skills, and difficulties with delaying gratification (Ceballo et al. 2010; Hill and Craft 2003). Not surprisingly, a lack of parental involvement in children's education was yet another explanation proffered for Latino youth's lower academic attainment. Strikingly absent from these explanations was any accounting of the socioeconomic and institutional disadvantages that many Latino families face as well as a blatant confounding of race/ethnicity with socioeconomic class, such that poor Latinos came to represent all Latinos. Poor, Latino parents, for example, may be less active in their children's schools due to demanding work schedules (e.g., working night shifts and multiple jobs), language barriers, unfamiliarity with the American school system, and difficulties with transportation rather than a lack of concern or investment in their children's education (Ceballo et al. 2010; Garcia Coll et al. 2002).

In response to such deficit approaches, one alternative perspective proposed by some researchers was a cultural discontinuity perspective (Reese and Gallimore 2000; Tyler et al. 2008), highlighting a cultural mismatch between home practices and school norms such that poor Latino parents may not understand the parental roles and practices expected by American teachers and school staff. From this perspective, the lack of congruence between Latino family norms (e.g., deferring to teachers' academic authority) and the expectations of American schools (e.g., valuing parental participation in school) may serve as barriers to parental school involvement. Additionally, the high emphasis placed on individual rights and assertive self-expression in American schools may be inconsistent with Latino values promoting harmonious social relationships and the importance of obedience and respect toward elders and authority figures. In fact, the Spanish word for education, *educación,* encompasses more than mere academic attainment, it also broadly incorporates acquiring strong moral values, integrity, and responsibility (Halgunseth et al. 2006; Tyler et al. 2008). These types of cultural differences may promote feelings of uncertainty and discomfort among some Latino parents about the parental roles and practices expected from them in American schools (Reese and Gallimore 2000); yet, by the same token, many schools may not accommodate their parental outreach practices to adopt to new immigrant groups.

However, the academic underachievement of some racial/ethnic minority students cannot be entirely explained by a cultural discontinuity perspective, as some racial/ethnic minority children succeed academically despite experiencing cultural differences between their home and school contexts. Another theoretical approach

was proposed by Ogbu's (1981, 1992) cultural-ecological theory. According to Ogbu, awareness of racially discriminatory practices in education and employment may dissuade many racial/ethnic minorities from adopting mainstream beliefs and socialization norms. Ogbu theorized that this was particularly true for African Americans whose ancestors were involuntarily brought to the United States as slaves. However, Ogbu's distinction between racial/ethnic groups with "voluntary" versus "involuntary" histories of migration to the United States seems far less applicable to Latino families. Many Latinos voluntarily immigrate to the U.S. for economic and educational opportunities, especially for the advancement of future generations (Perreira et al. 2006). In spite of these "voluntary" decisions to migrate, structural factors that include, but are not limited to, poverty, limited maternal education, low literacy levels, attendance in low-quality under-resourced schools, placement into lower track classes, limited neighborhood resources, discrimination, and acculturative stress may nevertheless compromise the academic performance of many Latino youth (Zambrana 2011). Across several studies, for instance, low-income Latino adolescents report facing high levels of racial/ethnic discrimination, and experiences of discrimination are, in turn, associated with worse academic performance and school engagement (Benner and Graham 2011; Delgado et al. 2011). Further, Latino parents and children may feel discouraged from investing in educational pursuits, because they are aware of the educational barriers and lack of opportunities afforded to them (Becerra 2012). Thus, even though Latinos were not involuntarily brought to the U.S. as slaves (a crucial factor in Ogbu's theorizing), many Latino families face severely restrictive social and economic conditions that cannot be easily overcome in this country.

A more expansive theoretical model was presented by Okagaki's (2001) triarchic model of minority children's school achievement. According to Okagaki (2001) three factors are critical in explaining the academic performance of poor, racial/ethnic minority students: (1) the form and perceived function of education, (2) family cultural norms and beliefs about education and development, and (3) child characteristics. For example, awareness of discriminatory practices and lack of opportunities in education and employment may dissuade some minority students from putting effort into their schoolwork, whereas the belief in the long-term benefits of education (e.g., as a means to improve their family's social and economic condition) may encourage others to do well in school. Although cultural discontinuity may inhibit some parents' involvement in schools, for instance, Latino parents may promote academic success in other ways, as in the case of a Latino parent working multiple jobs to ensure that their child has ample time and resources to study (Suarez-Orozco 1993, as cited in Okagaki 2001). Finally, familial, school, and cultural influences on academic achievement should always be considered in conjunction with individual child characteristics, like intelligence and temperament.

A past focus on the academic underachievement of poor Latino youth and their familial deficiencies effectively suppressed work on the strengths and resources of academically successful Latino children. Consequently, far less theory and research, to date, has focused on factors that promote academic achievement and resilience among Latino youth. While resilience research is fraught with complex definitional issues, "resilience" generally refers to the ability to maintain positive functioning despite experiencing significant adversity (Zolkoski and Bullock 2012). From a resilience perspective, a compelling research question would be: what are the parenting values and behaviors that foster the academic success of some Latino children despite numerous socioeconomic constraints and life stressors? Recently, more researchers have approached empirical investigations from a resilience perspective. Rather than examine factors accounting for academic underperformance, researchers have begun to investigate factors that promote academic success among Latino youth, such as parental involvement in education

(Alfaro et al. 2006; Ceballo 2004; Ceballo et al. 2014; Cruz-Santiago and Ramirez Garcia 2011; Sánchez et al. 2005).

Relatedly, placing this work in a developmental context provides a critical grounding for studying parental involvement. Developmental perspectives underscore changes in the nature of parental involvement as children move through different developmental transitions and stages of schooling. As children move from preschool to high school, for instance, some evidence indicates that parental educational involvement declines (Dearing et al. 2006; Hoover-Dempsey et al. 2005). In so doing, parental involvement strategies are also likely to shift from checking homework to providing motivational support at home, and from helping in classrooms to attending school initiated events at school (Seginer 2006). Although parents may adopt different strategies during different developmental periods, parental educational involvement continues to be related to positive educational outcomes throughout high school. For instance, a small body of quantitative and qualitative research, reveals a positive influence of parental involvement, specifically reading-supportive behavior and beliefs, on older children's and adolescents' (4th through 12th grades) reading motivation and activity (Klauda 2009).

The types of educational outcomes that are typically studied in relation to parental involvement become broader and more complex across later developmental periods. In particular, studies on preschool-aged children highlight school readiness and early literacy skills (e.g., Kingston et al. 2013), whereas studies on elementary and middle school youth often investigate a larger set of school-related outcomes such as grades, reading and math achievement, academic motivation, and degree completion (Hill and Tyson 2009; Jeynes 2007). Perhaps most importantly, it is quite possible that the strength of the relations between parental involvement and school achievement change across different developmental stages. In other words, certain parenting strategies like school-based practices may decline in effectiveness from elementary to middle school-aged children, whereas other aspects of parental involvement (e.g., reading-supportive behaviors) may have an increasingly positive impact on achievement (Hill and Tyson 2009). Yet again, a paucity of work examines Latino parents' educational involvement from a developmental perspective. Hence, in the present chapter, we use a developmental approach to organize our review of the existing literature while relying upon a resiliency framework to examine parental educational involvement in Latino children's academic performance from elementary through the secondary schools years.

Current Research Questions

Going forward, it is important to relinquish a deficit-oriented approach and instead, examine the parental values and behaviors that promote positive academic performance despite the adverse social and economic conditions that many poor, Latino children encounter. Rather than simplifying our investigations of these relations, we argue for the incorporation of greater complexity and contextualizing in this field. Firstly, broadening our definition of what "counts" as parental educational involvement will mean expanding our focus beyond traditional measures of parents' school-based participation to identify other parenting approaches used by Latino parents to promote academic achievement. Secondly, we must examine how the effects of parental educational involvement vary across different developmental periods and are moderated by different familial factors, such as socioeconomic class, immigrant and generational status, and the endorsement of culturally-specific values. Relatedly, research must now attend to the vast heterogeneity within Latino groups by specifying how parental educational involvement functions in specific Latino ethnic subgroups, residing in specific geographical locations, and of particular generational cohorts.

Definitional Issues, Research Measurement, and Methodology

Despite growing scholarly acknowledgement that parental involvement in education is a multidimensional construct, measures of parental involvement remain remarkably unidimensional (Fan et al. 2012; Garcia Coll et al. 2002). Grolnick and Slowiaczek (1994) define parental involvement as the resources that parents dedicate to their children's education. In other words, parental involvement in education encompasses, "parents' interactions with schools and with their children to promote academic success" (Hill and Tyson 2009, p. 741). Even with such clear and straightforward definitions, no exact and consistent operationalization of parental educational involvement exists in the literature. Consequently, measures of parental involvement differ drastically across studies, ranging from parental valuing of education to parental assistance with homework to parent-child discussions about school.

Traditional frameworks for studying parental involvement typically distinguish between two major types of parental involvement strategies: school-based involvement and home-based involvement (Epstein and Sanders 2002; Hill and Tyson 2009; Seginer 2006; Shumow and Miller 2001). *School-based involvement* consists of practices such as attending parent-teacher conferences, talking with school personnel, and participating or volunteering in school activities and governance. *Home-based involvement* includes provision of educational activities and support for learning at home by, for example, engaging in cognitively stimulating activities, helping with homework, or discussing school activities. To date, the bulk of existing research on school-age children, regardless of children's developmental levels, assesses only school-based forms of parental involvement, adopting a narrow, unidimensional conceptualization of parental involvement (Cooper and Crosnoe 2007; Henry et al. 2011; Hill et al. 2004). Among

Latino families, high levels of parental school involvement are associated with more parental education, English language proficiency, and welcoming responsive school systems (Zambrana 2011).

In a recent meta-analysis on the types of parental involvement associated with achievement in middle school that included studies with diverse samples, Hill and Tyson (2009) confirmed the importance of parental involvement via another type of activity: academic socialization. *Academic socialization* refers to parents who have discussions about educational expectations, values, or utility with their children, link school subjects to current events, discuss learning strategies and future goals, and foster academic aspirations. The latter component, parents' academic aspirations and/or expectations, is consistently found to have strong associations with children's educational outcomes (Ceballo et al. 2014; Fan and Chen 2001; Fan et al. 2012; Juang and Silbereisen 2002). By many accounts, researchers report that Latino parents express high educational aspirations for their children (Garcia Coll et al. 2002; Hill and Torres 2010); only negative social stereotypes, unsupported by empirical evidence, profess otherwise (Seginer 2006). Still, parental aspirations regarding educational attainment appear to be all the more effective when they are directly communicated to children and when parent-child discussions broadly encompass many school-related topics, as documented in measures of academic socialization.

Beyond the parental strategies discussed thus far (e.g., home- and school-based involvement, academic socialization, and parents' academic expectations), viewing parental involvement in education as a multidimensional construct means expanding our conceptualization of this construct even further (Fan et al. 2012; Garcia Coll et al. 2002; Henry et al. 2011). Extending our conceptualization of parental involvement is especially important given that some studies report that more traditional, school-based forms of parental involvement are less effective with racial/ethnic minority youth. Specifically, using data from the National Education Longitudinal Study (NELS), researchers found that traditional measures of school-based involvement were better predictors of achievement for European American students than for Latino youth (Desimone 1999; Valadez 2002). Whereas parents' PTO participation increased the odds of taking algebra and advanced math classes for European American students, PTO participation had no such effect for Latino students in a large nationally representative sample of European American and Latino eighth graders (Valadez 2002). Likewise, parental monitoring of school behavior and progress positively affected European American students' enrollment in algebra but not Latino students' enrollment in algebra classes (Valadez 2002). Thus, it behooves researchers to rely upon a multidimensional framing of parental educational involvement, incorporating cultural, social, and familial factors that may impact parental involvement among different racial/ethnic groups.

Additionally, qualitative and ethnographic researchers have made important contributions to broadening our notions of parental educational involvement and thereby illuminating non-traditional strategies practiced by poor, Latino parents in support of their children's educational pursuits (Ceballo 2004; Lopez 2001; Menard-Warwick 2007; Sy 2006). Non-traditional strategies of parental involvement in education, particularly in homes where there are limited resources, may include finding children a quiet place to work in small, overcrowded homes, excusing children from certain family obligations in order to focus on school work or school activities, providing realistic examples of the types of jobs available without a high school degree, and making personal or economic sacrifices in support of children's schooling. Further, parental involvement in Latino families may include drawing upon complex and rich networks of extended family members and fictive kin (Ryan et al. 2010). Compared to non-Latino parents, Ryan et al. (2010) reported that Latino parents were more likely to draw upon assistance from significant others (e.g., older siblings, godparents) in addressing the academic needs of their children. An important next step, then, is to test the relations between such extended network support and children's academic achievement. In sum, broadening notions of what "counts" as parental involvement in children's education may be essential to understanding the ways in which Latino parents influence their children's academic performance. We turn now to a discussion of the effects of parental educational involvement across different levels of schooling among Latino parents and children specifically.

Empirical Findings

Elementary School-Aged Children

In samples with few or no Latino families, support for the protective role of parental educational involvement is revealed in associations between parental involvement and better academic orientations among young, economically disadvantaged children (Dearing et al. 2006; Englund et al. 2004). However, research on parental educational involvement and its relation to the academic achievement of Latino elementary school-aged children, in particular, is exceedingly sparse. With elementary school aged children, school-based forms of parental involvement, such as classroom assistance and providing help with schoolwork, are the most frequently assessed parental strategies (Seginer 2006). In a representative sample of 415 third through fifth graders (representing 7 public elementary schools in a southeastern U.S. community), parental school involvement (e.g., volunteering in classrooms and attending parent-teacher conferences) was greater among European American parents as compared to both Latino and African American parents (Lee and Bowen 2006). Further, in this same sample that included 62 Latino children, school-based parental involvement was related to higher academic achievement, but educational discussions at home about things learned at school and things that happened during the school day were not (Lee and Bowen 2006). Although Latino parents may face numerous obstacles to becoming involved in children's schools (e.g., language

barriers, stressful life demands, nuanced or overt discrimination), Lee and Bowen (2006) underscored that the benefits of school-based parental involvement on children's academic achievement occurred for all children—regardless of social class and racial/ethnic group.

Furthermore, some researchers have found associations between home-based parental involvement and positive academic outcomes among Latino elementary school children (Cooper et al. 2010). Utilizing nationally representative data from the kindergarten cohort of the Early Childhood Longitudinal Study (ECLS-K), Cooper et al. (2010) reported that home-learning activities predicted reading achievement in Latino families. Home learning activities included engaging children in activities related to art, building, games or puzzles, chores, nature or science, reading, singing, physical exercise, and telling stories at home. In this study, the effects of home learning activities were greater for Latinos, in comparison to African American and European American families. The benefits of home-based involvement are all the more important given the authors' finding that traditional forms of school-based involvement (e.g., attending open houses, PTA meetings, class events, and parent-teacher conferences) were not positively linked to achievement for Latino children, as they were for African American and European American children.

In a large, multiethnic sample (with Latino children) drawn from the National Institute of Child Health and Human Development (NICHD) Study of Early Child Care and Youth Development (SECCYD), El Nokali et al. (2010) did not find any significant associations between engagement in a number of different parental involvement strategies and children's academic achievement over time, from first through fifth grades. The unexpected lack of associations, in this case, may be due to the breadth of the parental involvement measure used; their measure encompassed traditional school-based involvement, parental investment in education, as well as educational attitudes and values. The authors speculate that parent involvement may be more efficacious when it is subject-specific. Yet another possible explanation may be that parental educational involvement is linked to more global achievement outcomes but not to the more domain-specific measures of achievement (reading, math, and vocabulary scores) that were used in this study. Support for the latter hypothesis is provided by Fan and Chen's (2001) meta-analysis where the relation between parental involvement and academic achievement was stronger in studies that represented academic achievement with global indicators (e.g., GPA) rather than subject specific indicators, like math or English grades.

Middle School Students

Most children transitioning to middle school deal with multiple physical, cognitive, social, and identity changes associated with early adolescence (Lerner and Steinberg 2009) while simultaneously adjusting to larger, more complex, and typically less supportive school environments (Roeser et al. 2000). Documented declines in students' academic performance and motivation during middle school are partially attributed to the mismatch between middle school structures (e.g., larger classes with more restrictions) and children's changing developmental needs (e.g., desires for greater autonomy and individual expressiveness) during early adolescence (Eccles et al. 1993; Wigfield et al. 2015). Moreover, for Latino students, the transition to middle school may bring additional stressors related to racial/ethnic discrimination and cultural barriers to participation in school activities (Martinez et al. 2004). Among 564 Latino and non-Latino middle school and high school students, Latino students reported higher rates of racial/ethnic discrimination and institutional barriers to school participation, such as prohibitive fees, missing events because of work schedules, and not receiving necessary information. Likewise, Latino parents also reported more unwelcoming encounters at their children's schools than the non-Latino parents (Martinez et al. 2004). Despite the challenges encountered by many Latino middle school children, parental

involvement and educationally-supportive practices may, nonetheless, enhance academic performance, especially if parental strategies fit the changing developmental needs of early adolescents.

It is not surprising, however, that traditional forms of parental involvement in education decline during children's middle school and high school years (Crosnoe 2001; Hill and Tyson 2009). This may be a response to adolescents' growing needs for autonomy or it may be due to parents' own lack of comfort with more difficult or complex school material (Crosnoe 2001; Martinez et al. 2004). Alternatively, declines in parental involvement, in some cases, may be driven by academically successful students, such that parents see less need to monitor children who are doing well academically (Crosnoe 2001). In general, parental involvement tends to shift from providing assistance within classrooms and help with homework for younger children to attending school-sponsored events and providing academic encouragement for young adolescents in middle school (Seginer 2006). Nevertheless, some evidence reveals positive relations between traditional school-based parental involvement and better academic functioning among Latino youth in middle school (Kuperminc et al. 2008).

Overall, parental involvement in middle school students' education is related to positive academic outcomes for children; further, Hill and Tyson's (2009) previously mentioned meta-analysis revealed that academic socialization had an even stronger and more positive relation to academic achievement in middle school than other forms of parental involvement, including both school- and home-based involvement. Based on 50 articles (representing 127 correlations), their meta-analysis included longitudinal and cross-sectional studies as well as articles using nationally representative datasets with European American, African American, Latino, and Asian youth. Across all racial/ethnic groups, academic socialization is one of the most likely forms of in-home parental involvement, encompassing parent-child discussions about school subjects, about educational values and utility, and about future plans. Further, academic socialization may be one of the most beneficial parenting strategies—precisely because it is compatible with young adolescents' advancing cognitive and decision-making skills, it facilitates the internalization of educational values, and it is not likely to interfere with students' needs for autonomy at school and with peers (Hill and Tyson 2009).

Accordingly, for Latino middle school students, home-based parental involvement strategies, especially parent-child discussions or parents' investment in academic socialization, are related to higher academic functioning. Several studies report that discussions regarding school-related matters were significantly related to better academic outcomes among Latino middle school students specifically (Eamon 2005; Valadez 2002; Woolley et al. 2009). Relying on a large, nationally representative data set, Valadez (2002) reported that parent-child discussions about school predicted Latino eighth graders' enrollment in algebra and advanced math classes. (Conversely, school-based parental involvement, like attendance at PTO meetings, increased the likelihood that European American students would enroll in advanced math classes.) Likewise, using data with a national sample of 388 Latino early adolescents, Eamon (2005) similarly found that parent–child discussions (about school-related issues and events outside of school) and cognitive stimulation in the home were associated with higher reading and math achievement. Additionally, while accounting for emotional support from parents and peers, Woolley et al. (2009) reported that parents' educational monitoring, including discussions about school-related activities and homework, was indirectly related to Latino middle school students' higher grades via increases in teacher support, positive school behaviors, and school satisfaction. Of note, these results differ from Lee and Bowen's (2006) findings with elementary school children and perhaps indicate that the importance of academic socialization increases with children's age.

High School Students

Several studies indicate that Latino parents' school-based involvement continues to play an influential role in adolescents' academic functioning throughout the high school years. In a study of 324 mostly Mexican, middle school and high school students, Kuperminc et al. (2008) reported significant associations between school-based parental involvement specifically and students' academic adjustment and reported that the association between parental involvement and academic functioning was stronger for students in high school than in middle school. Commenting on this unexpected finding, the authors noted the relative absence of a developmental perspective in this research area. In their sample, Latino middle school students reported higher levels of parental involvement than did high school students. Given the lower levels of parental involvement in high school, Kuperminc et al. (2008) speculate that parental involvement may be more salient for students when it occurs in high school, compared to middle school. In another study with 223 Latino, mostly Dominican American, ninth graders, school-based parental involvement and parental assistance with schoolwork at home were significantly and positively related to adolescents' educational expectations, academic values, and school effort (Ceballo et al. 2014). Ibañez et al. (2004) reported similar findings with a sample of 129 Mexican, mostly immigrant youth. School-based parental involvement was positively linked to adolescents' achievement motivation. More specifically, valuing school was related to adolescents' perceptions of traditional school-based parental involvement for high acculturated students, more so than for low acculturated students. Altogether, these findings confirm the influential role of school-based parental involvement during Latino adolescents' high school years.

Similar to school-based involvement, home-based forms of parental involvement and academic encouragement have also been associated with positive educational outcomes among Latino high school students (Alfaro et al. 2006; Ceballo et al. 2014; Fan et al. 2012; Martinez et al. 2004; Mena 2015). Once again, the potency of academic socialization to positively influence educational outcomes for Latino youth emerges in several studies. Relying upon data from the Educational Longitudinal Study with 1,919 Latino tenth graders, Fan et al. (2012) found that parental advice and communication about school matters was positively associated with Latino students' intrinsic motivation toward English and academic self-efficacy in English (but not Mathematics). These results remained while controlling for gender and socioeconomic class. More specifically, in this study, the researchers included questions tapping parental educational advice concerning a number of topics, such as selecting school courses, preparing for college entrance exams, applying to college, availability of jobs for high school graduates, current community, national or world events, and "things that are troubling your 10th grade student" (Fan et al. 2012, p. 25). In a similar fashion, using a scale of future-related discussions that tapped communication about different kinds of jobs, future career goals, and future interests, Ceballo et al. (2014) reported that such parent-adolescent discussions were significantly and positively related to adolescents' academic values and school effort. These results emerged while controlling for gender, immigrant status, and mothers' educational aspirations and while accounting for several other types of parental educational involvement.

To examine parental educational involvement as a multidimensional construct, Ceballo et al. (2014) surveyed a sample of Latino ninth grade high school students from low-income homes about an array of different types of parental involvement strategies. The results of an exploratory factor analysis identified six distinct and coherent components of parental educational involvement. Along with school-based involvement, home-based involvement, and future discussions (e.g., academic socialization), a fourth parental strategy was identified as "gift/sacrifice." The scale for "gift/sacrifice"

consisted of items assessing students' desire to succeed in school in order to help parents in the future, acquiring academic inspiration from parents' sacrifices, and wanting to do well academically because of parents' own hard work. While controlling for adolescents' age, gender, immigrant status, and mothers' educational aspirations, "gift/sacrifice" was positively related to higher academic values and school effort among Latino adolescents. Two of the identified parental involvement strategies that were associated with adolescents' academic outcomes—future discussions as well as "gift/sacrifice"—may be especially salient to low-income, Latino youth since they tap a desire to do well academically that is motivated by parents' hard work, sacrifice, and communication about the value of education for future opportunities. Moreover, such forms of parental involvement are not dependent upon learned knowledge or the accumulation of social resources. In essence, Latino parents and immigrant parents may effectively call upon non-traditional parental involvement practices, such as discussions of their own sacrifices, in order to bolster their children's academic functioning. Hence, a more comprehensive and culturally-specific understanding of parental educational involvement among poor, Latino families is highlighted by these findings and by researchers' efforts to expand our conceptualization of parental educational involvement.

Academic Performance of and Parental Involvement with Immigrant Latino Youth

According to demographers, immigrant youth, defined as those children (under 18 years of age) who are foreign-born or U.S.-born to immigrant parents, account for one-fourth of the nation's 75 million children (Passel 2011). Of these immigrant youth in the U.S., about 58 % are Latino. Typically, "first generation" refers to foreign-born children that immigrated to the U.S.; "second generation" consists of U.S.-born children with at least one immigrant parent; and "third generation" are U.S.-born children with two U. S.-born parents. Further, in 2009, there were approximately 1.1 million unauthorized, foreign-born children in the United States, and the majority of unauthorized children are children in Latino families (Passel 2011). "Unauthorized" immigrants are those who reside in the U.S. without the legal authority to do so. In some families, referred to as "mixed status" families, there may be both U.S.-born, citizen children as well as unauthorized, foreign-born children; similarly, different adults in the same family may have different legal statuses. In fact, an estimated 14.6 million people live in a mixed-status home with at least one unauthorized family member, and there are approximately 4 million citizen-children growing up with unauthorized parents, fearing deportation, in the United States (Suárez-Orozco et al. 2011). In families with unauthorized members, parents' ability to engage in school-based activities is restricted by a host of challenges, including severe economic hardship, grueling work conditions, and the fear of separation and deportation of family members. Consequently, immigrant Latino children in families with unauthorized members may face particularly elevated risks for academic underperformance; unfortunately, this highly vulnerable group also presents a uniquely challenging group for researchers to study because their very survival rests upon staying "in the shadows" (Suárez-Orozco et al. 2011).

By contrast, much more research has examined generational differences in the academic performance of Latino youth. Most recently, mounting evidence suggests that Latino youth of later generations, those whose families have been living in the U.S. for longer, perform worse academically than their earlier generation immigrant counterparts (foreign-born youth and children of foreign-born parents) (Hill and Torres 2010; Perreira et al. 2010; Portes and Rumbaut 2001). This pattern, whereby early generation youth exhibit more positive academic outcomes than their later generation peers, is referred to as the "immigrant paradox" (Garcia Coll and Marks 2009). It is strikingly counterintuitive, because as families acculturate

to the U.S., they typically gain social and economic resources such that we would expect children in these families to excel scholastically. Although the "immigrant paradox" cannot be explained by differences in socioeconomic status, self-esteem, or racial/ethnic identity, several alternative explanations have been offered. Researchers speculate that the immigrant paradox may be due to certain advantages associated with characteristics more commonly found in earlier immigrant generations such as fluency in multiple languages, the presence of strong parent-child bonds in immigrant families, immigrants' firm belief in the importance of education, or pre-migration factors that lead to immigrant selectivity (Crosnoe and Lopez Turley 2011). For example, some studies have linked bilingualism to higher academic performance, and parents with higher educational and professional training in their home countries may transmit strong educational values to their immigrant children (Crosnoe and Lopez Turley 2011).

In keeping with the immigrant paradox, some research indicates that the relation between parental educational involvement and academic outcomes is also stronger among Latino immigrant youth than among their later generation peers (Hill and Torres 2010; Plunkett et al. 2009). Ceballo et al. (2014) provide corroborating support for the immigrant paradox among a mostly Dominican American sample. In essence, the positive relation between parental involvement (e.g., school-based involvement and gift/sacrifice) and academic outcomes was stronger for immigrant, in comparison to non-immigrant, Latino youth. Perhaps, parental support for education assumes greater salience and import among immigrant adolescents who have experienced the hardships of moving to a new country and are therefore strongly motivated to make the most of new opportunities.

Undoubtedly, immigration poses an array of challenges for parents and children that include, but are not limited to, the loss of close relationships, inadequate and overcrowded housing conditions, isolation, legal uncertainty, English language barriers, renegotiation of ethnic identity, and adjusting to new school contexts (Perez et al. 2009). Some scholars report that immigrant parents prefer to engage in home-based parental involvement strategies, limiting their participation at children's schools (Seginer 2006). In their study of immigrant families, Garcia Coll et al. (2002) found that Dominican American parents cited language barriers, lack of education, long work hours, and lack of familiarity with the American school system as impediments to becoming involved in their children's American schools.

Policy Implications and Future Directions

While most parents engage in behavior to promote their children's academic success (perhaps a close to universal phenomena), our chapter focuses specifically on identifying culturally-salient mechanisms that foster academic achievement for Latino parents and children. As the largest and fastest-growing ethnic group in the United States, it can be no less than a national imperative that we find ways to improve the educational performance and attainment of Latino youth. On a practical level, we must invest in providing Latino youth with a sound education; our very future in maintaining a competitive work force and an engaged, productive citizenship depends upon these efforts. Collectively, a number of studies reviewed in this chapter illustrate the protective role of parental educational involvement—of various kinds and with different age groups of children—for promoting the academic performance of Latino youth (Alfaro et al. 2006; Ceballo et al. 2014; Cooper et al. 2010; Eamon 2005; Fan et al. 2012; Ibañez et al. 2004; Kuperminc et al. 2008; Lee and Bowen 2006; Martinez et al. 2004; Valadez 2002; Woolley et al. 2009). Yet, the immigrant paradox indicates that we need research on why these protective factors may decrease in effectiveness across generations.

Even more importantly, parental educational involvement is a malleable and viable target for prevention and intervention efforts (Henry et al. 2011). Relatedly, some scholars view parental involvement as key to closing the achievement gap across racial and socioeconomic divides with a clear necessity for providing culturally-sensitive programs to Latino populations (Henry et al. 2008; Hill and Tyson 2009). In a meta-analysis of 51 studies, Jeynes (2012) highlighted a significant relation between parental involvement programs and academic achievement for students from pre-elementary school through high school. Thus, increasing the ability of immigrant parents—authorized or unauthorized—to engage in their children's schools is good policy, as are policies that increase and support parental educational involvement in Latino families.

Research efforts should continue to expand and broaden our conceptualizations of parental educational involvement. A narrow, myopic, and unidimensional focus on traditional school-based involvement, such as participation in PTO meetings and attendance at parent-teacher conferences, will not broaden our knowledge base nor facilitate our ability to intervene as we move forward. In adopting a multidimensional approach to parental involvement, different dimensions of parental involvement should be measured separately, rather than combining factors into one summary composite score. Further, qualitative methods may be especially fruitful in revealing different forms of parental educational involvement that are contextually grounded in the life circumstances of poor, Latino families, as well as other immigrant families. In this regard, many qualitative studies underscore the role of parental sacrifice as a compelling source of inspiration and educational motivation for Latino, especially immigrant, children (Ceballo 2004; Lopez 2001; Sánchez et al. 2005; Suárez-Orozco and Suárez-Orozco 2001). Since parental migration stories are often plagued with hardship and adversity, it is not surprising that immigrant Latino children may view academic success as a means of returning their parents' investment and demonstrating appreciation for the opportunities that they were given. Indeed, Sánchez et al. (2005) found that scholastically high-achieving Mexican American youth often identified their academic success as a way of contributing to their families of origin. In this sense, then, family stories in which parents share experiences about their struggles with poverty, immigration, and a lack of education may provide a crucial and meaningful form of parental educational involvement—one that is typically unexamined in scholarly research.

As noted earlier, Latino families come from many different countries and cultural backgrounds even though the term "Latino" is used to describe them all. Despite the tremendous heterogeneity that exists among Latino families (e.g., immigration histories, countries of origin, socioeconomic statuses, acculturative stressors), cultural values, such as *educación*, *familismo*, and *respeto*, have been identified as shared commonalities across different Latino subethnic groups (Cruz-Santiago and Ramirez Garcia 2011). Accordingly, Latino parents often seek to instill in their children cultural values that emphasize diligent study (*estudios*), dedication and commitment to goals (*empeños*), and the drive to succeed (*ganas*) (Hill and Torres 2010). Yet, few researchers actually incorporate Latino cultural values when studying parenting and academic performance among Latino children. As deeply motivating aspects of family functioning, cultural values are likely to influence both Latino youth and parents. For instance, *respeto* refers to the valuing of decorum, politeness, deference to elders, and harmonious interpersonal relationships (Calzada et al. 2010). Acknowledging the importance that Latino parents give to inculcating the value of *respeto* in their children, Latino youth with higher endorsements of *respeto* may be more likely to pursue the educational goals and aspirations set by their parents. Indeed, in one study, the link between parental educational involvement and academic outcomes was stronger for Latino adolescents with higher endorsements of the traditional cultural value of *respeto* (Ceballo et al. 2014). Perhaps the endorsement of such cultural values declines in subsequent generations of more "Americanized" Latino children, contributing to the immigrant paradox.

Another illustrative example of how cultural values may enhance our understanding of Latino parenting is provided by the cultural value of *familismo*. In particular, *familismo* entails having a strong sense of family unity and loyalty, prioritizing family over personal needs, and relying upon family, first and foremost, for support (Calzada et al. 2010; Halgunseth et al. 2006). Scholarly evidence indicates that *familismo* can serve as a protective buffer for Latino youth (Kennedy and Ceballo 2013; Ojeda et al. 2010; Roche et al. 2012). In this way, a strong sense of familial obligations and closeness may be experienced by youth as a source of educational inspiration and motivation. In fact, Roche et al. (2012) reported that *familismo* positively predicted academic achievement among second generation Latino youth. Thus, youth who endorse a strong sense of *familismo* may be more likely to spend time at home with parents and other family members and wish to "give back" to their families by doing well academically. These reasons may be particularly salient to Latina girls. Additionally, *familismo* may motivate Latino youth to do well academically in efforts to reunite families separated by immigration.

Conversely, cultural values like *familismo* may incur vulnerabilities for youth and even impair academic functioning. Suárez-Orozco and Suárez-Orozco (1995) proposed that, for some adolescents, familial duty and obligations may assume priority over academic tasks, particularly in families facing severe financial difficulties. Moreover, in families with more traditional gender role scripts, parents may expect girls to be less focused on academics and more devoted to traditional household responsibilities. At present, according to Suárez-Orozco and Qin (2006), the effects of household responsibilities on academic outcomes among immigrant youth and immigrant girls, in particular, are inconclusive and contradictory. While there is some evidence that high-achieving Latinas report greater responsibilities at home, there are also studies showing that excessive home responsibilities hinder the educational performance of immigrant girls. It is important to note that changes in traditional gender role attitudes and behaviors have occurred in Latino families over time and with generational increases in educational attainment (Zambrana 2011).

As previously mentioned, Latino males tend to perform worse across numerous educational indicators compared to Latina females (Kena et al. 2015). Lower rates of academic achievement among Latino boys, in comparison to girls, are most likely determined by numerous factors, such as racial/ethnic stereotypes, teacher expectations, and familial demands. When Latino families face difficult economic circumstances, parents may expect adolescent males to seek employment more often than girls, perhaps partially explaining higher drop out rates and lower college attendance among Latino boys. Racial/ethnic stereotypes and discrimination may also contribute to lower academic performance among Latino males (DeGarmo and Martinez 2006). In a longitudinal study of 221 Latino adolescents, perceived discrimination was significantly associated with academic motivation a year later for boys, but not for girls (Alfaro et al. 2009). Moreover, cultural stereotypes of young Latino males portray them as lazy, unmotivated, unintelligent, and violent (Hudley and Graham 2001). When investigating adolescents' achievement-related cultural stereotypes, photos of African American, Latina, and European American females were selected most frequently for scenarios of achievement striving; whereas African American and Latino males were most often chosen for scenarios of academic disengagement (Hudley and Graham 2001). Even more telling for our purposes, Latino male adolescents were the most likely to be selected for low achievement striving scenarios by all adolescents —even Latinos themselves. Thus, negative stereotypes and expectations are quite likely to influence the motivation and academic performance of Latino boys.

As we noted at the beginning of this chapter, more research on Latino parents' educational involvement should adopt a developmental perspective, identifying what specific types of parental involvement are most strongly related to achievement and educational outcomes at different developmental periods and tracking changes in these relations over time. Additionally, future research should incorporate both qualitative and quantitative methodologies, include samples with different Latino subethnic groups, besides Mexican Americans with whom the majority of research has been done (Hill and Torres 2010; Ibañez et al. 2004), and investigate the differential and combined contributions of mothers' and fathers' involvement on children's academic achievement. Far too little work attends to fathers' educational involvement as well as potential gender differences in Latino parents' involvement and academic expectations for their sons and daughters. Moreover, future work should also address the experience of unauthorized youth, students who are academically under-achieving, as well as those who have dropped out of school altogether. Finally, we must look beyond the direct relations between parental educational involvement and academic outcomes to test potential moderating and mediating factors between parental involvement and children's educational outcomes.

References

Alfaro, E. C., Umaña-Taylor, A. J., & Bamaca, M. Y. (2006). The influence of academic support on Latino adolescents' academic motivation. *Family Relations, 55*, 279–291.

Alfaro, E. C., Umaña-Taylor, A. J., Gonzales-Backen, M. A., Bámaca, M. Y., & Zeiders, K. H. (2009). Latino adolescents' academic success: The role of discrimination, academic motivation, and gender. *Journal of Adolescence, 32*, 941–962.

Becerra, D. (2012). Perceptions of educational barriers affecting the academic achievement of Latino K-12 students. *Children & Schools, 34*(3), 167–177.

Benner, A. D., & Graham, S. (2011). Latino adolescents' experiences of discrimination across the first 2 years of high school: Correlates and influences on educational outcomes. *Child Development, 82*, 508–519.

Calzada, E. J., Fernandez, Y., & Cortes, D. E. (2010). Incorporating the cultural value of respeto into a framework of Latino parenting. *Cultural Diversity and Ethnic Minority Psychology, 16*(1), 77–86.

Ceballo, R. (2004). From barrios to Yale: The role of parenting strategies in Latino families. *Hispanic*

Journal of Behavioral Sciences, 26(2), 171–186. doi:10.1177/0739986304264572

Ceballo, R., Huerta, M., & Epstein-Ngo, Q. (2010). Parental and school influences promoting academic success among Latino students. In J. L. Meece & J. S. Eccles (Eds.), *Handbook of research on schools, schooling, and human development* (pp. 293–307). New York: Routledge.

Ceballo, R., Maurizi, L. K., Suarez, G. A., & Aretakis, M. T. (2014). Gift and sacrifice: Parental involvement in Latino adolescents' education. *Cultural Diversity and Ethnic Minority Psychology, 20*(1), 116–127.

Cooper, C. E., & Crosnoe, R. (2007). The engagement in schooling of economically disadvantaged parents and children. *Youth & Society, 38*(3), 372–391.

Cooper, C. E., Crosnoe, R., Suizzo, M., & Pituch, K. A. (2010). Poverty, race, and parental involvement during the transition to elementary school. *Journal of Family Issues, 31*(7), 859–883. doi:10.1177/0192513X09351515

Crosnoe, R. (2001). Academic orientation and parental involvement in education during high school. *Sociology of Education, 74*(3), 210–230.

Crosnoe, R., & López Turley, R. N. L. (2011). K-12 educational outcomes of immigrant youth. *The Future of Children, 21*(1), 129–152.

Cruz-Santiago, M., & Ramirez Garcia, J. I. (2011). "Hay que ponerse en los zapatos del joven": Adaptive parenting of adolescent children among Mexican-American parents residing in a dangerous neighborhood. *Family Process, 50*(1), 92–114.

Dearing, E., Kreider, H., Simpkins, S., & Weiss, H. B. (2006). Family involvement in school and low-income children's literacy: Longitudinal associations between and within families. *Journal of Educational Psychology, 98*(4), 653–664.

DeGarmo, D. S., & Martinez, C. R., Jr. (2006). A culturally informed model of academic well-being for Latino youth: The importance of discriminatory experiences and social support. *Family Relations, 55*, 267–278.

Delgado, M. Y., Updegraff, K. A., Roosa, M. W., & Umaña-Taylor, A. J. (2011). Discrimination and Mexican-origin adolescents' adjustment: The moderating roles of adolescents', mothers', and fathers' cultural orientations and values. *Journal of Youth and Adolescence, 40*(2), 125–139.

Desimone, L. (1999). Linking parent involvement with student achievement: Do race and income matter? *Journal of Educational Research, 93*, 11–31.

Eamon, M. K. (2005). Social-demographic, school, neighborhood, and parenting influences on the academic achievement of Latino young adolescents. *Journal of Youth and Adolescence, 34*(2), 163–174. doi:10.1007/s10964-005-3214-x

Eccles, J. S., Midgley, C., Wigfield, A., Buchanan, C. M., Reuman, D., Flanagan, C., et al. (1993). Development during adolescence: the impact of stage-environment fit on young adolescents' experiences in schools and in families. *American Psychologist, 48*(2), 90–101.

El Nokali, N. E., Bachman, H. J., & Votruba-Drzal, E. (2010). Parent involvement and children's academic and social development in elementary school. *Child Development, 81*(3), 988–1005.

Englund, M. M., Luckner, A. E., Whaley, G. J. L., & Egeland, B. (2004). Children's achievement in early elementary school: Longitudinal effects of parental involvement, expectations, and quality of assistance. *Journal of Educational Psychology, 96*(4), 723–730.

Epstein, J. L., & Sanders, M. G. (2002). Family, school, and community partnerships. In M. H. Bornstein (Ed.), *Handbook of parenting (Practical issues in parenting)* (Vol. 5, pp. 407–437). Mahwah, NJ: Erlbaum.

Fan, X., & Chen, M. (2001). Parental involvement and students' academic achievement: A meta-analysis. *Educational Psychology Review, 13*(1), 1–22.

Fan, W., Williams, C. M., & Wolters, C. A. (2012). Parental involvement in predicting school motivation: Similar and differential effects across ethnic groups. *The Journal of Educational Research, 105*(1), 21–35. doi:10.1080/00220671.2010.515625

Garcia Coll, C., & Marks, A. K. (2009). *Immigrant stories*. New York: Oxford University Press.

Garcia Coll, C., Akiba, D., Palacios, N., Bailey, B., Silver, R., DiMartino, L., et al. (2002). Parental involvement in children's education: Lessons from three immigrant groups. *Parenting: Science and Practice, 2*(3), 303–324.

Garcia Coll, C., Lamberty, G., Jenkins, R., McAdoo, H. P., Crnic, K., Wasik, B. H., et al. (1996). An integrative model for the study of developmental competencies in minority children. *Child Development, 67*, 1891–1914.

Grolnick, W. S., & Slowiaczek, M. L. (1994). Parents' involvement in children's schooling: A multidimensional conceptualization and motivational model. *Child Development, 65*, 237–252.

Halgunseth, L. C., Ispa, J. M., & Rudy, D. (2006). Parental control in Latino families: An integrated review of the literature. *Child Development, 77*, 1282–1297.

Henry, K. L., Cavanagh, T. M., & Oetting, E. R. (2011). Perceived parental investment in school as a mediator of the relationship between socio-economic indicators and educational outcomes in rural America. *Journal of Youth and Adolescence, 40*(9), 1164–1177. doi:10.1007/s10964-010-9616-4

Henry, C. S., Merten, M. J., Plunkett, S. W., & Sands, T. (2008). Neighborhood, parenting, and adolescent factors and academic achievement in Latino adolescents from immigrant families. *Family Relations, 57*(5), 579–590. doi:10.1111/j.1741-3729.2008.00524.x

Hill, N. E., Castellino, D. R., Lansford, J. E., Nowlin, P., Dodge, K. A., Bates, J. E., et al. (2004). Parent academic involvement as related to school behavior, achievement, and aspirations: Demographic variations across adolescence. *Child Development, 75*(5), 1491–1509.

Hill, N. E., & Craft, S. A. (2003). Parent-school involvement and school performance. *Journal of Educational Psychology, 95*(1), 74–83.

Hill, N. E., & Taylor, L. C. (2004). Parental school involvement and children's academic achievement: Pragmatics and issues. *Current Directions in Psychological Science, 13*, 161–164.

Hill, N. E., & Torres, K. (2010). Negotiating the American dream: The paradox of aspirations and achievement among Latino students and engagement between their families and schools. *Journal of Social Issues, 66*(1), 95–112. doi:10.1111/j.1540-4560.2009.01635.x

Hill, N. E., & Tyson, D. F. (2009). Parental involvement in middle school: A meta-analytic assessment of the strategies that promote achievement. *Developmental Psychology, 45*(3), 740–763. doi:10.1037/a0015362

Hoover-Dempsey, K. V., Walker, J. T., Sandler, H. M., Whetsel, D., Green, C. L., Wilkins, A. S., et al. (2005). Why do parents become involved? Research findings and implications. *The Elementary School Journal, 106*(2), 105–130. doi:10.1086/499194

Hudley, C., & Graham, S. (2001). Stereotypes of achievement striving among early adolescents. *Social Psychology of Education, 5*, 201–224.

Ibañez, G. E., Kuperminc, G. P., Jurkovic, G., & Perilla, J. (2004). Cultural attributes and adaptations linked to achievement motivation among Latino adolescents. *Journal of Youth and Adolescence, 33*(6), 559–568. doi:10.1023/B:JOYO.0000048069.22681.2c

Jeynes, W. H. (2007). The relationship between parental involvement and urban secondary school student academic achievement a meta-analysis. *Urban education, 42*(1), 82–110.

Jeynes, W. H. (2012). A meta-analysis of the efficacy of different types of parental involvement programs for urban students. *Urban Education, 47*(4), 706–742.

Juang, L. P., & Silbereisen, R. K. (2002). The relationship between adolescent academic capability beliefs, parenting and school grades. *Journal of Adolescence, 25*, 3–18. doi:10.1006/jado.2001.0445

Kena, G., Musu-Gillette, L., Robinson, J., Wang, X., Rathbun, A., Zhang, J., et al. (2015). *The condition of education 2015* (NCES 2015-144). U.S. Department of Education, National Center for Education Statistics. Washington, DC. Retrieved June 24, 2015 from http://nces.ed.gov/pubsearch

Kennedy, T. M., & Ceballo, R. (2013). Latino adolescents' community violence exposure: After-school activities and *familismo* as risk and protective factors. *Social Development, 22*(4), 663–682.

Kingston, S., Huang, K. Y., Calzada, E., Dawson-McClure, S., & Brotman, L. (2013). Parent involvement in education as a moderator of family and neighborhood socioeconomic context on school readiness among young children. *Journal of Community Psychology, 41*(3), 265–276.

Klauda, S. L. (2009). The role of parents in adolescents' reading motivation and activity. *Educational Psychology Review, 21*, 325–363.

Kuperminc, G. P., Darnell, A. J., & Alvarez-Jimenez, A. (2008). Parent involvement in the academic adjustment of Latino middle and high school youth: Teacher

expectations and school belonging as mediators. *Journal of Adolescence, 31*(4), 469–483. doi:10.1016/j.adolescence.2007.09.003

Lee, J., & Bowen, N. K. (2006). Parent involvement, cultural capital, and the achievement gap among elementary school children. *American Educational Research Journal, 43*(2), 193–218. doi:10.3102/00028312043002193

Lerner, R. M., & Steinberg, L. (2009). The scientific study of adolescent development: Historical and contemporary perspectives. In R. M. Lerner & L. Steinberg (Eds.), *Handbook of adolescent psychology: Vol. 1. Individual bases of adolescent development* (3rd ed., pp. 3–14). Hoboken, NJ: Wiley.

Lopez, G. R. (2001). The value of hard work: Lessons on parent involvement from an (im)migrant household. *Harvard Educational Review, 71*(3), 416–443.

Martinez, C. R., DeGarmo, D. S., & Eddy, J. M. (2004). Promoting academic success among Latino youth. *Hispanic Journal of Behavioral Sciences, 26*, 128–151.

Mena, J. A. (2015). Latino parent home-based practices that bolster student academic performance. *Hispanic Journal of Behavioral Sciences, 33*, 490–506.

Menard-Warwick, J. (2007). Biliteracy and schooling in an extended-family Nicaraguan immigrant household: The sociohistorical construction of parental involvement. *Anthropology & Education Quarterly, 38*(2), 119–137.

National Center of Educational Statistics. (2007). *Status and trends in the education of racial and ethnic minorities*. Washington, DC: U.S. Department of Education, Office of Educational Research and Improvement.

Ogbu, J. U. (1981). Origins of human competence: A cultural-ecological perspective. *Child Development, 52*, 413–429.

Ogbu, J. U. (1992). Understanding cultural diversity and learning. *Educational Researcher, 21*, 5–14.

Ojeda, L., Navarro, R. L., & Morales, A. (2010). The role of la familia on Mexican American men's college persistence intentions. *Psychology of Men & Masculinity*. Advance online publication. doi:10.1037/a0020091

Okagaki, L. (2001). Triarchic model of minority children's school achievement. *Educational Psychologist, 36*, 9–20.

Passel, J. S. (2011). Demography of immigrant youth: Past, present, and future. *The Future of Children, 21*(1), 19–41.

Perez, W., Espinoza, R., Ramos, K., Coronado, H. M., & Cortes, R. (2009). Academic resilience among undocumented Latino students. *Hispanic Journal of Behavioral Sciences, 31*(2), 149–181.

Perreira, K. M., Chapman, M. V., & Stein, G. L. (2006). Becoming an American parent: Overcoming challenges and finding strength in a new immigrant Latino community. *Journal of Family Issues, 27*(10), 1383–1414.

Perreira, K., Fuligni, A., & Potochnick, S. (2010). Fitting in: The roles of social acceptance and discrimination in shaping the academic motivations of Latino youth in the Southeast. *Journal of Social Issues, 66*(1), 131–153.

Plunkett, S. W., Behnke, A. O., Sands, T., & Choi, B. Y. (2009). Adolescents' reports of parental engagement and academic achievement in immigrant families. *Journal of Youth and Adolescence, 38*, 257–268. doi:10.1007/s10964-008-9325-4

Portes, A., & Rumbaut, R. G. (2001). *Legacies: The story of the second generation*. Berkeley: University of California Press.

Rasinski, T., & Stevenson, B. (2005). The effects of fast start reading: A fluency-based home involvement reading program on the reading achievement of beginning readers. *Reading Psychology, 26*, 109–125.

Reese, L., & Gallimore, R. (2000). Immigrant Latinos' cultural model of literacy development: An evolving perspective on home-school discontinuities. *American Journal of Education, 108*, 103–134.

Roche, K. M., Ghazarian, S. R., & Fernandez-Esquer, M. W. (2012). Unpacking acculturation: Cultural orientations and educational attainment among Mexican-origin youth. *Journal of Youth and Adolescence, 41*, 920–931.

Roeser, R. W., Eccles, J. S., & Sameroff, A. J. (2000). School as a context of early adolescents' academic and social-emotional development: A summary of research findings. *Elementary School Journal, 100*(5), 443–471. doi:10.1086/499650

Ryan, C. S., Casas, J. F., Kelly-Vance, L., Ryalls, B. O., & Nero, C. (2010). Parent involvement and views of school success: The role of parents' Latino and White American cultural orientations. *Psychology In The Schools, 47*(4), 391–405.

Sánchez, B., Reyes, O., & Singh, J. (2005). Makin' it in college: The value of significant individuals in the lives of Mexican American adolescents. *Journal of Hispanic Higher Education, 5*(1), 48–67.

Seginer, R. (2006). Parents' educational involvement: A developmental ecology perspective. *Parenting: Science and Practice, 6*(1), 1–48.

Sheldon, S. B., & Epstein, J. L. (2005). Involvement counts: Family and community partnerships and mathematics achievement. *The Journal of Educational Research, 98*, 196–206.

Shumow, L., & Miller, J. D. (2001). Parents' at-home and at-school academic involvement with young adolescents. *Journal of Early Adolescence, 21*(1), 68–91.

Suárez-Orozco, C., & Qin, D. B. (2006). Gendered perspectives in psychology: Immigrant origin youth. *International Migration Review, 40*, 165–198.

Suárez-Orozco, C., & Suárez-Orozco, M. (1995). *Transformations: Migration, family life, and achievement motivation among Latino adolescents*. Stanford, CA: Stanford University Press.

Suárez-Orozco, C., & Suárez-Orozco, M. (2001). *Children of immigration*. Cambridge, MA: Harvard University Press.

Suárez-Orozco, C. A., Yoshikawa, H., Teranishi, R. T., & Suárez-Orozco, M. M. (2011). Growing up in the shadows: The developmental implications of unauthorized status. *Harvard Educational Review, 81*(3), 438–620.

Sy, S. R. (2006). Family and work influences on the transition to college among Latina adolescents. *Hispanic Journal of Behavioral Sciences, 28*(3), 368–386.

Tyler, K. M., Uqdah, A. L., Dillihunt, M. L., Beatty-Hazelbaker, R., Conner, T., Gadson, N., et al. (2008). Cultural discontinuity: Toward a quantitative investigation of a major hypothesis in education. *Educational Researcher, 37*(5), 280–297.

U.S. Bureau of the Census. (2007). *2005–2007 American community survey 3-year estimates: Hispanic or latino origin by specific origin*. Retrieved May 26, 2012, from http://factfinder.census.gov/servlet/ACSSAFFPeople?_submenuId=people_10&_sse=on

Valadez, J. R. (2002). The influence of social capital on mathematics course selection by Latino high school students. *Hispanic Journal of Behavioral Sciences, 24*(3), 319–339.

Wigfield, A., Eccles, J. S., Fredricks, J., Simpkins, Roeser, R., & Schiefele, U. (2015). Development of achievement motivation and engagement. In R. Lerner (Series Ed.) & M. Lamb (Vol. Ed.), *Handbook of child psychology* (7th ed., Vol. 3). New York: Wiley.

Woolley, M. E., Kol, K. L., & Bowen, G. L. (2009). The social context of school success for Latino middle school students: Direct and indirect influences of teachers, family, and friends. *Journal of Early Adolescence, 29*, 43–70.

Zambrana, R. E. (2011). *Latinos in American society*. Ithaca, NY: Cornell University Press.

Zolkoski, S. M., & Bullock, L. M. (2012). Resilience in children and youth: A review. *Children and Youth Services Review, 34*(12), 2295–2303.

Using Self-Regulated Learning as a Framework for Creating Inclusive Classrooms for Ethnically and Linguistically Diverse Learners in Canada

Nancy Perry, Nikki Yee, Silvia Mazabel, Simon Lisaingo, and Elina Määttä

Abstract

Canada is rich in ethnic and linguistic diversity. For example, in 2011 more than 200 ethnic origins were reported in Canada's National Household Survey. Similarly, those surveyed identified more than 200 languages as their home language or mother tongue. Most of this diversity is concentrated in Canada's largest urban centers: Montreal (Quebec), Toronto (Ontario), and Vancouver (British Columbia). Canadian classrooms reflect this diversity, which is a challenge for our predominantly Euro-Canadian and monolingual teaching force. This chapter for the *Handbook of Positive Development of Minority Children* describes the demographic characteristics and experiences of diverse groups of students in Canadian classrooms, with a particular focus on immigrant, Aboriginal, and language minority (LM) learners. Then we consider self-regulated learning (SRL) as a framework for creating inclusive and culturally responsive contexts that accommodate multiple pathways to knowing and learning and foster productive approaches to learning in *all* children.

Portrait of Canadian Classrooms

Canada is rich in ethnic and linguistic diversity. In 2011 more than 200 ethnic origins were reported in Canada's National Household Survey (NHS; Statistics Canada 2013a) and those surveyed identified more than 200 languages as their home language or mother tongue. Compared with other G8 countries, Canada had the largest proportion of foreign-born citizens—just over 20 % of the total population. Many Canadians identify with cultural groups from around the world, including: South Asians, Chinese, Afro-Caribbeans, Filipinos, Latin Americans, Arabs, Koreans, and Japanese (Statistics Canada 2013a). Most of this diversity is concentrated in Canada's three largest cities: Montreal, Toronto, and Vancouver. Also, data from the NHS indicate Aboriginal

N. Perry (✉) · N. Yee · S. Mazabel · S. Lisaingo
University of British Columbia, Vancouver, Canada
e-mail: nancy.perry@ubc.ca

E. Määttä
University of Oulu, Oulu, Finland

© The Editor(s) 2017
N.J. Cabrera and B. Leyendecker (eds.), *Handbook on Positive Development of Minority Children and Youth*, DOI 10.1007/978-3-319-43645-6_22

peoples—including First Nations Peoples, Metis, and Inuit—represent 4.3 % of Canada's total population (Statistics Canada 2013b). Importantly for educators, the NHS indicates Aboriginal peoples are a young and growing population (up by 20 % from the previous survey in 2006). Aboriginal communities are distributed across Canada and are highly diverse.

Canada's classrooms reflect this diversity. For example, Nadia (a pseudonym) teaches grade 1 in a suburban school district in British Columbia (BC), Canada. In her class of 23 students, 17 are language minority (LM) learners—they speak a language other than English or French at home, 20 are members of South Asian groups, and two have Aboriginal ancestry. This portrait of Nadia's classroom personifies the ethnic and linguistic diversity in many Canadian classrooms.

Canada does not have a national department of education, so information about children in schools is mainly located in provincial Ministry of Education documents. In BC, where Nadia teaches and where we live and work, the Ministry of Education's *Summary of Key Information* (2011/12) indicates 10.8 % of students attending public schools are of Aboriginal ancestry, 10.9 % are designated "English Language Learners" (ELLs) or "English as a Second Language" (ESL) learners. As a consequence of having this designation, these students receive additional support to increase their English language proficiency, but 23.8 % of students speak a language other English in their homes (BC Ministry of Education 2012). In several of the large urban school districts, the proportion of children who speak languages other than English in their homes is more than 50 % (Skelton 2014). In Nadia's classroom these children represent 74 % of the students. The Vancouver School Board (2014) reports more than 125 home languages for its student body. Our point is that, in some schools, students from so-labeled minority groups actually constitute a majority of the school's population.

Understandably, educators in BC and across Canada are challenged with teaching and meeting the needs of this diverse student body. As a group, teachers are predominantly Euro-Canadian, middle-class, female, and monolingual (Hodgkinson 2002). Our teacher preparation programs do little to prepare them to meet the diverse language and learning needs of children in their classrooms (Guo 2012; Deer 2013). Furthermore, our curriculum and evaluation processes continue to privilege European Enlightenment principles, which favor rational and objective over more holistic and subjective epistemologies. This prioritization has the effect of marginalizing Aboriginal and other groups of learners (Battiste 2013). Thus, there is need to examine the current educational environment with a view to creating inclusive teaching and learning contexts and promoting positive outcomes for *all* students.

In our chapter for the *Handbook of Positive Development of Minority Children* we consider how teachers can build on the strengths and diversity of students in Canadian classrooms by supporting self- and socially shared regulation of learning. "Self-regulated learning" (SRL) focuses on how learners, individually and socially, can exercise autonomy and function in complex learning contexts to meet personal and shared goals (Perry 2004; Zimmerman 2008). First we elaborate on the characteristics of three diverse groups of Canadian learners—immigrant, Aboriginal, and LM learners—and describe their experiences in school. Then we consider how SRL and SRL promoting practices might inform optimal teaching and learning approaches for these and other groups of learners. We conclude the chapter with recommendations for future research and practice aimed at supporting the positive development of minority learners.

Immigrant, Aboriginal, and Language Minority Learners

Immigrant Learners

Some immigrant learners are born in a different country (first generation), others are born in Canada to parents who originally emigrated from another country (second generation) (Areepattamannil and Freeman 2008; Onchwari 2013). Immigrant learners are a diverse population, not just in terms of their languages, cultural traditions, and religious affiliations, but also in terms of their experiences as immigrants. In Canada, most immigrant families choose to come to Canada, seeking new opportunities, or to join other family members (Organization for Economic Co-operation and Development (OECD) 2006). Relatively few come as refugees (10–12 %), leaving their homelands to escape economic, political, or religious turmoil. Some families arrive with substantial resources while others have very little social or economic support. And although some immigrants are already fluent in English, many are learning English (or French) and adapting to a new culture at the same time (Elizalde-Utnick 2010; Kugler and Price 2009). Whatever their circumstance, helping immigrant children make a positive adjustment in Canadian society and schools should be a high priority.

Even immigrant learners from the most affluent, educated, and socially connected families are likely to experience some degree of stress because of the differences between their heritage cultures and new communities (van Geel and Vedder 2011). Challenges for immigrant learners can include: lack of familiarity with the new culture and its educational system (Deyhle and Swisher 1997); learning a new language (Shields and Behrman 2004); expectations surrounding the process of acculturation (Elizalde-Utnick 2010); experiences of marginalization, racism, and discrimination (Lansford et al. 2007; Suárez-Orozco and Suárez-Orozco 2001; van Geel and Vedder 2011); and lowered socioeconomic status (Capps et al. 2005; Fuligni and Fuligni 2007; Shields and Behrman 2004).

Canada's official policy on multiculturalism (Citizen and Immigration Canada 2012), positions diversity as a national asset—citizens are encouraged to keep their individual and cultural identities while experiencing a sense of belonging in Canadian culture. Ideally, acculturation involves two or more groups exchanging culture characteristics (Acculturation 2014), such that the mainstream Canadian culture becomes increasingly informed by diversity while immigrants are able to integrate useful aspects of

Canadian culture with their culture. Unfortunately, this positive process of acculturation (characterized by reciprocity) has not been the experience for all immigrant learners. For some, the process of acculturation can feel like forced assimilation—they feel pressed to adopt Canadian customs. For example, the "Fresh Voices Youth Advisory Team" (2013), appointed by the Vancouver Foundation and BC's Representative for Children and Youth, interviewed more than 200 "newcomer" youth in communities throughout BC to understand what their experience of immigration had been (Fresh Voices Youth Advisory Team 2013). While many youth described positive experiences in schools and "finding helpful allies in teachers, support workers, and students," others described feeling stigmatized, devalued, and discriminated against within the school system. In particular, these youth perceived a stigma associated with being an English language learner and emphasized how the newcomer experience differs depending on the pathway to immigration (i.e., choosing to come versus coming as a refugee). Unfortunately the Fresh Voices report did not provide quantitative data, so it is not possible to know how widespread and representative these impressions were, or to identify particular groups of immigrants who may experience more discrimination than others.

However, this disenfranchisement deserves our attention. Marginalization and discrimination at school can inhibit students' sense of pride in culture and may be deleterious to their achievement and educational aspirations (Elizalde-Utnick 2010). It can cause learners to withdraw from school both socially and emotionally, perform poorly, and adopt maladaptive/anti-social behaviors (Dovidio et al. 2010; Elizalde-Utnick 2010). It has been associated with negative outcomes, such as increased levels of depression, anxiety, and identification with negative stereotypes. Interestingly, immigrant youth interviewed by the Fresh Voices Youth Advisory Team (2013) identified a strong connection between themselves and the Aboriginal peoples of Canada. Specifically, they perceived many immigrant communities "have similar values that could set a common ground to connect with indigenous communities" (p. 12). Building bridges and working in solidarity across these groups was one of the main themes emerging from their community dialogue process.

Finally, financial hardship and poverty can be significant issues for immigrants. According to the National Longitudinal Study of Children and Youth (NLSCY; Krahn and Taylor 2005) the total income for more than 30 % of all immigrant families in Canada falls below the poverty line. Poverty, especially if combined with other risk factors, can have major debilitating effects on immigrant learners' academic performance and life outcomes (Onchwari 2013). Previous studies have suggested that a low socio-economic status is related to poor social-emotional functioning, poor health, increased substance use, low cognitive performance, and low academic achievement in children and youth (Bradley and Corwyn 2002; McLoyd 1998).

Despite the potential to experience significant challenges, immigrant learners, on average, perform as well (first generation) or better (second generation) than their Canadian-born peers on standardized achievement tests (Organization for Economic Cooperation and Development, OECD 2006). This could be the result of a selective immigration policy, but there also is a good deal of research identifying familial and personal protective factors that support their learning, achievement, and positive life outcomes (Krahn and Taylor 2005; Onchwari 2013; van Geel and Vedder 2011). Adult immigrants to Canada have similar levels of education and employment as their Canadian born peers. Perhaps for this reason, they place high value on education, believing it is the most significant way for their children to improve their status in life (Anisef et al. 2000). In addition, immigrant learners are motivated learners and tend to have higher personal aspirations than their Canadian-born peers (Krahn and Taylor 2005; OECD 2006; Onchwari 2013; van Geel and Vedder 2011). Often they are more optimistic about the future (Kao and Tienda 1995; Suárez-Orozco and Suárez-Orozco 2001). Finally, immigrant families draw strength from a variety of resources in their communities—these strong social and cultural connections help them to flourish in a new society (Onchwari 2013; Park-Taylor et al. 2007).

We were not able to locate school performance data that distinguished between particular groups of immigrant learners. It could be informative, for example, to know how parents' income and education, ethnicity, and the circumstances that led to immigration are associated with students' success in school. However, making these distinctions may also risk the promotion of stereotypes and expectations that will not apply to every member of every group. Research along these lines should proceed with caution.

Aboriginal Learners

The term "Aboriginal peoples" is used to refer to diverse cultural, linguistic, and political groups living in rural and urban communities across Canada who were the first inhabitants of this country (Royal Commission on Aboriginal Peoples 1996). As indicated in our introduction, Aboriginal peoples correspond to 4.3 % of Canada's total population (Statistics Canada 2013b) and, because they are a young and growing population, there are a considerable number of Aboriginal children and youth in Canada's schools. In 2012/13, they comprised approximately 11 % of BC's public school students (BC Ministry of Education 2013a). Most Aboriginal children live and attend school off reserve (Statistics Canada 2006).

Although Aboriginal groups vary in terms of nuanced social and political structures, languages, and other cultural features, they share many foundational beliefs and experience similar social and economic challenges resulting from Canada's historically colonial policies and practices (Brayboy et al. 2012; Royal Commission on Aboriginal Peoples 1996). Aboriginal families face social, economic, and health challenges at rates that far exceed those of non-Aboriginal families (Truth and Reconciliation Commission of Canada 2012). Poverty, poor living conditions, and comparatively poor health inhibit opportunities for learning for many Aboriginal children and youth. In school, Aboriginal students are not performing as well as their non-aboriginal peers (Aboriginal Affairs and Northern Development Canada 2013). In BC, Aboriginal students have substantially lower graduation rates than their non-Aboriginal peers; score lower on standardized tests across subject areas; and are over-identified for special education programs, with the exception of gifted education programs, where they are under-identified (BC Ministry of Education 2013a). These outcomes have long-term implications for their pursuit of further education, training, and employment (Canadian Council on Learning (CCL) 2009).

Understanding and addressing these differences has become a priority for governments, school systems and Aboriginal organizations across Canada. Importantly, these statistics need to be interpreted in light of historically colonial approaches to curriculum and instruction in Canada's schools, which have resulted in a multitude of barriers for Aboriginal children and youth (CCL 2007; Royal Commission on Aboriginal Peoples 1996). Often, pedagogical approaches, and curricular topics and materials do not resonate with the unique histories and cultures of Aboriginal peoples, so learning lacks meaning for Aboriginal youth. Worse are materials that portray negative stereotypes of Aboriginal peoples, reinforcing negative self-images and disengagement (Congress of Aboriginal Peoples 2010).

First Nations, Inuit, and Métis have long advocated for learning opportunities that affirm their cultural traditions and values, but they also desire Western education that can equip their children with the knowledge and skills they need to participate in Canadian society (CCL 2007). Toward these ends, governments, schools and Aboriginal stakeholders across Canada are collaborating to develop frameworks for curricula that align with Aboriginal learners' needs and aspirations (e.g., CCL 2007). These frameworks recognize how vital Aboriginal languages and cultural traditions can be to the positive development and learning of Aboriginal youth, and

they seek to create opportunities for Elders to share knowledge and culture with youth. They also highlight the social and relational aspects of learning that recent research demonstrates are important for *all* learners (Oberle et al. 2014).

In fact, much of what we are learning from decolonizing and Aboriginal pedagogies can be applied to teaching other minority groups. In general, teachers and schools should do more to reach out to parents and other leaders in communities and encourage their meaningful involvement in areas where they have expertise. Increases in the quantity and quality of communication between parents and teachers, for example, could address misunderstandings on the part of teachers, and feelings of discomfort and distrust on the part of parents. Similarly, Faculties of Education, Ministries of Education, and school districts should do more to increase the diversity of Canada's teachers, and to build their confidence and competence in teaching diverse groups of learners (e.g., through all levels of professional learning and by providing material resources).

Language Minority Learners

LM learners speak a language at home that is different from the societal language—English or French in the Canadian context—and have attained some level of proficiency in their home language (August and Shanahan 2006). Their level of proficiency can vary from not speaking to being fully proficient in the societal language. The labels English language learners (ELL) or English as a second language learners (ESL) are used in BC to refer to a subset of LM learners whose English language proficiency is not sufficient to participate fully in English education programs (August and Shanahan 2006). This designation qualifies them for additional language instruction for up to five school years (British Columbia Ministry of Education 2013b). The number of LM learners in Canadian schools continues to increase, with 20 % of the Canadian population speaking a language other than English or French at home (Statistics Canada 2012).

This statistic refers to immigrant and Aboriginal learners, but it is important to note that not all LM learners in Canada are immigrants or have Aboriginal Ancestry. In Quebec, English speakers are in the minority and there are French enclaves across Canada, where children may speak French at home, but learn in English at school. Also, French immersion programs are very popular in English speaking Canada. These programs can include children who speak French at home and school, as well as English speaking children who are LM learners in school.

Bilingualism has clear benefits for learning. It is associated with increased creativity and cognitive flexibility, and enhanced metalinguistic awareness about how language works (Bialystok and Craik 2010). In fact, monolingual children who attend bilingual programs have performed better on measures of phoneme awareness and reading comprehension than peers educated in English-only programs (Petitto 2009). These findings appear to hold so long as there is no stigma attached to being bilingual and so long as children are not expected to abandon their first language in order to learn the second (Woolfolk et al. 2015; Bialystok et al. 2003).

Unfortunately, many immigrant children and adults lose their heritage language in the process of acculturation (Montrul 2010). As well, Aboriginal youth today are less likely to speak an Indigenous language than their Aboriginal ancestors, and immigrant learners report feeling that "English is the only language valued in Canada" (Fresh Voices Advisory Team 2013). We know that language plays an important role in maintaining cultural practices and paradigms (Battiste et al. 2010), and that learning multiple languages provides cognitive and educational benefits to students. Thus the loss of heritage languages not only diminishes the culture and diversity of Canada, but results in missed opportunities for individual learners as well.

LM learners may gain proficiency for communicating in everyday informal situations quite quickly. However, a challenge for them in school is the need to acquire a more complex set of oral and written language skills, including: language for general communication; academic discourses;

and academic content (Gunderson 2006; Leventhal et al. 2006). When LM learners do not master these processes quickly, there is potential for an achievement gap between them and their majority language-speaking peers to grow, leaving them at risk for academic failure (Lesaux and Geva 2006; Lesaux et al. 2006a, b). In fact, research indicates LM learners are disproportionately receiving special education services due to inaccuracies in distinguishing between language differences and learning disabilities in this population (Samson and Lesaux 2009). Failure to attain a level of language proficiency commensurate with majority language-speaking peers has been associated with high rates of school drop-out, reduced job expectations, and poverty among LM learners (August and Shanahan 2006; Gunderson 2006, 2008).

The challenges LM students who are also cultural minority students face in school and with learning are not only about speaking the mainstream language. Their familiarity with the dominant culture (i.e., understanding of beliefs, values, models of agency, and goals) is also an issue in becoming "school literate" (Orosco and O'Connor 2014; Trommsdorff 2009). LM learners who are also immigrant learners or Aboriginal learners may be challenged by a mismatch between home and school expectations. For example, school and classroom norms in North America reflect our relatively individualistic cultures, where direct interactions and independent learning are more prevalent. LM learners may come from homes and societies where learning is a more collectivist pursuit (Orosco and O'Connor 2014; Trommsdorff 2009). Moreover, rules for help giving and seeking, asking questions, group versus individual work, and social learning can vary across cultures (McInerney and Ali 2013). In some cultures, it is appropriate to ask questions and seek help from teachers (or other adults in 'power' roles), but this is not the practice in others.

Learning the societal language and becoming school literate can be stressful for LM and other minority learners and research shows that high levels of stress over long periods of time hinder learning and cognitive development (Joels et al.

2006). Therefore, educational systems should find ways to support LM learners to achieve academically and participate meaningfully in both their home and school communities. Ideally, schools and communities should work together to support "balanced bilingualism," whereby home languages connect children to their families and cultural traditions, and the school/societal language provides them with academic, social and economic opportunities outside their homes (Borrero and Yeh 2010). This approach to language learning also fits with views of acculturation that emphasize reciprocity (Acculturation 2014).

In this section we have focused on immigrant, Aboriginal, and LM learners, elaborating on who they are and the challenges they face, but also identifying protective factors and positive initiatives that can support them in school. Although we have described them separately above, we want to emphasize here that these groups are not mutually exclusive (e.g., immigrant and Aboriginal learners can also be LM learners) and children across groups such as these experience many of the same challenges in school (e.g., acculturation or assimilation, marginalization and discrimination, language acquisition, poverty and family stress). Moreover, as individuals, these learners are likely to face the same motivational, achievement, and overall adjustment issues as all other children.

Earlier, we described how teachers and schools are challenged by the extent of diversity in Canada's/BC's classrooms, but also alluded to some frameworks and approaches that could support teaching and learning by building on the strengths of diversity in a more inclusive context. We expand on this topic next.

Supporting Diverse Learners Through Promoting Their Self-Regulated Learning

In writings about competencies *all* learners need to acquire to become skilled workers and engaged citizens in twenty-first Century global and knowledge-based societies, emphasis is placed on: (a) applying knowledge meaningfully, flexibly, and creatively; (b) relating schoolwork to daily life; (c) formulating possible futures; and (d) continuously learning—i.e., committing to life-long learning (Dumont et al. 2010). Reflecting these goals, BC's Ministry of Education is implementing a new curriculum they suggest will "better engage students in their own learning". Specifically, their vision is of a school system that privileges "personalized learning … enabled and supported by quality teaching … flexibility and choice, and high standards" (p. 5). This system recognizes that no two students learn in the same way or at the same pace, and for students to become actively engaged in learning, teaching needs to focus on their individual interests and abilities. We see clear potential for building on the strengths of a diverse student body in this system—that's the goal! We also see clear connections between this vision and research on SRL. In particular, we believe helping teachers to develop SRL promoting practices can support them to better meet the needs of minority learners by first considering student characteristics and then designing instruction to meet their needs at school. We elaborate below.

Defining SRL

"Self-regulated" approaches to learning involve students controlling thoughts and actions to achieve personal goals and respond to environmental demands (Zimmerman 2008). As this description implies, an emphasis on SRL has the capacity to support diverse learning goals, help learners attend to key features of their environment (e.g., instructions and/or social norms for carrying out tasks and interacting with others), and consider how responses (e.g., asking for help; expressing of dislike or frustration) will serve them in particular situations (Blair and Razza 2007; Ponitz et al. 2009). Self-regulated learners use metacognition to consider personal characteristics (strengths and weaknesses) relative to task demands ("What am I being asked to do?") and, where gaps exist, identify strategies that will help them succeed (Winne and Perry 2000). Their motivation for learning reflects a "growth mind-set" (Dweck 2007)—they focus on personal progress and deep understanding, and they realize that challenge is inevitable in any learning opportunity. These qualities make them willing to engage with new and challenging tasks, which is necessary for learning and SRL (Hadwin et al. 2011). Furthermore, self-regulation is associated with self-determination, which reflects the ful-fillment of fundamental needs for autonomy (choice and control), belonging, and competence, and is associated with adaptive functioning, self-esteem, pro-social behavior, and personal well-being (Deci and Ryan 2002; Ryan and Deci 2000).

Significance of SRL for Diverse Groups of Learners

While research about SRL in culturally and lin-guistically diverse groups is scarce, what research does exist suggests "… self-regulation is an asset that cuts across socio-demographic boundaries and remains predictive of develop-mental outcomes" (McClelland and Wanless 2012, p. 292). For example, in their longitudinal study of children's transition from prekinder-garten to kindergarten, McClelland and Wanless found self-regulation was a statistically signifi-cant predictor of children's academic achieve-ment regardless of "demographic risk" (ELL and socioeconomic status), and that high self-regulation was positively associated with school adjustment and academic success. Simi-larly, Garrido-Vargas (2012) found a significant relationship between SRL motivational strategies and middle school ELL (Hispanic) students' academic performance. Finally, published descriptions of Aboriginal approaches to educa-tion can be facilitated through the use of SRL promoting practices (e.g., Barnhardt and Kawa-gley 2005; Brayboy and Maughan 2009; Cajete 1994; Deloria 1999; Newhouse 2008; Okakok 1989).

Both Aboriginal and SRL approaches to teaching and learning emphasize the importance

of making learning personally relevant and practical (Battiste 2013; Brayboy and Maughan 2009; Deloria 1999). Learning becomes mean-ingful when students are supported to achieve personal goals, consistent with their cultural values and community priorities. Well-known models of SRL are cyclical (Winne and Hadwin 1998; Zimmerman and Campillo 2003), describing processes learners use to guide their thoughts and actions before, during, and after they engage with tasks and activities. Likewise, Aboriginal epistemologies see knowledge as a holistic process involving careful planning, deliberate and strategic action, and ongoing assessment (e.g., Brayboy and Maughan 2009).

With regard to motivation, Aboriginal approaches tend to value learning from experi-ence and persisting to accomplish tasks that are difficult but meaningful or important (CCL 2007). This is consistent with the growth minded motivational orientation we described for self-regulated learners above (Dweck 2007). Both perspectives value self-discipline and self-knowledge (Deloria 1999). Also consistent with self-determination theory's emphasis on fundamental needs fulfillment (i.e., sense of autonomy, belonging, and competence), Abo-riginal epistemologies build from a foundation of: (a) individual responsibility within a collec-tive; (b) interconnectedness with all of the natural world; and (c) contributions of expertise from all people and the natural world (Deloria 1999; Phillips 2010; Marker 2011). Finally, Aboriginal ways of knowing are inherently social and research on students' regulation of learning is increasingly focusing on the social and situated aspects of it (Hadwin et al. 2010; Hurme and Järvelä 2005; Volet et al. 2009). We turn to social forms of self-regulation next.

Social Forms of Self-Regulation

The notion that self-regulation supports social as well as independent forms of learning (Zimmerman 2008) is particularly relevant for understanding how it might function in classrooms that include diverse groups of students. In these contexts, regulation of and for learning is rarely a solo event (Winne et al. 2013) and theories of co- and socially shared regulation of learning are relevant.

Co-regulation builds on Vygotskian and neo-Vygotskian frameworks for learning that emphasize the importance of instrumental interaction and activity to support SRL (McCaslin and Good 1996; McCaslin 2009). Co-regulation reflects a transitional phase whereby learners gradually develop SRL through, for example, instrumental feedback or metacognitive prompts. In classrooms, adults can co-regulate students and students can co-regulate peers, but students can also co-regulate adults by signaling how adults might tailor or adjust instruction or support to better meet their needs (e.g., by asking questions, providing incorrect answers, or showing confusion or frustration). Co-regulation presumes one or more actors have knowledge or skills that others need or want to acquire. This feature may be used strategically to value the diverse knowledge of country, culture, and language children bring with them to school. Also, parents' and community leaders' expertise might be used to elevate key perspectives within the classroom.

Shared regulation describes how learners regulate activity in collaborative tasks by co-constructing understandings about tasks and pooling metacognitive, motivational, and strategic resources (see Hadwin et al. 2010, 2011). It is highly relevant for students who come from countries or cultures that stress communal and relational aspects of learning. Conceptions of shared regulation are also highly suited to developing a "community of learners" in classrooms where individual responsibility is coupled with group support (Brown and Campione 1994; Marker 2011). In the classroom, sharing knowledge and resources allows students and teachers to fully appreciate one another's backgrounds and experiences. This kind of cultural sharing can help students learn and share multicultural thinking tools (e.g., holistic thinking, non-linear thinking, place-based knowledge), and also help them match particular tools with specific situations or learning tasks.

Furthermore, shared regulation of learning implies sharing goals and jointly monitoring progress toward a shared outcome (Winne et al. 2013), which helps students understand that, sometimes, individual preferences need to be compromised for the collective outcome. Therefore, productive co- and shared regulation of learning require *socially responsible self-regulation* (SRSR), which refers to how students regulate their actions in pro-social, socially competent ways (Hutchinson and Perry 2012). It reflects self and other awareness plus a desire to see others succeed. This aligns well with Aboriginal and other paradigms of learning that similarly emphasize responsibility and mutual respect (Deloria 1999).

SRL Promoting Practices

For 20 years, Perry's research has focused on how classroom tasks, instructional practices, and interpersonal relationships create opportunities for *all* learners to develop and engage in SRL (see Perry 2013 for a synthesis). Her in-depth classroom observations of predominantly elementary aged learners reveal opportunities for students to regulate learning in classrooms where they are engaged in meaningful work and where support for student autonomy (e.g., opportunities to make choices, control challenge, self-assess, and feed into assessments of learning) is provided through highly effective forms of co-regulation. Moreover, Perry's research has demonstrated how a focus on SRL promoting practices can support more student-centered instruction and higher levels of meaningful inclusion for students with diverse interests and abilities (Perry 2004; Perry et al. 2006b). Here we consider how SRL promoting practices might benefit the diverse learners who are the focus of this chapter, using an example from Nadia's classroom, which we described at the beginning of the chapter.

In particular, tasks that are complex by design create opportunities for students to engage in *meaningful work* (Perry 2013). Complex tasks address multiple goals, focus on large chunks of meaning, and extend over long periods of time. Typically, they engage learners in a wide range of processes and allow students to create diverse products as evidence of learning. As one example, Nadia addressed goals related to SRL and social problem-solving through language and literacy tasks. At the beginning of the school year, she read a popular pattern book to the class, titled "Pete the Cat: Rocking in My School Shoes" (Dean and Litwin 2011). In the book, Pete the cat encounters a wide range of challenges, but rather than succumb to adversity, he demonstrates resilience by identifying and then applying effective strategies to solve problems. After reading the book, whenever a problem occurred or a student seemed anxious about completing a task, Nadia asked, "What would Pete do?..."

Subsequently, Nadia used the patterned language of the Pete the Cat book to prompt her students to reflect on the problems they experience in school and then to generate strategies to solve them. These problems might reflect the particular challenges the children experienced as LM, immigrant, or Aboriginal learners, but often they were problems common across groups of students in grade 1. Solutions, likewise, could reflect shared and diverse experiences of children within the classroom. They role-played the problems and solutions and Nadia took pictures to use in a personalized version of the book. Following the language pattern in the book, examples that Nadia's students came up with included:

> Division XX loves learning at school! But sometimes there are problems! [Student 1] was playing on the playground and she tripped and fell! Did [Student 1] cry? Goodness no! She just found Miss [name], the supervisor, and asked for her help!

> [Student 2] was playing with blue playdough, but he really wanted [Student 3's] red playdough! Did [Student 2] cry? Goodness no! He just used his words and asked to share!

> [Student 4] was trying to finish his math, but his group just kept talking! Did [Student 4] cry? Goodness no! He just said, "Excuse me, can you please stop talking?" and they did!

> …

> Division XX knows that problems come and problems go. Do they cry? Goodness no! They just keep rocking in their school shoes!

They read and discussed their version of the book together and then Nadia put it on a bookshelf so that students could access it when they wanted. Throughout the year, they generated other books on social and motivational topics (e.g., "Playing with Friends," "Nobody's Perfect"). Then when they were learning and problems occurred, Nadia could prompt students to recall or consult their book: "Remember in our book when [Student] had the same problem? What did he do?" In this way, Nadia could provide culturally responsive cues to students, without being an expert in the culture herself.

This example incorporates many of the characteristics we've attributed to *complex tasks* that support SRL. It addressed multiple goals (social and academic), was meaningful to students (involved them in addressing their problems), and extended over time (the activity generated materials and strategies that students could reference and use throughout the year). Also, it engaged learners in a wide range of processes (e.g., reflection, role playing—perhaps perspective taking, reading, writing) and allowed them to demonstrate learning in diverse ways (speaking, acting, and writing). A key goal for Nadia was supporting students' *autonomy* in social problem solving. Consequently, she gave them choices about which problems and strategies to focus on, and encouraged students to solve their social problems without involving her by using the ideas in their books as a resource (control over challenge). As a follow up activity, Nadia had students write about problems they encountered in their learning journals. Again, working with a language pattern, children wrote, "I had a problem at school," followed by a description of their problem and an explanation of how they solved it (self-reflection/assessment). Two of the children's journal entries are shown in Fig. 1. The first is from a student who is designated ELL and the second is from a student with Aboriginal ancestry. Both students identify an instance in which there was a problem successfully solved

I had a problem at school ...

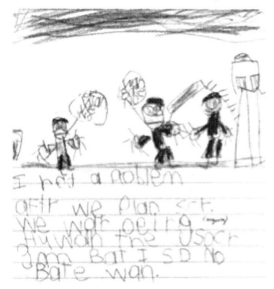

Nadia's feedback: "Was it a tie?"

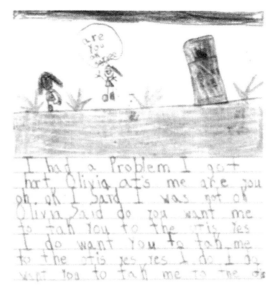

Nadia's feedback: "I'm glad Olivia helped you!"

Fig. 1 Excerpts from Nadia's grade 1 students' learning journals

and receive feedback from Nadia that supports positive interpersonal relationships among students in her classroom.

Reflecting on this activity, Nadia said she spent a lot of time at the start of the school year *co-regulating* students' social problem solving through activities like the one we have described above. She provided extensive scaffolding at the start of the school year to ensure students acquired respectful language and strategies for solving problems without involving her. Then she faded teacher support as students became more independent with the strategies for they developed together (e.g., how to ask for help; how to ask nicely). According to Nadia, having the book to refer to "helps [students] to remember the strategies we've talked about and gives them an idea about how to proceed with the problem." Taking time to establish norms for participation and a community of learners through tasks like the one we describe from Nadia's class is characteristic of teachers who are

committed to supporting SRL and creating inclusive classroom contexts with positive social and emotional climates.

Respecting the diverse learners who are the focus of this chapter, Nadia's social problem-solving activity has many features in common with tasks/activities characterized as culturally relevant and culturally responsive. Because it was built on children's experiences and personalized resources, children could recognize themselves in the problems and pictures (of them) that became the content of the books. The work was collaborative (they co-constructed the problem categories as well as the strategies), but they also were invited to write about their own problems and solutions (in their learning journals), so they could introduce problems that presented particular barriers to their learning and contribute or identify problem-solving strategies emphasized in their own cultures and families. Learning involved oral as well as written language and the patterned language and role-play provided models that likely benefitted all learners, but particularly linguistically and culturally diverse learners. Finally, Nadia's overarching focus on social and emotional learning likely helped to nurture a community of learners in which students could voice ideas and concerns and get support for learning and problem-solving from their teacher and peers.

Nadia's social problem-solving task is just one example of how diverse students' needs for autonomy, belonging and competence can be met through tasks that support self-, co-, and shared regulation of learning. In general, SRL promoting practices accommodate learning and motivational differences among students because they create spaces for multiple zones of proximal development to co-exist in a task environment (Brown and Campione 1994; Englert and Mariage 2003; Perry 2013). Moreover, they support a dynamic view of task environments (Perry et al. 2006a), one that recognizes novelty, meaningfulness, and challenge are not inherent properties of tasks. These features are open to interpretation (i.e., not every student interprets the same task in the same way) and interact with other features of a task environment, such as instructional supports and assessment practices (McCaslin 2009; Oyserman 2007; Perry and Rahim 2011). Ideally, teachers use SRL promoting practices (i.e., complex tasks, autonomy support, and co-regulation) to attend to complex and dynamic relationships between curricula and student characteristics and experiences.

What Is Next: Extending SRL Promoting Practices to Benefit Culturally and Linguistically Diverse Learners

Although SRL promoting practices can do a lot to build on the strengths of culturally and linguistically diverse groups of learners in classrooms, they will not necessarily increase understanding (in teachers and students) about particular cultures (their own or others), unless they are used to create opportunities for students to use their knowledge of heritage languages and

cultures in the classroom. For example, the task that Nadia implemented in her classroom could provide even stronger incentives for diverse learners if students were encouraged to share how their families and communities solve problems that are the same or similar to the problems they experience in their classrooms. How might their experiences outside of school inform their experiences in school? Also, when considering solutions and strategies, students might be encouraged to make choices that are responsible in the context of their communities. How might their choice reflect a community value or tradition? And teachers might seek out material and/or people to learn about ways of making particular tasks more responsive to the unique needs and traditions of their students.

More research is needed to validate the use of SRL promoting practices as appropriate pedagogical approaches for culturally and linguistically diverse learners. As one example of this kind of work, McIntyre (2010) asked elementary aged ELLs how their teacher helped them to learn, and they reported practices known to support SRL, but also diverse groups of students. They described opportunities to engage in collaborative work (shared regulation); teacher support in the form of instrumental feedback, modeling, and scaffolding (co-regulation); meaningful tasks; and having a sense of control over challenge (e.g., they had opportunities to demonstrate their knowledge and learning in different ways). These findings suggest, at the very least, SRL promoting practices offer a good deal of flexibility for adapting classroom tasks and guiding interpersonal interactions in diverse learning communities. More research is needed to understand how these practices might be adapted or expanded to increase their value as culturally responsive teaching tools.

Summary and Conclusions

Our chapter had two main goals. First we wanted to paint a portrait of the cultural and linguistic diversity in Canadian schools and communities, with a particular focus on schools and communities in BC, where we live and work. Second, we wanted to examine how a focus on SRL and SRL promoting practices might be used to support these diverse groups of learners in classrooms and schools. Regarding the first goal, we focused on three groups of learners: immigrant, Aboriginal, and LM learners. Our synthesis of the available demographic and research information about these groups emphasizes how culturally and linguistically rich Canada is as a nation. As a nation, we benefit enormously from our diversity, but the rate at which this diversity is increasing also poses some challenges, especially for our school systems. Our predominantly white, middle-class, female, and monolingual teachers often feel overwhelmed and ill-prepared to meet the diverse needs of the students in their classrooms. Access to professional learning opportunities and material resources to support culturally responsive approaches to learning are increasing (e.g., several Canadian universities include Indigenous teacher education programs, and incorporate approaches to teaching and learning for Aboriginal peoples into general teacher education programs as well), but are still limited. Education systems, curriculum and evaluation processes, to a large extent, continue to reflect the colonizing principles that marginalize Aboriginal and other groups of learners. Thus, we perceive a need to identify general approaches to teaching and learning that are flexible enough to accommodate a wide range of learner needs and interests.

Along these lines, we indicated how BC's new education plan, with its emphasis on personalized learning and the development of competencies that cut across knowledge domains (i.e., thinking, personal, social, and communication competencies), has potential to create a more inclusive school context for learners. Also we tried to show how SRL and SRL promoting practices might contribute to realizing the potential of a vision like the one the BC government is promoting. Specifically, we described how Nadia designed a complex task and carefully co-regulated her grade 1 students' engagement in self, shared, and socially responsible regulation of social problem-solving. The nature

of her task and the interpersonal interactions involved created relevant and supportive learning experiences for her students. Moreover, her emphasis on collaboratively co-constructing solutions for problems likely created an environment in which students felt included and a high level of efficacy for successfully solving their own problems and problems with peers.

However, the examples from Nadia's classroom do not provide a full validation of how SRL and SRL promoting practices may positively impact outcomes for the diverse learners in Canadian schools. There is need for more research about SRL and the efficacy of SRL promoting practices for supporting culturally and linguistically diverse groups of students to thrive academically, motivationally, emotionally, and socially. For example, most of the research about SRL reflects Western, Eurocentric, and psychological views about learning and being in the world. The relevance of SRL for diverse cultures needs to be examined. Recent advances in research concerning co- and shared forms of regulation hold promise in this regard, but a challenge remains for researchers to examine these constructs in ways that are culturally responsive and valid in specific contexts and with particular groups. With regard to Aboriginal cultures, for example, the positioning of non-Aboriginal researchers (or teachers) as experts is problematic (Smith 2012). Ideally, researchers might collaborate across cultures (e.g., Aboriginal with non-Aboriginal researchers) and disciplines (psychology and anthropology).

As an approach to pedagogy, SRL promoting practices do not attend to culture as explicitly as, for example, Aboriginal pedagogies do. One consideration for teachers and researchers is the extent to which SRL promoting practices are "flexible enough" to accommodate a wide range of cultural perspectives, as we have argued here. In practice, educators need to be intentional about efforts to bring culture into classrooms. Students need to perceive their heritage languages and home cultures are valued and reflected in their school/learning experiences. Teachers should actively look for ways to involve family and community members in creating opportunities for students to explore identities and examine cultures in deep and meaningful ways. Systemically, ministries of education and school districts need to find ways to support multilingual and multicultural approaches to learning. Decolonizing curriculum and, over the long term, diversifying teaching faculties are two strategies that can support these shifts.

In summary, we offer SRL and SRL promoting practices as one approach to creating more inclusive classrooms and supporting the positive development of diverse groups of students. In BC, this approach is appealing because it relates to initiatives already underway. Also, within the limitations of the current system, where teachers feel overwhelmed and ill-prepared to meet the diverse socio-demographic needs of students in classrooms, concentrating on SRL promoting practices provides teachers with a framework that is concrete and student-centered. In general, SRL promoting practices fit well with efforts to support knowledge and skills *all* learners need to succeed in increasingly global and knowledge-based societies.

References

Aboriginal Affairs and Northern Development Canada. (2013). *Fact sheet—2011 national household survey Aboriginal demographics, educational attainment and labour market outcomes*. Retrieved November 23, 2014, from https://www.aadnc-aandc.gc.ca/eng/1376329205785/1376329233875

Acculturation. (2014). In *Encyclopedia britannica*. Retrieved from http://www.britannica.com/EBchecked/topic/3083/acculturation

Anisef, R., Axelrod, R., Baichman-Anisef, E., James, C., & Turrittin, A. (2000). *Opportunity and uncertainty: Life course experiences of the class of '73*. Toronto, ON: University & Toronto Press.

Areepattamannil, S., & Freeman, J. G. (2008). Academic achievement, academic self-concept, and academic motivation of immigrant adolescents in the greater Toronto area secondary schools. *Journal of Advanced Academics, 19*, 700–743.

August, D., & Shanahan, T. (Eds.). (2006). *Developing literacy in second-language learners: Report of the National Literacy Panel on language-minority children and youth*. Mahwah, NJ: Lawrence Erlbaum.

Barnhardt, R., & Kawagley, A. O. (2005). Indigenous knowledge systems and Alaska Native ways of knowing. *Anthropology & Education Quarterly, 36*, 124–148.

Battiste, M. (2013). *Decolonizing education: Nourishing the learning spirit*. Saskatoon, SK: Purich Publishing Ltd.

Battiste, M., Kovach, M., & Balzer, G. (2010). Celebrating the local, negotiating the school: Language and literacy in Aboriginal communities. *Canadian Journal of Native Education, 32*, 4–12.

Bialystok, E., & Craik, F. I. (2010). Cognitive and linguistic processing in the bilingual mind. *Current Directions in Psychological Science, 19*, 19–23.

Bialystok, E., Majumder, S., & Martin, M. M. (2003). Developing phonological awareness: Is there a bilingual advantage? *Applied Psycholinguistics, 24*, 27–44.

Blair, C., & Razza, R. P. (2007). Relating effortful control, executive function, and false belief understanding to emerging math and literacy ability in kindergarten. *Child Development, 78*, 647–663.

Borrero, N. E., & Yeh, C. J. (2010). Ecological English language learning among ethnic minority youth. *Educational Researcher, 39*, 571–581.

Bradley, R. H., & Corwyn, R. F. (2002). Socioeconomic status and child development. *Annual Review of Psychology, 53*, 371–399.

Brayboy, B. M. J., Fann, A. J., Castagno, A. E., & Solyom, J. A. (2012). Framing the conversation. In B. M. J. Brayboy, A. J. Fann, A. E. Castagno & J. A. Solyom (Eds.), *Postsecondary education for American Indian and Alaska Natives: Higher education for nation building and self-determination* (pp. 11–30). San Francisco, CA: Jossey-Bass.

Brayboy, B. M. J., & Maughan, E. (2009). Indigenous epistemologies and teacher education: The story of bean. *Harvard Educational Review, 79*, 1–21.

British Columbia Ministry of Education. (2012). *2011/12 Summary of key information*. Retrieved February 19, 2015 from https://www.bced.gov.bc.ca/reporting/docs/SoK_2012.pdf

British Columbia Ministry of Education. (2013a). *Aboriginal report 2008/09–2012/13: How are we doing?*. Victoria, BC: BC Ministry of Education, Information Department.

British Columbia Ministry of Education. (2013b). *English language learning: Policy and Guidelines*. Retrieved on October 27, 2014 from http://www.bced.gov.bc.ca/ell//

Brown, A. L., & Campione, J. C. (1994). *Guided discovery in a community of learners*. Cambridge: The MIT Press.

Cajete, G. (1994). *Look to the mountain: An ecology of Indigenous education* (1st ed.). Durango, CO: Kivaki Press.

Canadian Council of Learning. (2007). *Redefining how success is measured in First Nations, Inuit, and Metis Learning*. Retrieved February 18, 2015 from http://www.ccl-cca.ca/pdfs/RedefiningSuccess/Redefining_How_Success_Is_Measured_EN.pdf

Canadian Council on Learning. (2009). *The state of Aboriginal learning in Canada: A holistic approach to measuring success*. Retrieved February 15, 2015 from http://www.ccl-cca.ca/CCL/Reports/ StateofAboriginalLearning.html

Capps, R., Fix, M., Ost, J., Reardon-Anderson, J., & Passel, J. S. (2005). *The health and well-being of young children of immigrants*. Washington, DC: The Urban Institute.

Citizenship and Immigration Canada. (2012). *Canadian multiculturalism: An inclusive citizenship*. Retrieved February 9, 2015 from Citizenship and Immigration Canada. http://www.cic.gc.ca/english/multiculturalism/ citizenship.asp

Congress of Aboriginal Peoples. (2010). *Staying in school: Engaging Aboriginal students*. Retrieved July 9, 2015 from https://neaoinfo.files.wordpress.com/ 2014/07/aboriginal-education-congress-of-aboriginal-peoples.pdf

Dean, J., & Litwin, E. (2011). *Pete the cat: Rocking in my school shoes*. New York: HarperCollins.

Deci, E. L., & Ryan, R. M. (2002). Overview of self-determination theory: An organismic-dialectical perspective. In E. L. Deci & R. M. Ryan (Eds.), *Handbook of self-determination research* (pp. 3–33). Rochester, NY: University of Rochester Press.

Deer, F. (2013). Integrating Aboriginal perspectives in education: Perceptions of pre-service teachers. *Canadian Journal of Education, 36*, 175.

Deloria, V. (1999). If you think about it, you will see that it is true. In B. Deloria, K. Foehner, & S. Scinta (Eds.), *Spirit and reason: The Vine Deloria Jr. reader* (1st ed., pp. 40–60). Colorado: Fulcrum Press.

Deyhle, D., & Swisher, K. (1997). Research in American Indian and Alaska Native education: From assimilation to self-determination. In M. W. Apple (Ed.), *Review of research in education* (Vol. 22, pp. 113–194). Washington, DC: American Educational Research Association.

Dovidio, J. F., Gaertner, S. L., & Kawakami, K. (2010). Racism. In J. F. Dovidio, M. Hewstone, P. Glick, & V. M. Esses (Eds.), *The SAGE handbook of prejudice, stereotyping and discrimination* (pp. 312–327). Thousand Oaks, CA: SAGE Publications Ltd.

Dumont, H., Istance, D., & Benavides, F. (Eds.). (2010). *The nature of learning: Using research to inspire practice*. OECD: Centre for Educational Research and Innovation.

Dweck, C. (2007). *Mindset: The new psychology of success*. New York: Random House.

Elizalde-Utnick, G. (2010). *Immigrant families: Strategies for school support*. Retrieved March 6, 2015 from National Association of Secondary School Principals. http://www.nasponline.org/resources/principals/ Immigrant_FamiliesJan10_NASSP.pdf

Englert, C. S., & Mariage, T. (2003). The sociocultural model in special education interventions: Apprenticing students in higher-order thinking. In Swanson, H. L., Harris, K. R., & Graham, S. (Eds.), *Handbook of learning disabilities* (pp. 450–467). New York, NY: Guilford press.

Fresh Voices Youth Advisory Team. (2013). *Fresh Voices report 2013*. Retrieved May 10, 2015 from https://www.vancouverfoundation.ca/sites/default/ files/documents/FreshVoices-Web-report-2013.pdf

Fuligni, A. J., & Fuligni, A. S. (2007). Immigrant families and the educational development of their children. In J. E. Lansford, K. Deater-Deckard, & M. H. Bornstein (Eds.), *Immigrant families in contemporary society: Duke series in child development and public policy* (pp. 231–249). New York: Guilford Press.

Garrido-Vargas, M. (2012). Relationship of self-regulated learning and academic achievement among English language learners (Doctoral dissertation, The University of Arizona). Retrieved from http://gradworks.umi. com/35/26/3526417.html

Gunderson, L. (2006). But she speaks English. In R. T. Jiménez & V. Ooka Pang (Eds.), *Race, ethnicity, and education (volume 2): Language and Literacy in Schools* (pp. 3–20). Wesport, CT: Praeger.

Gunderson, L. (2008). The state of the art of secondary ESL teaching and learning. *Journal of Adolescent & Adult Literacy, 52*, 184–188. doi:10.1598/JAAL.5

Guo, Y. (2012). Exploring linguistic, cultural, and religious diversity in Canadian schools: Pre-service teachers' learning from immigrant parents. *Journal of Contemporary Issues in Education, 7*, 4–23.

Hadwin, A. F., Järvelä, S., & Miller, M. (2011). Self-regulated, co-regulated, and socially-shared regulation of learning. In B. J. Zimmerman & D. H. Schunk (Eds.), *Handbook of self-regulation of learning and performance* (pp. 65–84). New York, NY: Routledge.

Hadwin, A. F., Oshige, M., Gress, C. L. Z., & Winne, P. H. (2010). Innovative ways for using gStudy to orchestrate and research social aspects of self-regulated learning. *Computers in Human Behavior, 26*, 794–805.

Hodgkinson, H. (2002). Demographics and teacher education: An overview. *Journal of teacher education, 53*, 102.

Hurme, T. R., & Järvelä, S. (2005). Students' activity in computer-supported collaborative problem solving in mathematics. *International Journal of Computers for Mathematical Learning, 10*, 49–73.

Hutchinson, L. R., & Perry, N. E., (2012, August). *Examining the psychometric properties of the self-regulation in school inventory*. Poster presented at the annual meeting of the American Psychological Association, Orlando, Florida.

Joels, M., Pu, Z., Wieger, O., Oitzl, M. S., & Krugers, H. J. (2006). Learning under stress: How does it work? *Trends in Cognitive Science, 10*, 152–158. doi:10. 1016/j.tics.2006.02.002

Kao, G., & Tienda, M. (1995). Optimism and achievement: The educational performance of immigrant youth. *Social Science Quarterly, 76*, 1–19.

Krahn, H., & Taylor, A. (2005). Resilient teenagers: Explaining the high educational aspirations of visible minority immigrant youth in Canada. *Journal of International Migration and Integration, 6*, 405–434.

Kugler, K. E., & Price, O. A. (2009). *Helping immigrant and refugee students succeed: It's not just what happens in the classroom.* Centre for Health and Health Care in the Schools. Retrieved May 20, 2015 from http://www.healthinschools.org/immigrant-and-refugee-children/caring-across-Communities.aspx

Lansford, J. E., Deater-Deckard, K., & Bornstein, M. H. (2007). *Immigrant families in contemporary society: Duke series in child development and public policy.* New York: Guilford Press.

Lesaux, N., & Geva, E. (2006). Synthesis: Development of literacy in language—Minority students. In D. August & T. Shanahan (Eds.), *Developing literacy in second-language learners. Report of the national literacy panel on language-minority children and youth* (pp. 53–74). Mahwah, NJ: Lawrence Erlbaum Associates.

Lesaux, N. K., Koda, K., Siegel, L. S., & Shanahan, T. (2006a). Development of literacy. In D. August & T. Shanahan (Eds.), *Developing literacy in second-language learners. Report of the national literacy panel on language-minority children and youth* (pp. 75–122). Mahwah, NJ: Lawrence Erlbaum Associates.

Lesaux, N. K., Lipka, O., & Siegel, L. S. (2006b). Investigating cognitive and linguistic abilities that influence the reading comprehension skills of children from diverse linguistic backgrounds. *Reading and Writing, 19*, 99–131. doi:10.1007/s11145-005-4713-6

Leventhal, T., Xue, Y., & Brooks-Gunn, J. (2006). Immigrant differences in school-age children's verbal trajectories: A look at four racial/ethnic groups. *Child Development, 77*, 1359–1374.

Marker, M. (2011). Teaching history from an Indigenous perspective: Four winding paths up the mountain. In P. Clark (Ed.), *New possibilities for the past: Shaping history education in Canada* (pp. 97–112). Vancouver, BC: UBC Press.

McCaslin, M. M. (2009). Co-regulation of student motivation and emergent identity. *Educational Psychologist, 44*, 137–146.

McCaslin, M. M., & Good, T. L. (1996). *Listening in classrooms.* New York, NY: Harper Collins College Publishers.

McClelland, M. M., & Wanless, S. B. (2012). Growing up with assets and risks: The importance of self-regulation for academic achievement. *Research in Human Development, 9*(4), 278–297. doi:10.1080/15427609.2012.729907

McInerney, D. M., & Ali, J. (2013). Indigenous motivational profiles: Do they reflect collectivism? A cross-cultural analysis of similarities and differences between groups classified as individualist and collectivist cultures. In R. Craven, G. Bodkin-Andrews, & J. Mooney (Eds.), *Indigenous Peoples* (pp. 211–232). Charlotte, NC: Information Age Publishing.

McIntyre, E. (2010). Principles for teaching young ELLs in the mainstream classroom: Adapting best practices for all learners. In G. Li & P. A. Edwards (Eds.), *Best practices in ELL instruction* (pp. 65–83). New York, NY: Guilford Press.

McLoyd, V. C. (1998). Socioeconomic disadvantage and child development. *American Psychologist, 53*, 185–204.

Montrul, S. (2010). Current issues in heritage language acquisition. *Annual Review of Applied Linguistics, 30*, 3–23.

Newhouse, D. (2008). Ganigonhi: Oh: The good mind meets the academy. *Canadian Journal of Native Education, 31*, 184–197.

Oberle, E., Schonert-Reichl, K. A., Guhn, M., Zumbo, B. D., & Hertzman, C. (2014). The role of supportive adults in promoting positive development in middle childhood: A population-based study. *Canadian Journal of School Psychology, 29*, 296–313.

OECD. (2006). *Where immigrant students succeed: A comparative review of performance and engagement in PISA 2003.* OECD: Programme for International Student Assessement.

Okakok, L. (1989). Serving the purpose of education. *Harvard Educational Review, 59*, 405–422.

Onchwari, J. (2013). Protective factors immigrant children bring to the classroom. In J. Keengwe & G. Onchwari (Eds.), *Cross-cultural considerations in the education of young immigrant learners* (pp. 265–279). Hershey: IGI Global.

Orosco, M. J., & O'Connor, R. (2014). Culturally responsive instruction for English language learners with learning disabilities. *Journal of Learning Disabilities, 47*, 515–531. doi:10.1177/0022219413476553

Oyserman, D. (2007). Social identity and self-regulation. *Social psychology: Handbook of Basic Principles, 2*, 432–453.

Park-Taylor, J., Walsh, M. E., & Ventura, A. B. (2007). Creating healthy acculturation pathways: Integrating theory and research to inform counselors' work with immigrant children. *Professional School Counseling, 11*, 25–34.

Perry, N. E. (2004). Using self-regulated learning to accommodate differences among students in classrooms. *Exceptionality Education Canada, 14*, 65–87.

Perry, N. E. (2013). Classroom processes that support self-regulation in young children [Monograph]. *British Journal of Educational Psychology, Monograph Series II: Psychological aspects of Education—Current Trends, 10*, 45–68.

Perry, N. E., & Rahim, A. (2011). Studying self-regulated learning in classrooms. In Zimmerman, B., & Schunk, D. H. (Eds.), *Handbook of self-regulation of learning and performance* (pp. 122–136). New York, NY: Taylor & Francis.

Perry, N. E., Phillips, L., & Hutchinson, L. R. (2006a). Preparing student teachers to support for self-regulated learning. *Elementary School Journal, 106*, 237–254.

Perry, N. E., Turner, J. C., & Meyer, D. K. (2006b). Classrooms as contexts for motivating learning. *Handbook of Educational Psychology, 2*, 327–348.

Petitto, L. A. (2009). New discoveries from the bilingual brain and mind across the life span: Implications for education. *Mind, Brain, and Education, 3*, 185–197.

Phillips, R. (2010). "Try to understand us": Aboriginal elders' views on exceptionality. *Brock Education: A Journal of Educational Research and Practice, 20*, 64–79.

Ponitz, C. C., McClelland, M. M., Matthews, J. S., & Morrison, F. J. (2009). Touch your knees! Using a direct observation of behavioral regulation to predict math, literacy, and vocabulary achievement in kindergarten. *Developmental Psychology, 45*, 605–619.

Royal Commission on Aboriginal Peoples. (1996). *Report of the Royal Commission on Aboriginal Peoples* (Vol. 3). Ottawa, ON: Canada Communication Group.

Ryan, R. M., & Deci, E. L. (2000). Self-determination theory and the facilitation of intrinsic motivation, social development and well-being. *American Psychologist, 55*, 68–78.

Samson, J. F., & Lesaux, N. K. (2009). Language-minority learners in special education: Rates and predictors of identification for services. *Journal of Learning Disabilities, 42*, 148–161. doi:10.1177/0022219408326221

Shields, M. K., & Behrman, R. E. (2004). Children of immigrant families: Analysis and recommendations. *The Future of Children, 14*, 4–15.

Skelton, C. (2014, July 8). ESL students in the majority at more than 60 schools in Metro Vancouver. Retrieved March 3, 2015 from the Vancouver Sun. http://www.vancouversun.com/health/students+majority+more+than+schools+Metro+Vancouver/10005768/story.html#__federated=1

Smith, L. T. (2012). *Decolonizing methodologies: Research and Indigenous people.* New York: Zed Books.

Statistics Canada. (2006). Aboriginal Peoples in Canada in 2006: Inuit, Métis and First Nations, 2006 Census. Retrieved June 24, 2015 from http://www12.statcan.ca/census-recensement/2006/as-sa/97-558/pdf/97-558-XIE2006001.pdf

Statistics Canada. (2012). *Linguistic characteristics of Canadians: Language, 2011 census of population.* Retrieved from Statistics Canada: http://www12.statcan.gc.ca/census-recensement/2011/as-sa/98-314-x/98-314-x2011001-eng.pdf

Statistics Canada. (2013a). Immigration and Ethnocultural Diversity in Canada (pp. 1–23). Retrieved March 3, 2015 from Statistics Canada. http://www12.statcan.gc.ca/nhs-enm/2011/as-sa/99-010-x/99-010-x2011001-eng.pdf

Statistics Canada. (2013b). *Aboriginal Peoples in Canada: First Nations People, Métis, and Inuit.* (Catalogue number 99-011-X2011001). Retrieved

March 3, 2015 from Statistics Canada. http://www12.statcan.gc.ca/nhs-enm/2011/as-sa/99-011-x/99-011-x2011001-eng.pdf

Suárez-Orozco, C., & Suárez-Orozco, M. (2001). *Children of immigration.* Cambridge, MA: Harvard University Press.

Trommsdorff, G. (2009). Culture and development of self-regulation. *Social and Personality Psychology Compass, 3*, 687–701. doi:10.1111/j.1751-9004.2009.00209.x

Truth and Reconciliation Commission of Canada. (2012). *Truth and Reconciliation Commission of Canada: Interim Report.* Retrieved May 21, 2015 from http://www.myrobust.com/websites/trcinstitution/File/Interim%20report%20English%20electronic.pdf

van Geel, M., & Vedder, P. (2011). The role of family obligations and school adjustment in explaining the immigrant paradox. *Journal of Youth and Adolescence, 40*, 187–196.

Vancouver School Board. (2014). *Our District.* Retrieved from http://www.vsb.bc.ca/about-vsb

Volet, S., Vauras, M., & Salonen, P. (2009). Self-and social regulation in learning contexts: An integrative perspective. *Educational Psychologist, 44*, 215–226.

Winne, P. H., & Hadwin, A. F. (1998). Studying as self-regulated learning. In D. J. Hacker, J. Dunlosky & A. C. Graesser (Eds.), *Metacognition in educational theory and practice* (pp. 279–306). Hillsdale, NJ: Erlbaum.

Winne, P. H., Hadwin, A. F., & Perry, N. E. (2013). Metacognition and computer-supported collaborative learning. In Hmelo-Silver, C. E. (Eds.), *The international handbook of collaborative learning* (pp. 462–479). New York, NY: Routledge.

Winne, P. H., & Perry, N. E. (2000). Measuring self-regulated learning. In P. Pintrich, M. Boekaerts, & M. Seidner (Eds.), *Handbook of self-regulation* (pp. 531–566). Orlando, FL: Academic Press.

Woolfolk, A. E., Winne, P. H., & Perry, N. E. (2015). *Educational psychology* (6th ed.). Scarborough: Prentice Hall/Allyn and Bacon Canada.

Zimmerman, B. J. (2008). Investigating self-regulation and motivation: Historical background, methodological developments, and future prospects. *American Educational Research Journal, 45*, 166–183.

Zimmerman, B. J., & Campillo, M. (2003). Motivating self-regulated problem solvers. In J. E. Davidson & R. J. Sternberg (Eds.), *The psychology of problem solving* (pp. 233–262). Cambridge: Cambridge University Press.

Part VI

Policies/Prevention/Programs

Positive Development of Minority Children and Youth: Translating Theory to Action

Nancy Gonzalez

According to the positive developmental framework articulated in this volume and by others before (Lerner et al. 2009), children naturally possess strengths and the capacity for positive developmental outcomes, and this potential can be realized when there is alignment between these strengths and the resources for healthy development present in their environments. This perspective represents a significant shift for research on minority populations, from one that has focused almost exclusively on deficits and risks to one that is focused on the positive growth and inherent potential of minority youth (Guerra and Bradshaw 2008). What follows naturally from this shift is to question how children's developmental contexts and the policies that shape these contexts can be structured or improved to maximize this potential. Thus, this perspective also moves the social policy debate away from a dominant focus on remediation. It is not that "at-risk" youth need special treatment for their deficits; what is needed, rather, is to ensure the basic conditions for positive development are made accessible and equitable for all children and youth. This section considers how research on positive development can inform programs, practices and policies to meet this goal.

The chapters in this part address this question with respect to diverse populations of children and youth living in the United States (U.S.), England (UK), and Canada. Along with a focus on policy, these chapters include research on programs and practices that target varied developmental contexts (e.g., parents, families, youths, schools,

communities). This part also features research at different phases of translation (Spoth et al. 2013), including Type 1 translation (Umana-Taylor, Chapter "Developing an Ethnic-Racial Identity Intervention from a Developmental Perspective: Process, Content, and Implementation of the Identity Project") that attempts to use generative research and theory to design programs and practical applications (i.e., "bench to bedside", to use the medical metaphor), and Type 2 translation research (Chumak-Horbatsch, Chapter "Instructional Practice with Young Bilingual Learners: A Canadian Profile", and Evangelou et al., Chapter "Children's Centres: An English Intervention for Families Living in Disadvantaged Communities") that studies what happens when evidence-based programs are adopted and implemented in the real world (i.e., bedside to community). Each chapter draws on extant empirical evidence while raising several conceptual and practical challenges for moving from theory to practice in research on positive development in minority populations.

The most fundamental challenge for translational research on positive development of minority children and youth is to strategize what type of policy change and at what level in the ecodevelopmental system will make a difference in the lives of minorities. Although the majority of interventions developed for minority children and youth typically target microsystemic or local processes (i.e., in families, schools), chapters in this part illustrate why change also is needed at broader systemic levels (i.e., national policy). Rosario and

Yoshikawa (Chapter "Documentation Status and Child Development in the U.S. and Europe") examine common barriers experienced by children across two distinct historical and policy environments—undocumented children in the U.S. and the Roma in Europe—and illustrate how public policies tied to citizenship and documentation have pervasive effects on their developmental contexts and opportunities for positive development. As they explain, programs and policies can address the consequences of undocumented status by affecting the status directly (e.g., policies that provide pathways to citizenship, border enforcement and deportation policies), or by affecting access to the systems and institutions (i.e., education, housing, social services) in ways that can exclude the undocumented from mainstream life. In a chapter that highlights how the intersection of being male and an ethnic minority creates unique challenges for boys of color (BOC), Gaylord-Harden et al. (Chapter "Research on Positive Youth Development in Boys of Color: Implications for Intervention and Policy") articulate why a focus on positive development has become a national priority for BOC in the U.S. This chapter reflects a growing movement and an active network of scholars (Barbarin 2013) that have coalesced in response to a national initiative launched by President Barack Obama. The My Brother's Keeper Initiative' aims to provide opportunities for boys and young men of color to reach their full potential through coordinated philanthropic efforts and evidence-based community solutions that target critical intervention points in the lives of boys and young men of color. This initiative illustrates another way in which policy can direct needed attention and resources toward the positive development for minority youth.

Gaylord-Harden et al. raise another challenge in mounting comprehensive solutions that prioritize positive development over deficit or risk-reduction models, which is the reality that BOC and other cultural minorities are disproportionately exposed to under-resourced or high-risk settings in which ecological assets for positive development may be limited. As such, an emphasis on promotion of positive development may not be sufficient without broader policies or programs that also reduce ecological risks and inequalities. As well, Hope and Spencer (Chapter "Civic Engagement as an Adaptive Coping Response to Conditions of Inequality: An Application of Phenomenological Variant of Ecological Systems Theory (PVEST)") underscore that the positive development of minority youth, particularly those who have been disenfranchised socially, politically, and economically, is inexorably bound with their exposure to adversity and their need to make meaning of their experiences to achieve a positive adaptation. Drawing on Spencer's phenomenological variant of ecological systems theory (Spencer and Swanson 2015), they maintain that civic engagement functions as an adaptive coping strategy for disenfranchised minority youth which, in turn and recursively, facilities future positive development. Thus, like other culture-specific competencies (e.g., ethnic identity, protective cultural values) that become more salient in high-risk contexts in which they are needed to promote adaptation to culturally-linked stressors (e.g., ethnic and racial discrimination) (Gonzales et al. 2015a), strict separation of risk-resilience and positive development framework may neither be possible nor desired in practice.

The chapters in this part also highlight the need to consider developmental assets and processes that are either distinct or more salient for particular subgroups (e.g., dual language learning, ethnic identity development, critical civic engagement), as well as those that are more universally relevant for children's development (e.g., maternal well-being, food security, family stability). Several scholars have argued that culturally specific or segmented programs and services are necessary to address the needs of minority populations, particularly in light of the intersectionality of social categories (race, sex, linguistic ability, documentation status, sexual orientation) that create unique challenges for certain subgroups (Castro et al. 2004). However, when the goal is broad dissemination within multicultural settings, such as schools, culturally segmented strategies may not be feasible and may inadvertently undermine efforts to promote access for all youth (Gonzales et al. 2015b). They also may limit opportunities for greater cultural awareness and the potential for majority groups to derive benefits from inclusive programs and practices. Umaña-Taylor and Douglass (Chapter "Developing an Ethnic-Racial Identity Intervention from a Developmental Perspective: Process, Content, and Implementation of the Identity Project") address this issue head-on in their efforts to design the Identify Project Curriculum, a universal school-based program to engage high school aged youth in the developmental processes of ethnic-racial identity (ERI) exploration and resolution. Building on a strong base of evidence to support ERI as a critical, distinct pathway to positive development among minority youth (Umaña-Taylor 2015), Umaña-Taylor and Douglas designed a curriculum for universal delivery to all students in a school, irrespective of their cultural background or majority-minority status. The program aims to increase students' salience and understanding of their own and others' ethnic heritage(s) and background(s); increase students' awareness and understanding of multiple groups' experiences with contemporary and historic discrimination in the U.S.; expose students to the notion that differences within groups are oftentimes larger than differences between groups; engage students in activities designed to increase their understanding of their family heritage; clarify misconceptions students may have regarding a "right or wrong" way to identify with an ethnic group; provide students with tools with which to explore their ethnic heritage; and provide opportunities for students to discuss their heritage with others. In addition to increasing the likelihood that this program can be supported and sustained within public schools, their approach shifts the burden and potential benefits of increased cultural awareness to all groups within the school community, and also offers potential for positive impact on school culture and climate.

One final challenge for translational research on minority children's positive development is to ensure that programs and policies are implemented and sustained in ways that will produce the desired benefits when transported to communities and implemented at scale. Even well-supported programs may fail when implemented poorly or without attention to implementation factors such as quality delivery, training, systems of support, and the need for buy-in and adaptation to local contexts (Spoth et al. 2013). Evangelou, Goff, Sylva, Sammons, Smith, Hall and Eisenstadt (Chapter "Children's Centres: An English Intervention for Families Living in Disadvantaged Communities") describe the country-wide system of community-based Children's Centres in the UK that were established to reduce inequalities between poor and affluent young children living in the UK. Similar to the Head Start in the U.S., the initial goal of this national program was to provide a network of centers in high-risk communities across England that would offer integrated services (e.g., health, education, welfare) for all parents in the community and their young children, up to age 5. By placing centers in communities with greater need for such services, the intention was to elevate the whole community regardless of the family's level of risk or cultural background, therein providing non-stigmatizing access to services for the most disadvantaged families. However, following an early evaluation that showed they were producing greater benefits for moderately disadvantaged families than for more severely disadvantaged families (Melhuish et al. 2005), a new model was adopted in which a "core offer" of services was provided universally in the community, with more intensive or stepped-up services for those at greatest risk (Goff et al. 2013). A major consideration in ongoing program adaptations over time has been to maintain a balance in the offer of universal or "open access" versus targeted services to avoid the stigma attached to programs for "at-risk" or needy families. Local adaptation also has been important as a strategy to address culture-specific concerns within the context of the universal community delivery model.

Chumak-Horbatsch (Chapter "Documentation Status and Child Development in the U.S. and Europe") also examined implementation factors in research to train early childcare educators (ECEs) and teachers to adopt a new model of instructional practice for young bilingual learners (BLs) attending Canadian childcare centers and kindergartens with little or no proficiency in the language of program delivery. Due to rapid immigration and an upward trend for more immigrant women to work outside the home, BLs presents a significant challenge for early childhood professionals and teachers in Canada. Linguistically Appropriate Practice is a new multilingual or culturally inclusive, strength-based approach to classroom practice that is supported by development research on children's language acquisition. LAP views young BLs as "emergent bilinguals" that are capable, active dual language learners who use their entire linguistic repertoire to navigate the many communicative contexts they encounter. In contrast to "assimilative practice" that views BLs as language deficient and "supportive and inclusive practice" that acknowledges and values cultural differences yet still maintains the singular goal of English acquisition, inclusive practice integrates BLs home language(s) daily and directly into the classroom. However, Chumak-Horbatch found significant barriers in efforts to retool early childcare educators and teachers to move towards inclusive practice. Various personal, professional and curricular factors affected ECE professionals' instructional practice decision-making, and only a small number successfully made the transition. Further, a significant number held on to supportive practice "as tightly as possible" due to personal and professional beliefs, and were not interested in retooling their practice with BLs.

Against the backdrop of the diverse and complex experiences of children and youth that are cultural and political minorities within their communities, positive development emerges as a progressive approach towards providing more balanced programs and practices that encompass both promotion and protection. Collectively, the papers in this part highlight inherent challenges in operationalizing and implementing this approach in ways that will ultimately lead to effective and sustained solutions. Systemic policy change also will be needed to ensure that minority children and youth have access to resources and opportunities they need to reach their potential.

References

Barbarin, O. A. (2013). Development of boys of color: An introduction. *American Journal of Orthopsychiatry, 83*(2–3), 143.

Catalano, R. F., Hawkins, J. D., Berglund, M. L., Pollard, J. A., & Arthur, M. W. (2002). Prevention science and positive youth development: competitive or cooperative frameworks? *Journal of Adolescent Health, 31*(6), 230–239.

Castro, F. G., Barrera, M., Jr., & Martinez, C. R. (2004). The cultural adaptation of preventive interventions: Resolving tensions between fidelity and fit. *Prevention Science, 5*, 41–45.

Goff, J., Hall, J., Sylva, K., Smith, T., Smith, G., Eisenstadt, N., Sammons, P., Evangelou, M., Smees, R., & Chu, K. (2013). *Evaluation of Children's Centre's in England (ECCE) – Strand 3: Delivery of Family Services by Children's Centre's Research Report.* (DfE Research Report No. DFE-RR297). London: DfE.

Gonzales, N. A., Jensen, M., Montano, Z., Wynne, H. (2015a). The Cultural Adaptation and Mental Health of Mexican American Adolescents. In Y. M. Caldera & E. Lindsey (Eds.), Handbook of Mexican American Children and Families: Multidisciplinary Perspectives. Oxford, UK: Routledge.

Gonzales, N. A., Lau, A., Murry, V. M., Pina, A., Barrera, M.Jr. (2015b). Culturally Adapted Preventive Interventions for Children and Youth. Chapter to appear in D. Cicchetti (Ed.) *Developmental Psychopathology, Third Edition.* Hoboken, NJ: John Wiley & Sons.

García, O., Makar, C., Starcevic, M. & Terry, A., (2011). The translanguaging of Latino kindergarteners. In K. Potowski & J. Rothman (Eds.), *Bilingual youth: Spanish in English-speaking societies* (pp.33–55). Philadelphia: John Benjamin Publishing Co.

Guerra, N. G., & Bradshaw, C. P. (2008). Linking the prevention of problem behaviors and positive youth development: Core competencies for positive youth development and risk prevention. *New Directions for Child and Adolescent Development, 122*, 1–17.

Lerner, J. V., Phelps, E., Forman, Y. E., & Bowers, E. P. (2009). Positive youth development. In R. M. Lerner & L. Steinberg, L. (Eds.), *Handbook of Adolescent Psychology, Individual Bases of Adolescent Development* (Vol. 1). John Wiley & Sons, Inc.

Melhuish, E., Belsky, J., & Leyland, A. (2005). *Early Impacts of Sure Start Local Programmes on Children and Families.* London: DfES.

Spencer, M. & Swanson, D. (2015). Vulnerability and resilience: Illustrations from theory and research on African American youth. In D. Cicchetti (Ed.), *Handbook of developmental psychopathology.* New York: John Wiley & Sons.

Spoth, R., Rohrbach, L.A., Greenberg, M., Leaf, P., Brown, C.H., Fagan, A., Hawkins, J.D. (2013). Addressing the core challenges for the next generation of Type 2 translation research and systems: The translation science to population impact (TSci Impact) Framework. *Prevention Science, 14*, 319–351. doi: 10.1007/s11121-012-0362-6

Umaña-Taylor, A. J. (2015). Ethnic identity research: How far have we come? In C. E. Santos & A. J. Umaña-Taylor (Eds.), *Studying Ethnic Identity: Methodological and Conceptual Approaches across Disciplines* (pp. 11–26). Washington, DC: American Psychological Association.

Documentation Status and Child Development in the U.S. and Europe

Natalia Rojas and Hirokazu Yoshikawa

Abstract

Unauthorized status pertains to immigrants in countries around the world who do not have full inclusion and status as citizens. This chapter focuses on two examples—the Roma in Europe and the undocumented in the U.S.—that reflect groups at risk due to formal social exclusion. The United States and the European Union each face their own policy debates regarding unauthorized immigrants and its effects on child development. In each case, we briefly summarize the history of those with the status, including trends over recent years; evidence on whether lacking citizenship as represented in documentation affects child development; the mechanisms through which the status may affect access to contexts associated with positive child development; and then programs and policies that may affect the status itself, or access to developmental contexts linked to the status. Finally, we synthesize the emerging commonalities and distinct patterns across the U.S. and Europe from the relevant evidence, and future directions for theory and research.

Introduction Historical Overview and Theory

One of the central functions of public policy is to define what constitutes membership in and therefore inclusion in a nation (Bardach 2012). Defining conditions for legal entry into a country

and the pathway to citizenship represents a central process for social inclusion of outsiders in every nation. With large numbers of migrants crossing borders globally in recent years (roughly 40 million in the period 2005–2010; Abel and Sander 2014), issues of citizenship have become ever more urgent and vexed issues of national and international policy debate. Citizenship is proven and shown publicly through documents—with the international convention of proving citizenship, includes having a passport with name and photograph linked. Increasingly, biomarkers (e.g., fingerprints) are being integrated into the process of establishing citizenship

N. Rojas (✉) · H. Yoshikawa (✉)
NYU, New York, NY, USA
e-mail: nmr254@nyu.edu

H. Yoshikawa
e-mail: hiro.yoshikawa@nyu.edu

© The Editor(s) 2017   385
N.J. Cabrera and B. Leyendecker (eds.), *Handbook on Positive Development of Minority Children and Youth*, DOI 10.1007/978-3-319-43645-6_23

(Torpey 2001). Without a name registered to a passport or biomarker, access to the immigrant dream of social inclusion and mobility can be denied.

Children and youth are implicated centrally in issues of citizenship. The extent to which social integration of immigrants occurs, including their access to citizenship status, is closely linked to the future prosperity of generations (Alba and Nee 2009; Suárez-Orozco et al. 2015). Our thesis in this chapter is that policies related to citizenship affect positive child development through a set of developmental contexts (Yoshikawa and Kalil 2011). Citizenship and the documentation status (of identity; of residence) that proves it typically provide access to developmental contexts (e.g., schools) that may enhance children's positive development, particularly for disadvantaged newcomers. These developmental contexts include proximal contexts of child and youth development such as housing, public education, early care and education, and health care. When public policies exclude certain families by virtue of not having papers (i.e., not having citizenship), children and youth in those families (or unaccompanied children and youth) are excluded from these associated supports and may suffer in terms of their learning, health and development.

A recent conceptual model of how documentation status affects child and youth development (Yoshikawa 2011; Yoshikawa and Kalil 2011) suggests that non-citizens and those lacking documentation experience authorities and formal systems (e.g., health, education, social protection or poverty reduction) in different ways than citizens. These systems can influence children directly through the quality of their schooling, for example, or indirectly, through the social networks or well-being of their parents. There may be compounded effects on children's development when both children and their parents lack citizenship or documentation status (Gonzales 2011; Potochnick and Perreira 2010).

We examine the conceptual model for how lack of citizenship status—which we term "undocumented status"—may affect positive development and social inclusion of immigrant-origin children (born in a different country than they are currently residing) and youth in two contexts: the United States and Europe. We define positive development as encompassing academic, learning, socio-emotional and civic and community participation outcomes. We draw on the cases of recent waves of undocumented migration in the U.S., and the case of the Roma in Europe, particularly those who cross national borders, to illustrate how public policies related to citizenship and documentation may affect children and youth. As perhaps the most vulnerable social group in these countries with various forms of unauthorized status, Roma, especially children, are overrepresented in all categories in need of social protection. The most recent developments at European level show an increasing willingness to adopt minority rights documents and develop comprehensive approaches directed at Roma integration. The United States faces its own policy debates regarding unauthorized immigrants and its effects on child development.

Case Study I: The Undocumented in the United States

Today 5.27 million U.S. children reside with at least one undocumented immigrant parent. The vast majority of these children—4.5 million—are U.S.-born citizens; 775,000 are unauthorized themselves (note that the U.S. has birthright citizenship, unlike many of the European countries we discuss later in this chapter; Passel et al. 2014). Children with undocumented parents and undocumented children constitute roughly one-third of all immigrant-origin children.

The history of undocumented migration to the United States starts with the Chinese Exclusion Act of 1882 (Congress 1882). Prior to this law, which singled out a single racial/ethnic group for exclusion, there was no category of "undocumented" or "illegal" immigrant. The major immigration legislation passed in 1924, the Johnson-Reed Act, retained racially determined quotas, with northern European favored over Jews, Eastern and Southern Europeans, and Asians in quotas for legal migration to the U.S (Act 1924). Not until the landmark Hart-Celler

Act of 1965 (Congress 1965) were these country-based quotas replaced by hemispheric quotas (although with particular numbers for the country of Mexico, which has had a unique role and prominence in U.S. legislation related to the undocumented; Ngai 2004). The total number of undocumented immigrants in the U.S. was estimated to be roughly 2 million in 1980, with growth of between 100,000 and 300,000 per year between 1980 and 1983 (Passel 1986). The Immigration Reform and Control Act of 1986 both restricted employment opportunities of the undocumented and provided a pathway to citizenship, resulting in 70 % of the undocumented in the country in 1986 becoming documented by 1988.

Beginning in the early 1990s and stretching through the beginning of the Great Recession, economic crises in Mexico and elsewhere increased the number of undocumented arriving in the U.S., such that by 2000–2005, 800,000 a year arrived in the U.S. After 2005 that number fell to 500,000 and after the Great Recession of 2008–2009, the number plunged further (Passel and Cohn 2008). However, it is estimated that roughly 11 million undocumented reside in the U.S., an historic high.

Case Study II: The Roma in Europe

The Roma people are the largest marginalized minority group in Europe and one of the most heterogeneous, encompassing many different religious affiliations, cultures, historical experiences, and dialects. It is difficult to get an accurate count of the Roma population due to fear of registering this identity and other factors. Currently, the Roma population across Europe is estimated to be roughly 12 million. The population of Roma children under the age of 15 is 35.7 % compared to 15.7 % of the EU population overall, which is considerably higher than the rest of Europe (UNICEF 2007). There are few official estimates of poverty among the Roma population but all estimates clearly indicate that Roma are among the poorest in the region.

The Roma have been among the poorest people living in Europe and live in nearly all the countries in Europe and Central Asia. Lacking a historic homeland, they are at particular risk of undocumented status. Traditionally, they maintained a nomadic lifestyle but since the 1900's they have become more settled (Migration Policy Institute 2004). However, since the Middle Ages, they experienced low social status and exclusion from the mainstream population. During the Second World War, the Roma population was the object of Nazi repression. Following the collapse of the Iron Curtain in 1989, political liberalization allowed increased international and national awareness of the Roma, including human rights violations and humanitarian concerns related to worsening socio-economic conditions and discrimination. Though, over the last two decades, there has been a movement away from viewing Roma as a disadvantaged social category and towards recognition as an ethnic minority and distinct cultural group (Svensson et al. 2007).

One of the common features across all Roma is risk for high levels of discrimination, poverty, and social exclusion. Many of them are forced to live partially or entirely segregated from the rest of the population. In many European countries, the Roma people are continuing to trail other ethnic groups in almost every characteristic that defines well-being. World Bank poverty assessments indicate that Roma "are almost entirely marginalized" and many "live in conditions below even the most minimal for survival" (World Bank 2003). The situation necessitates a strong focus on improving the well-being and future of poor and excluded Roma youth. The successful integration of Roma children and families into European society is critical to reducing the continuing and growing prevalence of intergenerational poverty.

The lack of a homeland makes Roma at particular risk regarding legal status, since there is no country to take responsibility for their specific protection, as often happens to particular migrant groups globally. For example, embassies in the United States have taken proactive steps to help incorporate groups (e.g., from Central America) with high levels of social exclusion—e.g., by providing consular identification and changing local laws so that such ID provides access in cases where the undocumented cannot get driver's licenses (e.g., for parents to access their children's schools). Roma children and adults often face serious challenges accessing important social services and programs when they lack citizenship.

As a transnational minority, Roma inclusion is no longer solely a national responsibility but a European one as well. Progress towards integration is being made. International and regional standards prohibit discrimination on the basis of race, ethnicity, and a variety of other criteria (Zoon 2001). In fact, the protection of minorities, such as Roma, has become an important feature of various international bodies, organizations and treaties. One of the first and most comprehensive documents for the protection and promotion of minority rights in the European Union is the Framework Convention for the Protection of National Minorities (1994) issued by the Council of Europe. Broadly, the treaty aims to ensure that the Council of Europe member states respect national minorities, combat discrimination, guarantee certain freedoms and promote equality. The intention of acknowledgement as a national minority is to create the necessary conditions for effective participation of national minorities in social, economic, cultural and public life. Unlike most international instruments that only contain political obligations, the Framework is legally binding for member states of the Council of Europe.

Legal and Documentation Status Among the Roma

Often times, the legal status of a Roma group is associated with the timing of their migration to their country of residence. Some groups of Roma who have been settled for many years are citizens of the country where they live. They may be considered national minorities or ethnic minorities but they have full citizenship with paperwork identifying them as citizens. Conversely, in the same countries, there could be other groups of Roma who are considered refugees or asylum-seekers, and they are not considered national or ethnic minorities. In this situation, most countries consider those Roma to be illegal immigrants. In Europe, there is general lack of pathways to citizenship for immigrants, particularly for those who cross borders from a non-EU country to an EU country. Unlike the United States, most countries do not offer birthright citizenship. Thus the Framework's failure to provide a strictly worded distinction between traditional national minorities or new minorities is more pronounced (Lipott 2012).

Current Research Questions

In the case of both the US and Roma in the E.U., after we briefly summarize the history of those with the status, including trends over recent years; empirical evidence on whether lacking citizenship as represented in documentation affects positive child development; the mechanisms through which the status may affect access to contexts associated with positive child development; and then programs and policies that may affect the status itself, or access to developmental contexts linked to the status. Finally, we synthesize the emerging commonalities and distinct patterns across the U.S. and Europe from the relevant evidence, and future directions for theory and research.

Research Measurement and Methodology

The evidentiary base for undocumented in the U.S. and in the E.U. is in its nascent stage. Much of what we know is based from large-scale secondary data analyses or findings that have emerged from data sets not specifically designed with the intent to consider the undocumented experience (Yoshikawa 2011; Suárez-Orozco et al. 2011). There is still a lot we do not know about how undocumented status affects developmental outcomes across domains, life stages, and contexts.

Empirical Findings

Undocumented Status in the U.S. and Positive Child Development

There is emerging evidence that children's and parents' undocumented status is associated with lower levels of positive development (Abrego 2014). Parents' undocumented status is associated with lower levels of cognitive development and educational progress across early and middle childhood (Brabeck and Xu 2010; Ortega et al. 2009; Yoshikawa 2011). By adolescence, having an undocumented parent is associated with higher levels of anxiety and depressive symptoms (Potochnick and Perreira 2010). Finally, a large-scale study of Mexican-origin young adults showed that having an undocumented mother, relative to an authorized one, was associated with between 1.25 and 1.5 fewer years of schooling (Bean et al. 2011). Being an undocumented youth limits educational attainment severely as well (Gonzales 2011). Thus, undocumented status restricts the ability of youth and young adults to participate fully in society both directly and indirectly through parental influences.

Legal and Undocumented Status Among Roma in the E.U. and Positive Child Development

Much policy attention has been put on improving education attainment. The participation rate of Roma children in preschool across Europe is likely around 20 % (UNICEF 2011). The rates of attendance and completion of primary school also remains staggeringly low. An estimate by UNICEF suggested that only one Roma child completes primary school for every four non-Roma child in Central and South Eastern Europe (Bennett 2012). In south-eastern Europe only 18 % of Roma children ever enroll in secondary school and less than 1 % attend university (UNICEF 2011).

More must be done once Roma children attend school. The Romani language is one of the most significant minority languages in the EU, encompassing several distinct dialects, but it is endangered. Given that many Roma children do not have the majority language as their mother tongue, that many do not complete primary education and that the children of illiterate parents are more likely to have limited literacy (RECI 2012). The few studies examining academic achievement find huge disparities among Roma and non-Roma children. Lazarová and Pol (2002) estimated that a Roma child coming to school possess the vocabulary of 400–800 Czech words, while the typical Czech child possess the vocabulary of 2000–3500 words. One study of first grade Roma children found that intellectual abilities, which are strongly influenced by a Roma child's family SES and family educational climate, are most predictive of scholastic achievement (Biro et al. 2009). Roma students in Serbia were on average 130 points behind the national average on a third grade national assessment and about 50 % of Roma students did not develop the very basic mathematical, language and literacy skills (Baucal 2006).

During adolescence, children continue to develop a firm personal identity and figuring out their place in society (Erikson 1959, 1968). Facing this identity task is vital to becoming responsible adults and active citizens (Havighurst,1952). Civic engagement is particularly important in the case of young people from ethnic minorities, like Roma youth, who face discrimination and socioeconomic disadvantages. Individuals who are engaged in society tend to feel that they are authorized to regulate the structures they are a part of (Zimmerman 1995) and this feeling contributes to a common sense of community (De Piccoli et al. 2002). Developing strong civic engagement among Roma youth potentially is beneficial because of the tendency of Roma's to be most seriously affected by an insensitive governance. Some research has been conducted examining civic engagement, citizenship and ethnic identity development among Roma youth. For instance, in one study, young Roma's tended to understand citizenship as working alongside nationality and rights (Ataman et al. 2012). Ataman et al. (2012), found that Roma youth associated poverty and unemployment with having a second class citizenship. Roma youth in their study felt that they lacked information about their rights and obligations as citizens and perceived a range of barriers against political participation. Possibly, differences in civic engagement between the Roma community and the majority group may not stem from differences in cultural values and norms, but rather from socioeconomic and educational inequalities (Lopez and Marcelo 2008). Civically engaged young Roma who participated in another study, often described their negative feelings associated with civic engagement (Šerek et al. 2011).

In a number of European countries, Roma demonstrate a remarkable ability to cope with unrelenting and marginalizing discrimination by creating energetic ethnic communities (European Commission 2010). Historically, the family has been the core component of the Roma community and the leading cause of preservation of Roma traditions and values. A strong identification with the family and Roma community can also act as a strength and resource for Roma to compensate for a lack of identification with mainstream society and culture as well as severe discrimination due to their Roma ethnic identification (Nunev 2000). Such resilience, referring to the achievement of positive developmental outcomes in the context of adversity (Luthar et al. 2000; Masten 2001), can be attributed to beneficial psychological and social resources that protect youth against the negative consequences of their ethnic identities. Research on ethnic minorities increasingly recognized that collective identity components, such as familial, ethnic and religious identity, have a significant influence on well-being (Dimitrova et al. 2013). However, the hostility, rejection, negative stereotypes, prejudice and discrimination faced by Roma can account for the tendency to internalize the negative image perpetuated by the majority groups. Little is known about the identity processes of Roma and several studies have shown lower levels of satisfaction with life among Roma youth (Dimitrova et al. 2013). Nonetheless, results are also consistent with our expectation that Roma youth who felt connected to their ethnic, religious and familial identity would exhibit greater well-being, irrespective of ethnic group membership (Dimitrova et al. 2013).

Universal Versus Cultural Specific Mechanisms

Mechanisms of Undocumented Status in the U.S

In the U.S., undocumented status can affect children's learning and positive development through a variety of proximal developmental contexts in their lives. These influences may occur above and beyond the high levels of poverty and low levels of education of those entering the U.S. without documents, relative to those who enter with documents. First, undocumented individuals are not eligible for a variety of elements of the U.S. safety net for the poor. For example, they are not eligible for publicly funded health care aside from emergency Medicaid and other emergency care; they are not eligible for public housing subsidies; they are not eligible for Food Stamps or SNAP; and they are not eligible for workforce development funds or subsidies for higher education provided by the federal government. Thus, access to health care, the safety net, and quality housing is severely restricted for undocumented parents and youth.

Second, undocumented parents appear reluctant to enroll their citizen children in programs for which their children are eligible (e.g., child-only TANF or cash welfare or Food Stamps; child care subsidies) because of the need to document earnings and therefore identify employers (Suárez-Orozco et al. 2011). This appears to result in lower levels of access to center-based care, the form of care most strongly associated with learning and cognitive skills in the first years of life (Yoshikawa 2011). In addition, children and youth who are undocumented themselves have no access to these programs.

Third, the undocumented experience substantially worse work conditions than documented low-wage workers. Exploitation of this workforce results in dramatically higher rates of illegally low wages (Bernhardt et al. 2009). These work conditions associated with undocumented status—low wages, and low levels of autonomy in the workplace—were linked to children's early cognitive skills in one study (Yoshikawa 2011).

Fourth, being undocumented and a newcomer to the U.S. can result in substantially lower levels of knowledge conveyed in social networks about opportunities for children. Ethnographic data suggest that the networks of recently arrived undocumented have high concentrations of other undocumented recent arrivals, with resulting lower levels of knowledge about resources for children such as public libraries, preschool education, and even laws and regulations related to migration. Undocumented parents, for example, are over-represented among those who have not applied (yet are eligible) for Deferred Action for Childhood Arrivals, the Obama administration regulation providing a temporary reprieve from deportation and legal worker status (New York Office of Immigrant Affairs 2014).

Finally, the fear of deportation has severely reduced community and civic participation among undocumented parents. In order to protect their families and children from the risk of deportation, undocumented parents have been much less likely than undocumented youth to become visible activists, thus reducing their positive roles in civic life. And in states with particularly harsh policies towards the undocumented, fear of being apprehended during one's daily routine can cut across all proximal contexts of family life and child development. Some states, such as Arizona, Tennessee and Alabama, have stronger norms of local law enforcement apprehending immigrants simply because of their legal status than other states or localities. The federal Secure Communities regulation varied in its implementation across the U.S., with some states and localities not implementing its linkage of federal with local law enforcement databases and others using these linkages to greatly increase stopping of immigrants and initiating deportation proceedings if they lacked proof of LPR or citizenship status. A racialized aspect of this process is the targeting of those who "look Mexican" for enforcement and deportation proceedings. Anti-Latino bias has increased substantially in recent years, with several highly prominent incidents of attacks in which groups of youth, for example, set out to find and kill "a Mexican" (e.g., the case of Marcelo Lucero in suburban New York; New York Times 2008).

Each threats to children's developmental contexts—their blocked access to the safety net, compromised work conditions, limited knowledge capital within their social networks, and parents' fear of deportation—can convey exclusion from the mainstream and lower the probability of educational progress, psychological well-being, and ultimately the ability to be a productive citizen among children and youth. The most proximal mechanisms for these contextual effects consist of the psychological distress and blocked community participation experienced by parents and by children who are aware of this status in their families (Yoshikawa et al. 2008), and growing awareness of one's own "illegality" and its implications for blocked opportunities, among youth who are undocumented themselves (Gonzales 2011).

Mechanisms of Legal and Undocumented Status Among Roma in E.U.

Across the European Union, Roma children have poorer developmental outcomes and educational attainment compared to non-Roma children. The inability of Roma to exercise their fundamental rights as EU citizens on equal footing as other Europeans may partly be responsible for the developmental disparities. The mechanisms of identifying an individual, as a citizen is a problem, both in terms of developing an identity and legally, particularly if an individual cannot access documents proving their citizenship. There are cases in which autochthonous Roma qualify for citizenship but they simply do not have the documents to prove it. The lack of documentation, such as identification documents, residence permits, and birth and marriage certificates, can leave Roma "stateless" and puts into question their legal status. Without clear identification as a citizen of their country, many Roma face barriers to accessing social and health services.

The inability to access social services because of a limited or lack of legal status within their own country may hinder positive development in several ways. First, Roma-origin children experience substantially worse quality of education than other children in Europe. One of the persistent problems is the failure of schools to recruit, include, and educate Roma children. Teachers' low expectations in dealing with Roma children and families, limited teacher training in diversity, ineffective governance of early education systems, incompatibility between traditional teaching practices and Roma learning styles, quality of teaching in schools with large Roma population, lack of competency in majority language, school readiness, and prejudice are just a few more of the many difficulties that Roma children face in order to get a quality education. However, above and beyond these factors Roma children are less likely to access education due to their increased risk of lacking documents and registration.

Second, many Roma families live in favela-like settlements, in shelters put together out of mud, cardboard, metal sheets, that are more likely to be located in hazardous areas even compared to other low-income populations in Europe. Often times, these settlements have poor access to public services, employment and schools. Roma families can be living without adequate access to public utilities like water, electricity, transportation or gas. In Serbia, there are estimated to be almost six hundred Roma settlements, half of which are considered unsanitary slums (UNICEF 2007). In Romania, about one third of Roma are estimated to live in compact homogenous communities.

Residents of slums suffer legal insecurity and typically do not have property rights and cannot register their home as a permanent address. This can lead to children not being called to school or being registered with a doctor. Poor living conditions are evident in both urban and rural areas.

Even if there are villages made up entirely of Roma, they are rarely represented in local councils and have no one advocating for their needs. The lack of official residence papers can result in the inability to access basic services, like water and electricity.

Poor housing conditions, including unhygienic and unsafe environments, have a direct impact on a young child's well-being, even prior to their birth (Evans 2004). Among researchers and policymakers, there is a consensus that housing has an impact on health. The fact that Roma children likely do not have adequate housing exasperates the likelihood that other aspects of their development are being compromised. For example, a child living far from transportation is likely to have difficulty going to school every day. By addressing the housing situation of Roma, countries should be integrating housing policies into social inclusion and desegregation programs.

Thirdly, Roma experience discrimination based on their perceived physical features. A recent case in Greece demonstrated the racialized treatment of Roma and assumptions regarding their physical appearance. Roma can be of any race; however, those who look stereotypically Roma face everyday harassment and discrimination (Kitsantonis and Bilefsky 2013).

Policy Implications

Policies and Programs Directly Affecting Undocumented Status

Programs and policies can address the consequences of undocumented status in two broad ways—by affecting the status directly, or by affecting access to the systems and institutions in ways that can exclude the undocumented from mainstream life.

Among policies that directly affect the status are deportation and border enforcement policies, as well as policies that provide temporary or permanent pathways to citizenship. Nearly two million people have been deported during the Obama administration; 96.7 % have been of

Latino descent, placing disproportionate stress and disruptions on Latino families (MALDEF 2014). It is important to understand the particular stress Latino children and youth face with family disruptions in the wake of deportations as well as in living in the shadow of undocumented status. It is also important to understand issues related to the undocumented of non-Latino groups, who have thus far been nearly invisible with regard to prevalence or specific needs (non-Latino groups with the highest proportions of undocumented status include those from China, the Philippines, India, Korea, and Vietnam; Hoefer et al. 2012).

Policies that provide a pathway to citizenship may bring children and youth out from the shadows of unauthorized status. As a federal system that provides unusual levels of discretion to the subnational level, the U.S. form of government can allow states to engage in some roles that are usually taken by central levels of government. States have taken a variety of policy directions in immigration enforcement and deportation, some in the harsher direction (Arizona's SB1070 legislation, e.g.) and some in the more generous direction (providing, for example, temporary reprieve from local deportation-related enforcement for certain categories of unauthorized workers, as in Utah). The effects of such state policy variation on youth have not been investigated. The Obama administration implemented Deferred Action for Childhood Arrivals year (DACA), a regulation providing temporary, 2-year reprieve from deportation and legal working status to certain unauthorized individuals under the age of 31 who came to the U.S. prior to age 15. Some research on the effects of this regulation has begun (Gonzales et al. 2014; Teranishi et al. 2015), finding positive associations of becoming "DACAmented" with employment, access to drivers' licenses, and higher education, yet at the same time high levels of worry about family members who are undocumented. A recent regulation expanding eligibility for DACA and adding undocumented parents of U.S. citizen children to its reprieve was announced in late 2014, but as of this writing has been blocked from implementation by state-level opposition.

U.S. Policies that Affect Access to Services and Programs

Other program approaches can increase access to publicly funded health, antipoverty and learning programs for affected children and youth (Crosnoe and Fuligni 2012; Yoshikawa et al. 2014). Not all organizational and policy approaches need to identify this group directly; some organizational practices can be implemented for low-income immigrant families. This includes simplifying paperwork so undocumented parents can enroll their citizen children; providing municipal identification to ease access to community resources (cf. New York City's recent initative and previous efforts in San Francisco and New Haven); offering legal services (in addition to social and educational services) in trusted settings like immigrant-serving organizations or schools. Universal public prekindergarten programs do not carry burdens of proof of low income that means-tested programs require—they may therefore increase the scope of the "protected period" that public education provides for undocumented parents and children alike. There is also evidence that quality universal preschool programs can reduce disparities between dual-language learner children and their English-speaking counterparts, and between Latino and White children's school readiness (Gormley et al. 2005; Weiland and Yoshikawa 2013).

Finally, efforts to improve the housing and work conditions of the unauthorized could improve parents' employment-related factors that have been shown to be associated with youth achievement and well-being in studies of the general low-wage working population. Employment-related factors include higher wages and wage growth; shorter and more standard work hours, relative to the very high work hours of many unauthorized individuals; greater complexity and opportunities for growth in job duties (Yoshikawa et al. 2006). Due to lack of access to housing subsidies, many of the undocumented live in doubled-up housing with little space for children to study. Alternative supports for housing such as better enforcement of housing quality laws and protections in low-income immigrant neighborhoods could address these developmental contexts.

E.U. Policies and Programs Directly Affecting Roma Documentation Status

As in the case of the undocumented in the United States, policies to address the role of legal and documentation status in the development of Roma-origin children may be of two types: those that affect the status directly, and those that affect access to the systems and institutions and comprise the social exclusion of the undocumented from mainstream life.

The Framework Convention for the Protection of National Minorities (1994) requires that Member States designate national minorities who would receive certain legal rights and protections. Some of the rights and protections include, the right of equality and equal protection under the law, right for equal opportunities to access to education, encouragement of mutual respect and tolerance, and freedom of expression and linguistic freedoms to be taught in their minority language. Thus, the Framework potentially provides an important, direct mechanism to address the status of Roma. However, one of the major shortcomings is the lack of a definition of what constitutes a national minority. Thus, despite the intention of the Council of Europe for its member states to recognize the minority status of Roma, the legal status of Roma now varies by country. The ambiguities around terminology makes it difficult to discern whether the Roma are considered national minorities who would receive legal status and protections, or as minorities with special (unprotected) status. The lack of a clearly defined description of a national minority allows each EU country the right to develop their own interpretation. Only a small number of EU countries give full legal recognition to Roma and, even in those countries, they are recognized as indigenous minorities.

Bulgaria, Romania, Spain, and Greece, a few of the countries with the largest numbers of Roma residing within their territory, do not consider Roma to be national minorities. Roma in Sweden are made up of various groups, including groups of Roma who are non-autochthonous, however, the country decided to not make a distinction among the groups and to confer them all to the status of national minorities (Lipott 2012). Under the Slovenian constitution, Roma are considered a minority community (Lipott 2012) but only autochthonous Roma are part of the minority community and considered citizens of Slovenia. However, autochthonous Roma is not defined in their law. This could be a real problem for the Roma community, particularly since non-autochthonous Roma have fewer rights.

Even when Roma are considered a national minority within a country, they often do not have supporting documentation. One example of a country trying to address the documentation problem directly is Romania. Their inter-ministerial commission has put on their agenda the need to address the lack of identification documents among Roma. However, the success of a program would depend on the cooperation among national and local authorities, Roma NGO's, the Roma community and funding organizations.

E.U. Policies that Affect Roma Access to Services and Programs

With the passing of the EU Framework for National Roma Integration Strategies up to 2020, the EU sent a signal that equal treatment and social inclusion must be a priority for all countries. Under the EU framework, all countries have developed their own Roma integration strategies. EU Roma policy requires member states to give ethnic minorities, such as Roma, equal access to education, housing, health, and employment (European Commission 2014). Several years after the passing of the Framework, it is evident that more still needs to be done. At present, only 12 countries have clearly identified funding and inclusion policy measures. Across the Member States, policy progress is being made but there still remains a large gap between policy and implementation. In general, the national legislations of Member States are weak. Rarely are explicit actions or measurable achievement specified in policies passed. Governments have failed to integrate external initiatives from the EU or other sources into national policy (UNICEF 2011).

Children in Roma families face many challenges that can be attributed to the hundreds of years of discrimination they have experienced. In particular, Roma parents and youth face numerous challenges affecting their inclusion into the labor market. Despite positive efforts by some countries, the levels of unemployment among Roma are at significantly higher levels than non-Roma. In fact, the income disparity between Roma and non-Roma has increased in the past 10 years. Poverty rates among Roma can be four times higher than among non-Roma. Oftentimes, employment in permanent jobs with benefits is denied based on discriminatory grounds (European Union Agency for Fundamental Rights 2014). Throughout Europe, the average life span of Roma is shorter than that of non-Roma and infant mortality rates are higher, indicating lower access to preventive and curative health care, especially prenatal and perinatal care. In terms of education, Roma tend to have much lower educational attainment and higher levels of illiteracy (especially among Roma women). These major barriers and factors contribute to the social exclusion and inability to access the widespread social services offered by EU countries.

Governments in Europe do provide a wide variety of benefits to those in need, including social support, monthly assistance for rent, food pantry distributions, support of heating, child allowances, additional benefits for families with children, maternity benefits and birth grants. However, the amount of each benefit is often insufficient to cover the overall needs of the Roma families. In most countries within the EU, beyond a certain number of children, there are no more increases in benefit levels. The higher number of children per Roma family means poor Roma are in greater need of receiving child benefits (Zoon 2001). In determining eligibility for benefits, governments impose a number of criteria, most of which have a disparate impact

on Roma. The inclusion and access criteria for services vary from country to country, but they can include: means tests, work responsibilities, ban on foreign travel, a domicile requirement, limitations on the size of living quarters, bans on corporate ownership, and housing sales. The means tests tend to disadvantage those, such as the Roma through discriminatory practices (i.e., caseworker discrimination); the domicile requirement, similarly, can disadvantage the Roma who have no official residences due to living in settlement areas.

According to the EU Framework, Member States must guarantee completion of primary school, increase access to quality early childhood education, eliminate segregation and discrimination experienced by Roma children and reduce the number of early school leavers. As a result of these and other rights-based frameworks, several countries have been taking important steps to remedy the situation. For instance, it has become more common for countries to pass laws that make preschool obligatory and universal, reducing barriers of documentation, registration and proof of citizenship. In Romania, as of the academic year 2012–2014, there will be one year of compulsory preschool, which is meant to equalize the level of preparation of children for primary school. In Hungry, obligatory pre-school from the age of three will be introduced in the 2014–2015 school year. The Hungarian legislation further stipulates that educational programs for minority children include the minority language, culture and history (Molnár and Dupcsik 2008). In the absence of reliable census data, Romani, the largest minority language in the European Union, is estimated to have a total population of 3.5 million speakers (Thompson 2013). Serbia passed two laws intended to improve the educational opportunities for children and increase fairness of access to disadvantaged children. The Law on the Fundamentals of the Educational System contains new regulations with specific implications for Roma children to improve the enrollment process (National Assembly of the Republic of Serbia 2009). Testing will occur after enrollment in the child's native language and the aim of testing is to ascertain what additional services a child may need. The Law on Preschool Education of 2010 proposes expanding the number of preschools and improving the quality (National Assembly of the Republic of Serbia 2010). In distant and rural regions, the law proposed traveling kindergartens or traveling preschool teachers.

Innovative policies and programs to increase and improve education for older children are increasing as well. In Demark, the project 'Hold On Tight Caravan', administered by the Ministry of Education, is focused on getting youth from ethnic minorities, including the Roma, to begin and complete a Vocational Education and Training program. The initiative is managed in schools by coordinators who ensure an individual approach to each young person at risk of school failure or drop out. Since it started in 2009, overall school and training drop-out rates have fallen from 20 % to fewer than 15 %, while the gap with ethnic Danish students has narrowed (European Commission 2014).

In order to close the gap in housing access and quality between the Roma and other groups, the EU framework calls on Member States to establish non-discriminatory access to housing, including social housing and public utilities. However, housing interventions and policies are often the weakest links in national strategies. The lack of progress tends to be due to grey areas concerning the legislation of existing housing laws, failure to establish a real dialogue with Roma communities, and lack of national public funds. Despite this challenging context, there are some examples of promising practices and policies. In Hungary, cities are required to develop local equal opportunity (desegregation) plans (European Commission 2014).The plans identify systematic intervention to stop or reduce segregation. In Germany, housing projects are also including measures that promote the integration of Roma in neighborhoods. The 'Maro Temm e.G' housing projects helps Roma of all generations preserve their culture and language by living together and not being segregated. Activities such as homework support, fun activities and cultural celebrations are offered. Additionally, they have a task force aimed to ensure Roma are accepted as neighbors in their community (European Commission 2014).

Many pioneering programs and policies are being developed across the region to tackle the exclusion of Roma children from education. The lessons from these programs need to be shared, replicated and scaled up. Governments need to be encouraged to take the lessons learned and create programs that can impact all Roma children and not rely so heavily on NGO initiatives. Progress is being made with positive results but much more work is required.

Future Directions

The undocumented in the U.S. and the Roma in Europe face some common barriers, yet also distinct historical and policy environments and experiences. Children in mixed-status families, or children and youth who are undocumented themselves, are some of the most disadvantaged in the U.S., showing evidence of substantially lower educational attainment and learning outcomes throughout childhood and adolescence (Bean et al. 2011; Yoshikawa 2011). Roma children likewise show persistently low levels of educational attainment throughout schooling, from preprimary through secondary and tertiary education (UNICEF 2007).

The mechanisms of such disadvantage include lack of access to formal systems of support that require registration, proof of residence, citizenship, or documentation of various kinds (not simply passports, but drivers' licenses in the U.S to birth registration and proof of residence in Europe). Thus the lack of official status of various kinds can impede access to quality education, housing, child care, and social services across these very different contexts. When a particular group is especially likely to lack these documents, children and youths' positive development can suffer.

To the extent that a marginalized population lacks the official documents that provide access to formal systems of support, the status of being undocumented may carry a universal set of disadvantages. These may however be weaker in societies whose social-sector supports, across health, education, social protection and child protection, are more universal in nature. The more means-tested and targeted such support systems are, such as in the U.S., the more a barrier being undocumented may constitute for well-being, educational progress and community participation (Yoshikawa et al. in press). Cultural factors such as the specificity and particularly long-lived historical features of discrimination that the Roma face (stretching across national and political boundaries, as well as across centuries) can make it more likely that members of this group will be undocumented in various ways. The racialized contexts of discrimination in the U.S. and Europe can further exacerbate the disadvantages of undocumented or Roma status, when individuals share stereotyped physical features associated with these groups.

Future theoretical and empirical work may benefit from addressing the notion of lacking documents, registration or legal status in studies of child and youth development more generally. Theoretically, European notions of social exclusion may be more applicable to these populations than theories based on socioeconomic disadvantage. In the U.S., the primary theories explaining consequences of disadvantage are based on race or poverty. In Europe, the notion of social exclusion is both a theoretical construct (cf. Lenoir 1974) and has become the basis of policies to counter disadvantage (e.g., the UK Social Exclusion Unit, which was set up as part of the Cabinet and then the Deputy Prime Minister's office in 1997 and through the 2000's). The theory and policies surrounding exclusion are based in concepts of the universality of child rights (UN 1999).

Empirically, there has been very little linking the lack of official documentation or identification across nations and how that may affect human development. For example, birth registration is tracked in international development work, yet without much contribution from developmental science. Without registration at birth, enrollment

in many social programs—health, education, social protection—is threatened. In some regions of the world, over one-third of children are not registered before their 5th birthday, and millions remain unregistered throughout their entire lives (UNICEF 2013). The consequences for child and youth development are severe, yet remain unexplored by developmental scientists.

Finally, refugee immigrant populations in conflict-affected and emergency situations are another prominent population that is at risk due to lack of citizenship. Most studies focus on short-term effects of refugee status. The consequences of long-term lack of documentation or integration into host countries have been less investigated (Burde et al. 2014).

By drawing on the cases of recent waves of undocumented migration in the U.S., and the case of the Roma in Europe, particularly those who cross national borders, we have aimed to illustrate how policies and programs related to citizenship affect positive child development through a set of developmental contexts. Future research and policy should focus on further specifying the mechanisms through which legal status may affect access to contexts associated with positive child development. Such data would help improve and expand the policies and practices that can counter this severe form of social exclusion.

Acknowledgement Yoshikawa's effort on the chapter was partially supported by a grant from the NYU Abu Dhabi Research Institute to the Global TIES for Children Center at New York University.

References

A death in Patchoque. (2008). New York Times, A28.

Abrego, L. (2014). *Sacrificing families: Navigating laws, labor, and love across borders*. Palo Alto, CA: Stanford University Press.

Abel, G. J., & Sander, N. (2014). Quantifying global international migration flows. *Science, 343*(6178), 1520–1522.

Act, J. R. (1924). ch. 190. *Stat, 153*.

Alba, R., & Nee, V. (2009). *Remaking the American mainstream: Assimilation and contemporary immigration*. Cambridge, MA: Harvard University Press.

Ataman, A., Çok, F., & Şener, T. (2012). Understanding civic engagement among young Roma and young Turkish people in Turkey. *Human Affairs, 22*(3), 419–433.

Bardach, E. (2012). *A practical guide for policy analysis: The eightfold path to more effective problem solving.* Thousand Oaks, CA: CQ Press.

Baucal, A. (2006). Development of mathematical and language literacy among Roma students. *Psihologija, 39*(2), 207–227.

Bean, F. D., Leach, M. A., Brown, S. K., Bachmeier, J. D., & Hipp, J. R. (2011). The educational legacy of unauthorized migration: Comparisons across US-immigrant groups in how parents' status affects their offspring. *International Migration Review, 45,* 348–385.

Bennett, J. (2012). *The Roma early childhood inclusion overview report.* Budapest: UNICEF, Open Society Foundations and Roma Education Fund.

Bernhardt, A., Milkman, R., Theodore, N., Heckathorn, D., Auer, M., DeFilippis, J., et al. (2009). *Broken laws, unprotected workers. National employment law project.* New York: NELP.

Biro, M., Smederevac, S., & Tovilovic, S. (2009). Socioeconomic and cultural factors of low scholastic achievement of Roma children. *Psihologija, 42*(3), 273–288.

Brabeck, K., & Xu, Q. (2010). The impact of detention and deportation on Latino immigrant children and families: A quantitative exploration. *Hispanic Journal of Behavioral Sciences, 32*(3), 341–361.

Burde, D., Kapit, A., Wahl, R., Guven, O., & Skarpeteig, M. (2014). *Education in emergencies: A review of theory and research (manuscript under review).* New York: New York University.

Congress, U. S. (1882). Chinese Exclusion Act. In *47th congress, session I.*

Congress, U. S. (1965). Hart-celler act (Immigration and Naturalization Act of 1965).

Crosnoe, R., & Fuligni, A. J. (2012). Children from immigrant families: Introduction to the Special Section. *Child Development, 83*(5), 1471–1476.

De Piccoli, N., Colombo, M., & Mosso, C. (2002). Active participation as an expression of the sense of community. *Paper presented at the IV European Congress of Community Psychology,* Barcelona, Spain, 8–11 November.

Dimitrova, R., Chasiotis, A., Bender, M., & van de Vijver, F. (2013). Collective identity and wellbeing of Roma minority adolescents in Bulgaria. *International Journal of Psychology, 48*(4), 502–513.

Erikson, E. H. (1959). Psychological issues: identity and the life cycle. In Erikson E. H. (Ed.), *Growth and crises of the healthy personality* (Vol. 1, pp. 50–100). New York, NY: International Universities Press.

Erikson, E. H. (1968). *Identity: Youth and crisis (No. 7).* WW Norton & Company.

Evans, G. (2004). The environment of childhood poverty. *American Psychologist, 59*(2), 22–92.

European Commission. (2010). *Roma in Europe: The implementation of European Union Instruments and Policies for Roma Inclusions—Progress Report 2008–2010.* European Union.

European Commission. (2014). *Report of the implementation of the EU framework for National Roma Integration Strategies.* European Union.

European Union Agency for Fundamental Rights. (2014). *Poverty and employment: The situation of Roma in 11 EU Member States.*

Framework Convention for the Protection of National Minorities, adopted 10 Nov. 1994, opened for signature 1 Feb. 1995, entered into force 1 Feb. 1998, 2151 UNTS 243, ETS 157, reprinted in 34 ILM 351 (1995). http://conventions.coe.int/Treaty/en/Treaties/Html/157/htm.39statesparties.

Gonzales, R. G. (2011). Learning to be illegal: Undocumented youth and shifting legal contexts in the transition to adulthood. *American Sociological Review, 76*(4), 602–619.

Gonzales, R. G., Terriquez, V., & Ruszczyk, S. P. (2014). Becoming DACAmented assessing the short-term benefits of Deferred Action for Childhood Arrivals (DACA). *American Behavioral Scientist, 58*(14), 1852–1872.

Gormley, W. T., Jr., Gayer, T., Phillips, D., & Dawson, B. (2005). The effects of universal pre-K on cognitive development. *Developmental Psychology, 41,* 872–884.

Havighurst, R. J. (1952). *Developmental tasks and education.* New York: McKay.

Hoefer, M., Rytina, N., & Baker, B. C. (2012). *Estimates of the unauthorized immigrant population residing in the United States: January 2011.* Washington, DC: U. S. Department of Health and Human Services.

Kitsantonis, N., & Bilefsky, D. (2013). *Greek abduction case highlights Roma tensions.* The New York Times. Retrieved November 11, 2014, from http://www.nytimes.com/2013/10/22/world/europe/roma-couple-ordered-jailed-by-greek-authorities.html

Lazarová, B., & Pol, M. (2002). *Multikulturalita a rovné příležitosti v české škole [Multiculturality and equal opportunities in Czech school].* Praha: Institut pedagogicko-psychologického poradenství ČR.

Lenoir, R. (1974). *Les Exclus: Un Français sur dix [The excluded: One in ten French].* Paris: Le Seuil.

Lipott, S. (2012). Roma as a protected minority-policies and best practices in the EU. *The Romanian Journal European Affairs, 12,* 78.

Lopez, M. H., & Marcelo, K. B. (2008). The civic engagement of immigrant youth: New evidence from the 2006 Civic and Political Health of the Nation Survey. *Applied Developmental Science, 12*(2), 66–73.

Luthar, S. S., Cicchetti, D., & Becker, B. (2000). Research on resilience: Response to commentaries. *Child Development, 71*(3), 573–575.

Masten, A. S. (2001). Ordinary magic: Resilience processes in development. *American Psychologist, 56*(3), 227.

Mexican American Legal Defense and Educational Fund. (2014). *Detention, deportation, and devastation: The disproportionate effect of deportations on the Latino Community.* MALDEF.

Migration Policy Institute. (2004). The Roma of Eastern Europe: Still searching for inclusion. *Migration Information Source.*

Molnár, E., & Dupcsik, C. (2008). Country report on education: Hungary. *EDUMIGROM Background Papers.*

National Assembly of the Republic of Serbia. (2009). *Law on the fundamentals of the educational system.* Official Gazette of the Republic of Serbia.

National Assembly of the Republic of Serbia. (2010). *Law on preschool education.* Official Gazette of the Republic of Serbia.

New York Office of Immigrant Affairs. (2014). *Deferred action.* Retrieved November 16, 2014, from http://www.nyc.gov/html/imm/html/initiatives/defaction.shtml

Ngai, M. M. (2004). *Impossible subjects: Illegal aliens and the making of modern America.* Princeton: Princeton University Press.

Nunev, J. (2000). Current problems of ethno-cultural identification of Roma in Bulgaria. In V. Rusanov (Ed.), *Aspects of ethnocultural situation in Bulgaria* (pp. 273–281). Sofia: Open Society Foundation.

Ortega, A. N., Horwitz, S. M., Fang, H., Kuo, A. A., Wallace, S. P., & Inkelas, M. (2009). Documentation status and parental concerns about development in young US children of Mexican origin. *Academic pediatrics, 9,* 278–282.

Passel, J. S. (1986). Undocumented immigration. *The Annals of the American Academy of Political and Social Science, 487,* 181–200.

Passel, J. S., & Cohn, D. (2008). *Trends in unauthorized immigration.* Washington, DC: Pew Research Center.

Passel, J., Cohn, D., Krogstad, J. M., & Gonzalez-Barrera, A. (2014). *As growth stalls, unauthorized immigrant population becomes more settled.* Washington, DC: Pew Research Institute.

Potochnick, S. R., & Perreira, K. M. (2010). Depression and anxiety among first-generation immigrant Latino youth: key correlates and implications for future research. *The Journal of Nervous and Mental Disease, 198,* 470–477.

Roma Early Childhood Inclusion. (2012). *Roma early childhood inclusion: The RECI Overview Report.*

Šerek, J., Petrovičová, Z., & Macek, P. (2011). The civic life of young Czech Roma: Perceived resources, barriers, and opportunities. *Diversity is Reality: Effective Leadership of Diverse Teams in a Global Environment,* 143–152.

Suárez-Orozco, C., Yoshikawa, H., Teranishi, R. T., & Suárez-Orozco, M. M. (2011). Growing up in the shadows: The developmental implications of unauthorized status. *Harvard Educational Review, 81,* 438–473.

Suárez-Orozco, C., Yoshikawa, H., & Tseng, V. (2015). *Intersecting inequalities: Future directions for research with immigrant-origin children and youth.* Report, William T. Grant Foundation.

Svensson, A. L., Marojevic, S., Kovats, M., Surdu, M., & Rakocevic, N. K. (2007). *Breaking the cycle of exclusion: Roma children in South East Europe.*

Teranishi, R., Suarez-Orozco, C., & Suarez-Orozco, M. (2015). *In the shadows of the ivory tower: Undocumented undergraduates in the uncertain era of immigration reform.* Los Angeles: UCLA Graduate School of Education.

Thompson, I. (2013). *Romani.* Retrieved November 14, 2014, from http://aboutworldlanguages.com/romani

Torpey, J. C. (Ed.). (2001). *Documenting individual identity: The development of state practices in the modern world.* Princeton: Princeton University Press.

United Nations. (1999). *Convention on the rights of the child.* New York: Author.

UNICEF. (2007). *Breaking the cycle of exclusion–Roma children in South East Europe.*

UNICEF. (2011). *The right of Roma children to education: Position paper.*

UNICEF. (2013). *Every child's birth right: Inequities and trends in birth registration.* New York: Author.

Weiland, C., & Yoshikawa, H. (2013). Impacts of a prekindergarten program on children's mathematics, language, literacy, executive function, and emotional skills. *Child Development, 84,* 2112–2130.

World Bank. (2003). *Bosnia Herzegovina Poverty Assessment* (p. 21).

Yoshikawa, H. (2011). *Immigrants raising citizens: Undocumented parents and their young children.* New York, NY: Russell Sage.

Yoshikawa, H., Godfrey, E. B., & Rivera, A. C. (2008). Access to institutional resources as a measure of social exclusion: Relations with family process and cognitive development in the context of immigration. *New Directions for Child and Adolescent Development, 2008*(121), 63–86.

Yoshikawa, H., & Kalil, A. (2011). The effects of parental undocumented status on the developmental contexts of young children in immigrant families. *Child Development Perspectives, 5,* 291–297.

Yoshikawa, H., Suarez-Orozco, C., & Gonzales, R. (in press). Society for Research in Adolescence consensus statement on unauthorized status and youth development. *Journal of Research on Adolescence.*

Yoshikawa, H., Weiland, C., Ulvestad, K., Perreira, K., Crosnoe, R., Chaudry, A., et al. (2014). *Improving access of low-income immigrant families to health and human services: The role of community-based organizations* (Policy Brief No. 4, Immigrant Access to Health and Human Services Project). Washington, DC: The Urban Institute.

Yoshikawa, H., Weisner, T. S., & Lowe, E. D. (Eds.). (2006). *Making it work: Low-wage employment, family life, and child development.* New York: Russell Sage Foundation.

Zimmerman, M. A. (1995). Psychological empowerment: Issues and illustrations. *American Journal of Community Psychology, 23*(5), 581–599.

Zoon, I. (2001). *On the margins: Roma and public services in Romania, Bulgaria, and Macedonia; with a supplement on housing in the Czech Republic; a call to action to improve Romani access to social protection, health care, and housing.* Open Society Institute.

Research on Positive Youth Development in Boys of Color: Implications for Intervention and Policy

Noni K. Gaylord-Harden, Cynthia Pierre, Latriece Clark, Patrick H. Tolan, and Oscar A. Barbarin

Abstract

Boys of color (BOC) face unique challenges related to the intersection of being male and an ethnic minority in our society. There is an urgent need for a more balanced view of psychosocial functioning in BOC that highlights positive developmental trajectories. In response to this need, the current chapter provides an overview of the research on positive youth development (PYD) in BOC with a focus on implications for programs and policies. The chapter presents an historical overview and the theoretical perspectives on PYD, including the need for examining PYD in BOC and the current conceptualizations of PYD. Next, the empirical findings of studies that explicitly examine PYD in BOC are reviewed, with a discussion of the implications for programs and interventions, and research questions that are raised by findings in these studies. In conclusion, policy implications and future directions for research and intervention efforts in this area are discussed.

"Over the years, we've identified key moments in the life of a boy or a young man of color that will, more often than not, determine whether he succeeds, or falls through the cracks. We know the data. We know the statistics. And if we can focus on those key moments, those life-changing points in their lives, you can have a big impact; you can boost the odds for more of our kids."—President Barack Obama, *My Brother's Keeper Initiative*, February 24, 2014.

In February of 2014, President Barack Obama launched the My Brother's Keeper Initiative to provide opportunities for boys and young men of color to reach their full potential, noting that coordinated philanthropic efforts and enhancement of effective community solutions should target critical intervention points in the lives of boys and young men of color. Now, more than

N.K. Gaylord-Harden (✉) · C. Pierre · L. Clark
Department of Psychology, Loyola University
Chicago, 1032 W. Sheridan Rd., Chicago,
IL 60660, USA
e-mail: ngaylor@luc.edu

P.H. Tolan
The University of Virginia, Charlottesville,
VA, USA

O.A. Barbarin
The University of Maryland, College Park,
MD, USA

© The Editor(s) 2017
N.J. Cabrera and B. Leyendecker (eds.), *Handbook on Positive Development of Minority Children and Youth*, DOI 10.1007/978-3-319-43645-6_24

ever, adolescence can be regarded as a critical intervention point in development due to the increasing shifts in roles, responsibilities, expectations, and instability in the lives of today's adolescents (Tolan 2014). Boys of color face these challenges, as well as challenges unique to the intersection of being male and an ethnic minority in our society. Given that this intersection brings with it lower expectations and negative stereotypes, there is a need for a more balanced view of development of boys of color that can be informed by a positive youth development approach (Barbarin 2013). In response to this need, the current chapter provides an overview of positive youth development (PYD) in boys of color with a focus on implications for programs and policies. Since the launch of the My Brother's Keeper Initiative, over $300 million has been committed by corporations, foundations, and social enterprises to support programs and efforts that promote positive youth development in boys of color. As such, there is a need to ensure that there is a strong theoretical and empirical basis for these efforts (Catalano et al. 2004). In this chapter, boys of color (BOC) are defined as boys from African American, Latino, and American Indian ethnicities (Barbarin 2015). First, we provide an historical overview and the theoretical perspectives on PYD, including the need for examining PYD in BOC and a brief discussion of the current conceptualizations of PYD. Next, we review the empirical findings of studies that explicitly examine PYD in BOC, provide implications for programs and interventions, and discuss research questions that are raised by findings in these studies. Finally, we discuss policy implications and future directions for research and interventions in this area.

Historical Overview and Theoretical Perspectives

Historical perspectives on adolescent development characterized adolescence as a period of "storm and stress" (e.g., Hall 1904), in which adolescents experience significant difficulties characterized by conflictual parent–child relationships, mood disruptions, and risky behaviors (Arnett 1999). Misconceptions regarding adolescence are deeply embedded in our societal belief system, and these strongly-held beliefs have guided research inquiries and developmental theories for many years (Damon 2004; Offer and Schonert-Reichl 1992). A qualitative review synthesizing the content of over 2000 adolescent research articles over a ten-year period found that the majority of articles focused on adolescent turmoil, instability, and abnormality, leading the authors to characterize research on adolescent development as possessing an "obsession with the dark side of adolescence" (Ayman-Nolley and Taira 2000). The bias in basic research spills over into applied work, with pathogenic mental health models emphasizing psychopathology, disability, and distress (e.g., Antaramian et al. 2010), zero tolerance discipline policies criminalizing behavior in schools (e.g., Fenning and Rose 2007), and punitive models of juvenile justice emphasizing punishment over rehabilitation (e.g., Steinberg 2009).

In addition to the general preconceptions in adolescent research, a closer examination of how research with youth of color is approached reveals this bias is particularly characteristic of the literature about this population. Content analysis of single-ethnic group studies of adolescents showed that the most frequently examined topic for African American and Latino youth was "risk-taking behavior," compared to the topic "family" for White youth (Ayman-Nolley and Taira 2000). The stark contrast in research topic prevalence reflects an unfortunate pattern in research and theoretical perspectives of psychosocial development; to frame the development of youth of color, and particularly boys of color, in deficit-based models (García Coll et al. 1996; McLoyd and Randolph 1985; Tucker and Herman 2002). Deficit-based models emphasize the problems of youth of color as most informative, rather than focusing on normative development and cultural strengths. These models explain differences between ethnic groups as deficits, maladaption, or pathology among youth of color (García Coll et al. 2000; Gaylord-Harden et al. 2012; McLoyd 1990). This proclivity among researchers often couches these differences as due to an increased likelihood for maladaptive functioning as a result of exposure to more serious and frequent stressors. Consequently, the implication is that youth of color are at once pathologized (characterizing behavior as abnormal based on the assumption that youth of color differences from other youth are signs of stress-induced pathology) and also "idealized" (characterizing those boys of color who do not show these behavioral patterns as "exceptional" or "rare"). Capability and contextual variations in demands and resources are absent or at least overlooked in such models.

The intersection between misconceptions about adolescent development and the framing of development of boys of color in deficit models leads to these boys being overdiagnosed with "socially disruptive" psychiatric disorders, such as conduct disorder and oppositional defiant disorder (Mizock and Harkins 2011; Schwartz and Feisthamel 2009), being suspended and expelled from schools at disproportionately higher rates than other youth (Fenning and Rose 2007; Reynolds et al. 2008), and being overrepresented in the juvenile justice system where punitive policies and practices increase the rates of recidivism (Steinberg 2009). These same orientation features lead to a common belief that boys of color are a particularly problematic and pathology vulnerable population, spawning either villianizing them or rendering them tragic figures. Among the many harmful examples is the myth of BOC as super predators: a hardened, lawless violence prone group threatening to society (Jennings 2014). For example, recent research demonstrates that Black boys are perceived as older and less innocent by police officers (Goff et al. 2014) and Latino males are seen as threats to national security and American values (Chavez 2013; Fujioka 2011). Certainly, recent events in the United States involving the shootings of unarmed adolescent males of color highlight the firmly-held societal beliefs that BOC are problematic and threatening and their deficits and limitations are what is of most interest.

To counter misconceptions regarding development in youth of color, scholars have begun to argue that the paucity of focus on positive functioning is biasing or allowing biases to prevail (Cabrera 2013). Moreover, descriptive studies are showing that for youth of color, as for other children, capabilities and assets may explain functioning at least as well as risk factors (Tolan et al. 2013). Moreover, a range of factors that promote and maintain positive development are embedded in the families and communities that socialize these youth (e.g., Gaylord-Harden et al. 2012). A collective effort to highlight positive development in BOC is reflected in the recent work of the Boys of Color Collaborative (Barbarin 2013), developed to utilize existing longitudinal data sets to advance research on development in BOC. As noted in a 2013 special issue of the *American Journal of Orthopsychiatry* devoted to research on BOC, the purpose of the Collaborative is "to provide a more balanced view of the development of BOC by including a focus on strengths and resilience, not only to understand the problems that BOC face but also to place a spotlight on the fact that many are doing well in a way that helps us to figure out how to expand the numbers of these BOC who thrive (Barbarin 2013, p. 143)." As a consequence of this intention, research in the special issue emphasized the development of individual, family, and environmental characteristics, as well as trajectories that bring about positive development in BOC. It is important to highlight efforts such as the BOC collaborative, as they represent a critical shift in the narrative on development in a segment of youth who will soon be part of the majority of the U.S. youth population (Sesma and Roehlkepartain 2003). Thus, the intellectual and cultural climate is ripe to merge this burgeoning body of empirical research with theories on how positive development occurs in youth.

Conceptualization of Positive Youth Development

The field of Positive Youth Development (PYD) developed in response to the negative, deficit view of adolescent development that dominated theory and research on youth for several decades (Lerner et al. 2009a; Tolan 2014). Prior to the development of a literature on PYD, positive development was regarded as the absence of or decreases in risk, problems or mental health symptoms. The PYD framework changes the perspective on youth development from one that focuses on deficits and risks to one that focuses on strengths and potentiality for healthy development. According to the PYD perspective, all youth have strengths, and consistent with relational developmental theory, PYD is facilitated when there is alignment between the strengths of youth and the resources for healthy development present in the environments (families, school, communities) of youth (Lerner et al. 2009a, b). Rather than conceptualizing development as a process that is focused on overcoming deficits and risks, PYD posits that when there is alignment between strengths and resources, youth are poised to make significant contributions to themselves, their family, their community, and the society at large (Damon 2004).

While there is agreement that PYD is heavily related to environmental resources, termed assets, there is disagreement regarding whether specific assets are important, how many assets are needed for adequate functioning, and whether assets can be clearly differentiated from indicators of functioning (Lerner et al. 2009b). Among the various theoretical models of PYD, two approaches to defining assets have emerged as leading PYD models. Benson and colleagues at the Search Institute developed a framework of 40 developmental assets that they characterize as contextual and individual "building blocks" that

enhance positive developmental outcomes in youth (Leffert et al. 1998). These assets are categorized into 20 internal assets or personal characteristics of young people and 20 external assets or health-promoting features of the environment (Leffert et al. 1998). The 20 internal assets are further categorized into 4 groups: commitment to learning, positive values, social competencies and positive identity. Similarly, the 20 external assets are further categorized into 4 groups: support, empowerment, boundaries and expectations, and constructive use of time.

The Five C's Model of PYD, developed by Lerner and colleagues, is regarded as the most empirically-support framework in the literature (Bowers et al. 2010). Developed from the experiences of practitioners and comprehensive reviews of adolescent development, the Five C's include the following assets for PYD: competence (intellectual ability and social/behavioral skills), confidence (positive self-regard, and sense of self-efficacy), connection (positive bond with people and institutions), character (integrity and moral centeredness), and caring (human value and empathy) (Lerner et al. 2009a; Phelps et al. 2009). Recently, scholars have added an additional "C" of contribution (Lerner et al. 2009a). The Six C's have been linked to the positive outcomes of youth development programs, and can be widely applied because they are terms used by practitioners, adolescents, and parents.

Finally, there are other models that emphasize the role of engagement and agency as important indicators of positive youth development (Larson 2000). In particular, Larson discusses youth's engagement in development that results from their internal motivation (agency) being activated and sustained by challenges (Larson 2006). In this regard, youth become producers of their own growth and the role of adults is to support youth's experience of ownership and agency (Larson 2006). A key emphasis of this model is initiative—the ability for an adolescent to be motivated from within to direct attention and effort toward a challenging goal (Larson 2000). Researchers have discussed PYD programs and mentoring relationships as key contexts that facilitate the development of youth initiative (Larson 2000).

In addition to youth initiative, research suggests that the development of the assets presented in all of the PYD models above occurs in the context of youth development programs (Lerner et al. 2005; Roth and Brooks-Gunn 2003a). In fact, in a sample of 6000 adolescents across multiple ethnic groups, researchers examined the impact of 40 developmental assets on seven thriving outcomes (Scales et al. 2000). Of the 40 assets, time spent in youth programs showed the most pervasive positive effect on thriving indicators, predicting five out of seven thriving indicators and the composite index of thriving (Scales et al. 2000). As such, there is a need to synthesize research findings on PYD in BOC to ensure that evidenced-based goals can be established for PYD programs, and that the effectiveness of PYD programs or policies can be evaluated (Lerner et al. 2005).

Empirical Findings of PYD Studies with BOC

While the empirical research devoted to positive youth development in BOC is sparse, the potential for understanding how PYD manifests in BOC has been attracting increasing amounts of attention recently as researchers begin to take advantage of longitudinal data sets and advanced statistical analyses that highlight growth and change over time. To help facilitate the progressive development of the literature on PYD in BOC, a review of existing empirical studies in the area is presented below with three specific objectives. The first objective was to provide a brief summary of the current state of the research on PYD in BOC, as well as highlight methodological features of existing studies. The second objective was to discuss the implications of the existing research for intervention and programming efforts with BOC. The third objective was to identify unanswered questions that may assist in further advancing the application of PYD frameworks to BOC. Given the lack of empirical research examining the effectiveness of PYD

programs and interventions specifically for BOC, we focused our review on basic research studies that included the following: (1) an explicit focus on assessing positive youth development using existing PYD frameworks, and (2) a focus on boys of color, as defined by Barbarin (2015) or on youth of color with gender-specific findings reported.

Some of the earliest work on positive development in BOC is demonstrated in the Overcoming the Odds (OTO) study, a longitudinal study that examined characteristics of positive functioning and individual and ecological developmental assets among African American male youth either involved in gangs or in community-based organizations (CBO's) designed to promote positive development in youth (e.g., 4-H club, churches, and Boys and Girls Clubs). By employing the Search Institute framework of developmental assets (Benson 1997; Benson et al. 1998), the OTO study collected qualitative data from interviews with African American male adolescent gang-involved youth and CBO youth (Taylor et al. 2002a, b; 2004). Results showed CBO youth scored higher than the gang-involved youth on the presence of individual and ecological assets for positive youth development such as boundaries and expectations, constructive use of time, support, social competencies, empowerment, commitment to learning, and positive values; however, the contrast in assets between gang and CBO youth were not absolute (Taylor et al. 2002a, 2004). All gang-involved youth possessed at least one asset across the seven asset categories' studied in OTO and 15.6 % had total mean asset scores at the first wave of testing that were more positive than the average total asset score among CBO youth (Taylor et al. 2002a). Further, for gang-involved youth, the individual assets of commitment to learning, positive values, and social competencies, and the ecological assets of support and boundaries and expectations were associated with an increase in positive functioning over time. Thus, findings suggest that there are subsets of gang-involved youth that, despite high levels of environmental risk, possess individual and ecological assets that are associated with positive functioning (Taylor et al. 2002a). Further, when gang-involved youth maintain high levels of assets over time or show increases in the levels of assets over time, they show more positive youth development over time (Taylor et al. 2002b).

A more recent prospective study sought to understand PYD's role in mitigating HIV-related risk behaviors among rural African American male youth (Murry et al. 2014). Using 5 waves of data from middle childhood to young adulthood, the researchers tested a conceptual model in which positive parenting practices (e.g., involved-vigilant parenting; supportive relationships; parent–child communication regarding risky behaviors; racial socialization) led to PYD via future orientation and self-regulation skills. These skills represent the Competence and Confidence factors, respectively, in the Six Cs model of PYD (Lerner et al. 2009a; Phelps et al. 2009). These PYD factors were predicted to increase prosocial peer affiliation, and such affiliation was then predicted to increase the utilization of conventional norms and values in interpersonal relationships. Finally, these social norms were expected to mitigate HIV-related risk behaviors (e.g., unprotected sex; drug use). The results demonstrated that parenting strategies (vigilant parenting and racial socialization) during middle childhood predicted youth future orientation, which in turn, predicted self-regulation during early adolescence, which increased affiliation with prosocial peers during the transition from early to late adolescence. Affiliation with prosocial peers led directly to positive developmental outcomes of risk avoidance prosocial norms and values as these African American males transitioned to young adulthood. Profile analyses revealed that, in comparison to high-risk males, low-risk males were more likely to have positive experiences with parental socialization, to have like-minded peers and in turn, espouse more prosocial norms and values.

Another prospective study sought to examine a developmental-ecological framework of both positive development and risky development in a sample of 315 African American and Latino male adolescents from high-risk urban communities

(Tolan et al. 2013). In particular, the study examined how stress measured during early adolescence impacted two indicators of positive functioning (prosocial values and engagement to school) and two indicators of problems in functioning (depressive symptoms and external behavior) later in adolescence, as well as how family functioning, engagement in potentially protective prosocial activities, and individual coping skill might mitigate those outcomes. The results revealed that stress was a significant predictor of depressive symptoms and problem behaviors, but did not directly predict indicators of positive functioning. Instead, stress interacted with coping to predict engagement in prosocial values with a positive association between coping effectiveness and later endorsement of prosocial values when stress levels were low. Likewise, there was an interaction between stress and family functioning in the prediction of school engagement, with a positive association between family functioning and later school engagement when stress levels were low. Stress also interacted with coping effectiveness in the prediction of problem behaviors, such that there was an inverse association between coping effectiveness and later problem behaviors when stress was low. In sum, the pattern of results in this study demonstrate that positive and negative outcomes are not in direct opposition, underscoring the importance of examining both positive functioning and problem functioning in BOC to obtain a more holistic understanding of development in this population (Tolan et al. 2013).

A cross-sectional study examined the relationships between lifetime community violence exposure, family functioning, and PYD in a sample of 110 predominantly African American (>96 %) adolescents from urban communities (McDonald et al. 2011). Approximately 46 % of the sample was male. The researchers expected family functioning to act as a buffer or protective factor for the effects of community violence exposure on PYD outcomes, as assessed by the Six Cs model of PYD (Lerner et al. 2009a). In this study, youth were allowed to define family as "whoever they considered to be family" to account for the role of fictive kin and extended family relationships in African American families (McDonald et al. 2011). Although healthier family functioning was consistently predictive of PYD, there were some gender-specific findings for males that are worth noting. Specifically, PYD was significantly lower for boys reporting unhealthy family functioning in comparison to girls reporting unhealthy family functioning. Further, unlike girls, for boys in the study, the global dimensions of family functioning assessed were more important for PYD than the specific presence of a parental figure.

In sum, the results of these studies provide strong support for the applicability of the PYD model to boys of color and provide direct implications for PYD interventions and programs. First, the findings of these studies demonstrate that positive growth can occur over time in boys of color, and that this growth can be predicted by a number of individual and ecological assets. The range of assets linked to positive developmental outcomes across these studies bodes well for intervention efforts. A qualitative review of PYD programs revealed that effective programs targeted a minimum of five assets, with an average of eight assets across programs demonstrating positive effects on outcomes (Catalano et al. 2004). Thus, the findings across the studies reviewed above suggest that the number of potential intervention targets for BOC is sufficient for PYD programs to produce positive effects. In addition, the significant interaction effects and path models demonstrating relationships between various indicators of PYD in the studies above highlight the dynamic and interactive nature of individual and ecological assets in the lives of BOC. The range of assets coupled with the interactive associations between assets may boost the promotive effects of PYD interventions for BOC by increasing the range of outcomes that are impacted (Taylor et al. 2003). Third, the findings highlight the importance of parental socialization strategies and family relationships as predictors of PYD for BOC, with some findings showing that assets in the family are more important for BOC than for girls. The importance of family is particularly encouraging for intervention efforts with BOC,

as family relationships and processes are a flexible and malleable intervention target during adolescence (Granic et al. 2003). Thus, intervention efforts with BOC should focus both on building individual assets of youth and building support systems and interventions for the family unit (McDonald et al. 2011). Finally, the gender differences identified in these studies suggest that BOC may benefit from gender-tailored intervention programs (McDonald et al. 2011; Murry et al. 2014).

Research Methodology in PYD Research with BOC

The larger body of empirical literature on PYD encompasses a variety of research methodology, but interestingly, the emerging empirical PYD literature on BOC is predominantly longitudinal. Of the studies on BOC reviewed above, only one study utilized a cross-sectional research design (i.e., McDonald et al. 2011). Although cross-sectional research is informative, the inability to infer causality between constructs limits the utility of this work to inform prevention and intervention efforts. Longitudinal, prospective investigations of PYD using advanced statistical methods (e.g., growth modeling) help to identify specific developmental periods of growth and change, critical levels of individual and ecological risk and assets, and, consequently, determine when, where, and how to intervene with BOC. The existing longitudinal studies reviewed here (i.e., Murry et al. 2014; Taylor et al. 2004; Tolan et al. 2013) include variables at multiple levels of influence, such as youth, parenting, family and community factors, and there is a need for continued longitudinal research in this area that examines the dynamic transactions among these multiple levels of influences (Cabrera 2013; Lerner et al. 2011). Such ecological-transactional investigations of BOC can provide information regarding how assets in various contexts in the lives of BOC transact with each other over time to shape PYD outcomes. Further, when examining the transactional nature of ecological and individual assets, there is a need to include biological processes, as well as cultural processes (Cabrera 2013). The roles of culture and biology are often approached as separate lines of inquiry in developmental research, but recent work is beginning to show the dynamic interplay between biological processes and cultural experiences in youth, providing a more nuanced understanding of the complexity of youth development (Causadias 2013).

In addition, the existing research on PYD in BOC employs either survey methodology or structured interviews. Other methodologies may provide a deeper understanding of responses to survey items or interview questions, such as the use of mixed-methods designs that integrate qualitative and quantitative data collection approaches (Johnson et al. 2007). In PYD research, variables representing individual and ecological assets are most frequently assessed via youth self-report surveys (Leffert et al. 1998, Lerner et al. 2005). However, some researchers have called for less reliance on quantitative data as the sole source of information on youth of color (Cabrera 2013). For BOC, integrating survey approaches with in-depth interviews can provide a richer understanding of youths' perceptions of the availability of assets as a function of context, the sequential nature of assets and PYD outcomes, and transactional relationship between assets at various levels in youths' ecologies.

Current Research Questions

The results of the studies on BOC reviewed above also lead to questions regarding how PYD should be conceptualized in specific intervention efforts with BOC. In examining the utility of a PYD framework to BOC, each study included a focus on understanding how assets linked to PYD may operate under conditions of high levels of ecological stress, such as gang-involvement, community violence, and HIV risk. These studies provide critical insight into PYD in the lives of young men in settings marked by limited resources and developmentally-appropriate opportunities; however, such research may blur the line

between PYD and the concept of resilience, leading to questions regarding whether programs should be based on promotion effects models or preventive science and, relatedly, how to maximize the inclusion of context in PYD programs for BOC. Given this, there are a number of research questions that should be explored regarding the overlap between resilience and PYD, as well as the balance between promotive and preventive intervention models.

Are Resilience and PYD Conceptually Distinct or Overlapping Constructs for BOC?

While theorists make clear distinctions between PYD and resilience, the majority of research on PYD with boys of color is conducted from a resilience perspective, leading to questions of whether the conceptualization of PYD should be different for BOC or whether research on PYD in BOC should be more mindful of the distinctions between the two constructs. Often, in the developmental systems literature, the terms PYD and resilience are used interchangeably to refer to adaptive traits or assets observed in youth. As discussed below, these terms both place emphasis on a strengths-based approach to understanding youth development, but it is important, in the effort to develop a theoretically grounded and empirically supported operational definition of PYD, to carefully examine ways in which resilience both reflects this concept and diverges from it. In turn, a more clear understanding of the relationship between resilience and PYD can provide more direction with regard to interpreting these respective literatures.

Resilience has been defined broadly as the process of positive adaptation from or in the face of experiences of adversity (Ungar 2010). That is, the necessary components that come together to bring about resilience include experience of a significant adverse event or set of events or circumstances, the presence of assets or resources that blunt the impact of the adverse event, and therefore a positive adaptation to the stressor (Windle 2011). While similar to PYD concepts such as positive development indicators, specifically PYD factors are generally conceived as promotive main effects on development, not simply acting as protective in the face of threat or adversity. The blurring of lines between PYD and resilience appears to result from the similarity in interest of protective and directly promotive influences on functioning as well as frequent reference to developmental influences as assets that also serve as protective factors (e.g., positive parenting). These terms and their corresponding developmental influences have both been defined across the ecological context of youth, encompassing the individual, family, and community settings (Damon 2004). However, while researchers often use the terms protective factor and developmental assets interchangeably, they are conceptually-distinct concepts in that protective factors operate only in the presence of risk or adversity, whereas developmental assets operate without the influence of risk (Kia-Keating et al. 2011). Distinct from protective factors and more akin to conceptualization of PYD characteristics are promotive or main effect positive development promoting influences.

In resilience research, positive adaptation to stress may be conceptualized as maintaining or regaining mental health (or other indicators of adjustment) following adversity, but is often operationalized as the absence of deleterious outcomes that would be expected to result from exposure to adversity (e.g., mental health symptoms, problem behaviors, etc.) (Luthar et al. 2000). On the other hand, PYD is not typically discussed in the context of adverse events and risk, but is rather considered to be a general index of developmental success for all youth (Guerra and Bradshaw 2008). In fact, the relationship between PYD and problem behaviors or negative outcomes is not a linear inverse relationship, as very few youth show the assumed pattern of linear increases in PYD coupled with linear decreases in problem behaviors (Lerner et al. 2009b). According to PYD theorists, preventing problems or symptoms from occurring is not equivalent to promoting positive youth development and does not guarantee that youth are provided with the assets that are necessary for

positive development or that they will be capable of making positive contributions to family, community, and society (Lerner and Benson 2003; Lerner et al. 2000).

The ongoing theoretical and empirical exploration of PYD among boys of color is particularly warranted as it relates to the resilience and PYD literatures. African American, Latino, and Native American male youth are often described as facing disproportionate levels of adversity, and this emphasis reflects many disparities that ethnic minority youth face compared to White counterparts, such as poverty, community violence (Bellair and McNulty 2005; Sun and Li 2007), and racial stereotyping (Swanson et al. 2003). The majority of research, even PYD research, focuses on how these youth become successful "despite the odds" (Lerner and Steinberg 2004), which has positive implications for youth who present with a number of risk factors. However, the sparser emphasis on variables that might promote positive development and thriving, for boys of color *across* the continuum of adversity is concerning. Models of resilience incorporate a "deficit perspective", as represented by the expectation of susceptibility to stress and adversity. Further, resilience research and the perspective of "overcoming the odds" categorizes the trajectory of the young men who show resilient outcomes as "atypical" (Luthar et al. 2000; Roosa 2000), in stark contrast to PYD models that promote positive outcomes as normative for all youth (Lerner et al. 2009a, b). Given that youth of color are subject to negative bias and the "criminal justice" mentality described above, both intentionally and unintentionally, PYD researchers must be mindful not to paint the positive development of youth of color as always occurring within the context of adversity. This is not to suggest that researchers ignore the disproportionate levels of adversity experienced by BOC, but rather, to caution against the proclivity of research to view all BOC as high-risk.

As follows, the majority of developmental research on boys of color focuses on boys in "high-risk contexts," such as low-income, high-crime urban communities or low-income, rural communities that are predominantly or almost exclusively composed of populations of color. There is a need for PYD research on boys of color in communities that may be considered low-risk settings, such as middle and upper-middle class communities with low levels of crime, as well as under researched settings for BOC, such as suburban communities and communities with diverse racial and ethnic groups. When percentages are presented on BOC, research often highlights the small percentage of youth who are on challenging trajectories (dropping out of high school, teen parents, crime victims); however, PYD research is warranted on the larger percentage of BOC who are not on these trajectories (Cabrera 2013; Rozie-Battle 2002). Such research is needed to dispel the belief that being a male of color is synonymous with being disadvantaged and to highlight the variability within males of color as a group (Cabrera 2013). For example, educational aspirations in middle-class African American youth are strongly related to academic performance (Sirin and Rogers-Sirin 2004). However, a study with African American male adolescents from various SES backgrounds showed that SES significantly impacted educational aspirations, such that males from middle-class, suburban neighborhoods had significantly higher aspirations than males from low-income rural and urban communities (Strayhorn 2009), underscoring within-group variation. Also, recent research findings show that even in "high-risk contexts," the majority of boys of color are not categorized as "high-risk" (Copeland-Linder et al. 2010; Gaylord-Harden et al. 2015; Murry et al. 2013), challenging the existing notions of normative and atypical developmental trajectories for BOC (Gaylord-Harden et al. 2012) and underscoring the need for more emphasis on redefining positive development for all BOC (Barbarin 2013).

How Should Context Be Included in PYD Programs for BOC?

In light of the above discussion regarding resilience and PYD, questions remain as to how context should be incorporated into PYD intervention efforts with BOC without limiting the availability of these programs to a small subset of BOC, namely BOC in high-risk contexts. The development of BOC occurs in an ecological context and successful PYD interventions with BOC must incorporate an understanding of the role of context on developmental trajectories (Livingston and Nahimana 2006), along with the consideration of "contextual variability" across BOC. As noted earlier, a key component of the PYD framework is that youth are embedded in family, school, and community contexts that possess important ecological assets (Lerner et al. 2013). However, in under-resourced or high-risk settings the availability of ecological assets may be limited, posing a challenge for interventionists attempting to apply comprehensive models of PYD to BOC in these settings. Given this, some researchers propose that an integrative model be applied to guide such work with BOC. For example, context can be used determine whether an integrative model incorporating aspects of both resilience and PYD should be applied with BOC (Murry et al. 2014). For BOC *in under-resourced contexts*, the resilience perspective can be used as a framework for examining trajectories of BOC to support them in the face of adversity in these settings, *in conjunction with* the PYD framework to identify the *internal* assets that may help BOC show resilient outcomes in contexts with low external assets (Murry et al. 2014). In contrast, the integration of resilience and PYD may not be necessary or advantageous for BOC in contexts with higher levels of external assets or resources.

Still others propose integrative models that can be applied to all BOC, regardless of levels of contextual risk. One such model incorporates two main pathways toward positive development: the protecting pathway, which is influenced by resilience research and includes concepts of risk and protection; and the promoting pathway, which is influenced by positive youth development research and includes the concept of assets (Kia-Keating et al. 2011). Both pathways lead to positive development, but the protecting pathway leads to healthy development when risk factors are buffered by protective factors, whereas the promoting pathway leads to positive development directly from assets. In regards to the role of context, the protecting pathway and the promoting pathway are both influenced by individual, family, school, community, and cultural factors (Kia-Keating et al. 2011). While both pathways are active in this model, the relative influence of each pathway on a young man's positive development would depend on the level of risk that a young man's experiences in the contexts of family, school, and community. Similar to the findings of Tolan et al. (2013), this model may allow for the delineation of trajectories to both PYD and resilience for BOC in various contexts.

Can Intervention Efforts Integrate PYD and Prevention Science?

A discussion of context is critical for intervention efforts with BOC. A wealth of interventions exists for youth of color that are based on resilience models and target the prevention or reduction of emotional and behavioral problems that develop in risky contexts. However, advocates of the PYD approach assert that "problem-free" is not fully prepared (Pittman et al. 2011). In other words, while prevention is an important goal, in isolation, prevention is inadequate (Pittman et al. 2011). Similarly, research suggests that focusing solely on strengthening assets is insufficient, especially for youth exposed to very high levels of risk (Catalano et al. 2002).

How then should context be considered when PYD is applied to interventions and programs for BOC to ensure that programs are effective across various settings? One consideration is to include context through the integration of PYD promotion and prevention science approaches (Catalano et al. 2002; Guerra and Bradshaw 2008). Recent assertions are that if an exclusive focus on asset enhancement can mitigate the negative effects of risk factors, then youth development programs need not attend to contextual risk; however, if such an approach is ineffective, then intervention and

policy work in this area should focus on both the reduction of risk factors to prevent youth problems and the enhancement of assets to promote positive development (Catalano et al. 2002). Consistent with the integrative theoretical models that can be applied to all BOC, regardless of levels of contextual risk (Kia-Keating et al. 2011; Murry et al. 2014), this approach calls for a balance between risk reduction and promotive approaches to prevention and intervention. For example, a quasi-experimental examination of an after-school PYD program targeting both prevention of substance use and promotion of well-being among 304 urban adolescents of color (75 % African American and 19.7 % Latino) demonstrated that PYD provides a useful platform for preventive intervention delivery (Tebes et al. 2007).

Although such work represents an important step in utilizing an integrative framework in applied PYD research, it is not yet clear from the literature whether interventions that combine the reduction of the effects of risk factors and the enhancement of assets are more effective than interventions that focus solely on the enhancement of assets (Catalano et al. 2002). While continued exploration of this issue will be fruitful for applied work with BOC, interventionists must consider how an integrative approach may prove more challenging than traditional approaches. For example, linking prevention efforts with positive youth development efforts requires that interventionists expand their definitions of "problems" and goals for programs (e.g., moving from gang prevention to civic involvement), which in turn may require a shift in their intervention strategies (Pittman et al. 2011). This shift will be particularly important for work with BOC given that their development is often framed in deficit-based models that emphasize problems rather than strengths (García Coll et al. 1996; McLoyd and Randolph 1985; Tucker and Herman 2002). Similarly, a shift in definitions and goals may require interventionists to think beyond the models and approaches with which they have expertise and also consider how youth behaviors may be defined by other approaches (Small and Memmo 2004). Finally, the comprehensive nature of integrative models may make it difficult for communities or organizations to implement both PYD strategies and preventive strategies simultaneously at the start of a program. If this is the case, interventionists must attend to both the context (e.g., community support for programs) and focal issue to determine if prevention or promotion should occur first (Small and Memmo 2004).

Another approach to considering context in PYD programs and policy with BOC is the concept of community youth development (Hughes and Curnan 2000; Rozie-Battle 2002). Community youth development is based on both PYD models and risk and resilience models (Perkins et al. 2001). Community youth development is defined as "purposely creating environments that provide constructive, affirmative, and encouraging relationships that are sustained over time with adults and peers, while concurrently providing an array of opportunities that enable youth to build their competencies, and become engaged as partners in their own development as well as the development of their communities" (Perkins et al. 2001, p. 47). Consistent with concerns that the concept of resilience may overemphasize the responsibility of the individual in overcoming the effects of contextual risk (Small and Memmo 2004; Tolan 1996) and the notions that healthy communities are more likely to contribute to positive youth development (Hughes and Curnan 2000), the community youth development approach to intervention and programming focuses on developing community-wide efforts to promote positive youth development for all youth, while simultaneously addressing risk factors that impact specific subsets of youth (Perkins et al. 2001). Key to this approach is creating partnerships between youth and adults that focus on engaging youth to be active shapers of their communities (Perkins et al. 2001). Kirshner and Ginwright (2012) provide numerous examples of successful community youth development in which networks of African and Latino adolescents mobilized and connected with adult allies and policy-makers to create community- and city-level changes to public education, juvenile justice policies, interracial relationships, and to secure public funding for youth opportunities. While many examples of the community youth development approach are from under-resourced, urban communities (Rozie-Battle 2002), the approach can be applied to other types of communities in which BOC reside.

Universal Versus Culture-Specific Mechanisms for BOC

A final issue involves whether PYD interventions and programs for BOC should focus solely on promoting universal assets or if they should incorporate culturally specific asset development. Because PYD represents a framework for understanding development rather than a specific set of characteristics that mark positive development (e.g. each of the concepts in the 6Cs and many of the assets in the 40 assets model are general terms), it is seen as applicable to youth across populations and circumstances (e.g., Leffert et al. 1998; Lerner et al. 2009b). Specific forms of assets or of how positive developmental processes are promoted can and are thought to vary by population and social circumstances.

The empirical studies reviewed earlier in this chapter suggest that assets from both the Six C's model and the Search Institute help to promote PYD in BOC. In other words, the set of studies can be fit to a 6 C's or 40 assets framework for interpreting results. Specifically, from the Search Institute's model, the individual assets of commitment to learning, positive values, and social competencies, and the ecological assets of support and boundaries and expectations were important for gang-involved BOC (Taylor et al. 2002a, b). From the Six C's model, indicators for competence and confidence predicted positive developmental outcomes in BOC from rural communities (Murry et al. 2014) and indicators for connection predicted positive developmental outcomes for BOC from urban communities (McDonald et al. 2011).

It should be noted that research comparing assets across multiple racial/ethnic groups shows that, while some assets (e.g., support, social competencies) are important for youth from all racial/ethnic backgrounds, there are also clear differences between racial/ethnic groups on the importance of other assets (Scales et al. 2000; Sesma and Roehlkepartain 2003). Specifically, for American Indian youth, constructive-use-of-time assets were important for school success and other adult relationships, creative activities, and caring for important for overall thriving. Among African American youth, self-esteem and reading for pleasure assets were important for overall thriving, and empowerment was important for positive health outcomes for Latino youth. While these findings were not specific to boys, they suggest that some universal assets could be better suited for the cultural experiences of certain subgroups of BOC than other assets.

Given that the enhancement of particular assets for specific subgroups of youth in particular communities is a better predictor of PYD than increasing the quantity of all assets (Lerner et al. 2009b), the identification of universal assets that may be specific to the positive development of BOC is needed. However, such specificity research must also attend to within group variability with regards to contextual factors and boys' levels of identification with their racial/ethnic group. These findings may also suggest that definitions of risk, protection, promotion, and assets may vary across boys from various racial/ethnic groups (Kia-Keating et al. 2011). Similar to McDonald et al.'s (2011) approach of allowing participants to define "family" for themselves when examining how connections with others predicts PYD in BOC, PYD research with BOC should incorporate community engagement strategies and community-based participatory research strategies to ensure that conceptualizations of risk, protection, promotion, and assets are consistent with the cultural framework of BOC and their communities.

In addition to targeting particular universal assets, it may also be beneficial to consider the role of cultural assets that are specific to BOC. For example, research highlights the role of familism values as a predictor of PYD outcomes in Mexican youth (Knight and Carlo 2012). Also, engaging American Indian youth in Native cultural practices and reinforcing traditional Native worldviews is regarded as important for promoting the 6 C's of PYD (Kenyon and Hanson 2012). Another example is seen in the importance of racial socialization efforts of African American parents for PYD development in African American youth (Evans et al. 2012). In response to the exclusion of normative developmental processes and cultural strengths in youth of color from mainstream models of youth development (García Coll et al. 2000; Spencer and Markstrom-Adams 1990), models have been created that emphasize the importance of culturally-specific factors on the development and functioning of youth of color from a strengths-based perspective (e.g., García Coll et al. 1996; Harrell 2000; Miller 1999). For example, García Coll et al. (1996) proposed a comprehensive, integrative model of normative development that includes developmental factors unique to children of color (e.g., racial socialization), as well as mainstream developmental factors relevant to all populations (e.g., temperament). Other models like the Phenomenological Variant of Bronfenbrenner's model to attend to Black youth development (PVEST; Spencer 1995) demonstrate efforts to emphasize minority youth competencies. These models offer examples of cultural assets that can be incorporated into PYD interventions with BOC.

Very little empirical research examines the role of cultural assets as promotive for PYD. One notable exception is a recent study with boys of color (60 % African American and 39 % Latino) examining the role of ethnic identity as a PYD asset based on research showing ethnic identity is more salient for these youth (Williams et al. 2014). Results showed that the best fitting model was a two-factor PYD-ethnic identity model. The PYD factor related to a range of youth outcomes, while the ethnic identity factor related to fewer internalizing behaviors. The results suggest that establishing ethnic identity is an important means for minimizing the likelihood of negative mental health symptoms and counteracting the negative effects of discrimination. Across time, the model fit the better when the boys were ages 14–15, suggesting that ethnic identity may become more central to youth as they move through adolescence, and that ethnic identity is a psychosocial asset that is related to, but distinct from, general indicators of PYD. By highlighting the importance of culturally specific assets for BOC, this research provides empirical evidence to guide the development of interventions that are both contextually- and culturally-relevant for BOC.

Policy Implications

Positive youth development is not only an intervention approach, it has become a policy perspective that focuses on providing services and programs to support the healthy development of all youth. However, the historical emphasis on risk frameworks for youth development has resulted in policy initiatives that support separate problem-specific programs funded by independent agencies, rather than initiatives to support programs that consider the common risk, protective, and promotive factors of multiple youth behaviors (Guerra and Bradshaw 2008). As policy makers seek to incorporate a positive youth development approach for BOC, it will be important to ensure that funding is designated for research that seeks to identify common risk, protective, and promotive factors for targeted behaviors in BOC. Further, once these shared factors are identified, policy efforts should support the development of multidimensional and multi-institutional PYD interventions for BOC informed by this research.

It has been suggested that because program inputs for prevention, positive development, and engagement are largely the same, policy work related to PYD will benefit from a new set of questions that focus less on what BOC need and focus much more on (1) how to bring those conditions about and (2) how to ensure that BOC have access to opportunities (Pittman et al. 2011). The My Brother's Keeper Initiative may be an example of a policy initiative that focuses more on promoting solutions than outlining problems by identifying existing private and public intervention efforts that are effective and

supporting the expansion of those efforts, rather than supporting additional needs assessment. If successful, the goals of this initiative could serve as a model for policies than emphasize solutions to bring about conditions of change for BOC. Similarly, policy efforts must focus on understanding how BOC have access to these opportunities (Pittman et al. 2011). Research demonstrates that participation in youth development programs declines as youth enter adolescence, likely due to programs not meeting the needs or interests of adolescents, adolescents having more autonomy over their free time, and adults being more comfortable supervising younger children (Quinn 1999). The community youth development approach discussed above may be particularly helpful in ensuring that programs for BOC are developmentally appropriate, engaging, and contextually- and culturally-relevant by giving BOC a voice in the development of these programs. Other issues of access are more salient for subsets of BOC, such as those from low-income areas or rural areas. These issues include transportation issues, proximity to programs, participation fees, and whether youth will be made to feel welcome at the program (Quinn 1999). Thus, BOC will need, not just services, but also supports and opportunities to remain engaged with programs (Pittman et al. 2011). While programs can address these barriers to increase access to and engagement with programs for BOC, such outreach work is dependent upon policies to ensure that adequate funding is available from external sources (Quinn 1999).

While most policy makers would agree that early intervention is important, PYD research with BOC suggests that preventive intervention with BOC during adolescence is also critical for promoting their positive development as they transition to adulthood (Catalano et al. 2004; Rozie-Battle 2002). However, given the importance of early intervention to many policy makers, the call for longitudinal research may also lead to answers regarding how to promote healthy development in early childhood that can serve as a foundation for later development during adolescence and early adulthood. For example, Murry et al. (2014) included developmental stages from middle childhood to young adulthood to provide empirical evidence regarding how early life experiences with parents and peers predict positive, healthy development in BOC later in life. While interventions and policies based on this work can focus on asset building in early childhood, the aims would be to target assets with lasting effects and ensure that supports are in place to sustain assets into adolescence.

Also for BOC, it is important for policy makers to provide opportunities not just to the BOC on the extremes of developmental outcomes (i.e., high-achieving, problem-free BOC and low-achieving BOC with behavioral and/or emotional problems), but all BOC, including those "in the middle" who are often ignored when such opportunities are created (Rozie-Battle 2002). Even the My Brother's Keeper initiative is based on a resilience framework and runs the risk of leading to the identification of effective programs for only a subset of BOC. Given that BOC are disproportionately exposed to risk factors that predict problem behaviors, policies for BOC must be aimed at both the prevention of risks and problems and the promotion of PYD (Catalano et al. 2004). Further, policy makers have more influence over contextual risks than individuals have, and an overemphasis on making individuals more resistant to risk can divert attention or responsibility away from policy-level efforts to reduce this risk (Small and Memmo 2004; Tolan 1996). The prevention of risk by policy makers must focus on the reduction of risk factors such as poverty, joblessness, crime, and poor quality schooling at the community-level, in addition to ensuring that BOC in these communities are equipped with individual resources that buffer the effects of these risk factors. Consistent with a community youth development approach to PYD, policy advocates must work with BOC to identify issues that are pertinent to the lives of BOC, to develop contextually- and culturally-sensitive solutions, and to communicate ideas for potential legislation to policy-makers (Perkins et al. 2001).

Future Directions

The experience of boys of color in our society involves a unique and diverse range of experiences that are influenced by a myriad of social, historical, and political factors, as well as complex intersections of community, family, and individual factors. In light of these experiences, positive youth development emerges as a progressive approach towards providing more balanced and holistic intervention efforts with BOC that encompass both promotion and protection. The existing basic research on PYD in BOC provides evidence of assets that can be targeted in intervention efforts. As such, future research on the developmental trajectory, antecedents, correlates, and consequences of positive youth development in BOC has the potential to narrow the critical research gap in knowledge on variability in the experiences of BOC to inform the development of effective programs and preventive interventions to promote positive and healthy development in these youth. While basic research is necessary to ensure that there is a strong theoretical and empirical basis for intervention and policy efforts (Catalano et al. 2004), there is a critical need for *applied* research on PYD programs for BOC. From the existing reviews of PYD programs (e.g., Catalano et al. 2004; National Research Council 2002; Roth and Brooks-Gunn 2003a, b), it appears that very few programs are developed for specific subgroups of youth by race/ethnicity, gender, etc. This is likely due to the belief that PYD theory is universally applicable to youth across populations and circumstances (Lerner et al. 2009a, b). These reviews of PYD programs suggest that the overwhelming majority of programs serve multiple ethnic groups (Catalano et al. 2004; Roth and Brooks-Gunn 2003b). While this fact is encouraging, it remains unclear if these universal programs are equally effective for the youth from different backgrounds, and in particular, if they are effective for BOC. Further, given the role of culturally specific assets in the promotion of PYD, additional applied research is warranted to identify effective PYD programs that are developed specifically for BOC. While almost no examples exist in the existing PYD literature, it is likely that numerous small, grassroots, community-based programs exist for BOC, but due to funding concerns that render these programs unstable, there is a disconnect between research and small community-based programs. To fully understand the opportunities for BOC, research should be devoted to identifying and evaluating these programs. It should be noted that this level of understanding warrants deeper examination of within-group variability in the effectiveness of interventions for various subgroups of BOC, including a critical need for identifying effective programs for BOC across sociocultural backgrounds, socioeconomic statuses, communities, and emotional/behavior problem histories. The promise of a positive youth development approach for boys of color is a one that advances the narrative of BOC beyond risk and pathology to one that sees possibilities and potential and works to advance opportunities for health and positive development.

References

Antaramian, S. P., Huebner, E. S., Hills, K. J., & Valois, R. F. (2010). A dual-factor model of mental health: Toward a more comprehensive understanding of youth functioning. *American Journal of Orthopsychiatry, 80* (4), 462.

Arnett, J. J. (1999). Adolescent storm and stress, reconsidered. *American Psychologist, 54*(5), 317.

Ayman-Nolley, S., & Taira, L. L. (2000). Obsession with the dark side of adolescence: A decade of psychological studies. *Journal of youth studies, 3*(1), 35–48.

Barbarin, O. A. (2013). Development of boys of color: An introduction. *American Journal of Orthopsychiatry, 83*(2–3), 143.

Barbarin, O. A. (2015). Parental practices and developmental challenges of boys of color: Opportunities for early intervention. *Zero to Three, 35*(3), 9–18.

Bellair, P. E., & McNulty, T. L. (2005). Beyond the bell curve: Community disadvantage and the explanation of black–white differences in adolescent violence. *Criminology, 43*(4), 1135–1168.

Benson, P. (1997). *All kids are our kids: What communities must do to raise caring and responsible children and adolescents.* San Francisco: Jossey-Bass.

Benson, P., Leffert, N., Scales, P., & Blyth, D. (1998). Beyond the village rhetoric: Creating healthy communities for children and adolescents. *Applied Developmental Science, 2,* 138–159.

Bowers, E. P., Li, Y., Kiely, M. K., Brittian, A., Lerner, J. V., & Lerner, R. M. (2010). The five Cs model of positive youth development: A longitudinal analysis of confirmatory factor structure and measurement invariance. *Journal of Youth and Adolescence, 39*(7), 720–735.

Cabrera, N. (2013). Positive development of minority children. *Social Policy Report, Society for Research in Child Development, 27*(2), 1–29.

Catalano, R. F., Berglund, M. L., Ryan, J. A., Lonczak, H. S., & Hawkins, J. D. (2004). Positive youth development in the United States: Research findings on evaluations of positive youth development programs. *The Annals of the American Academy of Political and Social Science, 591*(1), 98–124.

Catalano, R. F., Hawkins, J. D., Berglund, M. L., Pollard, J. A., & Arthur, M. W. (2002). Prevention science and positive youth development: Competitive or cooperative frameworks? *Journal of Adolescent Health, 31* (6), 230–239.

Causadias, J. M. (2013). A roadmap for the integration of culture into developmental psychopathology. *Development and Psychopathology, 25*(4), 1375–1398.

Chavez, L. (2013). *The Latino threat: Constructing immigrants, citizens, and the nation.* Redwood City: Stanford University Press.

Copeland-Linder, N., Lambert, S. F., & Ialongo, N. H. (2010). Community violence, protective factors and adolescent mental health: A profile analysis. *Journal of Clinical Child and Adolescent Psychology, 39,* 176–186.

Damon, W. (2004). What is positive youth development? *The Annals of the American Academy of Political and Social Science, 591,* 13–24.

Evans, A. B., Banerjee, M., Meyer, R., Aldana, A., Foust, M., & Rowley, S. (2012). Racial socialization as a mechanism for positive development among African American youth. *Child Development Perspectives, 6* (3), 251–257.

Fenning, P., & Rose, J. (2007). Overrepresentation of African American students in exclusionary discipline the role of school policy. *Urban Education, 42*(6), 536–559.

Fujioka, Y. (2011). Perceived threats and Latino immigrant attitudes: How White and African American college students respond to news coverage of Latino immigrants. *The Howard Journal of Communications, 22*(1), 43–63.

García Coll, C., Ackerman, A., & Cicchetti, D. (2000). Cultural influences on developmental processes and outcomes: Implications for the study of development and psychopathology. *Development and Psychopathology, 12,* 333–356.

García Coll, C., Lamberty, G., Jenkins, R., McAdoo, H. P., Crnic, K., Wasik, B. H., et al. (1996). An integrative model for the study of developmental competencies in minority children. *Child Development, 67,* 1891–1914.

Gaylord-Harden, N. K., Burrow, A., & Cunningham, J. A. (2012). A cultural-asset framework for investigating successful adaptation to stress in African American youth. *Child Development Perspectives, 6*(3), 264–271.

Gaylord-Harden, N. K., Zakaryan, A., Bernard, D. L., & Pekoc, S. (2015). Community-level victimization and aggressive behavior in African American male adolescents: A profile analysis. *Journal of Community Psychology, 43*, 502–519.

Goff, P. A., Jackson, M. C., Di Leone, B. A. L., Culotta, C. M., & DiTomasso, N. A. (2014). The essence of innocence: Consequences of dehumanizing Black children. *Journal of Personality and Social Psychology, 106*(4), 526–545.

Granic, I., Hollenstein, T., Dishion, T. J., & Patterson, G. R. (2003). Longitudinal analysis of flexibility and reorganization in early adolescence: A dynamic systems study of family interactions. *Developmental Psychology, 39*(3), 606–617.

Guerra, N. G., & Bradshaw, C. P. (2008). Linking the prevention of problem behaviors and positive youth development: Core competencies for positive youth development and risk prevention. *New Directions for Child and Adolescent Development, 122*, 1–17.

Hall, G. S. (1904). *Adolescence: Its psychology and its relations to physiology, anthropology, sociology, sex, crime, religion, and education.* Englewood Cliffs, NJ: Prentice-Hall.

Harrell, S. P. (2000). A multidimensional conceptualization of racism-related stress: Implications for the well-being of people of color. *American Journal of Orthopsychiatry, 70*(1), 42–57.

Hughes, D. M., & Curnan, S. P. (2000). Community youth development: A framework for action. *Community Youth Development Journal, 1*(1), 7–11.

Jennings, M. E. (2014). Trayvon Martin and the myth of superpredator. In T. Martin (Ed.), *Race, and American justice* (pp. 191–196). Sense Publishers.

Johnson, R. B., Onwuegbuzie, A. J., & Turner, L. A. (2007). Toward a definition of mixed methods research. *Journal of Mixed Methods Research, 1*(2), 112–133.

Kenyon, D. B., & Hanson, J. D. (2012). Incorporating traditional culture into positive youth development programs with American Indian/Alaska Native youth. *Child Development Perspectives, 6*(3), 272–279.

Kia-Keating, M., Dowdy, E., Morgan, M. L., & Noam, G. G. (2011). Protecting and promoting: An integrative conceptual model for healthy development of adolescents. *Journal of Adolescent Health, 48*(3), 220–228.

Kirshner, B., & Ginwright, S. (2012). Youth organizing as a developmental context for African American and Latino adolescents. *Child Development Perspectives, 6*(3), 288–294.

Knight, G. P., & Carlo, G. (2012). Prosocial development among Mexican American youth. *Child Development Perspectives, 6*(3), 258–263.

Larson, R. W. (2000). Toward a psychology of positive youth development. *American Psychologist, 55*, 170–183.

Larson, R. (2006). Positive youth development, willful adolescents, and mentoring. *Journal of Community Psychology, 34*(6), 677–689.

Leffert, N., Benson, P. L., Scales, P. C., Sharma, A. R., Drake, D. R., & Blyth, D. A. (1998). Developmental assets: Measurement and prediction of risk behaviors among adolescents. *Applied Developmental Science, 2*(4), 209–230.

Lerner, J. V., Phelps, E., Forman, Y. E., & Bowers, E. P. (2009a). *Positive youth development.* In R. M. Lerner, & L. Steinberg, L. (Eds.), *Handbook of adolescent psychology, individual bases of adolescent development* (vol. 1). New York: Wiley.

Lerner, R. M., Abo-Zena, M., Bebiroglu, N., Brittian, A., Lynch, A. D., & Issac, S. (2009b). Positive youth development: Contemporary theoretical perspectives. In R. J. DiClemente, J. S. Santelli, & R. A. Crosby (Eds.), *Adolescent health: Understanding and preventing risk behaviors* (pp. 115–128). New York: Wiley.

Lerner, R. M., Agans, J. P., Arbeit, M. R., Chase, P. A., Weiner, M. B., Schmid, K. L., et al. (2013). Resilience and positive youth development: A relational developmental systems model. In S. Goldstein & R. R. Brooks (Eds.), *Handbook of resilience in children* (pp. 293–308). New York: Springer.

Lerner, R. M., & Benson, P. (Eds.). (2003). *Developmental assets and asset-building communities: Implications for research, policy, and practice* (Vol. 1). New York: Springer.

Lerner, R. M., Fisher, C. B., & Weinberg, R. A. (2000). Toward a science for and of the people: Promoting civil society through the application of developmental science. *Child Development, 71*(1), 11–20.

Lerner, R. M., Lerner, J. V., Almerigi, J., Theokas, C., Phelps, E., Gestsdottir, D., et al. (2011). *The positive development of youth: Report of the findings from the first seven years of the 4-H study of positive youth development.* Institute for Applied Research in Youth Development, Tufts University. Technical Report. Chevy Chase, Md.: National.

Lerner, R. M., Lerner, J. V., Almerigi, J. B., Theokas, C., Phelps, E., Gestsdottir, S., et al. (2005). Positive youth development, participation in community youth development programs, and community contributions of fifth-grade adolescents findings from the first wave of the 4-H study of Positive Youth Development. *The Journal of Early Adolescence, 25*(1), 17–71.

Lerner, R. M., & Steinberg, L. (Eds.). (2004). *Handbook of adolescent psychology* (2nd ed.). Hoboken, NJ: Wiley.

Livingston, J. N., & Nahimana, C. (2006). Problem child or problem context: An ecological approach to young black males. *Reclaiming Children and Youth, 14*(4), 209.

Luthar, S. S., Cicchetti, D., & Becker, B. (2000). The construct of resilience: A critical evaluation and guidelines for future work. *Child Development, 71*(3), 543–562.

McDonald, C. C., Deatrick, J. A., Kassam-Adams, N., & Richmond, T. S. (2011). Community violence exposure and positive youth development in urban youth. *Journal of Community Health, 36*, 925–932.

McLoyd, V. C. (1990). The impact of economic hardship on black families and children: Psychological distress, parenting, and socioemotional development. *Child Development, 61*, 311–346.

McLoyd, V. C., & Randolph, S. (1985). Secular trends in the study of Afro-American children: A review of *Child Development*. In A. B. Smuts, & J. W. Hagen (Eds.), *History and research in child development. Monographs of the society for research in child development, 50*, (4–5, Serial No. 211).

Miller, D. B. (1999). Racial socialization and racial identity: Can they promote resiliency for African American adolescents? *Adolescence, 34*, 493–501.

Mizock, L., & Harkins, D. (2011). Diagnostic bias and conduct disorder: Improving culturally sensitive diagnosis. *Child & Youth Services, 32*(3), 243–253.

Murry, V. M., Berkel, C., Simons, R. L., Simons, L. G., & Gibbons, F. X. (2014). A twelve-year longitudinal analysis of positive youth development among rural African American males. *Journal of Research on Adolescence, 24*(3), 512–525.

Murry, V. M., Simons, R. L., Simons, L. G., & Gibbons, F. X. (2013). Contributions of family environment and parenting processes to sexual risk and substance use of rural African American males: A 4-Year longitudinal analysis. *American Journal of Orthopsychiatry, 83* (2pt3), 299–309.

National Research Council. (2002). *Community programs to promote youth development*. Washington, DC: National Academy Press.

Offer, D., & Schonert-Reichl, K. A. (1992). Debunking the myths of adolescence: Findings from recent research. *Journal of the American Academy of Child and Adolescent Psychiatry, 31*(6), 1003–1014.

Perkins, D. F., Borden, L. M., & Villarruel, F. A. (2001). Community youth development: A partnership for action. *School Community Journal, 11*(2), 39–56.

Phelps, E., Zimmerman, S., Warren, A. E. A., Jeličić, H., von Eye, A., & Lerner, R. M. (2009). The structure and developmental course of positive youth development (PYD) in early adolescence: Implications for theory and practice. *Journal of Applied Developmental Psychology, 30*(5), 571–584.

Pittman, K. J., Irby, M., Tolman, J., Yohalem, N., & Ferber, T. (2011). *Preventing problems, promoting development, encouraging engagement*. Washington, DC: Forum for Youth Investment.

Quinn, J. (1999). Where need meets opportunity: Youth development programs for early teens. *The Future of Children, 9*(2), 96–116.

Reynolds, C. R., Skiba, R. J., Graham, S., Sheras, P., Conoley, J. C., & Garcia-Vazquez, E. (2008). Are zero tolerance policies effective in the schools? An evidentiary review and recommendations. *The American Psychologist, 63*(9), 852–862.

Roosa, M. W. (2000). Some thoughts about resilience versus positive development, main effects versus interactions, and the value of resilience. *Child Development, 71*(3), 567–569.

Roth, J. L., & Brooks-Gunn, J. (2003a). What exactly is a youth development program? Answers from research and practice. *Applied Developmental Science, 7*, 94–111.

Roth, J. L., & Brooks-Gunn, J. (2003b). Youth development programs: Risk, prevention and policy. *Journal of Adolescent Health, 32*(3), 170–182.

Rozie-Battle, J. L. (2002). Youth development: A positive strategy for African American youth. *Journal of Health & Social Policy, 15*(2), 13–23.

Scales, P. C., Benson, P. L., Leffert, N., & Blyth, D. A. (2000). Contribution of developmental assets to the prediction of thriving among adolescents. *Applied Developmental Science, 4*(1), 27–46.

Schwartz, R. C., & Feisthamel, K. P. (2009). Disproportionate diagnosis of mental disorders among African American versus European American clients: Implications for counseling theory, research, and practice. *Journal of Counseling & Development, 87*(3), 295–301.

Sesma, A., Jr., & Roehlkepartain, E. C. (2003). Unique strengths, shared strengths: Developmental assets among youth of color. *Search Institute Insights & Evidence, 1*(2), 1–13.

Sirin, S. R., & Rogers-Sirin, L. (2004). Exploring school engagement of middle-class African American adolescents. *Youth & Society, 35*(3), 323–340.

Small, S., & Memmo, M. (2004). Contemporary models of youth development and problem prevention: Toward an integration of terms, concepts, and models. *Family Relations, 53*(1), 3–11.

Spencer, M. B. (1995). Old issues and new theorizing about African–American youth: A phenomenological variant of ecological systems theory. In R. L. Taylor (Ed.), *Black youth: Perspectives on their status in the United States* (pp. 37–69). Westport, CT: Praeger.

Spencer, M. B., & Markstrom-Adams, C. (1990). Identity processes among racial and ethnic minority children in America. *Child Development, 61*(2), 290–310.

Steinberg, L. (2009). Adolescent development and juvenile justice. *Annual Review of Clinical Psychology, 5*, 459–485.

Swanson, D. P., Cunningham, M., & Spencer, M. B. (2003). Black males' structural conditions, achievement patterns, normative needs, and "opportunities". *Urban Education, 38*(5), 608–633.

Strayhorn, T. L. (2009). Different folks, different hopes the educational aspirations of black males in urban, suburban, and rural high schools. *Urban Education, 44*(6), 710–731.

Sun, Y., & Li, Y. (2007). Racial and ethnic differences in experiencing parents' marital disruption during late adolescence. *Journal of Marriage and Family, 69*(3), 742–762.

Taylor, C. S., Lerner, R. M., von Eye, A., Balsano, A. B., Dowling, E. M., Anderson, P. M., et al. (2002a). Individual and ecological assets and positive developmental trajectories among gang and community-based organization youth. *New Directions for Youth Development, 95*, 57–72.

Taylor, C. S., Lerner, R. M., Von Eye, A., Balsano, A. B., Dowling, E. M., Anderson, P. M., et al. (2002b). Stability of attributes of positive functioning and of developmental assets among African American adolescent male gang and community-based organization members. *New Directions for Youth Development, 95*, 35–55.

Taylor, C. S., Lerner, R. M., von Eye, A., Bobek, D. L., Balsano, A. B., Dowling, E. M., et al. (2003). Positive individual and social behavior among gang and nongang African American male adolescents. *Journal of Adolescent Research, 18*, 547–574.

Taylor, C. S., Lerner, R. M., von Eye, A., Bobek, D. L., Balsano, A. B., Dowling, E. M., et al. (2004). Internal and external developmental assets among African American male gang members. *Journal of Adolescent Research, 19*(3), 303–322.

Tebes, J. K., Feinn, R., Vanderploeg, J. J., Chinman, M. J., Shepard, J., Brabham, T., et al. (2007). Impact of a positive youth development program in urban after-school settings on the prevention of adolescent substance use. *Journal of Adolescent Health, 41*(3), 239–247.

Tolan, P. (2014). Forward thinking: Preparing our youth for the coming world. *Journal of Research on Adolescence, 24*(3), 411–416.

Tolan, P. T. (1996). How resilient is the concept of resilience. *The Community Psychologist, 29*(1), 12–15.

Tolan, P., Lovegrove, P., & Clark, E. (2013). Stress mitigation to promote development of prosocial values and school engagement of inner-city urban African American and Latino youth. *American Journal of Orthopsychiatry, 83*(2–3), 289.

Tucker, C. M., & Herman, K. C. (2002). Using culturally sensitive theories and research to meet the academic needs of low-income African American children. *American Psychologist, 57*(10), 762.

Ungar, M. (2010). What is resilience across cultures and contexts? Advances to the theory of positive development among individuals and families under stress. *Journal of Family Psychotherapy, 21*(1), 1–16.

Williams, J. L., Anderson, R. E., Francois, A. G., Hussain, S., & Tolan, P. H. (2014). Ethnic Identity and positive youth development in adolescent males: A culturally integrated approach. *Applied Developmental Science, 18*(2), 110–122.

Windle, G. (2011). What is resilience? A review and concept analysis. *Reviews in Clinical Gerontology, 21*(02), 152–169.

Civic Engagement as an Adaptive Coping Response to Conditions of Inequality: An Application of Phenomenological Variant of Ecological Systems Theory (PVEST)

Elan C. Hope and Margaret Beale Spencer

Abstract

In this chapter we use Phenomenological Variant of Ecological Systems Theory (P-VEST) to consider civic engagement as a coping response to systems of inequality faced by racial minority children. After a brief introduction we present a historical and theoretical overview of civic engagement with regard to children and adolescents and racially marginalized communities. We then introduce the P-VEST framework and examine civic engagement as a proactive reactive coping method to counteract the vulnerability and stress of systematic racial injustice. Following a discussion of the current empirical literature we explore the utility of civic engagement programs (e.g., Youth Participatory Action Research) as interventions to support positive development of minority youth. We conclude with policy implications and future directions for research to leverage civic engagement as a coping strategy for the positive development of minority children and their communities.

The United States functions as a participatory democracy, where citizens elect public officials who are expected to make decisions to govern based upon the views and needs of their constituents. As such, a critical method of growth for society and positive development of the citizenry is *civic engagement*. However, in the United States, there exists a history of political marginalization where the voices of some constituents are stifled through gerrymandering, voter suppression, and other forms of institutional oppression, which—although generally not formally acknowledged—nevertheless, serve to limit the political power of racial minorities. The imbalance of social power and opportunity among citizens assured the same rights contributes to and guarantees significant political vulnerability given the historical differences noted. The consequent myriad representations of social dissonance function as sources of challenge and social risk.

E.C. Hope (✉)
Department of Psychology, North Carolina State University, Raleigh, USA
e-mail: ehope@ncsu.edu

M.B. Spencer
Department of Comparative Human Development, University of Chicago, Chicago, USA

© The Editor(s) 2017
N.J. Cabrera and B. Leyendecker (eds.), *Handbook on Positive Development of Minority Children and Youth*, DOI 10.1007/978-3-319-43645-6_25

In this chapter, we consider what civic engagement means for youth who are members of racial groups that have been historically and contemporarily disenfranchised socioculturally, politically, and economically. We propose that civic engagement is an adaptive coping strategy for racial minority youth, which functions as a source of support given the political imbalance described. As such, civic engagement provides an active form of resistance to protest inequitable conditions and to promote positive well-being for self and community. In a quest for positive development, minority youth move beyond the altruistic nature of community service and democratic purpose of political participation towards *critical civic engagement*—i.e., *civic engagement as a revolutionary act of self preservation in direct response to broadly under-acknowledged conditions of sociopolitical inequality.*

Historical Overview and Theoretical Perspectives

Civic engagement activities may look the same but serve different purposes. Certainly an examination of youths' functional use of community involvement suggests this phenomenon. For example, privileged youth may consider civic engagement as a strategy for increasing chances of admission to selective colleges or as an altruistically motivated endeavor. At the same time, racially marginalized youth may view their civic engagement efforts as acts of resistance against conditions of inequality. Framing such perceptual differences theoretically is important to fully understand youth civic engagement.

Civic Engagement from a Youth Development Perspective

Civic engagement is a widely used term with a range of definitions that encompass individual and collective civil and political participation (Adler 2005). Throughout psychology, education, and political science literatures civic engagement is referred as community service, activism,

volunteerism, social action, and political participation. One commonality among most definitions is that a citizen performs civic engagement and, his or her actions, whether individual or collective, interact with society, and more often address problems or concerns of the public. When considering civic engagement among children and young people, we adopt a broad definition of civic engagement offered by Adler (2005): "Civic engagement describes how an active citizen participates in the life of a community in order to improve conditions for others or to help shape the community's future." Scholarship on youth civic development supports the use of a comprehensive definition, suggesting:

> Perhaps the fairest conclusion is that there is not a definite demarcation between political and civil realms. Rather there is a continuum between formal political acts such as voting, political actions such as protesting for a moral cause, and performing a service such as working in a rural literacy campaign. Scholarship concerned with young people's preparation for civic participation as adults would be wise to take into account the whole range.
>
> Youniss et al. (2002)

Amnå (2012) asserts that the term civic engagement is often used to indicate the social, civic, and political dimensions of engaged citizenship. As such, Ekman and Amnå (2012) developed a typology of civic engagement that considers both individual and collective forms of civic engagement, while also accounting for non-participation, civic participation, and political participation. The first category, non-participation, is divided into active/anti-political forms and passive/apolitical forms of inaction, which include non-voting. Active or anti-political actions are motivated by dissatisfaction or disgust while passive or apolitical actions are related to disinterest in politics and feelings that politics are not important. Civic participation is the second category and consists of social involvement—attention to and interest in politics and society, and civic engagement—actions with attention to social and political issues. Finally, political participation includes formal political participation such as voting and contacting political representatives. Political participation also includes extra-parliamentary actions—legal activism such as boycotts and involvement in social movements and illegal activism in the form of civil disobedience or politically motivated violence. By considering distinct types of civic engagement, scholars can have a common framework and language to understand mechanisms of action relevant for voting versus volunteering, while acknowledging both as equally important components of civic engagement.

Another dimension of civic engagement that scholars consider as part of a comprehensive approach to citizenship and civic participation, particularly among children not yet eligible for some formal civic activities (e.g., voting), is pro-social behavior (Sherrod and Lauckhardt 2008; Sherrod et al. 2010). Pro-social behaviors include helping behavior, sharing, concern for others, and tolerance (Metzger and Smetana 2010; Wentzel et al. 2007). During childhood and adolescence, young people may not have physical access, logistical resources, or cognitive and developmental capacity to participate in other types of community and political actions. However, they act as citizens through accessible community spaces, such as classrooms, playgrounds, neighborhoods, and schools (Astuto and Ruck 2010; Flanagan 2013). These spaces function as microcosmic reproductions of broader society, where democratic processes and principles are learned and practiced. In these spaces, pro-social behavior is a developmentally relevant form of civic engagement. For instance, while an adult might help the community by participating in a "Meals-on-Wheels" program, children might share their lunch with a hungry classmate. In fact, these pro-social behaviors in childhood are proposed as antecedents to long-term civic engagement (Astuto and Ruck 2010) and relate positively to social responsibility (Metzger and Smetana 2010). These pro-social behaviors, such as helping, can be considered as a unique type of civic engagement relevant during childhood and adolescence.

Typically, research on civic engagement considers performed behavior as an indicator of civic engagement without giving proper attention to the intention of the individual to become civically engaged in the future. However, some theorists contend that commitment to civic engagement without action is a relevant consideration, particularly for groups such as youth who may not have access to opportunity structures that promote civic engagement (Diemer and Li 2011; Watts and Flanagan 2007; Watts and Guessous 2006). *Civic Commitment* is emotional and intellectual resolution to future action that may serve as a proxy for performed civic engagement. During adolescence, particularly in early adolescence, individuals may have barriers to engagement beyond their control, and what may appear to be civic dis-engagement may in fact be a reflection of poor resources, access to resources, or insufficient scaffolding to support the development of civic knowledge and agency towards civic engagement. By considering civic commitment as a component of civic engagement, we can understand what factors relate to commitment to future civic engagement, as well as past civic engagement.

A History of Civic Engagement in Racially Marginalized Communities

The history of political activism among racial minority youth runs as deep as the history of racism and political disenfranchisement. For example, during the 1960s, Black Americans and many allied groups worked through the Civil Rights Movement to counteract systemic political and social injustice and to demand equal political rights under the Constitution. Through the Civil Rights Movement and other grassroots movements (e.g., the Black Power Movement), racial segregation, political disenfranchisement, and racial violence were constitutionally outlawed, granting all citizens equal protection under the law. Black Americans were no longer subject to legally sanctioned voter suppression, private acts of race-based violence, and separate and unequal public education without legal recourse in the face of those injustices. With these policy changes that were fueled by political and social activism that included sit-ins, protests, and marches, began the slow decline of overt mainstream racism and discrimination. The systemic constraints that precluded all Americans from exercising their civil rights were challenged under the law. Discrimination that was once legally sanctioned, as well as socially expected, was no longer tolerated as a barrier to engaged citizenship. However, racism and discrimination still function as cultural norms that run through the fabric of American society.

The long-standing history of institutional violence against people of color, though *constitutionally illegal*, still impacts the lived experiences of people today. In the past 50 years since the Civil Rights Act of 1964, many minority youth still report experiences of racial discrimination and systematic inequality in schools, communities, and institutions (Cohen 2005; Fine et al. 2004; Hope et al. 2014; Williams, et al. 2012). To counteract these negative experiences, many individuals and programs are dedicated to decreasing discrimination, increasing respect of diversity and difference, and promoting critical analysis of social issues (Bowman 2011; Ginwright 2010; Kumagai and Lypson 2009). Modern sociopolitical movements seek to help maintain the system changes that have occurred through the Civil Rights era and to encourage further systemic social evolution to challenge contemporary injustice. For example, sociopolitical movements are made manifest through protests of police brutality and racially biased policing practices, grassroots movements that target educational inequity in public schools, and unprecedented mobilization of citizens exercising their right to vote, among other issues.

With a changing social and political landscape, the nature of civic behavior for minority youth is also evolving. Like the youth of the civil rights movement who were an integral part of sit-ins and other forms of protest, politically engaged minority youth are a key demographic in modern protests and elections. For instance, in the 2012 Presidential election, the political participation of young people proved a critical influence, as 29 % of youth ages 18–29 voted according to exit polls (Rogowski and Cohen 2012). Researchers at the Black Youth Project noted the specific impact of Black and Latino youth on the election results (emphasis original):

This new analysis shows that youth again increased their presence at the voting booth, and this increase was driven largely by *high levels of turnout among young Blacks and Latinos*... Because of the increased percentages of young people of color in the population and in the voting electorate, these populations have played an increasingly important role in selecting the nation's president, and will continue to do so.

Black Youth Project (November 9, 2012)

While the fight for constitutional equality was enacted into legislation 50 years ago with the Civil Rights Act of 1964, there is still work to be done towards supporting the continued civic participation and growing civic development of racial minorities, particularly given the racial history of political disenfranchisement and marginalization in America. The high numbers of young racial minority voters in the 2012 Presidential election is an example of how such change can occur and how civic engagement functions as a direct response to counter racial injustice. Social change is also created through grassroots movements, community organizing, and other forms of social and political participatory citizenship to counter interpersonal and institutional racial discrimination (Cohen 2005; Ginwright 2010).

Inspired and enlightened by a history of youth led resistance, minority youth continue to participate as citizens. Young people are re-imagining *critical civic engagement* as a social response to the remnants of injustice and racial bias that have yet to be eradicated from our social milieu. The work of civic engagement as a statement of humanity and equality in the lives of twenty-first century minority youth is not a new proposition. Freire (1970) suggested that disenfranchised groups of people are most ideally prepared to be active participants in their own liberation *when they pursue a critical analysis of the structural roots of bias and injustice that oppress them* (emphasis added). Contemporary and historical experiences of discrimination coupled with understanding the sociopolitical culture influence if, how, and why minority youth participate as members of society. Indeed, today's minority youth hold fast to the roots of youth-led resistance from social movements past as a mandate to actively invoke civic engagement as a form of resistance for the sake of the positive development of self and community. In this way, civic engagement can be used as a positive and proactive reaction to interpersonal and institutional discrimination.

An Inclusive Perspective of Human Vulnerability: Phenomenological Variant of Ecological Systems Theory (P-VEST)

A phenomenological variant of ecological systems theory (acronym pronounced "P-VEST") is a human development framework that acknowledges, from a traditional phenomenological stance, the critical role of the *individual's unavoidable cognition-based perceptions* (Spencer 1995, 2006; Spencer and Swanson 2015; Spencer et al. 2015). The theoretical standpoint emphasizes identity formation while simultaneously considering social structural forces and cultural influences—naming but a few contributors—along with an individual's recursive and reciprocal perceptual processes and responsive behavioral orientation. The latter includes those processes relevant for the self-system albeit also implicating the contributions of significant others and life events as one copes with normative developmental tasks while navigating across myriad social contexts and physical spaces. As such, the PVEST framework is conceptualized as *an identity-focused cultural ecological (ICE) perspective.* Consistent with Eriksonian (1968) psychosocial notions, identity formation takes place across the life course and, as generally understood, is especially salient during the fragile adolescent and young-adulthood transitions, given both periods' foundational associations with heightened self-consciousness.

Accordingly, PVEST represents an emphasis on individual normative and unavoidable perceptual processes along with Bronfenbrenner's ecological systems perspective (1979). The consequent conceptual strategy indelibly links context character and social experiences with *individuals' meaning-making based perceptual process.* Thus, while Bronfenbrenner's model provides a conceptual strategy for describing the ways by which multiple levels of context can influence individual development, additionally, PVEST directly illustrates how normative life course tasks and adaptations (to multiple layers of the ecology and linked experiences) unavoidably impact how people make sense of the world. Consequent meaning-making and coping processes for individuals emanate both from *within and between* context experiences. Accordingly, as a conceptual device, PVEST emphasizes the individual's cognition and context-associated conceptual efforts, which link with obvious socio-emotional processes and motivational relevant outcomes. Together, these processes and consequences underlie *identity development; thus*, they have implications for behavioral outcomes and their stable character (see Spencer 1995, 1999, 2006; Spencer et al. 2006, 2015; Spencer and Swanson 2015).

These progressions and outcomes are linked with the developmental tasks and maturational themes concomitant with a particular developmental period. For example, given the psychosocial emphasis of Erikson's theory, an infant's *development of trust* as linked to needs, tasks and adaptations are related to the nature of identity achievement themes particularly critical for a successful adolescence. The supports available and challenges confronted have relevance *for the level of human vulnerability, thus, the successful engagement of ongoing adaptive requirements and needs.*

Also important is that inferences about identity formation and the interpretation of parallel behavioral orientations have been framed in patterned ways for particular individuals. Specific groups have been consistently portrayed as bereft of strengths and protective factors and, alternatively, are inferred to lead lives endorsed narrowly by significant risks and challenges; relatedly, published interpretations of behavior assume psychopathology and/or a deficit perspective for *highly vulnerable* populations (i.e., those individuals and groups which represent high risk status and low accessible resources). At the same time, these prevalent perspectives assume positive outcomes for low vulnerability individuals and populations (i.e., those assumed to have significant resources and few or low risk [s]). Yet such explanatory frameworks fail to clarify diverse outcomes for individuals sharing circumstances.

Examples of the latter include siblings developing within the same family, neighborhood and socioeconomic status although manifesting quite different life-stage specific outcomes (e.g., one sibling's graduation from high school versus another's incarceration in a juvenile facility). At the same time, youth appearing to represent mainly protective factors, strengths, and opportunities (i.e., versus those in situations characterized as high risk) produce heinous outcomes. With reference to the latter, level of vulnerability is not always apparent (i.e., the balance or imbalance between protective factor presence versus risk level). The youthful perpetrator of the relatively recent 2012 Newtown, Connecticut school carnage as well as the those responsible for the Littleton, Colorado, Columbine High School massacre—the commitment of mass murder versus the enactment and receipt of a successful career—had life experiences and outcomes quite different from the trajectory stereotypically expected for those living under high resourced situations. The examples suggest that too frequently supports and protective factors are misconstrued or ignored for some youth (e.g., youth for whom their social status is exclusively inferred as associated with risks and challenge) and others for whom daily life accomplishments are assumed to represent earned strengths and superior social status. We infer that civic engagement for youth of color, and sociopolitically marginalized young people more generally, functions as a protective factor. Thus civic engagement can be leveraged as an effective response to a myriad of developmental tasks and environmental challenges. Such proactive responses accumulate positive identifications and patterned identity processes which become linked with positive and/or resilient outcomes. Productive outcomes, subsequently, function to serve as more enhanced protective factors and facilitate positive and productive response to

more stressful challenges (and the recursive processes continue "playing forward").

The PVEST model (see Fig. 1) consists of five basic components that form a dynamic theoretical system and are applicable to any period of the life course; the nature of the protective factors and risks are specific to a particular period of development.

The first component, *Net Vulnerability Level*, consists of individual, family, and community characteristics that may serve as risk factors or provide protective functioning for an individual's development. The risks, of course, may be offset by protective factors (e.g., additional instrumental, emotional or financial support provided by family or non-blood "kin" and having opportunities to develop and hone civic engagement insights); thus, defining net vulnerability for a given individual. For marginalized individuals (e.g., immigrants, youth of color and low resource citizens), the noted risk factors can include socioeconomic conditions such as living in poverty, and may be challenged by imposed expectations based upon race, affluence and gender stereotypes, stigma, and assumptions about effort and ability. In sum, net vulnerability refers to the balance between risk factor versus protective factor presence. Accordingly, a highly vulnerable individual has an imbalance between the levels of evident risks (i.e., excessively high) versus the accessibility of protective factors (i.e., uncommonly low).

The second component of the PVEST framework, *Net Stress Engagement* (2), refers to the actual experience of stress; the degree of stress experienced is determined by the available challenges versus the available support. Accordingly, the balance of the two (i.e., level of challenge vs. myriad support) can affect an individual's well-being and decision-making process and its character. In contrast to the risk factors noted in the Net Vulnerability Level first component of PVEST, the challenges referred to represent actual *transformed risks* encountered and which, given their impact as stress, require a response. Available supports (i.e., personal, social, or structural) can help individuals negotiate experiences of stress in that they diminish

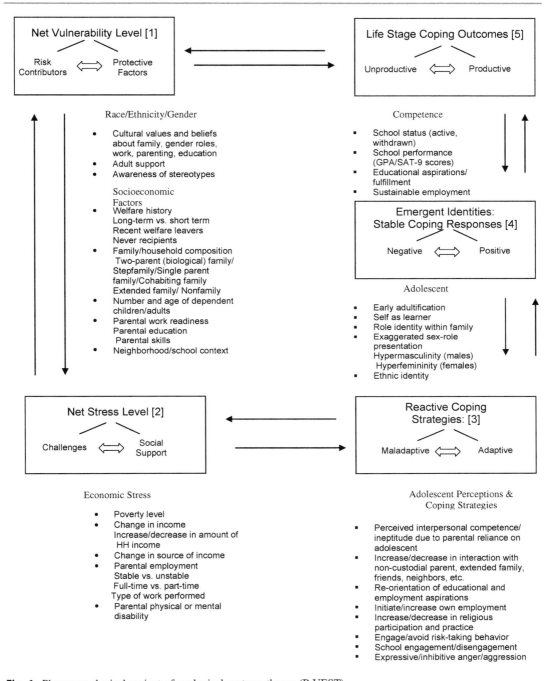

Fig. 1 Phenomenological variant of ecological systems theory (P-VEST)

the level of impact; in fact, supports function as actualized protective factors. Risk and protective factors denote potential entities within the individual, family or community as net vulnerability level; *however, challenges* and *support* refer to actual phenomenological experiences of risk and protection in context, which have implications for the character of stress (i.e., stress engagement). For example, youths' exposure to activist's historical explanations for contemporary behavioral orientation, may act as either a challenge or a support depending on the context. That is, an inclusive history of race-relations in the United States may be perceived as supportive socialization given the current racialized sociopolitical climate. However, this type of activist socialization might challenge internalized beliefs and "learning" and be stressful for adolescents who are negotiating racially hostile academic or vocational environments.

In response to stressors and in conjunction with supports, Reactive Coping Methods (3) are employed. Reactive coping responses include problem-solving strategies that can be either adaptive or maladaptive. For instance, in response to decreased time and attention from parents, adolescents may take on more familial responsibilities, engage in more risk taking behavior, seek greater interaction with other kin and non-kin adults or, like the Columbine massacre perpetrators, engage in highly anti-social behavior with similarly marginal and highly vulnerable youth. At the same time, youth's involvement with political youth forums may find the associations determinative of adaptive behaviors and outcomes.

As youth employ various coping strategies, self-appraisal continues, and those strategies yielding desirable results are repeated. Accordingly, they become *stable coping responses*, and, over time, yield Stable Emergent Identities (4). Emergent identities define how individuals view themselves within and between their various contexts of development (e.g., family, school, neighborhood, and peer group). The combination of such factors as cultural/ethnic background, understandings about gender roles, and self and peer appraisal all define one's identity. Given the youth activism of many during the Civil Rights era and suggestions for turning back principles of inequality, *proactive civic engagement makes a difference for coping and identity processes.*

Not unlike Eriksonian perspectives on the topic, identity processes provide behavioral stability over time and space and lay the foundation for future perception, self-appraisal, and behavior. The resulting behavior can yield productive or adverse Life-stage Coping Outcomes (5).

Productive outcomes can include school engagement, a sense of agency, positive family relationships, adequate employment preparation, parenting skills and low levels of risk behavior. On the other hand, adverse or unproductive outcomes can include school dropout, poor school performance, engagement in illegal means of earning income, and mistimed or unplanned child bearing. Untoward outcomes potentially function as risk contributors and thus impact subsequent levels of vulnerability whereas, on the other hand, success may function to contribute protective factors and decreased vulnerability.

The bidirectional, recursive, and dynamic process of negotiating the fulfillment of life course tasks is influenced by net vulnerability and continues throughout life (i.e., as individuals balance new risks against protective factors). The challenge associated with confronting normative and unique development specific tasks is offset by accessible supports and, together, impact stress engagement which, too frequently, can be highly uncomfortable and psychologically intrusive (e.g., as in the situation of stereotype threat). It is the level of discomfort, which establishes the use and need for expansive reactive coping strategies, which can be either adaptive or maladaptive. The implicit positive or negative character of the reactive coping responses possible may define or redefine how individuals are treated and viewed by others and, most salient, may impact how individuals view themselves or manifest a stable emergent identity as associated with particular settings and the performance of critical tasks (e.g., academic achievement). As noted by Erikson (1968), unresolved issues within one life stage influence future coping and identity formation processes. PVEST aims not only to capture this developmental process, but also to place it within its broader social contexts.

Current Research Questions

In light of PVEST, we situate civic engagement as a positive and proactive reactive coping strategy to unjust sociopolitical conditions that serve to reduce the net level of human vulnerability over time. Inequality is a stressful situation, which for many precipitates the need for civic engagement as a reactive coping strategy. The unavoidable bi-directionality between net vulnerability level, stress encountered, and reactive coping provides a good illustration of recursive processes. For example, *early cultural socialization* functions as an identity relevant protective factor that is recursively influential. Specifically, cultural socialization is theorized as impacting the character of links between stress engagement and reactive coping (i.e., PVEST components 2 and 3, respectively). Functioning in a recursive manner through socialization and context linked experience (i.e., given the protection provided as an *identity element*); early and/or ongoing cultural socialization *may reduce net vulnerability (functioning as a protective factor, PVEST component 1) and the character of bi-directional links between stress and reactive coping needs* (see McGee and Spencer 2013; Spencer and Swanson 2013).

Accordingly, as an adaptive reactive coping strategy, civic engagement has the potential to provide youth with a space for positive youth development and development of resilience through taking an active role in negotiating and changing the sociopolitical conditions that contribute to their net vulnerability. Further, through civic engagement, youth develop civic identities and further define racial/ethnic, gendered, and vocational identities, which contribute to civic engagement throughout the lifetime. The net vulnerability level dictates the nature of and necessity for civic engagement to challenge environmental distress. Equally, through civic engagement minority youth are positioned to contribute to larger structural changes and thus reduce the future net vulnerability level for themselves and the community at-large. The primary research question that emerges from this theoretical perspective is, how can civic engagement be leveraged as an intervention to support development of resilience and positive identity among minority children? Specifically, (1) how do net vulnerability and stress relate to civic engagement as an adaptive coping

mechanism? and (2) how does civic engagement relate to emerging identities and life stage coping outcomes?

Empirical Findings

Extant literature on the civic development of minority youth has emphasized the "civic achievement gap" where minority youth participate less in traditional politics, have more negative political attitudes, and have less knowledge of traditional political systems than their white and highly resourced (wealthy) counterparts (Levinson 2007). Further, empirical research shows that some minority youth are skeptical of traditional political participation given a history of political marginalization, lack of government trust, and perception that the government will not adequately respond to their political needs (Diemer and Li 2011; Watts and Flanagan 2007). However, civic engagement is related to positive development among minority youth beyond the civic domain. In a study of the long-term influence of adolescent civic engagement among African American and Latino youth, researchers found that civic engagement during adolescence is related to higher life satisfaction, greater civic participation, greater educational attainment, and lower rates of arrest in emerging adulthood (Chan et al. 2014).

Empirical research has begun to examine relationships between civic engagement and both interpersonal and institutional discrimination among racial minority youth. In a study of Black college students, White-Johnson (2012) considers the relationship between discrimination and within group civic attitudes and behavior. She finds that more frequent experiences of racial discrimination (e.g., not given service in a store) are related to more frequent civic engagement within the African American community (e.g., tutoring Black youth) and greater endorsement of prosocial attitudes within the African American community (e.g., responsibility to contribute to the Black community). Similarly, among Latino college students, experiencing discrimination is related to a commitment to activism on behalf of the Latino community (e.g., demonstrating, petitioning), and this relationship works through positive ethnic identity (Cronin et al. 2012).

Perceptions of institutional discrimination are also related to civic engagement. In a study of Black youth ages 15–25, stronger endorsement of the presence of institutional discrimination against Blacks in America is related to a greater breadth of civic engagement including campaigning, boycotting, and volunteer community work (Hope and Jagers 2014). Among minority and low-income high school students, researchers found that experience with journalism illuminated an understanding of discrimination in media and promoted civic engagement among the students (Marchi 2012). While in its infancy, this research provides empirical evidence that establishes civic engagement as a positive and proactive coping response to negative experiences of discrimination, particularly in the case of *critical civic engagement* that emphasizes improving social conditions for members of one's own racial-ethnic group. Further, this research suggests that it may be meaningful to investigate both experiences of interpersonal discrimination and understanding of institutional discrimination. While interpersonal discrimination is related to within group civic engagement, understanding systematic forms of institutionalized discrimination is related to civic engagement broadly for racial and ethnic minority youth (Hope and Jagers 2014; White-Johnson 2012).

Civic Engagement Programs and Positive Youth Development

It is important to establish that civic engagement can truly be leveraged to enhance positive development among minority youth, disturbing the notion that minority youth who participate in civic engagement are simply youth who already manifest such positive development outcomes. Findings from applied intervention and evaluation research suggest that civic engagement is indeed an intervention strategy to promote positive youth development, especially when considering social justice based programs (e.g.,

Youth Participatory Action Research) that prepare minority youth to engage in dismantling structural inequality through facilitated discussion and action (Berg et al. 2009; Foster-Fishman et al. 2010).

Youth Participatory Action Research (YPAR) is typically an out-of-school time program established to facilitate discussions of community through a lens of systematic discrimination and hegemony. From a systems-based community perspective, the youth conduct a related community-based research project and establish an action plan to enhance the community given research findings (Berg et al. 2009; Schensul and Berg 2004). Participation in YPAR is related to positive youth development outcomes including reduced drug and sex risks, increased positive attitudes towards education, increased critical analysis and problem-solving skills, increased sense of self and positive identity formation, and increased self-efficacy (Berg et al. 2009; Morrell 2008; Morsillo and Prilleltensky 2007). For instance, compared to a control group, low-income Black and Latino high school students who participated in an afterschool YPAR program had increased analytic skills, increased educational expectations, stronger disapproval of drug use, and decreased marijuana use (Berg et al. 2009). Similarly, high school students of color who participated in a summer YPAR program in California reported greater critical thinking skills, increased self-confidence, and increase political efficacy (Morrell 2008). Further, among a class of diverse high school students, researchers found that participation in community action intervention led to increased sociopolitical awareness, enhanced social responsibility, and increased community participation skills (obtaining permits, organizing meetings) (Morsillo and Prilleltensky 2007). This growing body of research highlights the utility of civic engagement as a tool for simultaneously combating structurally based marginalization in communities of color and promoting positive life skills and developmental characteristics for minority youth. Analyzed theoretically, we posit that identity changing activities serve to decrease net vulnerability due to the psychological protection provided by "new identities" or altered perceptions of self (see McGee and Spencer 2012; Youngblood and Spencer 2010).

Policy Implications

The most fundamental policy implication from this line of research is that children and adolescents from racially marginalized backgrounds are civically engaged and this civic engagement can mitigate ecological stress and vulnerability. Thus, municipalities, schools, and local authorities might consider implementation of structured ways to include minority youth and their families in local civic and political activities. Prior research has shown when youth are systematically included in municipal public policy, there are benefits for youth and community: (1) youth knowledge and expertise contribute to policy decisions and community welfare, and (2) this structured participation prepares youth and excites youth for lifelong civic participation and leadership (Checkoway et al. 2005). Some local municipalities are beginning to consider these implications more seriously. For instance, in Takoma Park, Maryland, the city council voted to lower the voting age to 16 years old (Vela 2013). While Takoma Park residents under 18 will not be able to vote in state and national elections, this decision illustrates the importance of young people as Takoma Park citizens and allows the youth to have a voice in a democratic process and practice engaging an adaptive coping response to risk and vulnerabilities in their local environment. Other ways to include children and adolescents would be a primary and secondary school seat on local school boards, working groups or committees that cater to youth members, and workshops to teach petitioning, letter writing, and legal protesting skills.

Future Direction

In light of the proposed utility of civic engagement as *both positive adaptive coping* for individual minority youth development (to reduce stereotypically framed net vulnerability assumptions), as well as a method of enacting *systematic changes* in the broader communities that minority youth are a part of, there are several meaningful research directions and questions that remain. These research directions complicate the pervasive assumption that civic engagement functions uniformly across racial groups by attending to the historical and contemporary sociopolitical positioning of racial minorities. With more nuanced interpretations of patterns in civic beliefs and participation that account for contextual experiences we can ask, how can civic engagement be leveraged for positive development of minority children? One line of research should seek to understand more deeply the relationship between net vulnerability and stress level (including experiences of discrimination and bias) and critical civic engagement as an adaptive coping strategy. It is important to investigate how ecological stressors (e.g., *experiences* of discrimination) promote or deter civic engagement for minority youth. On one hand, youth may experience interpersonal or institutional discrimination and become withdrawn from political systems, becoming cynical of the utility of engaging with formal institutions to address the needs of their communities. Alternatively, experiences of discrimination may prompt a desire to seek systematic changes within current systems to ensure that other members of the community do not experience the same bias and unfair treatment.

In a similar line of research, we need to investigate how racial minority youth are developing a cognitive and phenomenological *understanding* and *internalization* of their ecological vulnerability and risk within the context of a broader socio-historical landscape. For instance, as Freire and scholars of sociopolitical development (SPD) suggest, a critical understanding of discrimination and inequity is a principal contributor to critical civic engagement among racial minority youth (Freire 1970; Watts et al. 2011). By developing an understanding of inequitable social conditions, marginalized youth are in turn empowered to act politically and civically to express their own political voice. SPD theory contends that an achieved critical analysis reflects critical consciousness and serves as a potent catalyst to meaningful justice-oriented civic engagement (Watts et al. 2003). Simply put, when a young person understands that margins of society exist, that they are living in the margins, and that systematic policies and practices exist to maintain those margins, they are motivated to work to deconstruct those systematic agents of marginalization. Research supports this assumption, finding that individual characteristics that reflect aspects of a critical analysis, such as civic knowledge and political trust, are related to political activism among youth (Hart and Gullan 2010) and minority youth who believe the world is unjust have a stronger commitment to civic engagement (Watts and Guessous 2006). Given the prevalence of identity exploration, adolescence marks a critical period for scholars to consider phenomenological variation in the development of critical analysis of ecological risk and its relation to civic engagement.

Finally, as we explore the cognitive and phenomenological dimensions of ecological risk and vulnerability and how that relates to civic preparation and participation, we must turn attention to education as a primary socialization space. Schools reinforce the expectation that youth become engaged citizens through social studies curricula, and according to the Center for Information and Research on Civic Learning and Engagement, ten states still do not require students take at least one American Government or Civic course prior to high school graduation (Godsay et al. 2012). While citizenship is taught and reinforced through schools, racial minority youth also experience discrimination in schools and receive messages from curriculum and teachers on the inherent value and expected sociopolitical role of ethnic minorities (Hope et al. 2014). Scholars posit that schools serve as "mini-polities" that replicate the civic and political structures and practices of broader society (Fine et al. 2004; Flanagan 2013). This positions schools as unique socialization agents that can both teach students citizenry but simultaneously undermine that citizenry through the reinforcement of broader systemic and interpersonal discrimination.

Thus, the quality and content of civic education is an equally important line of inquiry to strengthen our understanding of civic engagement as an intervention towards ameliorating the negative consequences of bias for racial minority youth. Research has found that presence of civic education is directly related to civic engagement among Black youth and strengthens the relationship between political efficacy and civic engagement (Hope and Jagers 2014). However, less is known about how the quality, quantity, and content of civic education teach citizenship to minority students, particularly those with a history of political marginalization in America. Equally, research should investigate how minority students interpret the civic curriculum in relation to their experiences within the broader school and community culture. Sanchez-Jankowski (2002) posits that minority youth are encouraged toward or deterred from civic participation as a result of ethnic specific "transfer stations" that are shaped by the sociopolitical culture and history of one's racial-ethnic group. For example, while a Black student may be taught that voting is important, the history of voting rights in the Black community is a "transfer station" that further shapes that student's interpretation of the value of Black voters in America. Thus, it is important to understand what minority students are learning about both being a citizen and about being a citizen from a minority group through the curriculum, classroom dynamics, and informal interactions in the hallways. Research might also distinguish school practices that not only teach civics to minority youth, but empower those youth to become active and engaged citizens towards social change in their communities.

Taken together, critical civic engagement can be a powerful tool of intervention to enhance the development of minority children and protect against ecological risks and vulnerabilities. By using civic engagement to challenge systematic norms of marginalization, minority children engage in an adaptive coping strategy that supports individual and community well-being.

Civic engagement enriches the development of minority youth through promoting skill building and identity development. Civic engagement also provides means for young people to be directly involved in altering the ecological system that causes and perpetuates those very risks and vulnerabilities. By attending to civic engagement as an intervention researchers, practitioners, and policy makers are better positioned to strengthen the lives of minority children, their communities, and societies at-large.

References

Adler, R. (2005). What do we mean by "civic engagement"? *Journal of Transformative Education, 3*(3), 236–253.

Amnå, E. (2012). How is civic engagement developed over time? Emerging answers from a multidisciplinary field. *Journal of Adolescence, 35*(3), 611–627. doi:10.1016/j.adolescence.2012.04.011

Astuto, J., & Ruck, M. (2010). Early childhood as a foundation for civic engagement. In L. Sherrod, J. Torney-Purta, & C. Flanagan (Eds.), *Handbook of research on civic engagement in youth* (pp. 249–276). Hoboken, NJ: Wiley.

Berg, M., Coman, E., & Schensul, J. (2009). Youth action research for prevention: A multi-level intervention designed to increase efficacy and empowerment among urban youth. *American Journal of Community Psychology, 43*(4), 345–360. doi:10.1007/s10464-009-9231-2

Bowman, N. (2011). Promoting participation in a diverse democracy: A meta-analysis of college diversity experiences and civic engagement. *Review of Educational Research, 81*(1), 29–68. doi:10.3102/0034654310383047

Bronfenbrenner, U. (1979). *The ecology of human development*. Cambridge, MA: Harvard University Press.

Chan, W. Y., Ou, S.-R., & Reynolds, A. J. (2014). Adolescent civic engagement and adult outcomes: An examination among urban racial minorities. *Journal of Youth and Adolescence.* doi:10.1007/s10964-014-0136-5

Checkoway, B., Allison, T., & Montoya, C. (2005). Youth participation in public policy at the municipal level. *Children and Youth Services Review, 27*(10), 1149–1162. doi:10.1016/j.childyouth.2005.01.001

Cohen, C. (2005). *Democracy remixed: Black youth and the future of American politics*. New York, NY: Oxford University Press.

Cronin, T., Levin, S., Branscombe, N., van Laar, C., & Troop, L. (2012). Ethnic identification in response to perceived discrimination protects well-being and promotes activism: A longitudinal study of Latino college students. *Group Processes & Intergroup Relations, 15*(3), 393–407. doi:10.1177/1368430211427171

Diemer, M. A., & Li, C. H. (2011). Critical consciousness development and political participation among marginalized youth. *Child Development, 82*(6), 1815–1833. doi:10.1111/j.1467-8624.2011.01650.x

Ekman, J., & Amnå, E. (2012). Political participation and civic engagement: Towards a new typology. *Human Affairs, 22*(3), 283–300.

Erikson, E. (1968). *Identity, youth and crisis*. New York: W.W. Norton Company.

Fine, M., Burns, A., Payne, Y., & Torre, M. E. (2004). *Civics lessons: The color and class of betrayal* (pp. 53–74). Working method: Research and social justice.

Flanagan, C. (2013). *Teenage citizens: The political theories of the young*. Cambridge, MA: Harvard University Press.

Foster-Fishman, P., Law, K., Lichty, L., & Aoun, C. (2010). Youth ReACT for social change: A method for youth participatory action research. *American Journal of Community Psychology, 46*, 67–83. doi:10.1007/s10464-010-9316-y

Freire, P. (1970). *Pedagogy of the oppressed*. New York: Continuum Publishing Co.

Ginwright, S. (2010). Peace out to revolution! Activism among African American youth: An argument for radical healing. *Young: Nordic Journal for Youth Research, 18*(1), 77–96.

Godsay, S., Henderson, W., Levine, P., & Littenberg-Tobias, J. (2012). *State civic education requirements fact sheet*. Medford, MA: Center for Information and Research on Civic Learning and Engagement.

Hart, D., & Gullan, R. (2010). The sources of adolescent activism: Historical and contemporary findings. In L. Sherrod, J. Torney-Purta, & C. Flanagan (Eds.), *Handbook of research on civic engagement in youth* (pp. 67–90). Hoboken, NJ: John Wiley & Sons Inc.

Hope, E., & Jagers, R. (2014). The role of sociopolitical attitudes and civic education in the civic engagement of Black youth. *Journal of Research on Adolescence, 24*(3), 460–470. doi:10.1111/jora.12117

Hope, E., Skoog, A., & Jagers, R. (2014). "It'll never be the white kids, it'll always be us": Black high school students' evolving critical analysis of racial discrimination and inequity in schools. *Journal of Adolescent Research, 30*(1), 83–112. doi:10.1177/0743558414550688

Kumagai, A., & Lypson, M. (2009). Beyond cultural competence: Critical consciousness, social justice, and multicultural education. *Journal of Academic Medicine, 84*(6), 782–787.

Levinson, M. (2007, January). *The civic achievement gap (CIRCLE working paper 51)*. College Park, MD: Center for Information and Research on Civic Learning and Engagement.

Marchi, R. (2012). From disillusion to engagement: Minority teen journalists and the news media. *Journalism,* *13*(6), 750–765. doi:10.1177/1464884911431379

McGee, E., & Spencer, M. B. (2012). Theoretical analysis of resilience and identity: An African American engineer's life story. In E. J. Dixon-Román & E. W. Gordon (Eds.), *Thinking comprehensively about education: Spaces of educative possibility and their implications for public policy* (pp. 161–178). New York, NY: Routledge.

McGee, E. O., & Spencer, M. B. (2013). The development of coping skills for science, technology, engineering, and mathematics students: Transitioning from minority to majority environments. In C. C. Yeakey, V. S. Thompson, & A. Wells (Eds.), *Urban ills: Post recession complexities of urban living in the twenty first century* (pp. 351–378). Lanham, MD: Lexington Books.

Metzger, A., & Smetana, J. (2010). Social cognitive development and adolescent civic engagement. In L. Sherrod, J. Torney-Purta, & C. Flanagan (Eds.), *Handbook of research on civic engagement in youth* (pp. 221–248). Hoboken, NJ: Wiley.

Morrell, E. (2008). Six summers of YPAR: Learning, action, and change in urban education. In J. Cammarota & M. Fine (Eds.), *Revolutionizing education: Youth participatory action research in motion* (pp. 155–184). New York: Routledge.

Morsillo, J., & Prilleltensky, I. (2007). Social action with youth: Interventions, evaluation, and psychopolitical validity. *Journal of Community Psychology, 35*(6), 725–740. doi:10.1002/jcop.20175

Rogowski, J. C., & Cohen, C. J. (2012, November 9). The political impact of young people of color in the 2012 election. www.blackyouthproject.com. Retrieved November 10, 2012, from http://research.blackyouthproject.com/files/2012/11/PolitImpactofYouthofColor.pdf

Sanchez-Jankowski, M. (2002). Minority youth and civic engagement: The impact of group relations. *Applied Developmental Science, 6,* 237–245.

Schensul, J., & Berg, M. (2004). Youth participatory action research: A transformative approach to service-learning. *Michigan Journal of Community Service Learning, 10*(3), 76–88.

Sherrod, L., & Lauckhardt, J. (2008). The development of citizenship. In R. Lerner & L. Steinberg (Eds.), *Handbook of adolescent psychology* (3rd ed., Vol. 2, pp. 372–408). Hoboken, NJ: Wiley.

Sherrod, L., Torney-Purta, J., & Flanagan, C. (2010). Research on the development of citizenship: A field comes of age. In L. Sherrod, J. Torney-Purta, & C. Flanagan (Eds.), *Handbook of research on civic engagement in youth* (pp. 1–22). Hoboken, NJ: Wiley.

Spencer, M. (1995). Old issues and new theorizing about African–American youth: A phenomenological variant of ecological systems theory. In R. L. Taylor (Ed.), *Black youth: Perspectives on their status in the United States* (pp. 37–69). Westport, CT: Praeger.

Spencer, M. (1999). Social and cultural influence on school adjustment: The application of an identity-focus cultural ecological perspective. *Educational Psychologist, 34*(1), 43–57. doi:10.1207/s15326985ep3401_4

Spencer, M. (2006). Phenomenology and ecological systems theory: Development of diverse groups. In W. Damon & R. Lerner (Eds.), *Handbook of child psychology: Theoretical Models of Human Development* (6th ed., Vol. 1, pp. 829–893). New York: Wiley.

Spencer, M., & Swanson, D. (2013). Opportunities and challenges to the development of healthy children and youth living in diverse communities. *Development and Psychopathology, 25*(4pt2), 1551–1566.

Spencer, M., & Swanson, D. (2015). Vulnerability and resilience: Illustrations from theory and research on African American youth. In D. Cicchetti (Ed.), *Handbook of developmental psychopathology.* New York: John Wiley & Sons.

Spencer, M., Swanson, D. & Harpalani, V. (expected 2015). Conceptualizing the self: Contributions of normative human processes, diverse contexts and social opportunity. In Lamb, M., Coll, C. G., & R. Lerner (Eds.), *Handbook of child psychology and developmental science.* New York: Wiley.

Spencer, M. B., Harpalani, V., Cassidy, E., Jacobs, C., Donde, S., Goss, T., et al. (2006). Understanding vulnerability and resilience from a normative developmental perspective: Implications for racially and ethnically diverse youth. In D. Cicchetti & D. Cohen (Eds.), *Developmental Psychopathology: Theory and method* (2nd ed., Vol. 1, pp. 627–672). Hoboken, NJ: Wiley.

Vela, H. (2013, May 14). Takoma Park lowers voting age to 16. *ABC7 WJLA.* Retrieved from http://www.wjla.com

Watts, R. J., & Flanagan, C. A. (2007). Pushing the envelope on youth civic engagement: A developmental and liberation psychology perspective. *Journal of Community Psychology, 35*(6), 779–792. doi:10.1002/jcop.20178

Watts, R., & Guessous, O. (2006). Sociopolitical development: The missing link in research and policy on adolescents. In S. Ginwright, P. Noguera, & J. Cammarota (Eds.), *Beyond resistance! Youth activism and community change: new democratic possibilities for practice and policy for America's youth.* New York: Routledge.

Watts, R. J., Diemer, M. A., & Voight, A. M. (2011). Critical consciousness: Current status and future directions. In C. A. Flanagan & B. D. Christens (Eds.), *Youth civic development: Work at the cutting edge* (Vol. 134). San Francisco: Josey-Bass.

Watts, R. J., Williams, N. C., & Jagers, R. J. (2003). Sociopolitical development. *American Journal of Community Psychology, 31*(1), 185–194.

Wentzel, K., Filisetti, L., & Looney, L. (2007). Adolescent prosocial behavior: The role of self-processes and contextual cues. *Child Development, 78*(3), 895–910.

White-Johnson, R. (2012). Prosocial involvement among African American young adults: Considering racial discrimination and racial identity. *Journal of Black Psychology, 38*, 313–341. doi:10.1177/0095798411420429

Williams, D., John, D., Oyserman, D., Sonnega, J., Mohammed, S., & Jackson, J. (2012). Research on discrimination and health: An explanatory study of unresolved conceptual and measurement issues. *American Journal of Public Health, 102*(5), 975–978. doi:10.2105/AJPH.2012.300702

Youngblood, J., & Spencer, M. B. (2010). Understanding culture and context: The start-on-success scholars program (S-O-S). In K. E. Hoagwood, P. S. Jensen, M. McKay, & S. Olin (Eds.), *Children's mental health research: The power of partnerships* (pp. 118–121). New York: Oxford University Press.

Youniss, J., Bales, S., Christmas-Best, V., Diversi, M., McLaughlin, W., & Silbereisen, R. (2002). Youth civic engagement in the twenty-first century. *Journal of Research on Adolescence, 12*(1), 121–148.

Developing an Ethnic-Racial Identity Intervention from a Developmental Perspective: Process, Content, and Implementation of the Identity Project

Adriana J. Umaña-Taylor and Sara Douglass

Abstract

This chapter describes the process of developing an intervention grounded in developmental theory and focused on increasing adolescents' ethnic-racial identity exploration and resolution. We begin by describing the impetus for the focus on ethnic-racial identity as a target for intervention, which includes a brief overview of prior research identifying consistent associations between developmental features of ethnic-racial identity and adolescents' positive adjustment. We then review existing intervention efforts focused on identity, generally, and ethnic or cultural identity, specifically. In the second part of the chapter we present our approach for working with a community partner toward the development of the *Identity Project* intervention, discuss the mixed method (i.e., quantitative and qualitative) approach we used to develop the curriculum, and describe the curriculum. The chapter ends with a discussion of considerations for implementation, including the universal nature of the program and ideas regarding transportability.

Historical Overview and Theoretical Perspectives

Identity development is a significant developmental task that gains momentum and prominence during the developmental period of adolescence (Erikson 1968). Although individuals construct and revisit the conceptualization of their identities throughout the lifespan, it is during adolescence that individuals have the cognitive maturity and social exposure that enables them to more thoroughly explore their goals, values, and beliefs that inform how they define themselves and who they perceive themselves to be in relation to others (Erikson 1968). Individuals' identities are defined by many social identities, such as those informed by one's ethnicity, race, or gender (Umaña-Taylor 2011).

In the context of the United States (U.S.), which has a complex history with respect to

A.J. Umaña-Taylor (✉) · S. Douglass
Arizona State University, Tempe, AZ, USA
e-mail: adriana.Umana-Taylor@asu.edu

© The Editor(s) 2017
N.J. Cabrera and B. Leyendecker (eds.), *Handbook on Positive Development of Minority Children and Youth*, DOI 10.1007/978-3-319-43645-6_26

immigration, racism, and ethnic-racial tensions, ethnicity and race are salient social identities (Umaña-Taylor 2011). Although ethnicity refers to one's cultural heritage as informed by factors such as traditions and language that get passed on from one generation to the next (Phinney 1996), and race captures sociohistorically-defined phenotypic distinctions based on factors such as skin color and other observable features that have been arbitrarily used to classify individuals in an effort to justify the unfair distributions of resources and power among groups in the US (Helms 1990), these two aspects of individuals' identities cannot be easily disentangled (Umaña-Taylor et al. 2014). As such, the construct of *ethnic-racial identity* (ERI) captures individuals' identities as informed by both ethnic features of their ancestral heritage (e.g., cultural traditions, language) and the racialized nature of their group in a particular sociohistorical context (e.g., marginalization as a function of ethnic minority status; Umaña-Taylor et al. 2014). The current chapter focuses on ERI, and follows a developmental conceptualization of the construct, such that ERI is defined as a multifaceted construct that includes the extent to which individuals have explored their ethnic background (i.e., ERI exploration), and the degree to which they have achieved a sense of resolution regarding what this aspect of their identity means to them (i.e., ERI resolution; Phinney 1993; Umaña-Taylor et al. 2004). Specifically, the current chapter provides a brief overview of prior work on ERI that provided the impetus for the development of an intervention curriculum focused on this construct as a target for intervention; presents a summary of existing intervention efforts focused on identity, generally, and ERI specifically; describes the mixed-method approach that was used to develop the curriculum for the ERI intervention (i.e., the *Identity Project*); and provides an overview of the resulting curriculum that was developed. Finally, we end with a discussion of considerations for implementation, including the universal nature of the program and ideas regarding transportability.

Ethnic-Racial Identity Development and Adolescent Adjustment: An Overview

Drawing largely from Erikson's (1968) psychosocial theory of development, the developmental process of ERI is captured by individuals' *exploration* of their ethnic-racial background and their sense of *resolution* regarding this aspect of their identity. Consistent with conceptualizations of general identity formation (e.g., Erikson 1968), ERI development is believed to evolve throughout the lifespan (Phinney 1996; Syed et al. 2007) but to be particularly salient during the developmental period of adolescence (Phinney 1993). Interest in studying ERI rose dramatically in the early 1990s and has continued to date (Umaña-Taylor 2015); this research activity has resulted in a significant literature base in which scholars have examined the associations between different aspects of adolescents' ERI and numerous indicators of adjustment (e.g., self-esteem, depressive symptoms, academic adjustment, life satisfaction; see Umaña-Taylor 2011, for a review). Generally, this work has led to the conclusion that, consistent with developmental theory (e.g., Erikson 1968; Marcia 1980), adolescents who have explored the meaning of their ethnic-racial background and have a clearer sense of what this aspect of their identity means for their lives tend to demonstrate better adjustment (e.g., Rivas-Drake et al. 2014). Conceptually, as adolescents have a clearer sense of their identity and have gained this sense of clarity as a result of meaningful exploration of their background, this achieved sense of identity is expected to provide psychological benefits to youth (Phinney and Kohatsu 1997; Umaña-Taylor et al. 2004). Moreover, ERI development is considered a normative developmental task in which youth are expected to engage as part of the process of identity formation, particularly in the context of US where ethnicity and race are salient (Umaña-Taylor et al. 2014; Williams et al. 2012).

Given this background, the Identity Project was conceptualized as a universal mental health promotion intervention program. Mental health promotion interventions are typically targeted to a whole population and are designed to enhance individuals' ability to achieve key developmental competencies (National Research Council and Institute of Medicine 2009). The Identity Project was designed to be delivered to the general population of youth (i.e., universal), rather than specific to youth identified as being at high risk (i.e., selected) or those showing minimal but detectable signs of problems (i.e., indicated; National Research Council and Institute of Medicine 2009). Furthermore, the curriculum was designed to be universal with respect to its relevance to youth from diverse backgrounds, rather than being specific to any one single group; and it is expected to be efficacious for youth from ethnic minority and majority backgrounds. However, because it focuses on a feature of normative development that is particularly salient to ethnic minority youth (Umaña-Taylor et al. 2014), it is expected to be especially useful for promoting positive adjustment among ethnic minority youth.

A focus on a normative developmental process such as ERI (Umaña-Taylor et al. 2014) as a target for intervention is necessary for several reasons. First, scholars have emphasized the need to capitalize on naturally occurring strengths within ethnic minority communities in efforts to develop more efficacious prevention programming (Case and Robinson 2003); because ERI has been identified as a promotive factor among ethnic minority youth (e.g., Rivas-Drake et al. 2014), it is an ideal source of strength on which to focus. Second, the field of prevention science is limited in its prevention efforts with ethnically diverse populations (Knight et al. 2009), yet a focus on prevention efforts that are particularly relevant to ethnic minority populations is important due to their higher risk for maladjustment coupled with a greater ambivalence regarding seeking services (Case and Robinson 2003; Hollon et al. 2002). Finally, ERI symbolizes a non-stigmatizing and developmentally normative process (Umaña-Taylor et al. 2014; Williams et al. 2012), which enables researchers to move away from deficit-focused approaches when intervening with ethnic minority populations.

Current Research Questions

The Prevention Research Cycle and the Development of an ERI Intervention

The prevention intervention research cycle can be divided into four general stages: generative, program development, implementation, and dissemination (Knight et al. 2009; Mzarek and Haggarty 1994; Roosa et al. 1997). The *Identity Project* is currently reaching the end of the program development stage. Thus, the discussion that follows focuses on the *generative stage* of the prevention research cycle in which a problem is identified and researchers consider the risk and protective processes that inform the problem or disorder, and the *program development stage* in which the curricular components of an intervention are developed and refined (see Knight et al. 2009, for a review of the prevention research cycle). Our focus on promoting youths' engagement in a *normative developmental process*, which has been linked with positive outcomes among youth and has been demonstrated to buffer the negative impact of risk factors on youth adjustment (Umaña-Taylor et al. 2014), is recognized as an important component of the mental health intervention spectrum. Specifically, prevention scientists suggest that promotion efforts focused on the achievement of developmental competencies are crucial because they can strengthen individuals' ability to cope with adversity, serve as a foundation for future competencies that are necessary for positive adjustment, and ultimately aid in the prevention and treatment of disorders (National Research Council and Institute of Medicine 2009).

The Generative Stage

Extensive reviews of existing theoretical and empirical work on ERI and youth adjustment (e.g., Rivas-Drake et al. 2014; Smith and Silva 2011; Umaña-Taylor 2011; Umaña-Taylor et al. 2004) characterized the generative stage of the Identity Project. A large body of prior theoretical and empirical work has suggested that engagement in exploration and resolution promotes positive adjustment (e.g., psychological well-begin, academic achievement) among ethnic minority (e.g., Neblett et al. 2012; Rivas-Drake et al. 2014) and ethnic majority (e.g., Yasui et al. 2004) youth. Based on a review of this evidence, the first author concluded that there was sufficient consensus to suggest that ERI is a normative developmental process that, importantly, confers psychological benefits for youth when there is evidence of significant engagement in exploration and resolution of one's ERI. Because of the focus on positive youth development, rather than pathology, there was not a specific problem that was identified, but rather a set of positive outcomes that the literature had identified as ideal for positive youth development (e.g., academic engagement, self-esteem).

The generative stage of this process also involved developing a theoretical model that described the proximal program mediators that would be targeted in the proposed intervention; the development of this theoretical model was based on prior theoretical and empirical work that has consistently emphasized the importance of operationalizing and measuring ERI exploration and resolution as distinct, yet interrelated, aspects of the ERI formation process (e.g., Supple et al. 2006; Umaña-Taylor et al. 2004, 2014). This prior work informed ERI exploration and resolution as the specific constructs to target in the program (i.e., the modifiable mediators); the initial ideas for the types of activities that would be essential for an ERI intervention; and the age group (i.e., developmental period) that would be targeted with the proposed program (see Fig. 1). The small theory of intervention (i.e., theoretical model guiding the intervention development; Roosa et al. 1997) suggests that a program that effectively provides youth with strategies and tools with which to explore and consider the relevance of their ERI for their general self-concept will, in effect, result in youth engaging in higher levels of ERI exploration and reporting a greater sense of ERI resolution. In turn, engagement in these processes will ultimately be associated with increases in adjustment as indexed by factors such as greater self-esteem, higher school engagement, and more positive

orientation toward other ethnic-racial groups. Drawing from Erikson's (1968) psychosocial theory of development, a possible mechanism by which these positive benefits are conferred is via youths' more secure sense of self as evidenced by less identity confusion and greater identity cohesion.

The Program Development Stage

After defining the targeted focus of the program, the first author convened a research team that would contribute to the development of the Identity Project curriculum and devise the study design to pilot test the program and examine whether ERI exploration and ERI resolution were, indeed, modifiable mediators. The team included three faculty researchers, a postdoctoral fellow, and several graduate research assistants; together, members of the team represented significant expertise in intervention research, ERI development, and adolescent development. During the early stages of program development, members of the research team met regularly to discuss the type of program and the types of activities that were envisioned, the feasibility of developing and disseminating (i.e., selling to interested stakeholders) a program that targeted normative developmental processes, and the elements of intervention programming that would be essential to consider to ensure that the program was universal (i.e., not targeted to a specific group) and transportable (i.e., the program could be easily implemented as intended in various school settings without major adaptations).

A strong emphasis was placed on certain design elements due to the substantive focus on ERI. First, delivery in a school-based setting, as part of the regular school day, was important to avoid selection bias into the program; if participation were optional, youth who were interested in learning about their ERI may participate and engage with the program in a different manner than their less-interested counterparts. Second, a universal rather than ethnic-racial group-specific approach was important for conceptual and logistical reasons. Conceptually, because ERI development is associated with positive youth adjustment, this is an important developmental

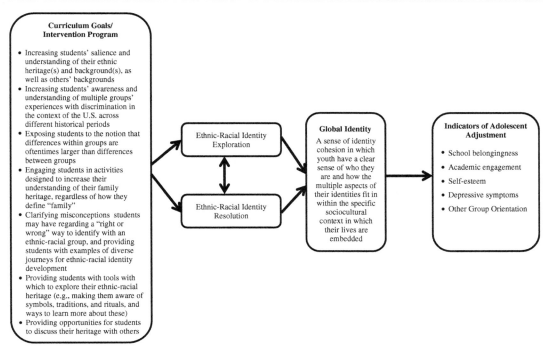

Curriculum Goals/Intervention Program

- Increasing students' salience and understanding of their ethnic heritage(s) and background(s), as well as others' backgrounds
- Increasing students' awareness and understanding of multiple groups' experiences with discrimination in the context of the U.S. across different historical periods
- Exposing students to the notion that differences within groups are oftentimes larger than differences between groups
- Engaging students in activities designed to increase their understanding of their family heritage, regardless of how they define "family"
- Clarifying misconceptions students may have regarding a "right or wrong" way to identify with an ethnic-racial group, and providing students with examples of diverse journeys for ethnic-racial identity development
- Providing students with tools with which to explore their ethnic-racial heritage (e.g., making them aware of symbols, traditions, and rituals, and ways to learn more about these)
- Providing opportunities for students to discuss their heritage with others

Ethnic-Racial Identity Exploration

Ethnic-Racial Identity Resolution

Global Identity
A sense of identity cohesion in which youth have a clear sense of who they are and how the multiple aspects of their identities fit in within the specific sociocultural context in which their lives are embedded

Indicators of Adolescent Adjustment
- School belongingness
- Academic engagement
- Self-esteem
- Depressive symptoms
- Other Group Orientation

Fig. 1 Theoretical model guiding intervention development for the identity project, an intervention focused on engaging youth in the developmental processes of ethnic-racial identity formation

competency that should be promoted among all youth, regardless of ethnic-racial background. Furthermore, because ERI is a normative developmental process that is relevant to all youth in ethnically diverse contexts such as the US, the development of a program designed to provide youth with tools, strategies, and ideas for how to explore and consider their commitment toward this aspect of their identity is most consistent with a universal approach; put differently, although the *content* of one's exploration may vary across ethnic-racial groups (e.g., learning a specific language, specific group history), the strategies and tools that youth would learn for engaging in exploration activities should not vary across groups. Thus, a universal approach was preferred because it would increase the reach of the program with respect to promoting this important developmental competency among all youth.

With respect to logistics, the ethnic-racial composition of the US is diverse (i.e., 62.6 % White, 17.1 % Latino, 13.2 % Black, 5.5 % Asian and Pacific Islander, 1.2 % American Indian and Alaska Native; US Census 2015) and, likewise, schools in the US vary in their ethnic-racial student body composition. In our experience with school partnerships, school administrators are hesitant to adopt programs that single out a specific ethnic-racial group due to concerns regarding unequal treatment of students, stigmatization of specific groups, and the logistical scheduling difficulties this can present for school personnel. Thus, it was important to develop a program that could be delivered to all youth, regardless of specific ethnic-racial background, which we also believed was more consistent with the ethnic-racial diversity that characterizes the US population. Finally, a universal approach would facilitate the transportability of the program (i.e., the ability for the program to be easily implemented in schools across the US), and this was an important goal given that ERI is an important developmental competency and programs designed to promote ERI should be accessible to youth across the nation.

Overview of Existing Identity Intervention Programming

In addition to determining the design elements noted above, a critical preliminary step in the program development stage involved conducting an exhaustive review of the literature on existing programs to ensure that the envisioned program had not already been developed. Toward this end, an exhaustive review of existing intervention programs was conducted via *PsycInfo* using 52 unique search queries (detailed table available upon request). Results were screened to identify interventions that targeted identity directly or as a mediating mechanism to affect change in a distal outcome (e.g., academic achievement, psychological health). Results also were screened according to the following criteria: (a) the intervention described was conducted in the US; (b) the work was published in English, though the intervention could be delivered in non-English; and (c) the work appeared in a published source (i.e., dissertations were excluded). Initial screening resulted in 74 results; 14 of these were excluded because they were: (a) conceptual or theoretical papers that did not describe an actual intervention ($n = 8$), (b) descriptions of curriculum to teach college students about ethnic-racial identity theory rather than curriculum to promote identity processes ($n = 2$), (c) case studies describing therapeutic approaches ($n = 2$), (d) recommendations for integrating ethnic and racial readings into literacy curriculum ($n = 1$), or (e) a parenting intervention designed to promote socialization behaviors within families ($n = 1$).

The final 60 results were categorized by the target of the program as either general identity interventions (i.e., focus on global identity formation, rather than specifically on ethnic-racial identity) or culturally relevant interventions. General identity interventions ($n = 6$) included those where specific aspects of social identities were not targeted, whereas culturally relevant interventions ($n = 54$) included those where issues of ethnicity, race, and/or culture were directly addressed. Although some of the general identity interventions targeted ethnic-racial minority *populations* through their programming, the programs had to include specific curricular components that directly addressed ethnic, racial, or cultural experiences in order to be considered a culturally relevant intervention.

We also classified the interventions based on specific themes identified within each curriculum to determine if any of the existing programs would be suitable candidates for modification for the Identity Project. Specifically, a basic content analysis of the stated goals of the 60 interventions and their respective curricular components was undertaken, and the interventions could generally be categorized by five fundamental themes: *socialization, affirmation, cultural awareness, exploration,* and *resolution. Socialization* programs included those aiming to increase participants' knowledge of their group, including cultural awareness of one's own background, socialization, mentoring, transmission of values, and enculturation. *Affirmation* programs included those aiming to promote positive feelings about one's identity, including pride and empowerment programs. *Cultural awareness* programs included those aiming to promote cultural awareness of many groups simultaneously, such as multicultural education programs. *Exploration* programs included those aiming to promote youths' self-exploration of their own identity. Finally, *resolution* programs included those aiming to help youth establish an explicit understanding of their identity. Of note, socialization and exploration themes were distinct in that socialization programs included the explicit sharing and/or providing of information and experiences related to individuals' ethnic, racial, or cultural heritage, whereas exploration programs included opportunities for youth to seek out such information or create such experiences of their own accord. Each intervention was classified by these themes, and when multiple themes were reflected within a single intervention, the program was jointly classified by all themes reflected in the program. Any interventions that targeted exploration or resolution were carefully reviewed to determine whether they could be modified to meet the goals of the envisioned Identity Project intervention.

Below is an overview of the program themes reflected in the *General Identity* and *Culturally Relevant* categories of interventions.

Interventions Focused on General Identity

Among the six general identity interventions, two were classified as exploration programs; three were classified as joint exploration and resolution programs; and one could not be classified into any of the five themes because of its unique and exclusive focus on modifying complex cognitive processes (i.e., perspective-taking) with the expectation that this would eventually inform identity formation. Four of the programs (i.e., Berman et al. 2008; Eichas et al. 2010; Ferrer-Wreder et al. 2002; Schwartz et al. 2005) had similar curricular components because all were based on Freire's (1970/1983) participatory and transformational learning model. The programs were guided by the notion that self-selecting personally important issues and being given the supportive structure to generate solutions to these issues would build feelings of competency which, in turn would promote "informational identity styles" characterized by active exploration (Berzonsky 1989). Although there were slight variations in implementation, the programs were largely consistent in their use of "mastery experiences" in which participants were challenged to identify a problem in their community or their life, and then encouraged to generate a solution with guidance and support from intervention leaders.

Program participants were typically assigned to small groups consisting of 6–9 students, and each small group was facilitated by at least two leaders (in some cases, a clinician; Berman et al. 2008). The groups met once per week, with extensive small group discussions of self-identified problems, and one participant's problem discussed in depth each week. Generally, participants worked on generating a solution to a self-identified problem, considering multiple strategies or options with which to tackle the problem. The programs varied in their length of time, because the program was designed to end after each group participant had worked through his or her problem solving process. Thus, some programs lasted only 8 weeks (e.g., Eichas et al. 2010), whereas others lasted 15 weeks (e.g., Berman et al. 2008).

Findings from three of the four studies that used the mastery experiences approach suggested that identity exploration was modifiable via curricula designed to engage youth in seeking information in a supportive context. Although these programs did not focus specifically on exploration of ethnicity or race, and the design features of the curriculum (e.g., low leader to participant ratio; small group setting; delivery of the program by a trained clinician; participant-led sessions) were not feasible given the goals of the Identity Project to develop a program that could be delivered in a classroom setting by a single teacher, the findings were encouraging with respect to whether identity exploration was a modifiable target for intervention.

The fifth program within the *general identity* category (i.e., Howard and Solberg 2006) exclusively targeted exploration among high school students, and was heavily tailored toward students' academic identities. Its curriculum, which was delivered approximately once every 2 weeks over the course of two grading periods, focused on the interface of student identities and school settings. A four-part series of activities were implemented to: (a) allow students to share their own life perspectives in a safe and validating environment, (b) provide individual assessment of their academic issues and barriers to success, (c) teach youth how to set achievable, concrete academic goals, and (d) promote positive social interactions. Program effects for high school students in an urban, low-income community included benefits in grades, attendance, and credit earnings (Howard and Solberg 2006). The curricular component within this program and the aforementioned programs that focused on providing a safe space within which to share and consider their own life perspectives was consistent with a goal of the Identity Project to provide students with a safe context within which to explore and consider the multifaceted nature of their identity. Other than this, however, our review revealed that a relatively simple modification of an existing program was not possible to achieve the goals of the Identity Project focused on targeting exploration and resolution of ERI.

Interventions Focused on Culturally Relevant Dimensions of Identity

The 54 culturally relevant interventions identified in our review were classified based on the following foci: socialization ($n = 28$), cultural awareness ($n = 8$), affirmation ($n = 6$), and exploration ($n = 1$). Several programs captured two foci: socialization and affirmation ($n = 7$), cultural awareness and exploration ($n = 2$), socialization and cultural awareness ($n = 1$), and affirmation and exploration ($n = 1$). Thus, no culturally relevant interventions captured both intended processes for the Identity Project (i.e., exploration and resolution). Nevertheless, we carefully reviewed the curriculum and program effects for the four interventions that included exploration in considering the Identity Project curriculum. Because these programs, relative to the *general identity* programs, were more directly related to the substantive topic on which the Identity Project focused (i.e., *ethnic-racial* identity), several aspects of program content were relevant to our goals and we ultimately adopted modified versions of these, as described below.

Of the four programs we reviewed in depth, one was an experience-based intervention designed to facilitate African American and Mexican American adolescents' exploration through civil rights education (Bettis et al. 1994). Students received direct instruction on the history of African American and Mexican American civil rights in the United States that included watching civil rights documentaries, reading civil rights literature, and writing essays. The main focus of the program was a 2-week field trip through the Southern US that included visits to prominent civil rights sites such as Little Rock, Arkansas, and San Antonio, Texas. In addition to visiting historical sites, participants also interviewed individuals who were directly involved in the civil rights movement. The program was evaluated qualitatively, with students reporting themes that reflected a broadened perspective on civil rights, a personal connection to the civil

rights movement, and a greater personal awareness of the meaning of ethnicity in their lives after taking part in the program; overall, findings suggested that the program had achieved its goals. Although the program's culture-specific approach (i.e., African American and Mexican American adolescents) and the time and cost-intensive nature of the program were incompatible with our goals for the Identity Project, the component of the curriculum in which students interviewed individuals with whom they shared an ethnic background was a compelling activity that we believed could be implemented in the Identity Project to facilitate ERI exploration; furthermore, this could be easily adapted to our proposed setting (e.g., participants could interview someone with whom they shared an ethnic background as part of a homework assignment). Therefore, a modified version of this activity was subsequently included in the Identity Project curriculum.

A second program used an intergroup dialogue framework in which discussion of ethnic and racial issues between groups was used to facilitate development of youths' own ERI (Aldana et al. 2012). In this program, youth from various ethnic-racial backgrounds (i.e., African American, Asian American, European American, Latino American, and Middle Eastern American) came together to discuss issues within and across their communities over the course of 8 weeks, culminating in a weekend retreat focused on youth activism and social advocacy skills. Program effects included significant increases in ERI exploration among youth from low socioeconomic families, but not among youth from high socioeconomic families, and no overall changes in ERI identity resolution. The program also appeared to influence awareness of racial issues, as youth participants reported significant increases in awareness of privilege, discrimination, and blatant racial issues. The intervention relied on intergroup dialogue as a proxy for self-exploration, which was a natural fit with the overall framework of the Identity Project and its envisioned universal approach; thus, this program element was incorporated into the Identity Project curriculum.

The third program was a graduate school curriculum that targeted exploration among therapists-in-training, with the assumption that promoting exploration would improve cultural competencies in therapeutic settings (Spears 2004). It was tested with a predominantly White sample of graduate students, and focused largely on understanding bias, prejudice, and discrimination. The curriculum included lectures, guest speakers, videos, readings, journaling, class discussion, and self-disclosure around issues of inequality. Although the goal of the program (i.e., therapeutic cultural competencies) and program contents were largely incompatible with our focus on the developmental period of adolescence, one program component appeared relevant and easily adaptable to the Identity Project. Specifically, in a Heritage Photo Sharing exercise, students created visual representations of their cultural selves through pictures, drawings, or paintings, and shared their creation with others. The activity was designed to increase awareness of cultural and racial identity of both the self and others; qualitative findings suggested that the activity resulted in increased sensitivity and knowledge about people from different ethnic backgrounds. Given its relevance, a modified version of this activity was incorporated into the Identity Project curriculum.

The final program was a therapy-based intervention designed to promote racial identity of White adults in the context of racial consciousness (i.e., Regan and Scarpellini Huber 1997). Components of the program included recognizing matters of privilege afforded by Whiteness, identifying and connecting to components of White culture, making implicit racial experiences explicit, and racism education. Although its culture-specific content, focus on adults, and therapeutic approach limited its relevance to the Identity Project, the authors' reflection of the effects of the program suggested that the program was effective in engaging individuals in the process of exploration of their ERI.

In sum, the review of the culturally relevant interventions targeting exploration revealed that while there were a select number of curriculum components that would be appropriate for the

Identity Project, there was no single program that was developmentally appropriate or that targeted both ERI components of interest. Taken together, however, findings from both the general identity and culturally relevant programs did support targeting ERI exploration. The focus on resolution was more limited and the review provided little information in this regard.

Research Measurement and Methodology

The Identity Project Curriculum: Engaging a Community Partner

After determining that we would indeed be developing a curriculum and pilot testing a new program, we initiated the process of finding a community partner. As noted above, a primary goal was to develop a universal school-based program; thus, we searched for schools that had high rates of ethnic diversity in their student body, with school diversity being operationalized by Simpson's Index of Diversity (see Juvonen et al. 2006). This index of diversity gives higher scores to schools with a more diverse representation of ethnic backgrounds, rather than focusing exclusively on the ethnic majority to ethnic minority student ratio to classify a school's degree of diversity. The school with which we eventually partnered for the development of the Identity Project curriculum and pilot testing had a Simpson's Index of Diversity score of 0.66, which is considered a school with high diversity (Juvonen et al. 2006). Specifically, the ethnic composition of the student body was 46.8 % White, 26.5 % Latino, 15.6 % Black, 4.6 % Asian, 2.6 % American Indian/Native American, and 3.9 % other.

After identifying potential partner schools (i.e., based on the ethnic diversity of the student population), we scheduled appointments with school administrators to discuss the goals of our project. When meeting with administrators, we explained that our purpose was to partner with their school to develop an intervention program focused on providing students with tools and strategies with which to explore their ethnic background and gain a clearer sense of the personal meaning that their ERI has for them. For each school with which we had scheduled meetings, we researched the school's mission statement and academic goals and made sure to explain how our focus in the Identity Project was related to advancing the school's stated goals and/or mission statement.

In our meetings with administrators, we also emphasized that we viewed our work together as a collaborative effort. Because we were aiming to develop a program that could be administered in the school setting (eventually as part of the school curriculum and to be delivered by teachers), fully engaging with our community partner of school administrators and teachers was essential for developing a program that would ultimately meet the intended goals of the program (see Bogart and Uyeda 2009, for a review). Furthermore, this initial groundwork, in which school administrators and teachers are involved at the onset of program development, is critical for increasing the sustainability of programs after the research team leaves (Jenson et al. 1999). After the community partner had been identified (and agreed to partner with our research team), we initiated the data collection process that would inform the development and refinement of the Identity Project curriculum.

The Identity Project: Phases of Curriculum Development

In the current section we describe the mixed-method approach that we used to inform the specific features of the Identity Project curriculum. Because the primary goal of the Identity Project intervention was to increase adolescents' ERI exploration and resolution, we sought information directly from adolescents regarding the best ways to engage young people of their same age group in a program designed to involve youth in the process of ERI development. This required gathering data from adolescents who were already reporting high levels of exploration and resolution (i.e., to better understand

adolescents' own perceptions of how they might have achieved their high levels of exploration and resolution), as well as gathering data from adolescents who were reporting low levels of exploration and resolution (i.e., to better understand potential barriers that they may have faced in the context of exploring or coming to a sense of resolution regarding their ERI). Toward this end, we followed a two-step mixed-method approach in which we initially gathered quantitative data on adolescents' levels of ERI exploration and resolution, and then used the data from the survey responses to purposefully recruit adolescents into focus groups where we would gather more in-depth information regarding adolescents' experiences with ERI.

Survey Data Collection

In the quantitative survey phase of this process, we gathered data from over 1500 adolescents from our target school. The purpose of the large-scale data collection was to quantitatively assess adolescents' ERI exploration and resolution and basic demographic characteristics, and to use this information to selectively recruit youth (based on their ethnicity, grade level, and ERI scores) into the qualitative portion of the study. We gathered data from the entire student body during school hours to minimize selection bias in this initial quantitative phase of the study. This design feature was important because, in an effort to develop a universal program, it was necessary to engage youth from all ethnic backgrounds and youth at all levels of the ERI formation process. Furthermore, data were collected during school hours to minimize barriers against participation (e.g., requiring students to stay after school or come early, conflicting with extracurricular activity involvement).

In the quantitative phase we assessed students' ERI exploration and resolution using the Ethnic Identity Scale (EIS; Umaña-Taylor et al. 2004). The aim of the focus groups was to purposefully target youth who were at different stages of the ERI formation process. To inform recruitment for the focus groups, therefore, we followed a three-step procedure to stratify the sample by ethnicity, grade level, and finally ERI.

First, participants were stratified by ethnic-racial self-identification based on the four largest groups represented in the sample (Latino, Black, White, and Asian). Next, within each ethnicity, participants were stratified based on grade level, with 9th and 10th grade students grouped together and 11th and 12th grade students grouped together. These two levels of stratification resulted in eight distinct groups (i.e., for each ethnicity there was a 9th/10th grade group and a 11th/12th grade group). Finally, to classify individuals into *high* versus *low* ERI exploration and resolution groups, cluster analyses were conducted individually for each group (with the exception of Asian 9th/10th grade students, as there were only 16 students who fell into this category, which was an inadequate sample size for cluster analysis).

Both exploratory (two-step) and confirmatory (k-means) cluster analyses were conducted to optimize the chance of finding the best-fitting solution for each grouping. With cluster analysis, we identified students within each ethnic group and grade stratification that scored *low* on both ERI exploration and resolution, and those who scored *high* on both dimensions. This resulted in a total of 14 categories (Table 1).

Focus Group Data Collection

The targeted sample size for each focus group was 7–8 participants; however, a larger number of students fell into each of the 14 categories that would be used to populate each focus group. Therefore, a random number generator was used to produce a unique set of 20 numbers for each of the fourteen groups. Within each group, these numbers were matched to the data file row to identify participants for recruitment. A total of 20 possible participants were selected for each focus group in case students refused to participate or did not respond to recruitment attempts. During recruitment, the first eight participants were contacted through phone calls and letters distributed through the schools. If participants indicated that they did not want to participate or if they did not respond to any of the recruitment attempts, the next person on the list was contacted. We attempted to contact 170

students for participation in the focus groups. We were unable to reach 46 students (i.e., 27 %); of the 124 students who we reached, 79 % participated ($n = 98$), 8 % refused participation ($n = 10$), and 13 % agreed to participate but did not arrive at the scheduled time ($n = 16$).

Focus groups took place during a study period during regular school hours, to minimize barriers to participation. Furthermore, as recommended by Morgan (1997), group composition was carefully considered with respect to homogeneity on a number of demographic factors. Specifically, focus groups were homogeneous with respect to developmental period to minimize younger students (e.g., 9th graders) feeling uncomfortable speaking up in the presence of significantly more advanced students (e.g., 12th graders). For logistical reasons, we were unable to conduct focus groups for each distinct grade; however, we grouped middle adolescents with one another (i.e., 9th and 10th graders) and late adolescents (11th and 12th graders) with one another. Similarly, focus groups were homogeneous with respect to ethnicity, given that the discussions were focused on ethnic-related experiences and we wanted to minimize potential barriers to speaking up about personal experiences in the context of peers from other ethnic groups. Due to sample size constraints for smaller groups (e.g., Asians), we were unable to make groups homogeneous with respect to gender. Group discussions lasted 60–90 min, and were audiotaped and transcribed verbatim. All focus groups were moderated by the first or second author; in addition, a note taker was present during each focus group to facilitate later transcription. At the end of each focus group, each adolescent received $10 for their participation.

The focus group protocols were tailored to the ERI exploration and resolution experiences of participants based on their responses to the survey questions. This phase of the process was critical because it enabled students to voice their opinions and experiences with respect to exploring and resolving issues surrounding their ERI, in their own words. Using this information to develop and refine the Identity Project

Table 1 Focus group stratification and sample overview ($N = 98$)

Ethnic-racial identity classification	Ethnicity[c]	No of focus groups	Participants' grade	n
Achieved ethnic identity[a]	Black	1	9th/10th grade	7
		1	11th/12th grade	5
	Latino	1	9th/10th grade	8
		1	11th/12th grade	8
	White	1	9th/10th grade	7
		1	11th/12th grade	7
	Asian	1	11th/12th grade	7
Diffused ethnic identity[b]	Black	1	9th/10th grade	8
		1	11th/12th grade	7
	Latino	1	9th/10th grade	6
		1	11th/12th grade	5
	White	1	9th/10th grade	10
		1	11th/12th grade	10
	Asian	1	11th/12th grade	3

[a]High scores on both ethnic-racial identity exploration and ethnic-racial identity resolution
[b]Low scores on both ethnic-racial identity exploration and ethnic-racial identity resolution
[c]Based on ethnic self-identification

curriculum was essential for creating a program that was relevant, meaningful, and empowering to high school students. Specifically, adolescents who scored high on ERI exploration and resolution were recruited to take part in a focus group that focused on what their experiences had been with respect to learning about their ethnicity and having a sense of clarity about the meaning that their ethnicity had for them. We asked adolescents to think about how they had learned about their ethnic background and to discuss experiences that were salient to them. Additionally, adolescents who scored low on ERI exploration and resolution were recruited to participate in focus group discussions designed to inquire about potential barriers to engaging in processes of exploration and resolution regarding ERI. Finally, adolescents in all groups were asked to generate and share ideas regarding activities that (from their perspective) would inform youth about their ethnic background and that students in high school would be interested in doing. The focus group setting was ideal for gathering these data because students bounced ideas off of each other; sometimes a comment made by one

student prompted another student to remember something they had not yet shared, and other times students disagreed with one another and offered varied perspectives on the topic of interest.

Development and Refinement of Curriculum

Data gathered during the focus group discussions were used in conjunction with prior research to inform the lessons that would eventually make up the curriculum for the Identity Project. We began with a general idea of the types of activities that would be included in the program and global objectives based on theoretical and empirical literature, including our review of existing intervention programs; but the information gleaned from adolescents in the focus groups helped to finalize the primary objectives for each lesson and to provide specific ideas for activities to include in the program. As one example, during our focus group discussions, students consistently raised the concern that there are many misconceptions about specific ethnic groups, and that there are many generalizations made about pan-ethnic groups (e.g., generalizations about Asians, versus understanding the diversity that exists within Asian subgroups). This was consistent with program content we had identified in our review (e.g., discussions of discrimination or racism; Aldana et al. 2012). Thus, the focus group data supported our inclusion of this program element in the curriculum and, as described below, one of the eight sessions in the Identity Project program focuses on defining and discussing terms such as stereotypes and discrimination, as well as on understanding within and between group differences.

As a second example, many focus group participants noted that they had learned about their ethnicity by being exposed to information about others' ethnic groups; learning about others' ethnicity often led students to examine or think about their own ethnic backgrounds in relation to what they had learned or been exposed to about someone else's ethnic group. This mirrored a program component that emerged in our review (i.e., Spears 2004), in which participants learned about the self and others via various activities in which they explored their backgrounds, and presented the information they had learned to other participants in the program. Accordingly, as we developed and refined the Identity Project curriculum, we integrated many opportunities for students to share the information that they were learning about their own ethnic background(s) with their classmates.

In other instances, findings from the focus group provided novel ideas with respect to activities that would promote the ERI formation processes of exploration and resolution. For example, focus group participants noted that learning about race and ethnicity from the perspectives of other young people who came to their schools as guest speakers or visitors, or who were telling their stories in movies, was very informative and interesting. Based on this information, we developed a video in which we presented interviews with several young adults who represented different ethnic-racial backgrounds and experiences, and chronicled their individual journeys with respect to their ERI development from when they were young children until the present time. Thus, the focus group data were used to refine ideas that we developed based on reviewing existing programs, considering the theoretical literature, and to develop new ideas that would be incorporated into the Identity Project curriculum.

After carefully revising and finalizing the curriculum based on the focus group data, the second author delivered each lesson to a small ethnically diverse group of 8 graduate research assistants and staff, which represented a group with varied levels of education (e.g., high school graduate, bachelor's degree, master's degree) as well as varied expertise in adolescent development and ERI. All sessions were videotaped, and we asked research staff to engage with the program as fully as possible, including completing all of the homework assignments. At the end of each lesson, the members of the research team discussed aspects of the lesson that seemed to work well, aspects that may not work well with the targeted population of high school students, and any other observations about the program or specific activities. Each session was videotaped and the first author carefully reviewed the videos and revised the curriculum content based on observations of how the lesson went, as well as based on the feedback that emerged during the research team's large group discussion at the end of each lesson. All lessons were reviewed at least two more times independently by both authors; the authors met regularly to discuss revisions and to decide on the final changes necessary before pilot testing. In the section that follows, we provide an overview of the curriculum.

Introduction to the Identity Project Curriculum

The Identity Project curriculum consists of an 8-week program designed to engage youth in the developmental processes of ERI exploration and ERI resolution by increasing students' salience and understanding of their ethnic heritage(s) and background(s), as well as others' backgrounds;

increasing students' awareness and understanding of multiple groups' experiences with discrimination in the context of the US across different historical periods; exposing students to the notion that differences within groups are oftentimes larger than differences between groups; engaging students in activities designed to increase their understanding of their family heritage, regardless of how they define "family;" clarifying misconceptions students may have regarding a "right or wrong" way to identify with an ethnic group, and providing students with examples of diverse journeys for ERI development; providing students with tools with which to explore their ethnic heritage (e.g., making them aware of symbols, traditions, and rituals, and ways to learn more about these); and providing opportunities for students to discuss their heritage with others. These goals are achieved via 8 lessons.

The Identity Project was designed to be a school-based intervention program that is delivered over an 8-week period, with weekly lessons that last approximately 55 min each. We developed all activities and lesson plans in a manner such that they could be delivered and implemented by a single leader, given that the ultimate goal is to have this program delivered in the school setting by a teacher or other school personnel. Starting in Week 2, students have homework assignments that relate to content they have learned about in the lesson, or in which they are gathering information and/or preparing materials that will be used in a subsequent lesson.

Throughout the 8 weeks, students participate in small group activities, large group activities, and complete individual work that is almost always shared in a larger group setting. Program materials include PowerPoint slides with key terms and definitions, video clips, worksheets, and ice breakers designed to help students feel comfortable sharing their experiences with their classmates and the instructor. Finally, the program also includes opportunities for students to explore their ethnic backgrounds by interviewing family members or members of their communities.

Future Directions

The Identity Project is currently in the pilot testing phase, which captures the final stages of program development within the prevention research cycle. We are piloting the program in 9th grade classrooms within our partner high school. A total of 8 classrooms have been randomized into the treatment condition (i.e., Identity Project curriculum) or an attention control condition in which the authors are delivering a curriculum that is focused on exposing students to educational and career opportunities after obtaining a high school degree. The classrooms were selected in consultation with our school partner and reflect all freshmen who are enrolled in an elective course focused on providing students with skills that will help them adapt to and succeed in the high school setting (e.g., computer skills, developing good study habits). Targeting 9th grade students is ideal for developmental reasons (i.e., middle adolescence has been identified as a period in which ERI processes are heightened; Umaña-Taylor et al. 2014), but also because 9th grade students will not have participated in any of the preliminary data collection efforts that took place the year prior when the research team was gathering survey and focus group data to inform the development of the curriculum.

In the pilot testing phase, we are examining the feasibility of delivering the program in an ethnically diverse school setting, assessing the extent to which students engage with the program content, and evaluating whether the content appears developmentally appropriate. With this small-scale efficacy trial, we are testing whether there are trends suggesting that participation in the program is indeed leading to greater changes in ERI exploration and resolution among youth in the treatment versus attention control conditions. Furthermore, the effect sizes we identify in the pilot testing phase will enable us to determine the sample size necessary to have sufficient power to test effects in a large-scale efficacy trial. We also will be able to examine whether effect sizes appear to vary based on demographic characteristics (e.g., student ethnicity, generational status). These preliminary data will be essential for informing the development of a large-scale efficacy trial of the program.

Given that the program is in its initial stages of development and implementation, we are limited in what we can say with respect to future implementation and feasibility of transportability. However, in developing the program, we have focused on ensuring that the activities and the lessons are relevant and accessible to students with diverse ethnic backgrounds (e.g., multiethnic) and diverse family constellations (e.g., youth being raised by one parent and having limited to no knowledge about a second parent; youth being raised by extended family members or by adoptive parents). We also developed the lessons to be relevant to participants regardless of the ethnic composition of the students in the classroom (e.g., many examples in the lessons are generated by student participants' experiences and backgrounds, rather than being predetermined in the curriculum). Because our program is designed to engage youth in the process of ERI formation, which focuses on increasing exploration and developing a clearer sense of resolution regarding one's background, the program does not focus on teaching students about any particular group. Thus, the focus on providing tools with which to engage in the process, rather than providing content about any specific group, lends itself well to delivering the program in multiple settings. We expect that the program will be relevant and easy to administer without adaptations in ethnically diverse school settings where many different ethnic-racial groups are represented as well as in school settings that are less diverse.

Finally, as we consider efficacy testing and further development of the Identity Project, an important idea to consider is whether program effects might be moderated by contextual factors that could strengthen the program's efficacy. For example, because greater salience of ethnicity is expected to increase adolescents' engagement in ERI development processes (Umaña-Taylor et al. 2014), and prior work has demonstrated that ethnicity is more salient in contexts in which one's ethnic group is a numerical minority (Umaña-Taylor 2004), it will be interesting to examine moderation of program efficacy by context. Perhaps program effects will be strongest in settings that are increasingly ethnically diverse, as ethnicity may be especially salient in such settings. Similarly, given the significant role that families play in socializing youth about ethnicity (Hughes et al. 2006; Umaña-Taylor et al. 2009), it will be interesting to examine if youths' experiences with family ethnic socialization modify program effects such that youth who report high levels of family ethnic socialization demonstrate relatively stronger program effects than youth reporting lower levels of family ethnic socialization.

References

Aldana, A., Rowley, S. J., Checkoway, B., & Richards-Schuster, K. (2012). Raising ethnic-racial consciousness: The relationship between intergroup dialogues and adolescents' ethnic-racial identity and racism awareness. *Equity and Excellence in Education, 45*(1), 120–137. doi:10.1080/10665684.2012.641863

Berman, S. L., Kennerley, R. J., & Kennerley, M. A. (2008). Promoting adult identity development: A feasibility study of a university-based identity intervention program. *Identity: An International Journal of Theory and Research, 8*(2), 139–150. doi:10.1080/15283480801940024

Berzonsky, M. D. (1989). Identity style: Conceptualization and measurement. *Journal of Adolescent Research, 4*(3), 268–282.

Bettis, P. J., Cooks, H. C., & Bergin, D. A. (1994). "It's not steps anymore, but more like shuffling": Student perceptions of the civil rights movement and ethnic identity. *Journal of Negro Education, 63*(2), 197–211.

Bogart, L. M., & Uyeda, K. (2009). Community-based participatory research: Partnering with communities for effective and sustainable behavioral health interventions. *Health Psychology, 28*, 391–393.

Case, M. H., & Robinson, W. L. (2003). Interventions with ethnic minority populations: The legacy and promise of community psychology. In G. Bernal, J. E. Trimble, A. K. Burlew, & F. T. L. Leong (Eds.), *Handbook of racial and ethnic minority psychology* (pp. 573–590). Thousand Oaks: SAGE.

Eichas, K., Albrecht, R. E., Garcia, A. J., Ritchie, R. A., Varela, A., Garcia, A., et al. (2010). Mediators of positive youth development intervention change: Promoting change in positive and problem outcomes? *Child and Youth Care Forum, 39*(4), 211–237. doi:10.1007/s10566-010-9103-9

Erikson, E. H. (1968). *Identity: Youth and crisis.* New York: Norton.

Ferrer-Wreder, L., Lorente, C. C., Kurtines, W., Briones, E., Bussell, J., Berman, S., et al. (2002). Promoting identity development in marginalized youth. *Journal of Adolescent Research, 17*(2), 168–187. doi:10.1177/0743558402172004

Freire, P. (1970/1983). *Pedagogy of the oppressed.* New York: Herder & Herder.

Helms, J. E. (1990). Introduction: Review of racial identity terminology. In J. Helms (ed.), *Black and white racial identity* (pp. 3–8). Westport, CT: Praeger Publishers.

Hughes, D., Rodriguez, J., Smith, E. P., Johnson, D. J., Stevenson, H. C., & Spicer, P. (2006). Parents' ethnicracial socialization practices: A review of research and directions for future study. *Developmental Psychology, 42*, 747–770. doi:10.1037/0012-1649.42.5.747

Hollon, S. D., Muñoz, R. F., Barlow, D. H., Beardslee, W. R., Bell, C. C., Bernal, G., et al. (2002). Psychosocial intervention development for the prevention and treatment of depression: Promoting innovation and increasing access. *Biological Psychiatry, 52*, 610–630.

Howard, K. A. S., & Solberg, V. S. (2006). School-based social justice: The achieving success identity pathways program. *Professional School Counseling, 9*(4), 278–287.

Jenson, P. S., Hoagwood, K., & Trickett, E. J. (1999). Ivory towers or earthen trenches: Collaborations to foster real-world research. *Applied Developmental Science, 3*(4), 206–212.

Juvonen, J., Nishina, A., & Graham, S. (2006). Ethnic diversity and perceptions of safety in urban middle schools. *Psychological Science, 17*, 393–400.

Knight, G. P., Roosa, M. W., & Umaña-Taylor, A. J. (2009). *Methodological challenges in studying ethnic minority or economically disadvantaged populations.* Washington, DC: American Psychological Association.

Marcia, J. E. (1980). Identity in adolescence. In J. Adelson (Ed.), *Handbook of adolescent psychology* (pp. 159–187). New York: Wiley.

Morgan, D. L. (1997). *Focus groups as qualitative research* (2nd ed.). Thousand Oaks: Sage.

Mzarek, P. J., & Haggerty, R. J. (1994). *Reducing risks for mental health disorders: Frontiers for preventive intervention research.* Washington, DC: National Academy Press.

National Research Council & Institute of Medicine (2009). *Preventing mental, emotional, and behavioral disorders among young people: Progress and possibilities.* Committee on the prevention of mental disorders and substance abuse among children, youth, and young adults: Research advances and promising interventions. M. E. O'Connell, T. Boat, & K. E. Warner (Eds.). Board on Children, Youth, and Families, Division of Behavioral and Social Sciences and Education. Washington DC: National Academies Press.

Neblett, E. W., Jr., Rivas-Drake, D., & Umaña-Taylor, A. J. (2012). The promise of racial and ethnic protective factors in promoting ethnic minority youth development. *Child Development Perspectives, 6*, 295–303.

Phinney, J. S. (1993). A three-stage model of ethnic identity development in adolescence. In M. E. P. Bernal & G. P. Knight (Eds.), *Ethnic identity: Formation and transmission among Hispanics and other minorities* (pp. 61–79). NY: SUNY Press.

Phinney, J. S. (1996). When we talk about American ethnic groups, what do we mean? *American Psychologist, 51*, 918–927.

Phinney, J. S., & Kohatsu, E. L. (1997). Ethnic and racial identity development and mental health. In J. Schulenberg, J. L. Maggs, & K. Hurrelmann (Eds.), *Health risks and developmental transitions during adolescence* (pp. 420–443). New York: Cambridge University Press.

Regan, A., & Scarpellini Huber, J. (1997). Facilitating White identity development: A therapeutic group intervention. In C. Thompson & R. Carter (Eds.), *Racial identity theory: Applications to individual, group, and organizational interventions* (pp. 113–126). Mahwah, NJ: Lawrence Erlbaum Associates

Rivas-Drake, D., Seaton, E. K., Markstrom, C., Quintana, S., Syed, M., Lee, R., et al. (2014). Ethnic and racial identity in adolescence: Implications for psychosocial, academic, and health outcomes. *Child Development, 85*, 40–57.

Roosa, M. W., Wolchik, S. A., & Sandler, I. N. (1997). Preventing the negative effects of common stressors: Current status and future directions. In S. A. Wolchick & I. N. Sandler (Eds.), *Handbook of children's coping: Linking theory and intervention* (pp. 515–533). New York: Plenum.

Schwartz, S. J., Kurtines, W. M., & Montgomery, M. J. (2005). A comparison of two approaches for facilitating identity exploration processes in emerging adults: An exploratory study. *Journal of Adolescent Research, 20*(3), 309–345. doi:10.1177/0743558404273119

Smith, T. B., & Silva, L. (2011). Ethnic identity and personal well-being of people of color: A meta-analysis. *Journal of Counseling Psychology, 58*, 42–60.

Spears, S. S. (2004). The impact of a cultural competency course on the racial identity of MSWs. *Smith College Studies in Social Work, 74*(2), 272–288. doi:10.1080/00377310409517716

Supple, A. J., Ghazarian, S. R., Frabutt, J. M., Plunkett, S. W., & Sands, T. (2006). Contextual influences on Latino adolescent ethnic identity and academic outcomes. *Child Development, 77*, 1427–1433.

Syed, M., Azmitia, M., & Phinney, J. S. (2007). Stability and change in ethnic identity among Latino emerging adults in two contexts. *Identity An International Journal of Theory, 7*, 155–178.

Umaña-Taylor, A. J. (2011). Ethnic Identity. In S. J. Schwartz, K. Luyckx, & V. L. Vignoles (Eds.), *Handbook of identity theory and research* (pp. 791–809). New York: Springer.

Umaña-Taylor, A. J. (2015). Ethnic identity research: How far have we come? In C. E. Santos & A. J. Umaña-Taylor (Eds.), *Studying ethnic identity: methodological and conceptual approaches across disciplines* (pp. 11–26). Washington, DC: American Psychological Association.

Umaña-Taylor, A. J., Alfaro, E. C., Bámaca, M. Y., & Guimond, A. B. (2009). The central role of familial ethnic socialization in Latino adolescents' cultural orientation. *Journal of Marriage and Family, 71*, 46–60.

Umaña-Taylor, A. J., Yazedjian, A., & Bámaca-Gómez, M. Y. (2004). Developing the ethnic identity scale using Eriksonian and social identity perspectives. *Identity: An International Journal of Theory and Research, 4*, 9–38.

Umaña-Taylor, A. J., Quintana, S. M., Lee, R. M., Cross, W. E., Rivas-Drake, D., Schwartz, S. J., et al. (2014). Ethnic and racial identity revisited: An integrated conceptualization. *Child Development, 85*, 21–39.

U.S. Census Bureau (2015). State and County Quick-Facts. Data derived from Population Estimates, American Community Survey, Census of Population and Housing, State and County Housing Unit Estimates, County Business Patterns, Nonemployer Statistics, Economic Census, Survey of Business Owners, Building Permits. Last Revised: March 31, 2015. Retrieved from: http://quickfacts.census.gov/qfd/states/00000.html

Williams, J. L., Tolan, P. H., Durkee, M. I., Francois, A. G., & Anderson, R. E. (2012). Integrating racial and ethnic identity research into developmental understanding of adolescents. *Child Development Perspectives, 6*, 304–311.

Yasui, M., Dorham, C. L., & Dishion, T. J. (2004). Ethnic identity and psychological adjustment: A validity analysis for European American and African American adolescents. *Journal of Adolescent Research, 19*, 807–825.

Children's Centres: An English Intervention for Families Living in Disadvantaged Communities

Maria Evangelou, Jenny Goff, Kathy Sylva,
Pam Sammons, Teresa Smith, James Hall,
and Naomi Eisenstadt

Abstract

The role of the parent has been clearly defined in the literature as having a positive influence on children's emotional, behavioural and educational development, more so than other factors such as maternal education, poverty, peers socio-economic status and schooling (DfES in Every child matters (Green Paper). DfES, London, 2003; Desforges and Abouchaar in The impact of parental involvement, parental support and family education on pupil achievement and adjustment. A literature review. DfES, London, 2003). Supporting the capacity to parent is of prime interest when considering how to improve opportunities for the most disadvantaged families and their children. This chapter focuses on one particular English intervention entitled the 'children's centre'. Drawing on international literature and definitions of parenting support, this chapter will explore some of the research evidence collected by the Evaluation of Children's Centres in England (ECCE) study which focuses on how children's centres conceptualise, choose and deliver parenting and family support services to families. A number of characteristics of effective interventions have been identified within the literature as having the greatest impact on improving child outcomes (Glass in Child Soc 13(4): 257–264 1999; Sure Start in The aim of sure start. http://www.surestart.gov.uk, 2001; Johnson in Impact of social science on policy. http://www.esrc.ac.uk/_images/Sure_Start_final_report_tcm8-20116.pdf, 2011). These include the following: a two-generational focus that targets both the parent and child together; multifaceted approaches that include amongst others, enhancing family relationships; services which are non-stigmatising, lasting long enough to make a difference, locally driven, culturally appropriate, sensitive to user needs and centre-based. This chapter will explore these findings in order to address three research

M. Evangelou (✉) · J. Goff · K. Sylva · P. Sammons ·
T. Smith · J. Hall · N. Eisenstadt
Department of Education, University of Oxford,
Oxford, UK
e-mail: maria.evangelou@education.ox.ac.uk

© The Editor(s) 2017
N.J. Cabrera and B. Leyendecker (eds.), *Handbook on Positive Development of Minority Children and Youth*, DOI 10.1007/978-3-319-43645-6_27

questions: (1) *Who are children's centres serving?* (2) *What are children's centres doing?* and (3) *How are children's centres approaching their work?* The chapter will conclude with policy implications and future directions for programmes that share similar characteristics to English children's centres.

Historical Overview and Theoretical Perspectives

The role of the parent has been clearly defined in the literature as having a positive influence on children's emotional, behavioural and educational development, more so than other factors such as maternal education, poverty, peers socio-economic status and schooling (DfES 2003; Desforges and Abouchaar 2003). Children of families living in disadvantaged circumstances are often referred to as 'at-risk' because they are considered to be at increased risk of 'learning delay' while their parents are perceived to be in greater need of interventions to enhance their child's life chances.

The English model of parenting support conceptualises 'at-risk' families broadly as those in need of parenting support to improve their child's developmental and learning outcomes; and those demonstrating a number of risk factors (Evangelou et al. 2008). Risk factors might include a lack of self-esteem or confidence as a result of isolation (geographical, economic and social), poor housing, ethnic minority status combined with low income, a lack of awareness of their needs, barriers in communication (literacy and additional language needs), and health issues (mental health). Parental life trajectories are also a contributing factor to family vulnerability in terms of drug or alcohol abuse, domestic violence and child abuse; or their transient lifestyles (traveller communities). 'At-risk' families have been the focus of parenting support in England for many years as demonstrated through a government initiative entitled the Sure Start Children's Centres programme.

Sure Start Children's Centres aim to provide integrated services (e.g. health, education, welfare) for all young children up to the age of five,

and their families. They have a long history dating back to 1999, and at their peak in 2004 a network of 3500 were in operation. A complex multi-layered evaluation, *the Evaluation of Children's Centres in England* (ECCE: 2009–2017) was commissioned by the Department for Children, Schools and Families (DCSF, now Department for Education: DfE), and led by a consortium of three organisations: NatCen Social Research, the University of Oxford and Frontier Economics. This chapter will explore some of the ECCE findings against features known to be characteristic of effective family interventions in the literature. In particular, this chapter will address three research questions: (1) *Who are children's centres serving?* (2) *What are children's centres doing?* and (3) *How are children's centres approaching their work?*

The chapter will first address definitions of parenting support, and family/parenting support programmes that provide the basis for practices used in English children's centres. It will also briefly consider national and international parenting policies and services to enable the readers to understand how children's centres compare to programmes developed in other countries. Research evidence collected by the ECCE study will have implications for policy and future directions for programmes that share some of the characteristics of the children's centres.

What Is Parenting Support?

Given the importance of the parental role on children's development, early interventions for children frequently position their focus on parenting when attempting to reduce later effects of disadvantage (Goff et al. 2012). More recently, parenting support has been considered a social investment to promote children's health and well-being, improved behaviour, and school achievement (Molinuevo 2013). The definition, availability, and offer of parenting support vary greatly across different countries and communities, and are influenced by societal priorities (Moran et al. 2004; Molinuevo 2013). In this chapter, we use the definition of parenting support offered by Evangelou et al. (2014, p. 1), which was drawn from a definition first posited by Pugh et al. (1994) and Smith (1996).

> A range of measures which support parents in their efforts to socially and culturally adjust to their surroundings, access appropriate economic resources and services, understand the social, emotional, psychological, educational, and physical needs of themselves, their children, and their families as a whole, and engage families with their communities.

While definitions of parenting support vary, there are similarities regarding intended users and needs, and the aims of the services on offer (Evangelou et al. 2014; Molinuevo 2013). The type of parenting support is dependent on country-specific opportunities, cultural priorities and constraints. Countries face similar challenges regarding their offer of parenting support, including *service uptake* (parental reluctance to engage with services due to associated stigma; low rates of father involvement); *service delivery* (varied staff job roles; high staff turnover and prioritisation of evidence-based programmes; and *service evaluation* regarding study designs and difficulty to establish control groups (Molinuevo 2013).

The 'ecological perspective' of human development described by Bronfenbrenner (1979) is often taken as a starting point when conceptualising parenting support. He described it as being akin to a nested structure such as 'Russian Dolls' (1994). When considering the development of a child, five systems shaping a child's development exist: microsystem, meso, exo, macro and chronosystem. Moran et al. (2004) recognised that parenting support typically caters towards the *microsystem* layer of the child, supporting their relationships with immediate family, parenting and individual characteristics. By focusing parenting support initiatives specifically on a child's *microsystem* there is

little consideration of more distal ecological factors such as their social environments, lifestyle, culture, community, and wider family. The parenting support intervention on which this chapter focuses takes a more holistic view to family support. The *Sure Start Children's Centre* programme considers distal elements of the child's ecological system alongside their immediate environment, including services to tackle family poverty, community integration, physical environment and housing, parental education and employment, and family relationships.

One way of reconceptualising parenting support is to place the parent, instead of the child, in the centre of the Bronfenbrenner model and consider the importance of parental needs in terms of their relationship with their child as well as with other adults. One dimension explores and supports how parents interact with their own child. The other dimension addresses the personal needs of parents, their role as a member of their local community, and their relationship with their partners. Parenting support is offered in multiple ways across the international spectrum, and parenting programmes or family interventions are a common means of offering such support. Other countries embed parenting policies or practices within their daily provision of services to children and families, to enable parenting support to reach greater numbers of families. Both methods of intervention will now be addressed.

Parenting and Family Support Approaches

A parenting programme is a well defined course of work aiming to support varied concepts and dimensions of parenting with clearly delineated principles and aims: it is focused on supporting parental understanding and enhancing awareness, underpinned by a set of implicit or explicit underlying theories that typically utilise a number of different strategies with both short and long-term outcomes for children and/or parents. Often such parenting programmes are referred to in the literature as parenting interventions and the terms are used interchangeably here. There appear to be commonalities in the target recipients of parenting interventions, in the foci of their offer and in the ways that the services are delivered. A number of programmes in the US and Canada support families with children aged under five, families living in poverty or in low income, young or first time parents, or families defined as being most 'at-risk' (for example the STEEP programme in the US (Erickson et al. 1992); Nobody's Perfect in Canada (Kennett and Chislett 2012); and Head Start in the US (ECLKC 2014).

The delivery of parenting support also varies internationally, with some programmes focusing on the parent-child dyad (STEEP); some on parenting development and wider family need (Nobody's Perfect); and others more heavily on child development (Head Start). Other models used internationally include parental peer support (REAAPS in France; Daly 2013), individualised parenting support through universally accessible services (Denmark, France, Germany, Italy and the Netherlands; Bobby et al. 2009); standardised parental support interventions (for example, Triple P, HIPPY and the German PEKiP programme), and area based support (Welsh Flying Start centres; Knibbs et al. 2013).

Parenting support is often embedded within the mainstream services of a country, and offered through a mix of overarching policies, universally accessible services and country-specific priorities and restraints. Examples of national approaches to parenting support include parenting advisory groups, research centres or national organisations, or institutions which support the development of future policy and parenting frameworks (for example, the CICC in the US (Alvy 2005); national parenting and family support bodies in France (Molinuevo 2013)).

The United Kingdom takes a strong interest in parenting support (and specifically on improving parenting practices) as a route to narrowing the gap in child outcomes between rich and poor, or those from a majority compared to a minority, background. The emphasis is commonly on reaching the most disadvantaged families, driven by a policy discourse suggesting that inadequate parenting will have an influence on poorer outcomes for children, as opposed to limited financial resources (Field 2010; Allen 2011). England was described by Daly (2013, p. 164) as having "the most elaborate architecture anywhere for parenting support". A number of institutions were in place including the existence of a National Academy for Parenting Practitioners which focused on professional development of practitioners (although this has since closed); a Family and Parenting Institute; and a national network of children's centres which are the focus of this chapter.

There is recent widespread international interest in the use of standardised 'evidence-based' programmes for parenting support and family intervention, although definitions and terminology of what constitutes 'evidence' vary by discipline (Williams-Taylor 2007). Many authors agree that robust scientific research methods such as evaluations using experimental designs (Randomised Control Trials: RCTs) and longitudinal evaluations should be conducted to test the sustainability and replicability of outcomes (Williams-Taylor 2007; Moran et al. 2004; Seibel et al. 2011). Moran et al. (ibid) however recognise that RCT designs are not well-suited to evaluating particular programmes (such as community-based parenting support) due to a lack of matched comparison groups or ethical reservations; and may be at the detriment of discarding promising practices (Molinuevo 2013).

The use of rigorously evaluated programmes with replicable outcomes has become more apparent with increased interest in the area. Well-evidenced parenting programmes and interventions have been promoted in the US since the early 1960s (Nurse Family Partnership, HighScope, Incredible Years and Parents as Teachers) (Williams-Taylor 2007; Small and Mather 2009). Interest in evidence-based programmes is similarly high in the UK: a Government report was commissioned to identify promising early interventions for children against strict criteria and standards of evidence (Allen 2011). The defining characteristics of an evidence-based programme include an evaluation that has been peer reviewed by knowledgeable experts, an endorsement by a respected governing agency with inclusion on their list of effective programmes and different ratings of effectiveness (Seibel et al. 2011; Huser et al. 2009).

Sure Start Children's Centres: A Community-Based Intervention in England

A major review in 1998 found that families tended to be poorer when children were very young, and that early poverty had lasting effects into adulthood (Glass 1999; Wagmiller and Adelman 2009). Sure Start Local Programmes (SSLPs) were established in England in 1999, and were area-based; that is, located in the most disadvantaged areas across England but open to all families with children aged four and under in that area. They aimed to follow the UK parenting agenda of narrowing the gap in outcomes between poor children and their more affluent peers, through the provision of new services for families and integration with existing public services. The centres bore a close resemblance to the earlier community-based family centres, aiming to integrate early education, childcare, healthcare, and family support services while preparing children to be academically, socially, and occupationally successful in their adult lives (Melhuish et al. 2010a, b).

In 2004, SSLPs were revised towards a network of 3500 children's centres across England, with the aim of one per community. The initial goal of children's centres resembled the original SSLPs: to provide integrated services (e.g. health, education, welfare) for all young children up to the age of five, and their families. In 2005, early findings from an evaluation of SSLPs suggested that benefits were greater for *moderately* disadvantaged families than for more *severely* disadvantaged families (Melhuish et al. 2005). As a result, children's centre aims were further revised to follow a 'core offer' of services: information and advice to parents; open-access sessions; outreach and family support; child and family health services and access to specialist services; links with *JobCentre Plus*

for training and employment advice; and support for local childminders. Centres in the 30 % most disadvantaged areas were additionally required to offer early education and childcare.

The original 'core offer' of services which centres were tasked to provide in 2005 was revised yet again in 2012 towards a 'core purpose', which removed the requirement for centres to support parents in finding employment, or early education and childcare for their children (Department for Education 2013):

> ...to improve outcomes for young children and their families and reduce inequalities between families in greatest need and their peers in: child development and school readiness; parenting aspirations and parenting skills; and child and family health and life chances.

The children's centre programme can be considered as following a *risk and protection-focused prevention model*, as it aims to tackle both the *risk* factors associated with later undesirable outcomes (such as poverty, poor home learning environments and poor parenting) as well as enhancing *protective* factors which are consistently associated with positive outcomes in later life (such as stronger families and social networks, healthy neighbourhoods and higher employment: France and Utting 2005). Evangelou et al. (2008) suggest early intervention to be an important element of successful preventative work; and high economic returns of early intervention have been recognised for promoting school, reducing crime, workforce productivity and reducing teenage pregnancy (Heckman 2008). Children's centres feature a number of characteristics which are common of preventative programmes: their community-based nature, their aim to increase community capacity and partnership, their target audience of economically deprived families, and their use of 'evidence-based' work (France and Utting 2005).

Building Evidence and Knowledge from Other Evaluations

Evaluation findings from similar community-based programmes in the United States have been mixed. Programmes aimed towards children classified as 'at-risk' such as Head Start, have generally shown positive impacts in the short term on increased IQ (Barnett and Hustedt 2005). A study carried out with families who were randomly assigned to Head Start treatment and waiting-list groups showed that children in the Head Start group were quicker to improve on receptive vocabulary and phonemic awareness than children in the comparison group; and children in the Head Start treatment group were significantly more likely to have parents address their children's health needs (Abbott-Shim et al. 2003). Results concerning the longer term outcomes of Head Start however vary, suggesting that there may be differences due to variations in populations, programmes and context across different evaluations (Barnett and Hustedt 2005).

A number of family-based intervention programmes in the UK have demonstrated benefits for families through their evaluations. For example, the National Evaluation of Sure Start (NESS) evaluated the original SSLP programme (from which children's centres were drawn) using an integrated cross-sectional, longitudinal design. The NESS evaluation intended to examine any effects of SSLPs on children, families, and communities, and any conditions under which Sure Start was most effective in improving outcomes (NESS Research Team 2012). NESS had a number of strands including implementation, impact, local context analysis, cost effectiveness and support for local evaluations. Within the implementation strand, a number of sub-studies were carried out to investigate the parenting focus of SSLPs: empowering parents; fathers; employability of parents; maternity services; outreach and home visiting; black and minority ethnic populations; and family and parenting support.

The impact strand of the NESS evaluation addressed parenting and family outcomes at the ages of 3, 5 and 7. For the parenting evaluation, the NESS team found some evidence towards SSLP parenting support programmes being effective when 'good practice' was apparent (Barlow et al. 2007). The impact study (Melhuish et al. 2012) followed over 5000 families of 7 year olds (also studied at 9 months; 3 and

5 years old) in 150 SSLP areas. A few positive effects of SSLPs related to improved maternal wellbeing and family functioning were displayed within the families of 7 year olds. Lone parent families and workless households were reported to have greater life satisfaction, and families of 7 year old boys were reported to have a less chaotic home environment. SSLPs were also associated with families engaging in less harsh discipline and providing a more stimulating home learning environment. There were, however, no effects on child outcomes such as "school readiness" (their cognitive, social and socio-emotional development) and positive effects regarding child health outcomes were only visible at age five (lower BMIs and better physical health: Melhuish et al. 2010b).

An evaluation of the Welsh Flying Start intervention compared parents living in Flying Start areas (more disadvantaged areas) to parents living in matched comparison areas (relatively less disadvantaged). The evaluation suggested that the Flying Start programme might have been successful in bringing families in disadvantaged areas up to the conditions experienced in relatively less disadvantaged comparison areas (Knibbs et al. 2013). Families in Flying Start areas reportedly had better awareness of parenting and language support programmes, better contact with health visitors, and more confidence as parents. There were however no statistical differences between the two areas when considering key parent outcomes (parental behaviour regarding child immunisation rates, parenting self-confidence, mental health, or home environment) or child outcomes (cognitive and language skills, social and emotional development and independence, self-regulation) (Knibbs et al. 2013).

Current Research Questions Addressed by This Chapter

Guidance regarding effective interventions in the UK is fairly limited. UK family interventions (Sure Start and Flying Start) have demonstrated significant improvements to family functioning, health and well-being, showing that interventions can develop parents' understanding of child behaviour and development. Importantly however, evaluations of such UK interventions have not shown any long-term improvements to child cognitive outcomes (Melhuish et al. 2010a; Knibbs et al. 2013). Indeed, evaluations of a similar community-based intervention in the US (Head Start) have shown mixed long-term effects on child outcomes.

A number of characteristics of effective interventions have been identified within the literature as having the greatest impact on improving child outcomes and were discussed within a UK comprehensive spending review (CSR) (Sure Start 2001; Johnson 2011). Characteristics of effective programmes include the following: a two-generational focus that targets both the parent and child together; use of multifaceted approaches that include, among others, enhancing family relationships; provision that is non-stigmatising, locally driven, culturally appropriate or sensitive to user needs; and centre-based provision. This chapter will explore these findings in order to address three research questions: (1) *Who are children's centres serving?* (2) *What are children's centres doing?* and (3) *How are children's centres approaching their work?*

Research Methodology

The evaluation comprised of five sub-studies: a survey of children's centre leaders; a survey of families using children's centres; visits to the children's centres to evaluate their service delivery; the impact of children's centres and a cost-benefit analysis. The study had a nested evaluation design, with children's centres participating in a large survey of over 500 children's centres leaders, being used to draw samples for the remaining four sub-studies.

The data reported within this chapter is taken from visits to 121 children's centres across 2012 and 2013, drawn from the first two phases of children's centres and located in the 30 % most disadvantaged areas of England. The evaluation used a mixed methods approach and collected data via questionnaires, interviews with staff and parents, documentation review and rating scales.

Empirical Findings

ECCE researchers conceptualised *parenting* and *provision for parents* within children's centres by placing the parent as the central focus. Researchers recognised that children's centres provide a range of services which address the wider needs of families (moving from the parents' immediate situation towards larger needs or societal demands). Figure 1 displays how ECCE researchers categorised children's centres support for families according to their parental needs; taking a more holistic view of other individuals in their lives. There are four *areas of parental lives* that are described within the model: two of these represent needs which relate to individuals that are close to them, i.e. children and family/partners, and two reflect the parent as an individual, i.e. in terms of their own personal needs and their community.

Who Are Children's Centres Serving?

Children's centres were targeting many of the 'at-risk' groups focused on by other international parenting support programmes, while keeping in mind UK Government guidance focusing their work on *families in greatest need, child development and school readiness* and *health and life chances*. Effective interventions are known to take the parent and child together as a focus (Sure Start 2001; Johnson 2011), and children's centres included both parents and wider family members in their approach towards intervention. Importantly, children's centres were also clearly moving beyond the child's *microsystem* of individual, parental and family needs to consider the needs of both the child's *mesosystem* and their *exosystem* (factors associated with the family location and neighbourhood characteristics).

Children's centres were reaching both extremely vulnerable and targeted families (for

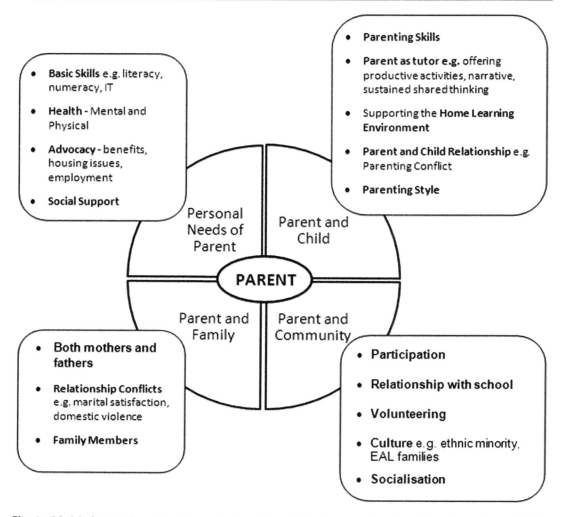

Fig. 1 'Model of parental needs' which may be targeted by children's centres (reproduced from Evangelou et al. 2014)

example, those on care plans which were part of the legal system), as well as less vulnerable families with particular needs. Lone parent families were reported most frequently, along with young parents, fathers, minority ethnic families living in poverty, or those from other cultures, and extended families. Deprivation and poverty was a frequent feature of family lives. Staff were interviewed from children's centres located in the most disadvantaged areas of England and therefore it was of little surprise that centres often aimed to provide services for *all* families in their area, offering open-access services to '*get*

families in' and support any families with needs. The nature of area deprivation meant that a number of families were living in geographical isolation, experiencing a lack of socialisation and reduced support networks, and often living in unsuitable or temporary accommodation. Families were described as facing issues such as substance abuse and obesity; or living in areas of multi-culture, gang culture, rurality, and poor transport.

Looking beyond the needs of the child's *microsystem*, staff recognised that a holistic offer of provision must first tackle parents' immediate needs (which can have a substantial impact on the quality of life for the child) before supporting their parenting role. In particular, staff recognised the need for parents to develop parenting skills and to become more knowledgeable about their child's development. Focusing more on the distal elements of the child's ecological system and moving away from the individual, staff were focused on the complete holistic ecology of the child's environment, and aware of the vast range of issues that need to be considered to support child development such as family poverty, location, parental education and security.

What Are Children's Centres Doing?

Children's centres in 2012 were offering a range of services centred on both the child and their family (parents and extended family). These services were largely consistent to those offered within children's centres in 2011 (Hall et al. 2015). Some of these services focused on adults' needs and skills, while others focused more strongly on the child or capacity-building in the community (Goff et al. 2013).

The Parent and Child Microsystem

Effective interventions tend to concentrate on enhancing family relationships through the provision of practical guidance on parental attachment, sensitivity and responsiveness to the child (Sure Start 2001). In line with Moran et al.'s (2004) findings that parenting support programmes commonly focus on the *microsystem* of the child, centres placed the greatest importance on targeting services towards the needs of 'parents and children' as a unit, which reflect more traditional conceptualisations of parenting support, specifically, the improvement of parenting skills and the parents' ability to look after their child. As shown in the ECCE *model of parental needs* (Fig. 1) ECCE researchers envisaged parent and child needs to include parenting skills, supporting their role as their child's first educator, developing a more supportive home learning environment, improving the parent-child relationship and parenting style. Centres provide a

number of services for children and families to access together (i.e. stay and play groups), along with positive parenting opportunities (developing attachment and positive interactions).

Multi-faceted Approaches

There was substantial variation in terms of the level and type of support offered, with centres offering a combination of generalised and personalised information, personalised support, and centre sessions, catering their level of support to meet the needs of attending parents. Children's centres offer a great variety of services targeting both parent and family needs including services aimed at partner emotional support (i.e. advice and support regarding separation, domestic violence and anger management), improving children's health and lifestyle, and family services (such as outreach or home-based support, and groups for fathers). This holistic approach follows the finding that effective early interventions are known to be multi-faceted and target several factors (Kumpfer 2009; Johnson 2011). The approach also supports more distal child ecology including family poverty, community integration, physical environment and housing, parental education and employment. Moran et al. (2004, p. 20) note that "few services are able to tackle directly the background to many problems—poverty, lack of community integration, degraded physical environments, inadequate education, poor housing": yet this is exactly what children's centres aim to accomplish. Children's centres recognise that children should be supported to live in a secure and safe home environment (before considering immediate parenting needs), and that families often face a multitude of complex intertwined difficulties.

Evidence-Based Intervention

The importance of using well-evidenced interventions has been clearly documented within the literature as a basis for replicating positive outcomes within controlled environments. ECCE researchers understood evidence-based programmes to mean those which met the strict standards of evidence and evaluation set down in a Government report by Allen (2011), which was taken as a guide for which programmes had rigorous research evidence, often through randomised control trials, for effectiveness. There was widespread use of well-evidenced programmes across the sample of children's centres between 2012 and 2013 (with centres particularly offering Incredible Years, Triple P and Family Nurse Partnership). Indeed, over half of the age-appropriate evidence-based family programmes defined by Allen (2011) were reported by staff as being implemented by these children's centres. The well-evidenced programmes however, differed in terms of their aims and the degree to which they were implemented with fidelity (Sylva et al. 2015).

The widespread offer of evidence-based programmes was alongside recognition of other promising practices (a challenge reportedly faced by other countries when planning parenting support; Molinuevo 2013). Children's centres staff reported implementing a wide range of other 'named' programmes which were deemed suitable for their families (for example Baby Massage, Every Child a Talker and the Solihull Approach) even though the evidence for their effectiveness was less secure as the programmes identified by Allen (2011).

Children's centres appear to be a successful vehicle for providing families with access to evidence-based family interventions and parenting programmes, a popular method of parenting support across a number of countries.

How Are Children's Centres Approaching Their Work?

Children's centres were using a wide range of supportive strategies with families. ECCE researchers recognised that the supportive strategies resembled and were heavily focused on the 'Opportunities, Recognition, Interaction and Model' (ORIM) framework developed by Hannon (1995), which positively acknowledges ways in which parents support their children's learning, and how staff might be working with the families. Staff from the majority of centres reported examples of providing *Opportunities* for

the parents (awareness of a variety of activities for use with their children, support to improve their financial situation, and employability); *Modelling* of learning strategies and dispositions from adults (for example parenting skills, cookery skills and health advice); *Interactions* with other adults and children (encouraging social interaction and trusting relationships); and finally *Recognition* and valuing of their early achievements (including praise and encouragement). Additional strategies used with parents included encouragement (presenting a welcoming, supportive, accessible and inclusive environment; developing independence, responsibility and participation); parental empowerment; focusing on meeting individual needs and providing information and knowledge.

In contrast, the ORIM framework was not so apparent in the examples of supportive strategies that staff used with children (which focused more on meeting their individual needs and improving their environments). Centre staff particularly spoke of providing *opportunities* for children to learn; developing school readiness (including early language skills, social skills, appropriate behaviours and adjusting to separation); facilitating *interaction* with adults in learning situations (for example, to enhance the parent-child relationship); individualised experiences (ensuring child activities are age, ability and child-led); creating supportive environments (relaxing, friendly and accessible); and lastly, *role-modelling* (from other children and adults).

Non-stigmatising Services

Moran et al. (2004) describe a distinction between 'universal' interventions (those aimed at less severe parenting difficulties and available to whole communities) versus 'targeted' interventions (those aimed at more complex parenting difficulties and specific individuals deemed to be most 'at-risk'). 'Progressive universalism' is noted to be a more effective method of delivering intervention, as this allows everyone to access support but reserves targeted support for the most 'at-risk' families (Molinuevo 2013). Boddy et al. (2009) identified four levels of accessibility in parenting support: (1) support embedded within universal services; (2) support activated as part of a universal service; (3) universally accessible support; and (4) targeted specialist support.

Children's centres are one of the main vehicles for ensuring that integrated and good quality family services are located in accessible places and are welcoming to all; as such centres typically offer services at all levels of Boddy et al.'s accessibility model. Open-access family services such as Stay and Play (where parent remains in charge of their child but both adult and child can experience a rich array of resources in the context of other families and child care staff) is both an open-access service as well as a means to engage and support targeted families. Stay and play is used to identify hidden family needs which might be prohibiting centres from carrying out successful parenting support; and to support and model appropriate parenting strategies. Centres often use open-access services such as stay and play as a means to implement 'progressive universalism' i.e. staff signpost or refer families to other services as more immediate needs become apparent, and staff offer a targeted package of family support and outreach in homes when families are identified as having the greatest needs.

A common challenge for parenting support is how to engage parents who are reluctant to attend an intervention, due to associated stigma and concern about being labelled as a 'bad parent' (Molinuevo 2013). Services which are non-stigmatising and avoid labelling are said to be most effective (Sure Start 2001; Johnson 2011). Children's centres aim to break down parent and family barriers which make it more difficult for families to attend, by building up trust and reassuring parents that they will not be 'judged'. Children's centres are also known for their welcoming open-access approach and non-stigmatising nature: however, during the period of children's centre data collection reported in this chapter (2012–2014) there was a clear shift in focus away from open-access services towards more targeted work with a narrower focus on vulnerable families with very complex needs (Hall et al. 2015; Sylva et al. 2015). This streamlined targeting was in line

with the revised core purpose for children's centres (DfE 2013), which specified that children's centres were now required to reduce inequalities for families in greatest need. Children's centre staff were concerned that a reduction in the availability of open-access services might mean that families with more preventable lower-level needs may not receive any help, due to their ineligibility to access the service, or the withdrawal of open-access services (Sylva et al. 2015). This was a clear tension for centre staff who recognised the importance of their open-access work for all families in the community but also for encouraging reluctant or excluded families, making centres more accessible, and reducing stigma.

Locally Driven Interventions

Effective family interventions are often locally driven, taking into account parent and local community consultation (Sure Start 2001; Johnson 2011). Children's centre staff were able to consult with centre families through parent forums and feedback channels, evaluating this information against their current provision and the needs of local families. It was more challenging for centres to consult with parents who were not yet involved with centre services due to their relative invisibility: those centres who were most successful at parent consultation were able to actively consult potential families through local surveys, and maintained good links with health visitors and midwives carrying out new birth visits (taking this as an opportunity to locate non-attending families: Goff et al. 2013). Children's centres considered the needs of their local community through the delivery of a range of services targeted towards local needs, and a multi-agency response that drew upon signposting and referrals to local agencies. Staff built links with their communities by consulting with other organisations, visiting the community, seeking new venues for services and developing community outreach and events. Children's centres were also offering a variety of opportunities for parents to get involved in the running of their centre and feel empowered: parents attending these children's centres were most likely to volunteer as a playworker during centre sessions, and volunteer at community events.

Centre-Based Intervention

Brooks-Gunn (2003) suggested that centre-based programmes report positive results over home-based programmes. The primary course of service delivery for children's centres was originally intended to be a centre-based 'one-stop-shop' for services in disadvantaged communities (noted by Boddy et al. 2009 as the 'come'-structure in Germany). While children's centres do offer a range of services on their centre site, they also balance this with more targeted services in the home (the 'go'-structure) which are known to be successful for improving access to hard-to-reach families, in line with the revised core purpose of the children's centre intervention (Boddy et al. 2009).

Universal Versus Culture-Specific Mechanisms

The children's centre intervention is innovative given that it displays a number of characteristics known to be associated with effective interventions as well as a range of mechanisms used within parenting support interventions internationally. This section will address 'universality' which can be seen as a mechanism of both *what* and *how* services are offered: this will be discussed in relation to the idea of cultural-specificity as a characteristic of effective interventions. It will argue that the dichotomy drawn between universal and culturally specific mechanisms in terms of children's centres work is a false dichotomy.

There are two levels to universality which are relevant to children's centres. The first regards *what* makes a service universal, specifically in terms of the *availability* and legal entitlement of an intervention or service open to all families (for example, schools and health services). The second details *how* services can be universal in terms of their *accessibility* for attending families, for example through accessible course materials and service structure. In terms of the *availability* of universal provision, children's centres provide

a number of services which follow 'progressive universalism' in that they are open and non-stigmatising for all families, but also aim to engage and support the more targeted families. The ECCE study however argued for the term 'open-access' as opposed to 'universal' services, as children's centres were intended to be available to local families in the most disadvantaged areas (rather than universally in every community), and were 'open' primarily as a means to avoiding stigma and reaching families on the cusp of disadvantage who needed some form of support (Sylva et al. 2015). Regarding *accessibility* to universal services, children's centres aimed to ensure open-access provision was available to the most disadvantaged or minority families in multiple ways. The vast majority of centres were able to provide translation services during centre sessions which allowed families (from a variety of backgrounds) to interact and engage with others during the same session while receiving identical information and activities. Leaflets (such as centre timetables) were often available in other languages.

A characteristic of effective interventions is that they are culturally appropriate to individual families and sensitive to their needs (Sure Start 2001; Johnson 2011). Children's centres are recognisable for the plethora of services which they offer towards a wide range of family, child and parental needs and their varied manner of delivery according to the needs of individual families. What is offered through children's centre services is carefully chosen by staff in order to meet the needs of the local community, and is sensitive to the accessibility needs of individual families. While the majority of centre resources were spent on families with young children or those with specific needs (for example, young parents, lone parents and workless households), a moderate amount of centre resources were also targeted towards Black and Minority Ethnic (BME) communities and parents with limited English language skills. Many children's centres in the sample offered translation services and signs and leaflets in non-English languages. There were also sign-language sessions and specialist groups for particular minority ethnic families or for fathers. The majority of centres reported that they focus their work on the individual needs of each family. What is interesting is that such 'cultural specificity' is also a feature of *accessibility* to universal services as just described. The dichotomy drawn between universal and culturally-specific mechanisms in terms of children's centres work cannot be drawn, as the very nature of the intervention requires that the two types of mechanism work alongside one another.

The flagship element of children's centres is their holistic approach: while a key feature of their service delivery is a focus on the primary parenting unit (the 'parent and the child'), service provision looks beyond this *microsystem* to consider wider familial and community needs known to affect the child's environment and ultimately their future development. This multi-faceted approach to service delivery supports more distal ecology including family poverty, community integration, physical environment and housing, and parental education and employment. Unlike parenting programmes and support offered by other countries which often have clearly specified foci and purpose, the children's centre holistic approach makes it challenging to generalise the findings from the evaluation of children's centres to other countries, as the provision is often culturally specific and sensitive to the needs of local service users.

There are however lessons that can be taken forward by other countries. The evaluation of children's centres has shown that it is not enough for parenting support interventions to focus only on the parent and child *microsystem*. Children's centres face many similar challenges to other international parenting support interventions including encouraging the engagement of more reluctant families; their holistic approach to service delivery however, ensures that the intervention is available to as many family groups as possible.

Policy Implications

This chapter has demonstrated that taking a more holistic approach to parenting support bears a number of similarities in the foci of effective interventions within the literature. Parenting support in other countries might benefit from a wider consideration of the full spectrum of complex issues facing families, and a deeper investigation into distal areas of a child's and parents' characteristics. Where possible, future provision should consider the wider parental needs reported by Evangelou et al. (2008) in their 'model of parental needs': for example, the personal needs of the parents in terms of their basic skills, health, advocacy and social support; the needs of the family in terms of relationship conflicts; and the needs of the parent in their community in terms of their participation, relationship with schools, volunteering, culture and socialisation.

There are two important points raised by the children's centres evaluation team:

1. While parenting support should be focused on parent and child needs, interventions must recognise the full spectrum of complex needs displayed by parents (which extend beyond parenting skill concerns) and need to be considered before parenting programmes and strategies can be successfully implemented;
2. Children's development should be considered in terms of their more distal experiences and in particular the influence of wider parental needs on their *mesosystem* and *exosystem*.

The evaluation of English children's centres reported in this chapter was carried out during a period of uncertainty and turbulence for children's centres. The children's centre programme has encountered vast changes to funding arrangements (moving away from an originally ring-fenced budget, towards unprotected local authority-led budgeting); widely reported funding reductions and restrictions; and volatility in terms of staffing and centre organisational structure (Sylva et al. 2015). A change in the UK political context has also led to a number of revisions to children's centre guidance documents (Hall et al. 2015), although centre staff were striving to ensure that such changes had a limited impact on the families accessing centre services.

Children's centres are well-known for offering welcoming, open-access services, although a move towards targeted provision was in line with recent Governmental changes to the specified core purpose for children's centres (now focussed more squarely on meeting the needs of the most disadvantaged families). Centre staff voiced concerns regarding what a loss of open-access services would mean for those families who do not meet the new criteria or have preventable low-level needs, particularly if their needs could easily be met with open-access services. Many centre staff recognised the value of open-access provision for engaging the more 'at-risk' families, and making services accessible to more reluctant families; and this is of key importance to effective intervention.

Future Directions

Children's centres have encountered multiple revisions to guidance documents and a redefined 'purpose'. Each fundamental revision requires a detailed and strategic reconsideration of the services on offer for families, and a scrutiny over which family needs to prioritise under the constraints of limited funds. A characteristic of effective interventions is that the intervention can be locally driven and takes account of 'local voices' from parent consultations—it is however more difficult for centres to plan their services with the needs of their local communities in mind, when their service offer is governed by prescriptive legislation. Children's centres in general would benefit from more stability in terms of the aims of their intervention as well as secure longer term funding, which would allow centre staff to plan for the future.

Coinciding with a change in focus towards more targeted work, centre staff described working with families with very complex needs. There was an increase both in the volume of this work and the skills required to provide more specialised support to families who were living in very difficult circumstances. The changing political climate had also affected the partner agencies with which children's centres offered their services, and partner organisations were pulling back their support and services to reserve

their own limited resources. In some cases, this meant that centre staff were taking on intense work with families who displayed complex needs, that would normally be carried out by specialised staff (Sylva et al. 2015). Centre staff would benefit from further training to enable them to work with the higher level of needs they are now encountering. Such training will enable them to understand how parents can be supported. There is to date some evidence within the literature regarding characteristics of successful interventions within a UK context, however the planning and development of future interventions would benefit from more robust evidence on effective interventions.

References

Abbott-Shim, M., Lambert, R., & McCarty, F. (2003). A comparison of school readiness outcomes for children randomly assigned to a Head Start program and the program's wait list. *Journal of Education for Students Placed at Risk, 8*(2), 191–214.

Allen, G. (2011). *Early Intervention: The Next Steps. An Independent Report to Her Majesty's Government.* London: HM Government.

Alvy, K. T. (2005). *An effective parenting initiative: To make the United States of America a model child and family friendly Nation.* California: Center for the Improvement of Child Caring. Retrieved January 30, 2015, from http://www.ciccparenting.org/pdf/NPI.pdf

Barlow, J., Kirkpatrick, S., Wood, D., Ball, M., & Stewart-Brown, S. (2007). *Family and parenting support in sure start local programmes.* London: DCSF.

Barnett, W. S., & Hustedt, J. T. (2005). Head start's lasting benefits. *Infants & Young Children, 18*(1), 16–24.

Boddy, J., Statham, J., Smith, M., Ghate, D., Wigfall, V., & Hauari, H. (2009). *International perspectives on parenting support: Non-english language sources (Research Report DCSF-RR114).* London: DCSF.

Bronfenbrenner, U. (1979). *The ecology of human development: Experiments by nature and design.* Cambridge: Harvard University Press.

Brooks-Gunn, J. (2003). Do you believe in magic? What we can expect from early childhood intervention programs. *Social Policy Report, 17*(1), 3–15.

Daly, M. (2013). Parenting support policies in Europe. *Families, Relationships and Societies, 2*(2), 159–174.

Department for Education. (2013). *Sure Start children's centres statutory guidance.* (DfE Research Report No. DFE-00314-2013). London: DfE.

Department for Education and Skills. (2003). *Every child matters (Green Paper)*. London: DfES.

Desforges, C., & Abouchaar, A. (2003). *The impact of parental involvement, parental support and family education on pupil achievement and adjustment. A literature review*. (DfES Research Report No. RR433). London: DfES.

Early Childhood Learning and Knowledge Center. (ECLKC). (2014). *About Us*. Retrieved January 30, 2015, from http://eclkc.ohs.acf.hhs.gov/hslc/hs/about

Erickson, M. F., Korfmacher, J., & Egeland, B. R. (1992). Attachments past and present: Implications for therapeutic intervention with mother-infant dyads. *Development and Psychopathology, 4*, 495–507.

Evangelou, M., Sylva, K., Edwards, A., & Smith, T. (2008). *Supporting parents in promoting early learning: The evaluation of the early learning partnership project*. London: DCSF.

Evangelou, M., Goff, J., Hall, J., Sylva, K., Eisenstadt, N., Paget, C. et al. (2014). *Evaluation of children's centres in England (ECCE)—Strand 3: Parenting Services in Children's Centres*. (DfE Research Report No. DfE-RR368). London: DfE.

Field, F. (2010). *The foundation years: Preventing poor children becoming poor adults. The report of the Independent Review on Poverty and Life Chance*. London: HM Government. The National Archives.

France, A., & Utting, D. (2005). The paradigm of "Risk and Protection-Focused Prevention" and its impact on services for children and families. *Children and Society, 19*, 77–90.

Glass, N. (1999). Sure Start: The development of an early intervention programme for young children in the United Kingdom. *Children and Society, 13*(4), 257–264.

Goff, J., Evangelou, M., & Sylva, K. (2012). Enhancing parents' ways of supporting their children's early learning through participation in an early-intervention project in the UK: The Early Learning Partnership Project. *Journal of Family Research (Zeitschrift für Familienforschung), 24*(2), 160–177.

Goff, J., Hall, J., Sylva, K., Smith, T., Smith, G., Eisenstadt, N., et al. (2013). *Evaluation of Children's Centre's in England (ECCE)—Strand 3: Delivery of Family Services by Children's Centre's Research Report*. (DfE Research Report No. DFE-RR297). London: DfE.

Hall, J., Eisenstadt, N., Sylva, K., Smith, T., Sammons, P., Smith, G., et al. (2015). A review of the services offered by English Sure Start Children's Centres in 2011 and 2012. *Oxford Review of Education,*. doi:10.1080/03054985.2014.1001731

Hannon, P. (1995). *Literacy, home and school research and practice in teaching literacy with parents*. London: The Falmer Press.

Heckman, J. J. (2008). The case for investing in disadvantaged young children. In L. Darling-Hammond, R. Grunewald, J. Heckman, J. Isaacs, D. Kirp, A. Rolnick, & I. Sawhill (Eds.), *Big ideas for children: investing in our nation's future* (pp. 49–58). Washington, DC: First Focus.

Huser, M., Cooney, S., Small, S., O'Connor, C., & Mather, R. (2009). *Evidence-based program registries*. Madison, WI: University of Wisconsin-Madison/Extension.

Johnson, S. (2011). Impact of Social Science on Policy: Sure Start Case Study. Retrieved 13 March, 2015, http://www.esrc.ac.uk/_images/Sure_Start_final_report_tcm8-20116.pdf

Kennett, D. J., & Chislett, G. (2012). The benefits of an enhanced Nobody's Perfect Parenting Program for child welfare clients including non-custodial parents. *Children and Youth Services Review, 34*(10), 2081–2087.

Knibbs, S., Pope, S., Dobie, S., & D'Souza, J. (2013). *National evaluation of flying start: Impact report*. Cardiff: Welsh Government Social Research.

Kumpfer, K. L. (2009). *Strengthening America's families: Exemplary parenting and family strategies for delinquency prevention*. United States: the Office of Juvenile, Justice and Delinquency Prevention, Office of Juvenile Programs. U.S. Department of Justice.

Melhuish, E., Belsky, J., & Leyland, A. (2005). *Early impacts of sure start local programmes on children and families*. London: DfES.

Melhuish, E., Belsky, J., Macpherson, K., & Cullis, A. (2010a). *The quality of group childcare settings used by 3–4 year old children in Sure Start local programme areas and the relationship with child outcomes*. (DfE Research Report No. DFE-RR068). London: DfE.

Melhuish, E., Belsky, J., & Leyland, A. (2010b). *The impact of Sure Start Local Programmes on five year olds and their families*. (DfE Research Report No. DFE-RR067). London: DfE.

Melhuish, E., Belsky, J., & Leyland, A. (2012). *The impact of Sure Start Local Programmes on seven year olds and their families*. (DfE Research Report No. DFE-RR220). London: Birkbeck University of London.

Molinuevo, D. (2013). *Parenting support in Europe*. European foundation for the improvement of living and working conditions (Eurofound): Ireland.

Moran, P., Ghate, D., & van der Merwe, A. (2004). *What works in parenting support? A review of the international evidence*. (DfES Research Report No. RR574). Nottingham: DfES.

National Evaluation of Sure Start Research Team. (2012). *Methodology report executive summary*. London: Birkbeck University of London.

Pugh, G., De'Ath, E., & Smith, C. (1994). *Confident parents, confident children. Policy and practice in parent education and support*. London: National Children's Bureau.

Seibel, N. L., Bassuk, E., & Medeiros, D. (2011). *Using evidence-based programs to support children and families experiencing homelessness*. Washington: Zero to Three.

Small, S. A., & Mather, R. S. (2009). *What works, Wisconsin: Evidence based parenting program directory*. Madison, WI: University of Wisconsin-Madison/ Extension.

Smith, C. (1996). *Developing parenting programmes*. London: National Children's Bureau.

Sure Start UK (2001). *The Aim of Sure Start*. Retrieved May 18, 2001, from http://www.surestart.gov.uk

Sylva, K., Goff, J., Eisenstadt, N., Smith, T., Hall, J., Evangelou, M., et al. (2015). *Organisation, Services and Reach of Children's Centres: Evaluation of Children's Centres in England (ECCE, Strand 3)*. London: DfE.

Wagmiller, L. R., & Adelman, R. M. (2009). *Childhood and intergenerational poverty: The long-term consequences of growing up poor*. Columbia University Academic Commons. http://hdl.handle.net/10022/AC

Williams-Taylor, L. (2007). *Research Review. Evidence-based Programs and Practices: What does it all mean?*. Florida: Children Services Council of Palm Beach County.

Instructional Practice with Young Bilingual Learners: A Canadian Profile

Roma Chumak-Horbatsch

Abstract

The focus of this chapter is instructional practice with the growing number of young bilingual learners who arrive in Canadian childcare centres and kindergartens with little or no proficiency in the language of program delivery. The chapter begins by setting the context, briefly describing the Canadian linguistic landscape and outlining the linguistic profile of Canadian early care and learning programs. This is followed by a review of practices currently adopted by EC professionals in their work with bilingual learners. A new multilingual, strength-based direction in classroom practice is briefly described and recent initiatives are summarized. The highlights of one of these initiatives, Linguistically Appropriate Practice, are presented and the main findings of its implementation in two early learning contexts are discussed. These findings include the varied interest in practice retooling and the identification of categories of factors that affect early childhood professionals' practice decision-making. Instructional practice with young bilingual learners in the United States of America and in select regions of Europe is also briefly outlined. The chapter concludes with recommendations for designing a course of action to fuel EC professionals' interest in and commitment to linguistically responsive practice.

Introduction

> One of today's most misunderstood issues in education ... is how to educate students who speak languages other than English.
>
> (García et al. 2008)

R. Chumak-Horbatsch (✉)
School of Early Childhood Studies, Ryerson University, Toronto, Canada
e-mail: rchumak@ryerson.ca

© The Editor(s) 2017
N.J. Cabrera and B. Leyendecker (eds.), *Handbook on Positive Development of Minority Children and Youth*, DOI 10.1007/978-3-319-43645-6_28

This chapter reports on instructional practice with the growing number of children[1] who arrive in Canadian childcare centres and kindergartens with little or no proficiency in the language of program delivery. These children are a diverse group. Referred to here as bilingual[2] learners (hereafter BLs), they are mostly born in Canada to newly arrived immigrant parents. Some are acquiring one home language, while others grow up in multiple language households. Some arrive with little or no exposure to the majority language, while others have been exposed to the new language through siblings and older family members, community experiences and/or the media. Young BLs' connections with their parents' countries of origin also vary—from annual trips to regular electronic communication and extended visits from family members. In all cases, young BLs enrolled in majority language programs find themselves in a unique language-learning situation—the continued acquisition of their first or home language or languages and the learning of a new language.

This growing demographic presents a double challenge to Canadian early childhood professionals[3] (hereafter EC professionals). They find themselves ill prepared to work with children who do not understand the language of the classroom. Moreover, they describe available resources as falling short of providing concrete support and guidance. While most Canadian EC professionals acknowledge the fact that BLs are speakers of "other" languages, they view them first and foremost as learners of the classroom language. As a result, they opt for instructional practice that hurries them into the new language. Only in a small number of cases are young BLs' prior linguistic skills valued and extended and their bilingual potential facilitated and encouraged.

The chapter begins by setting the context and describing the current linguistic landscape of Canadian early care and learning programs. In Sect."A new direction" instructional practices currently adopted by EC professionals are presented. Section "Linguistically Appropriate Practice (LAP)" describes a new direction in instructional practice and provides examples of recent initiatives. In Sect. "LAP Studies: Findings and Discussion" the main findings of the implementation of a new instructional practice called Linguistically Appropriate Practice or LAP (Chumak-Horbatsch 2012) in two early learning contexts are presented and discussed. Section "Future Directions and Policy Implications" looks briefly at instructional practice with BLs in other countries. And lastly, Sect. "Conclusion and Next Steps" opens the door to the next level of instructional practice investigation by providing recommendations for early learning stakeholders.

The Canadian Linguistic Landscape

Immigration is central to Canadian history. Often viewed as the "land of immigration"[4] and "a choice destination",[5] thousands of immigrants arrive in Canada yearly. Generally supportive and welcoming of foreign residents, Canada views immigration as an economic and cultural benefit and accepts high numbers of people from many different parts of the world for work, study or for humanitarian and compassionate reasons (Nanos 2008). Currently, there are more foreign-born residents (6.8 million or 20.6 %) in Canada than ever before. Often called a "nation of many languages",[6] the more than two hundred languages spoken by one in five people in

Canada have been described as economic and

---

[1]These children are between the ages of 15 months and 6 years.

[2]For reasons of convention and brevity, the term "bilingualism" is used in this chapter as a cover term to include both bilingualism and multilingualism.

[3]Early childhood professionals include childcare staff and kindergarten teachers who work directly with young children and are responsible for all aspects of program planning and delivery.

[4]http://www.immigrationdirect.ca/immigration-articles/statistics-facts/?gclid=CJGT6reYp8ACFQcLaQodBzkABQ.

[5]http://www.statcan.gc.ca/pub/11-008-x/2008001/article/10517-eng.htm.

[6]http://www.cbc.ca/news/canada/bilingualism-growing-but-not-in-french-and-english-1.1176469.

cultural assets.[7]

Children who do not understand or speak the majority languages (French and English) make up a significant proportion of Canadian early learning settings. In the large, high-immigrant Canadian "gateway cities" of Ontario, Quebec, British Columbia and Alberta, 18–26 % speak a language other than English or French at home.[8] A recent language profile revealed that nearly half (43 %) of the children enrolled in Toronto childcare centres (Chumak-Horbatsch 2010) speak one or more (of a total of 129 different) heritage languages in the home, while the Toronto District School Board reports a slightly higher number,[9] where over half of kindergarteners come from homes where English is not spoken. In Vancouver schools, 126 different heritage languages are spoken by 60 % of the school population[10] and in Montreal's public French-language schools, 46 % of students do not speak French as their home language. In over one-third of Montreal schools, students of immigrant origin account for the majority of the population, and just under one in ten schools has an immigrant population of over 75 % (McAndrew et al. 2014).

Over the past 10 years, EC professionals working in urban areas in other Canadian provinces are reporting an ever-increasing number of children who do not understand the majority language. Two reasons help explain this. Firstly, newcomers are settling in urban areas of the "other" Canadian provinces that offer affordable housing, promise economic opportunities and provide settlement support. For example, between 2006 and 2011, immigration significantly increased in the urban areas of Saskatchewan, Newfoundland, Prince Edward Island, New Brunswick and Manitoba. The Saskatchewan Ministry of Education reported the

following between 2007 and 2012: the number of young immigrant children (between the ages of 1 and 5 years of age)[11] tripled, the number of children who did not speak an official language (English or French) more than doubled and the number of immigrant children attending kindergarten in the 5-year span more than doubled.[12]

Another example comes from the province of Manitoba's "readiness for school" report,[13] which shows an increase of young EAL (English as an additional language) children between 2005 and 2010.

A second reason for the increase of BLs in Canadian early learning programs is the growing change in traditional and cultural childcare arrangements or norms, where fewer immigrant women are staying at home to care for their young children and are instead joining the workforce. For example, the rate of increase (17 %) for immigrant women in the labour force between 2001 and 2006 was more than double that for Canadian-born women (7 %) (Saraswati 2000).

Current Instructional Practice with Young Bilingual Learners

A recent investigation of instructional practice (Chumak-Horbatsch 2012) identified three different kinds of practices adopted by EC professionals in their work with BLs: assimilative, supportive and inclusive (see Table 1). These practices differ from one another on two aspects: the attention paid to the majority language and the support provided to BLs' home languages and cultures. The monolingual focus of *assimilative practice* is driven by a deficit agenda, where BLs are labelled and identified by what they lack, namely proficiency in the majority language. This practice ignores their linguistic

---

[7]http://www.environicsanalytics.ca/blog/doug-norris/doug-norris-blog/2012/11/02/canadians-speak-in-many-tongues.

[8]http://www.statcan.gc.ca.

[9]http://www.tdsb.on.ca/HighSchool/YourSchoolDay/Curriculum/ESL.aspx.

[10]http://www.vsb.bc.ca/english-second-language-information.

[11]This number would be higher if infants (ages birth to 12 months) were included.

[12]Immigration Services Division, Government of Saskatchewan: Citizenship and Immigration Canada: Microdata, 2013.

[13]http://www.gov.mb.ca/healthychild/edi/edireport_MB_201011.pdf.

Table 1 Instructional practices with young BLs (From Chumak-Horbatsch, 2012)

Instructional practice	Assimilative	Supportive	Inclusive
Main features	Teaching and learning the majority language Absorbing BLs into the majority language and culture as quickly as possible	Teaching and learning the majority language Acknowledging home languages Celebrating cultural differences	Teaching and learning the majority language Validating and supporting children's home languages Integrating home languages into the curriculum Using children's language skills as a resource Working closely with families to promote bilingualism and biliteracy
Focus	Monolingual, mono-literate, mono-cultural	Monolingual, mono-literate, inter-cultural	Multilingual, multiliterate, and intercultural
Sample strategies	Limit the number of BLs in each classroom Discourage interaction between children who speak the same home language	Use key words and phrases in the home languages to ease communication: Come here; bathroom; Do you want some help? It's OK; sleep; stop; eat Organize multicultural celebrations	Greet children in their home languages Invite family members to share and author dual language books

background, discounts what they have encoded in their home language or languages, fails to recognize their bilingual potential and hurries them into the majority language and culture. *Supportive practices* have a similar monolingual focus, with an addendum: while the focus of instruction remains the majority language, home languages are acknowledged and cultural differences are celebrated. These two monolingual practices rest on erroneous and out-dated assumptions, such as the idea that young children can manage only one language at a time, require increased input to master the new language and experience competition and negative

transfer between their two languages. Ostensibly adopted in the best interests of BLs, these two practices fall short of meeting their language and literacy needs.

Unlike the two monolingual practices, *inclusive or linguistically responsive practice* rests on a positive, strength-based approach to home languages, recognizing the personal, social, cognitive, linguistic and economic advantages of bilingualism. Inclusive practice reflects and concretely responds to the linguistic diversity found in centres and classrooms. In line with current research findings, this practice views young BLs as bilinguals in the making or "emergent

Fig. 1 Overlap in instructional practices

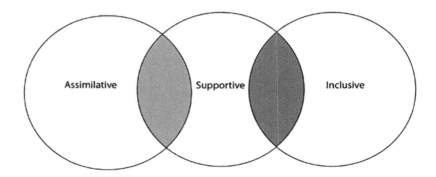

bilinguals" (García 2009), portraying them as capable, active dual language learners and acknowledging the fact that they, like all bilinguals, use their entire linguistic repertoire to navigate the many communicative contexts they encounter. Inclusive practice extends the knowledge that children have encoded in their home language(s) and views their prior experiences as important contributors to their identity formulation. Finally, inclusive practice bridges BLs' two language worlds, integrating their home language (s) daily and directly into the classroom.

Although the three practices can be characterized separately and may appear to be mutually exclusive, they are not. The shaded areas of Fig. 1 show that there is overlap between them. Indeed, numerous reports, classroom observations and accounts found in early learning resources reveal that in their work with BLs, Canadian EC professionals adopt strategies across all three practices. For example, general assimilative practice may include some supportive strategies such as acknowledgement and recognition of BLs' home languages, and inclusive strategies such as including home languages in the curriculum often accompany supportive practice. However, overlap is *not* found between the two kinds of instructional practices that are starkly different, assimilative and inclusive.

The majority of Canadian EC professionals find themselves ill prepared to work with children and families who have little or no proficiency in the language of program delivery (Meyers 2003; Webster and Valeo 2011; Pacini-Ketchabaw 2007). With little or no training in linguistic diversity, childhood bilingualism and linguistically responsive pedagogy, most remain unfamiliar with the importance of the language backgrounds and experiences of BLs and often feel that these children tax their busy and demanding agendas. As a result, they prefer supportive practice, a middle-of-the-road, accommodating approach that hurries BLs into the majority language, peripherally recognizes their home languages and celebrates their cultures.

Three factors help explain this choice of practice. Firstly, Canada is a country

characterized by linguistic and cultural diversity, where for the most part, its inhabitants have an open, respectful and positive attitude towards multiculturalism, diversity and immigration. As such, most EC professionals feel that a focus on the majority language, with a nod to children's linguistic and cultural differences, is the thing to do. The second reason is that many EC professionals, themselves speakers of heritage languages, view bilingualism positively and consider it appropriate to acknowledge home languages. Finally, as we will see in the next section, the majority of Canadian early learning resources promote and endorse supportive instructional practice.

Most Canadian early learning resources (curriculum guidelines and policy documents) include some information about BLs. This information varies in length, breadth, philosophy, developmental overview, theoretical framework and practicality. For example, some resources simply inform the reader about the presence of BLs, while others provide an overview of dual language learning in young children or offer strategies and suggestions for integrating BLs into their new language environment. Taken together, the resources characterize BLs in the following way:

- BLs are learners of the majority language. They are labelled as English Language Learners (ELLs), English as an Additional Language Learners (EAL), English as a Second Language (ESL) Learners or French as a Second Language (FSL) Learners.
- BLs will encounter some difficulties in learning the classroom language.
- In learning the classroom language, BLs will go through a silent stage.
- BLs' home languages and cultures are important.

With its focus on the majority language, this characterization of BLs is problematic and inequitable for four reasons. Firstly, majority language identification and labelling of BLs—as ELLs, EALs, ESLs, or FSLs—establishes the classroom language as the only language worth

Fig. 2 Typical photo found in early learning resources (Healthy Child Manitoba: http://www.gov.mb.ca/healthychild/ecd/index.html)

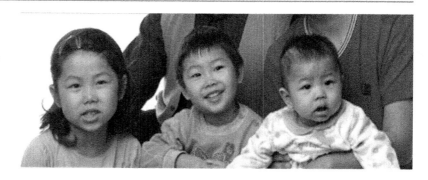

knowing, learning and speaking, solidifies majority language teaching as the goal of working with BLs, devalues their home languages and literacy experiences, skills and strengths and ignores their bilingual potential. Secondly, the deficit focus of the characterization—absence of the majority language and potential difficulties— stand in contrast to established principles of childhood bilingualism that portray young children as capable, active language learners. Thirdly, the silent stage, although widely accepted and expected by EC professionals, lacks research evidence (Roberts 2014), is artificially created and is damaging to BLs (Chumak-Horbatsch 2012). In reality, BLs are not silent, but are *silenced* by the monolingual classroom agenda. Finally, colourful celebrations and displays capture only one dimension of the many cultural experiences of BLs.

A close look at Canadian early learning resources often reveals a disconnect between the images and the message conveyed in the text. While the many photos of children and families from various ethnic groups, like the one in Fig. 2, reflect the diversity found in the childcare and kindergarten population, the message in the accompanying text promotes practice that focuses on the majority language, as seen in the characterization of BLs.

A particularly noteworthy example of image-text mismatch can be found in an Ontario ministry document entitled Supporting English Language Learners in Kindergarten: A practical guide for Ontario educators.[14] While the text

promotes inclusive practice, reminding EC professionals that young children "develop their knowledge by building on their past experiences and the learning they have already acquired" and encouraging the creation of "an inclusive learning environment that supports the success of every student" (p. 4), the title of the document and the tree images communicate a strong monolingual message. The purple tree foliage, trunk, ground and roots on the cover are filled with multi-coloured translations of the word ENGLISH (Fig. 3), while the purple borders (Fig. 4) with white translations of ENGLISH are found throughout the pages. Together, these images communicate not the many voices and roots of BLs but rather, the centrality and importance of one voice and one root—English.

In addition to the monolingual characterization of BLs, Canadian early learning resources remind EC professionals to be sensitive to cultures and languages, to "value, honour, and promote culture and language as integral components of programs, supports and services",[15] and to attend to home languages: "When educators are aware of and able to understand and respond to the many "languages" children use to communicate, they give every child a "voice".[16] While such reminders appear to promote children's home languages, their wording is broad, leaving EC professionals wondering, "How do I do this?"

---

[14]http://www.edu.gov.on.ca/eng/document/kindergarten/kindergartenell.pdf.

[15]Starting Early, Starting Strong: Manitoba's Early Childhood Development Framework, 2013.

[16]http://www.edu.gov.on.ca/childcare/HowLearning Happens.pdf.

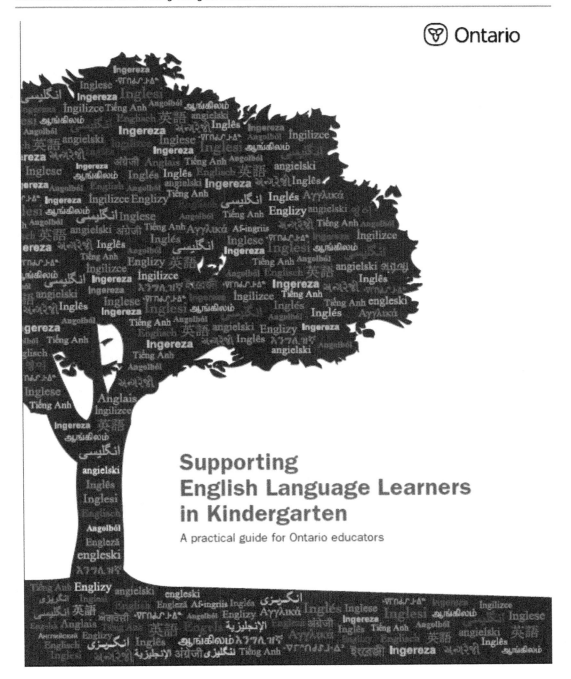

Fig. 3 Cover: supporting english language learners in kindergarten

The same is true of the widespread, inclusive-like home language word-phrase strategy, found in numerous early learning resources. Adopting this strategy, EC professionals learn and use key words in children's home languages (e.g., It's OK; Stop; Are you tired? Are you hungry?), to ease communication and help newly arrived BLs transition into their new language

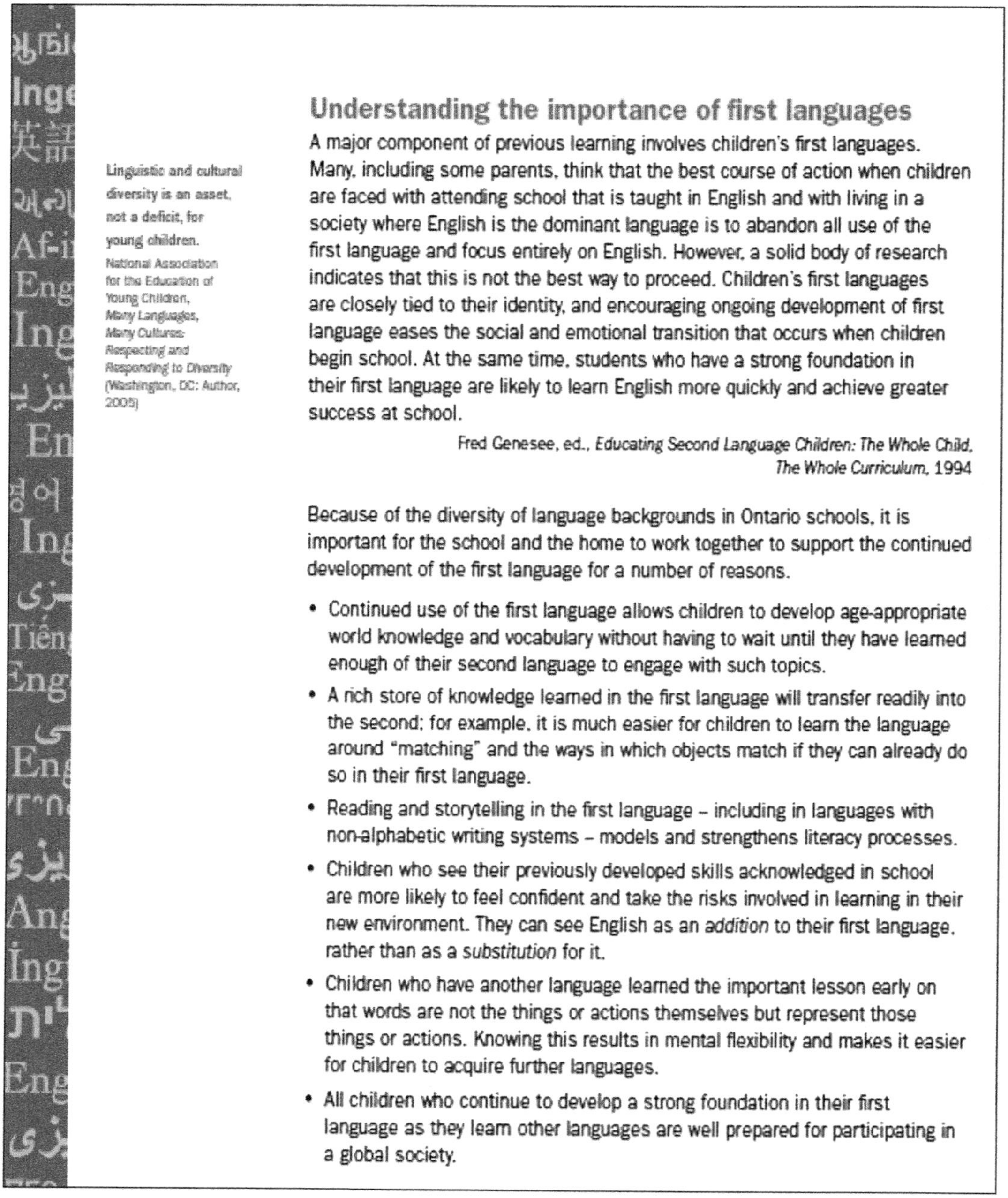

Linguistic and cultural diversity is an asset, not a deficit, for young children.

National Association for the Education of Young Children, *Many Languages, Many Cultures: Respecting and Responding to Diversity* (Washington, DC: Author, 2005)

Understanding the importance of first languages

A major component of previous learning involves children's first languages. Many, including some parents, think that the best course of action when children are faced with attending school that is taught in English and with living in a society where English is the dominant language is to abandon all use of the first language and focus entirely on English. However, a solid body of research indicates that this is not the best way to proceed. Children's first languages are closely tied to their identity, and encouraging ongoing development of first language eases the social and emotional transition that occurs when children begin school. At the same time, students who have a strong foundation in their first language are likely to learn English more quickly and achieve greater success at school.

Fred Genesee, ed., *Educating Second Language Children: The Whole Child, The Whole Curriculum*, 1994

Because of the diversity of language backgrounds in Ontario schools, it is important for the school and the home to work together to support the continued development of the first language for a number of reasons.

- Continued use of the first language allows children to develop age-appropriate world knowledge and vocabulary without having to wait until they have learned enough of their second language to engage with such topics.
- A rich store of knowledge learned in the first language will transfer readily into the second; for example, it is much easier for children to learn the language around "matching" and the ways in which objects match if they can already do so in their first language.
- Reading and storytelling in the first language – including in languages with non-alphabetic writing systems – models and strengthens literacy processes.
- Children who see their previously developed skills acknowledged in school are more likely to feel confident and take the risks involved in learning in their new environment. They can see English as an *addition* to their first language, rather than as a *substitution* for it.
- Children who have another language learned the important lesson early on that words are not the things or actions themselves but represent those things or actions. Knowing this results in mental flexibility and makes it easier for children to acquire further languages.
- All children who continue to develop a strong foundation in their first language as they learn other languages are well prepared for participating in a global society.

Fig. 4 Page 8: supporting english language learners in kindergarten

environment. In reality, this strategy is far from inclusive. Rather, it is simply used as a stepping-stone to the learning of the classroom language. Once children gain a basic proficiency in the new language, this home language strategy is no longer needed and is abandoned.

Overall, then, the majority of Canadian EC professionals adopt instructional practice that reflects the supportive directive endorsed and promoted in early learning resources. They view and label BLs as learners of the majority language, focus on the teaching of the majority language, peripherally acknowledge home languages and celebrate cultures.

A New Direction

Yet, the profile sketched in the previous section is not the full picture. Information gathered through the author's on-going work (research, teaching, classroom observation and school involvement) (Chumak-Horbatsch 2004, 2006, 2008, 2010, 2012) reveals a new direction in instructional practice with young BLs. Since 2000, a growing number of Canadian EC professionals, many of whom speak multiple languages and are aware of the benefits of bilingualism, are rethinking supportive practice, engaging in professional change behaviours and adopting various inclusive instructional strategies. According to Cummins (2014), this shift to linguistically responsive pedagogy, also referred to as "multi-literacies pedagogy" (Cummins 2006a, b) or "teaching with a multilingual lens" (Cummins and Early 2014) is still in its infancy. In line with a number of major learning and teaching frameworks, orientations and principles, it is fuelled by the growing number of collaborations between Canadian educators and university researchers, whose projects and initiatives are redefining multilingual education.

Linguistically responsive practice is grounded in the strength-based orientation of learning (Ruíz 1984; González and Moll 1995; Moll et al. 1992; Moll and Greenberg 1990) that views children's family and community experiences as important building blocks for acquiring new knowledge. Consistent with empirical research findings from cognitive psychology on how learning happens (Bransford et al. 2000; Donovan and Bransford 2005; Cummins 2001, 2006; Reyes 2001), linguistically responsive pedagogy positions teachers as supportive guides who activate learners' prior language and literacy

understandings, help learners formulate their identity, provide opportunities for age-appropriate levels of understanding and allow learners to take control of and self-regulate their language and literacy learning. In line with the social constructivist orientation on learning and teaching put forward by Piaget (1929) and Vygotsky (1978) and elaborated by numerous scholars (Coelho 2012; Cummins 2001, 2004, 2006; Skourtou et al. 2006; Cummins and Early 2011, 2014; Norton 2000; Siraj-Blatchford and Clarke 2000; Toohey 2000; Wardle and Cruz-Janzen 2003), linguistically responsive pedagogy emphasizes the joint construction of knowledge and the importance of the social context in supporting and enabling learning, literacy engagement and the affirmation of learners' identities. Finally, inclusive pedagogy is founded on three psycholinguistic and sociolinguistic principles that underlie educational success: strong and effective promotion of fluency and literacy in both the home and the classroom languages; sustained multi-literacy engagement where literacy is understood in a wide-ranging way and the collaborative creation of power within the classroom (Cummins 2001, 2009).

In the sections that follow, recent examples of multilingual initiatives with BLs undertaken by Canadian researchers and educators are briefly described. The highlights of one of these initiatives, Linguistically Appropriate Practice or LAP, are presented and the main findings of the implementation of this instructional approach in two early learning contexts are discussed.

Dual Language Reading Project

In the Dual Language Reading Project,[17] a partnership between the University of Calgary and the Calgary Board of Education, teachers, family and community members shared dual language books with young BLs in mainstream classrooms and in a Spanish–English bilingual

---

[17]www.rahatnaqvi.ca.

program. This collaboration bridged the school and the home, extended BLs' linguistic skills, improved early literacy skills, positively affected their identity development and helped all children develop awareness and understanding of linguistic diversity.

ELODIL

The ELODIL[18] project, developed at the Université de Montreal and also undertaken in Vancouver, concretely supports teachers who work with BLs. The goals of the project are to "legitimize the language of origin of students from immigrant families" and help, in age-appropriate ways, "to promote language awareness and openness to linguistic diversity in the classroom." The ELODIL resources (publications, book lists and videos) link to similar European initiatives, and the many classroom activities are intended to stimulate children's interest in and extend their knowledge about different language groups. Response to the ELODIL activities shows that giving home languages a place in the classroom motivates and excites BLs and helps them to understand linguistic diversity.

ScribJab

ScribJab[19] is a website and iPad application developed at Simon Fraser University. Built on the premise that children learn second languages faster and better if they have a strong foundation in their first language, ScribJab invites children to read, create and share digital stories (text, illustrations and audio recordings) in any language: English and/or French or home languages. Space is provided for young readers and authors to discuss their stories with one another.

Teachers can monitor and organize children's contributions and create reading groups.

Home Oral Language Activities (HOLA)

The Home Oral Language Activities (HOLA)[20] program supports young BLs' development in their home languages and builds family-teacher partnerships. Developed by speech and language pathologists, Early Years and English as a Second Language staff of the Toronto District School Board, the program invites families to share a collection of thematic books (available in 12 languages) and related objects with their children, to develop vocabulary, content and background knowledge. Like the three initiatives described previously, the HOLA program concretely supports children's home languages and scaffolds new learning on prior strengths and skills.

Linguistically Appropriate Practice (LAP)

In this section, Linguistically Appropriate Practice or LAP is briefly described. This is followed by a summary of the main findings of the implementation of this new instructional practice in two early learning contexts.

What Is LAP?

LAP is an inclusive instructional approach that views young, non-majority-language-speaking children as BLs rather than simply as learners of the classroom language. LAP links BLs' home and classroom language and literacy experiences, encourages home language use in the classroom and promotes multilingualism. It brings linguistic diversity to life and prepares young children for the complex communication and literacy demands of the twenty first century (García

---

[18]Éveil au langage et ouverture à la diversité linguistique (Awakening to Language and Opening up to Linguistic Diversity), http://elodil.com.

[19]http://www.scribjab.com/en/about/about.html.

---

[20]http://www.equinoxpub.com/journals/index.php/JIRCD/article/view/15999.

2009a, b, c). Developed in response to the numerous requests for concrete guidance, LAP helps EC professionals to retool the way they work with BLs and to move from supportive to inclusive instructional practice.

LAP is grounded in dynamic bilingualism (García 2009a, c), a theory that reflects the current global and technological communication reality and focuses on languages that speakers *use* rather than on separate languages they *have*. García defines dynamic bilingualism as "language practices that are multiple and ever adjusting to the multilingual multimodal terrain of the communicative act" (García 2009a: 144). Dynamic bilingualism, García explains, is not about adding additional languages. It is about using one's entire linguistic repertoire to deal with communication circumstances or "developing complex language practices that encompass several social contexts" (García 2010: 96).

The implementation of LAP is a four-step sequential process. In the first step, EC professionals are introduced to dynamic bilingualism, (García 2009a, b, c). This is followed by a review of the principles of childhood bilingualism. Finally, EC professionals are encouraged to reflect on their current practice with BLs in relation to three different kinds of approaches and consider strategies for moving towards inclusive practice.

Building on their new understanding of childhood bilingualism, EC professionals are then ready for the next LAP step, familiarity with a language portrait of BLs. This pedagogical tool provides an accurate, research-based picture of BLs' linguistic reality and bilingual potential. Adapted from qualitative research methodology (Lawrence-Lightfoot and Hoffman Davis 1997; Lawrence-Lightfoot 2005; Hackman 2002) and guided by the question "What is good here?" the language portrait describes the language and literacy strengths, abilities and needs of BLs. It also includes troubling and challenging aspects of their language lives, including the inequities and hardships they face when they join a new language environment and encounter "unfamiliar practices and discourses" (Bligh 2014).

The third step in the LAP implementation process is to consider appropriate strategies for managing five important issues that EC professionals encounter in their work with BLs: transitioning them from home to the classroom; introducing them to their classmates; partnering with families; using home languages in the classroom; and documenting language and literacy behaviours.

In the last LAP step, knowledgeable and committed EC professionals are finally ready to implement inclusive practice. To get them started, LAP provides over 50 activities. Designed to be conducted in the classroom language, these activities include a home language component and cover a wide range of topics and subject areas. As they transform their classrooms into multilingual environments, EC professionals select, modify and extend the LAP activities to match the ages and needs of their children and put strategies in place that actively engage both children and families.

LAP Studies

Unlike previous instructional practice studies with select, like-minded participants (Toohey 2000; Naqvi et al. 2012), the two studies presented here were context-wide, with the participation of *all* members of the teaching staff. The goal of the studies was to help two groups of EC professionals, who met the same general condition of working directly with BLs, to retool their instructional practice. In the two studies, practice retooling (hereafter PR-ing) was defined as the process of reflecting on and reviewing one's current instructional practice with BLs, aligning it with evidence-based principles of childhood bilingualism and using the four-step LAP guide (Chumak-Horbatsch 2012) to move towards inclusive practice. The research question guiding the two studies was "How can LAP help EC professionals retool their current instructional practice with BLs and move towards inclusive practice?" Study documentation included field notes, documentation logs, home language questionnaires (children and teaching staff), LAP-related artefacts created by the children and final evaluations.

Study A

Study A was small-scale and was implemented over a 10-month period in an urban fee-based licensed childcare centre (hereafter UCC). The UCC serves upper middle-class families and accepts children from 18 months to 5 years of age. At the time of the study, there were eight EC professionals, fifty placement students,[21] a manager and 58 children, divided into three age groups.[22] Approximately half (48 %) of the children spoke one or more of fifteen different heritage languages at home, half of the EC professionals were speakers of four heritage languages and fourteen heritage languages were reported by the placement students.

The UCC staff enthusiastically accepted the invitation to explore a new instructional practice and expressed an interest in improving their practice with BLs and making their practice more inclusive. Study A started with three workshops[23] that introduced the four parts of LAP, provided the EC professionals with the opportunity to collectively reflect on and review their current practice with BLs and outlined the direction and scope of the study. EC professionals were invited to review, select, adapt and implement LAP activities according to their suitability, age-appropriateness and the interests of the children in their groups. They were also encouraged to keep a written record of the implementation process and progress. LAP was also introduced to the UCC families and to the placement students. The highlights of this new instructional practice were presented, the importance of family engagement was discussed and the plan of the study was explained. Throughout the study, the author conducted both group and individual validation meetings with the EC

professionals to foster reflection on and discussion of all aspects of the implementation of LAP. To keep record keeping to a minimum and make the documentation task lighter and less demanding, the author took on the role of on-site observer and recorder, working directly with the children, meeting with families and collecting and photographing LAP-related artefacts created by the children.

Study B

Study B was conducted over a 10-month period in a large publicly funded school (hereafter PFS) situated in an immigrant, high-density, low-income, high-unemployment area of Toronto. At the time of the study, enrolment stood at 567, with 313 (55 %) 5-year-olds and 254 (45 %) 4-year-olds. PFS staff included a principal, a vice-principal, 50 EC professionals (25 teachers and 25 early childhood educators), specialized teachers (music, drama, gym, language intervention, literacy support and special needs) and an administrative team. Each of the 25 classrooms included a two-member teaching team (a certified teacher and an early childhood educator[24]) and up to 30 children. The majority of the families (97 %) spoke one of 31 different heritage languages at home and only 3 % reported English as the home language. In addition to English, the majority (84 %) of the teaching staff were speakers of two or more heritage languages (24 different languages in total), while the remainder were monolingual speakers of English.

Unlike Study A, only one LAP workshop,[25] attended by the principal and approximately half of the teaching staff, was conducted in Study B. In the early weeks, the author prepared the groundwork for the implementation of LAP by familiarizing herself with the school community, visiting classrooms, directly interacting with the children, informally chatting with teaching teams and families and organizing an after-school event

---

[21]Placement students were enrolled in a university Early Childhood Studies undergraduate program.

[22]Toddlers: 18–30 months; preschoolers: 2½–4 years; kindergarteners: 4–5 years.

[23]The workshops were conducted by the author.

[24]Each kindergarten teaching team included an early childhood educator and a certified teacher who work collaboratively on the management of the kindergarten classroom.

[25]School logistics did not allow for additional workshops.

Table 2 Studies A and B: Level of interest in retooling instructional practice

Level of interest in PR-ing	A	B	C	D	E
	Study A N = 8	Study B N = 46	Studies A & B N = 54	Study B Teachers N = 23	Study B ECEs N = 23
High	1 (12 %)	9 (19 %)	10 (19 %)	3 (13 %)	6 (26 %)
Minimal	3 (38 %)	16 (35 %)	19 (35 %)	7 (30 %)	9 (39 %)
None	4 (50 %)	21 (46 %)	25 (46 %)	13 (57 %)	8 (35 %)

that focused on the importance of children's home languages. Following this, classrooms were assigned to one of four LAP coaches who visited the school on a weekly basis. The role of the LAP coaches was to facilitate the teaching teams and document the implementation of LAP. Teaching teams were also encouraged to record the implementation process and progress in LAP logs. As well, four professionally relevant after-school events were organized.

LAP Studies: Findings and Discussion

The LAP studies revealed three things about instructional practice with young BLs: interest in PR-ing varied across EC professionals; instructional practice decision-making was affected by three categories of factors; and LAP served as a valuable PR-ing resource.

Interest in Retooling Practice

As Table 2 illustrates, response to the invitation to retool current practice and move towards inclusive pedagogy varied across EC professionals, ranging from high interest to a total lack of interest. Column C shows that less than one-fifth (19 %) of participants from the two studies chose to retool their practice, showed high interest and moved towards inclusive practice. These participants were proactive and exhibited high professional curiosity or "initiative, interest and active wondering" (Nersessian 1995) as they adopted and implemented LAP. Minimal interest in PR-ing was noted in just over one-third (35 %) of all participants. In

Study A, these participants implemented LAP activities sporadically and infrequently while those in Study B exhibited little or no self-initiated effort and followed the suggestions and guidance of the LAP coaches. Finally, nearly half (46 %) of the Study A and Study B participants chose not to follow up on the invitation to retool their instructional practice with BLs.

A closer look at the Study B levels of PR-ing (columns D and E) shows a marked difference in the level of interest in PR-ing among the teachers and early childhood educators. Twice as many early childhood educators as teachers retooled their practice (26 vs 13 %). The number of early childhood educators who engaged in minimal PR-ing with the support and guidance of LAP coaches was also higher (39 vs 30 %), while the lack of interest in PR-ing was lower (35 vs 57 %). Also, more early childhood educators than teachers attended the after-school professional events.

Factors that Affected Instructional Practice Decision-Making

From the available models of instructional choice and change, the Model of Teacher Change (Ni and Guzdial 2008) was selected and adapted to the BLs context. An analysis of Study A and B documentation generated three different yet related categories of factors that affected EC professionals' instructional practice decision-making with BLs: personal, professional and curricular knowledge, attitudes and beliefs. Table 3 sets out the broad characteristics that define each category.

Table 3 Three categories of factors that affected EC professionals' instructional practice decision-making

Category 1: PERSONAL: Knowledge, attitudes and beliefs about self as language user
Personal language history: monolingual or bilingual, languages spoken, attempted, lost
Personal interest and investment in bilingualism
Attitudes towards immigration, societal language use and multilingualism
Level of self-confidence, risk-taking
Category 2: PROFESSIONAL: Knowledge, attitudes and beliefs about BLs
The language reality of BLs
The principles of childhood bilingualism
Professional curiosity: motivation to enhance knowledge of bilingualism
View of teaching: collaborative or personal enterprise
Professional curiosity, commitment and engagement
Category 3: CURRICULAR: Knowledge, attitudes and beliefs about curriculr directives
Curricular requirements re teaching BLs
Early learning resources: working with BLs

It is noteworthy that identifying general categories of factors as listed in Table 3 proved to be more straightforward than attempting to identify the factors that affected the decision-making of individual EC professionals.

With participants who enthusiastically talked about their work with BLs and exhibited a high interest in PR-ing, it was clear that both personal and professional factors guided their choice to move towards inclusive practice and adopt LAP. These EC professionals were mostly speakers of two or more languages, had multilingual experiences in their homes and families and viewed childhood bilingualism favourably. Their high level of professional curiosity led them to look beyond the mandated supportive approach and to integrate home languages into the classroom agenda. Included in this group were many of the Study B early childhood educators who, as a group, displayed a greater interest in PR-ing than did the teachers.

Attempts to identify factors that affected the practice choices of the EC professionals who displayed a minimal interest in PR-ing (just over one-third) were particularly challenging. Even though they agreed to collaborate with LAP coaches, their accommodating yet disengaged attitude, together with their unwillingness to complete the final evaluation questionnaire, made it difficult to profile their practice decisions.

It was clear, however, that all three factors, personal, professional and curricular, were at play when the decision was made to dismiss PR-ing. Some (but not all) of the English-speaking monolingual EC professionals rejected the idea of PR-ing due to personal factors, reporting that as single language speakers, they were ill equipped to concretely support children's home languages and foster multilingualism. Participants who (for various reasons) lost their family languages in their early years were not interested in PR-ing because they felt that young BLs would also eventually lose their home languages. In a small number of cases, a negative view of school multilingualism ("English is the language of Canada and home languages, although important, belong in the home.") was translated into the dismissal of PR-ing and the adherence to supportive practice. In addition, curricular factors affected the decision-making of some of the non-PR-ing group. Some of these participants reported directly, while others inferred, that inclusive practice generally and LAP specifically are not included in the early learning curricular guidelines and hence do not fit in with the play- and inquiry-based agendas that they are required to follow in their work with young children.

LAP: An Important Practice Retooling Resource

The EC professionals who retooled their instructional practice described LAP as an "invaluable resource" and a "helpful guide" in transforming their classrooms into multilingual environments and making linguistic diversity come to life. As LAP activities were implemented, children's initial reluctance to use their home languages in the classroom changed to confidence, enthusiasm and spontaneous multilingual play. They reached a language "comfort zone" (Brown 2008) and freely "translanguaged" (García et al. 2011) or used words and phrases in their home languages with each other and in group activities. All of the children—and not only the BLs—were fascinated by the discovery that their friends were speakers of different languages. They developed an awareness of languages and exhibited an interest in their own home languages and those of others: for example, a child holding up a toy cow reported: "I speak Arabic and my cow speaks Hebrew". They played and experimented with language rhythms and patterns and imitated and attempted words in each other's languages. They talked about languages with each other and used them as identity markers for themselves and their friends: "I speak Arabic and so does Waqas and Rayan". As BLs discovered that the adults in the classroom did not share their home languages, they took on a teaching role and offered to help their "students": "I'll help you and teach you, yes. Say it like this."

In addition to children's positive response to LAP, families and placement students' reaction to linguistic inclusion is noteworthy. As families witnessed their children's interest, excitement and pride in languages, their initial uncertainty changed to approval, gratitude ("Thank you for encouraging our language.") and engagement in LAP. In a similar way, placement students were motivated and encouraged when they saw children's willingness and excitement to showcase and share home languages. These students journeyed from uncertainty to personal and professional confidence ("I didn't like to talk about my being Chinese…but once we did LAP with the children, I was happy to share what I know in Chinese, so I taught them a song in Chinese.") and took on the role of home language advocates, creating and extending LAP activities and preparing home language resources for children and families.

Summary of LAP Studies

The findings of the two studies are, to some extent, generalizable and reflect current instructional practice with BLs in Canadian early learning settings. They reveal that various combinations of personal, professional and curricular factors affected EC professionals' instructional practice decision-making and that only a small number of EC professionals who retooled their instructional practice journeyed from supportive to inclusive practice. LAP proved to be a useful tool in guiding this practice change. It also helped BLs adjust to their new language environment, enriched the language and literacy experiences of all children, supported families in their language maintenance attempts and helped placement students understand the importance of home languages. Alongside this practice change, a significant number of EC professionals held on to supportive practice "as tightly as possible" (Katz and Dack 2013) and were not interested in retooling their practice with BLs. Taken together, these findings raise a question that continues to be investigated in contexts beyond education, namely how to generate interest in and commitment to change in practice among professionals.

Future Directions and Policy Implications

Young Bilingual Learners Beyond Canada

> In every corner of the world, young children are learning languages at home that differ from the dominant language used in their broader social world.
>
> (Ball 2011)

The above quote reminds us that young BLs are everywhere and that the challenge of appropriate practice with this particular demographic is not unique to the Canadian early learning context. The situation in the United States is in many ways quite similar to that found in Canada. For example, provision for children's home languages or a home language mandate is included in numerous policy and educational documents (Espinosa 2008, 2013), and linguistically responsive teaching is gaining increased attention (Lucas and Villegas 2010). Yet, general suggestions to be "culturally and linguistically responsive"[26] most often translate into the adoption of supportive practice.

Unlike the widespread adoption of supportive practice in Canada and the United States, response to linguistic diversity in many European regions is quite different. Tradition and exclusivity of the official language (or languages), a wariness of "other" languages and the view of multilingualism as a problem or obstacle, together with official language or languages policy, often stand behind the widespread adoption of assimilative practice. Yet like their Canadian colleagues, a growing number of education researchers and EC professionals in many European regions are responding to their increasing "super-diversity" (Vertovec 2007) by reviewing and re-interpreting language policies, exploring and documenting language attitudes and questioning the equity and educational value of assimilative practice with BLs. For example, the Multilingual Early Learning Transmission (MELT)[27] project, a partnership between four language communities (the Frisian language in Fryslân [the Netherlands], the Swedish language in Finland, the Welsh language in Wales [UK], and the Breton language in Brittany [France]) advocates for the promotion of cultural and linguistic diversity, the recognition and support of home languages and helping families understand the benefits of bilingualism.

Conclusion and Next Steps

The early learning practice profile provided in this chapter, speaks to the pressing need for broad based instructional practice retooling with BLs. This need raises two questions. Firstly, how can the current widespread adoption of monolingually focused practices, which fall short of meeting the language and literacy needs of young BLs be "intentionally interrupted" (Katz and Dack 2013)? Secondly, what course of action will serve to fuel EC professionals' interest in and commitment to linguistically responsive practice? In response to these questions, change is recommended for four different levels of early learning stakeholders.

The very first level of instructional practice change must occur at the curriculum and policy levels. Since EC practitioners rely on early learning resources for direction and guidance, these documents must accurately reflect the linguistic reality of Canadian classrooms, be aligned with evidence-based principles of childhood bilingualism and portray young BLs as capable, active language learners who require concrete support and validation to grow bilingually. The images and the accompanying messages in these resources must be synchronized in their promotion and endorsement of linguistically responsive practice.

A review of local, regional, and national leadership practices must follow the curricular and policy update and review proposed in the previous paragraph. Principals, directors and managers of early learning contexts must engage

---

[26]TK California: A project of early edge California: http://www.tkcalifornia.org/tk-experience.

[27]http://www.poliglotti4.eu/docs/MELT_research_paper.pdf.

in high-leverage leadership by taking a "visible and public" interest (Katz and Dack 2013) in BLs. Together with their staff, they must move beyond one-time professional development events, actively participate in professional learning and understanding about childhood bilingualism and take on the role of "gatekeepers or facilitators of change" (Fullan 2007).

To work effectively and equitably with young BLs, EC professionals must understand the principles of childhood bilingualism and the linguistic reality of BLs. To do so, they would do well to create their own context-specific communities of practice (Lave and Wenger 1991; Wenger 1998, 2007; Katz and Dack 2013), where they engage in on-going, collaborative learning, sharing and professional understanding. When EC professionals update their understanding, assumptions and beliefs about children who grow in two (or more) languages, they will be ready to retool their practice, position home languages as instructional assets and essential parts of BLs learning equation and teach through a multilingual lens (Cummins and Early 2014).

Finally, education researchers are encouraged to turn their attention to the large number of EC professionals who focus on the majority language and either remain hesitant to venture beyond a token acknowledgement of BLs' home languages or are committed to monolingual instructional practice. Understanding the language realities and subsequent practice behaviours of these professionals will serve to rework and update the factors that affect instructional choices identified in this chapter and will help to inform the development of practice reform strategies.

On an encouraging and promising note, the growing and steady interest in retooling instructional practice with young BLs serves as evidence that this new direction is far more than a passing in-vogue event. It is a pedagogical evolution that is supporting, validating and extending BLs' language and literacy skills and abilities, strengthening the understanding and respect for diversity of all young children and transforming early education in Canada and beyond.

References

Ball, J. (2011). *Enhancing learning of children from diverse language backgrounds: Mother tongue-based bilingual or multilingual education in early childhood and early primary school years*. Paris: Analytical review commissioned by the UNESCO Education Sector, UNESCO.

Bligh, C. (2014). *The silent experiences of young bilingual learners: A sociocultural study into the silent period*. Rotterdam: Sense Publishers.

Bransford, J. D., Brown, A. L., & Cocking, R. R. (2000). *How people learn: Brain, mind, experience, and school*. Washington, DC: National Academy Press.

Brown, M. (2008). Comfort Zone: Model or metaphor? *Australian Journal of Outdoor Education, 12*(1), 3–12.

Chumak-Horbatsch, R. (2004). Linguistic diversity in early childhood education: Working with linguistically and culturally diverse children. *Canadian Children, 29*(2), 20–24.

Chumak-Horbatsch, R. (2006). Mmmm … I like English! Linguistic behaviours of Ukrainian-English bilingual children. *Psychology of Language and Communication, 10*(2), 3–25.

Chumak-Horbatsch, R. (2008). Early bilingualism: Children of immigrants in an English-language childcare centre. *Psychology of Language and Communication, 12*(1), 3–27.

Chumak-Horbatsch, R. (2010). Toronto childcare centres: A language profile. In B. Bokus (Ed.), *Studies in the psychology of language and communication* (pp. 289–307). Warsaw: Matrix.

Chumak-Horbatsch, R. (2012). *Linguistically appropriate practice: A guide for working with young immigrant children*. Toronto: University of Toronto Press.

Coelho, E. (2012). *Language and learning in multilingual classrooms: A practical approach*. Toronto: Multilingual Matters.

Cummins, J. (2001). *Negotiating identities education for empowerment in a diverse society* (2nd ed.). Los Angeles, California: Association for Bilingual Education.

Cummins, J. (2004). *Language, power and pedagogy—bilingual children in the crossfire*. Clevedon: Multilingual Matters.

Cummins, J. (2006a). Identity Texts: The imaginative construction of self through multi-literacies pedagogy. In O. García, T. Skutnab-Kangas, & M. E. Torres-Gutzman (Eds.), *Imagining multilingual schools: Languages in education and globalization*. Clevedon Hall: Multilingual Matters.

Cummins, J. (2006b). Pedagogy. In J. Cummins, K. Brown, & D. Sayers (Eds.), *Literacy, technology, and diversity: Teaching for success in changing times*. Toronto: Allyn and Bacon, Pearson.

Cummins, J. (2009). Fundamental psycholinguistic and sociological principles underlying educational success for linguistic minority students. In T. Skutnabb-Kangas, R. Phillipson, A. K. Mohanty, & M. Panda (Eds.), *Social justice through multilingual education*. Toronto: Multilingual Matters.

Cummins, J. (2014). Mainstreaming plurilingualism: Restructuring heritage language provision in schools. In P. Trifonas & T. Aravossitas (Eds.), *Rethinking heritage language education*. Cambridge: Cambridge University Press.

Cummins, J., & Early, M. (2011). *Identity texts: The collaborative creation of power in multilingual schools*. Stoke-on-Trent: Trentham Books.

Cummins, J., & Early, M. (2014). *Big ideas for expanding minds: Teaching english language learners across the curriculum*. Toronto: Rubicon Publishing.

Donovan, M. S., & Bransford, J. D. (2005). *How students learn: History, mathematics, and science in the classroom*. Washington, D.C: The National Academies Press.

Espinosa, L. M. (2008). *Challenging common myths about young English language learners. Policy to action briefs*. New York: Foundation for Child Development.

Espinosa, L. M. (2013). PreK-3rd: Challenging common myths about dual language learners—An update to the seminal 2008 report. In: PreK-3rd Policy to Action Briefs. New York: Foundation for Child Development.

Fullan, M. (2007). *The new meaning of educational change* (4th ed.). New York: Teachers College Columbia University.

García, O. (2009a). Emergent bilinguals and TESOL: What's in a name? *TESOL Quarterly* 43(2): 322–326. (Special issue edited by Shelley Taylor).

García, O. (2009b). Education, multilingualism, and translanguaging in the 21st century. In A. Mohanty, M. Panda, R. Phillipson, & T. Skutnabb-Kangas (Eds.), *Multicultural education for social justice: Globalizing the local* (pp. 128–145). New Delhi: Orient Blackswan. former Orient Longman.

García, O. (2009c). *Bilingual education in the 21st century: A global perspective*. Malden, MA: Basil/Blackwell.

García, O. (2010). Latino language practices and literacy education in the US. In M. Farr, L. Seloni, & J. Song (Eds.), *Ethnolinguistic diversity and education Language, literacy, and culture* (pp. 193–211). New York: Routledge.

García, O., Kleifgen, J. A., & Falchi, L. (2008). From english language learners to emergent bilinguals. In: *Equity matters: Research review*, Vol. 1. New York: A Research Initiative of the Campaign for Educational Equity.

García, O., Makar, C., Starcevic, M., & Terry, A. (2011). The translanguaging of Latino kindergarteners. In K. Potowski & J. Rothman (Eds.), *Bilingual youth: Spanish in English-speaking societies* (pp. 33–55). Philadelphia: John Benjamin Publishing Co.

González, N. E., & Moll, L. C. (1995). Funds of knowledge for teaching in Latino Households. *Urban Education, 29*(4), 443–470.

Gonzalez, N. E., Moll, L. C., & Amanti, C. (2005). *Funds of knowledge: Theorizing practices in Households, Communities and Classrooms*. London: Lawrence Erlbaum.

Hackman, D. G. (2002). Using portraiture in educational leadership research. *International Journal of Leadership in Education, 5*(1), 51–60.

Katz, S., & Dack, L. A. (2013). *Intentional interruption: Breaking down learning barriers to transform professional practice*. Thousand Oaks, CA: Corwin, Sage.

Lave, J., & Wenger, E. (1991). *Situated learning: Legitimate peripheral participation*. Cambridge: Cambridge University Press.

Lawrence-Lightfoot, S. (2005). Reflections on portraiture: A dialogue between art and science. *Qualitative Inquiry, 11*(1), 3–14.

Lawrence-Lightfoot, S., & Hoffman Davis, J. (1997). *The art and science of portraiture*. San Francisco: Jossey-Bass.

Lucas, T., & Villegas, A. M. (2010). The missing piece in teacher education: The preparation of linguistically responsive teachers. *National Society for the Study of Education, 109*(2), 297–318.

McAndrew, M., Audet, G., & Bakhshaei, M. (2014). Immigration and diversity in Quebec's schools: An assessment. In S. Gervais, C. Kirkey, & R. Jarett (Eds.), *Quebec questions: Quebec studies for the 21st century*. Toronto: Oxford University Press.

Meyers, M. (2003). *Myths and delusions: The state of ESL in large Canadian school boards*. Toronto: Main Streams Publications.

Moll, L., & Greenberg, J. (1990). Creating zones of possibilities: Combining social contexts for instruction. In L. C. Moll (Ed.), *Vygotsky and education*. Cambridge: Cambridge University Press.

Moll, L., Amanti, C., Neff, D., & González, N. (1992). Funds of knowledge for teaching: Using a qualitative approach to connect homes and classrooms. *Theory into Practice, XXXI*(2), 132–141.

Nanos, N. (2008). Nation building through immigration: Workforce Skills Come Out on Top. *Policy Options, 29*(6), 30–32.

Naqvi, R., Thorne, K. J., Pfitscher, C. M., Nordstokke, D. W., & McKeough, A. (2012). Reading dual language books: Improving early literacy skills in linguistically diverse classrooms. *Journal of Early Childhood Research., 11*(1), 3–15.

Nersessian, E. (1995). Some reflections on curiosity and psychoanalytic technique. *The Psychoanalytic Quarterly, 64*, 113–135.

Ni, L., & Guzdial, M. (2008). What makes teachers change? Factors that influence post-secondary teachers' adoption of new computing curricula. In: *Proceedings of the 40th ACM technical symposium on computer science education*. Chattanooga, Tennessee, pp. 544–548.

Norton, B. (2000). *Identity and Language Learning: gender, ethnicity and educational change*. Harlow: Longman/Pearson Education.

Pacini-Ketchabaw, V. (2007). Child care and multiculturalism: A site of governance marked by flexibility and openness. *Contemporary Issues in Early Childhood, 8*(3), 222–232.

Piaget, J. (1929). *The child's conception of the world.* New York: Harcourt, Brace.

Reyes, M. L. (2001). Unleashing possibilities Bi-literacy in the primary grades. In M. L. Reyes & J. J. Halcón (Eds.), *The best for our children Critical perspectives on literacy for Latino students.* New York: Teachers College Press.

Roberts, T. A. (2014). Not so silent after all: Examination and analysis of the silent stage in childhood second language acquisition. *Early Childhood Research Quarterly, 29*, 22–40.

Ruíz, R. (1984). Orientations in language planning. *NABE Journal, 8*, 15–34.

Saraswati, J. (2000). Poverty and visible minority women in Canada. *Canadian Woman Studies, 20*(3), 49–53.

Siraj-Blatchford, I., & Clarke, P. (2000). *Supporting identity, diversity and language in the early years.* Philadelphia: Open University Press.

Skourtou, E., Kourtis Kazoullis, V., & Cummins, J. (2006). Designing virtual learning environments for academic language development. In J. Weiss, J. Nolan, & P. Trifonas (Eds.), *International handbook of virtual learning environments* (2nd ed.). Norwell, MA: Springer.

Toohey, K. (2000). *Learning English at School: Identity, social relations and classroom practice.* Clevedon: Multilingual Matters Ltd.

Vertovec, S. (2007). Super-diversity and its implications. *Ethnic and Racial Studies.* 30(6): 1024–1054. Special issue on New Directions in the Anthropology of Migration and Multiculturalism. http://www.tandfonline.com/doi/abs/10.1080/01419870701599465#.VJ8bcP8uRA. Accessed 29 August 2014.

Vygotsky, L. S. (1978). *Mind in society: The development of higher psychological processes.* Cambridge, MA: Harvard University Press.

Wardle, F., & Cruz-Janzen, M. I. (2003). *Meeting the needs of multiethnic and multiracial children in schools.* Boston: Allyn & Bacon.

Webster, N. L., & Valeo, A. (2011). Teacher preparedness for a changing demographic of language learners. *TESL Canada Journal., 28*(2), 105–128.

Wenger, E. (1998). *Communities of practice: Learning, meaning, and identity.* Cambridge: University Press.

Wenger, E. (2007). *Communities of practice. A brief introduction.* http://www.wenger-trayner.com/theory/. Accessed December 12, 2014.

Printed by Printforce, the Netherlands